competishun
Power of real gurus

NEET (UG)

PHYSICS

Team Competishun

Published by :

Invincible Publication Pvt. Ltd.

INVINCIBLE
Publication Private Limited

Published by

Invincible Publication Pvt. Ltd.

201A, SAS Tower, Sector 38, Gurugram – 122003
Phone: +91-124-4034247, +91 9599066061
www.invinciblepublishers.com

NEET (UG) PHYSICS

First Edition 2024
This edition can be exported from India only by Invincible Publication.

ISBN-13 : 978-93-58860-57-3

Invincible Publication Pvt. Ltd.

Sales Office : 4760-61/23, Basement, Pratap Street, Ansari Road,
Daryaganj, New Delhi - 110002
Phone: +91-11-40198405
Email: invinciblepublishers@gmail.com

CONTENT

Chapter: 1

UNITS AND MEASUREMENTS

The International System of Units

1. The unit of thermal conductivity is **(2019)**

(a) $Wm^{-1} K^{-1}$ (b) JmK^{-1}

(c) $Jm^{-1} K^{-1}$ (d) WmK^{-1}

2. The damping force on an oscillator is directly proportional to the velocity. The units of the constant of proportionality are **(2012)**

(a) $kgms^{-1}$ (b) $kgms^{-2}$

(c) kgs^{-1} (d) kgs

3. The unit of permittivity of free space, ε_0, is **(2004)**

(a) coulomb/newton-metre

(b) newton-metre ^{2} / coulomb ^{2}

(c) coulomb ^{2}/ newton-metre ^{2}

(d) coulomb ^{2}/(newton-metre $)^2$

Accuracy, Precision of Instruments and Errors in Measurement

4. The errors in the measurement which arise due to unpredictable fluctuations in temperature and voltage supply are **(2023)**

(1) Personal errors

(2) Least count errors

(3) Random errors

(4) Instrumental errors

5. A metal wire has mass (0.4 ± 0.002)g, radius (0.3 ± 0.001) mm and length (5 ±0.02) cm. The maximum possible percentage error in the measurement of density will nearly be : **(2023)**

(1) 1.3% (2) 1.6%

(3) 1.4% (4) 1.2%

6. A screw gauge gives the following readings when used to measure the diameter of a wire Main scale reading: 0 mm Circular scale reading: 52 divisions Given that 1 mm on main scale corresponds to 100 divisions on the circular scale. The diameter of the wire from the above data is **(2021)**

(a) 0.052 cm (b) 0.52 cm

(c) 0.026 cm (d) 0.26 cm

7. A screw gauge has least count of 0.01 mm and there are 50 divisions in its circular scale. The pitch of the screw gauge is **(2020)**

(a) 0.01 mm (b) 0.25 mm

(c) 0.5 mm (d) 1.0 mm

8. In an experiment, the percentage of error occurred in the measurement of physical quantities A, B, C and D are $1\%, 2\%, 3\%$ and 4% respectively. Then the maximum percentage of error in the measurement X, where $X = \frac{A^2 B^{1/2}}{C^{1/3} D^3}$, will be **(2019)**

(a) 10% (b) (3/13)%
(c) 16% (d) −10%

9. The main scale of a vernier callipers has n divisions /cm. n divisions of the vernier scale coincide with $(n-1)$ divisions of main scale. The least count of the vernier callipers is

(Odisha NEET 2019)

(a) $\frac{1}{(n+1)(n-1)}$ cm (b) $\frac{1}{n}$ cm
(c) $\frac{1}{n^2}$ cm (d) $\frac{1}{n(n+1)}$ cm

10. A student measured the diameter of a small steel ball using a screw gauge of least count 0.001 cm. The main scale reading is 5 mm and zero of circular scale division coincides with 25 divisions above the reference level. If screw gauge has a zero error of −0.004 cm, the correct diameter of the ball is **(2018)**

(a) 0.521 cm (b) 0.525 cm
(c) 0.053 cm (d) 0.529 cm

11. In an experiment, four quantities a, b, c and d are measured with percentage error 1%, 2%, 3% and 4% respectively. Quantity P is calculated as follows $P = \frac{a^3b^2}{cd}$. % error in P is **(2013)**

(a) 7% (b) 4%
(c) 14% (d) 10%

12. A student measures the distance traversed in free fall of a body, initially at rest, in a given time. He uses this data to estimate g, the acceleration due to gravity. If the maximum percentage errors in measurement of the distance and the time are e_1 and e_2 respectively, the percentage error in the estimation of g is

(Mains 2010)

(a) $e_2 - e_1$ (b) $e_1 + 2e_2$
(c) $e_1 + e_2$ (d) $e_1 - 2e_2$

13. If the error in the measurement of radius of a sphere is 2%, then the error in the determination of volume of the sphere will be **(2008)**

(a) 8% (b) 2%
(c) 4% (d) 6%

14. The density of a cube is measured by measuring its mass and length of its sides. If the maximum error in the measurement of mass and lengths are 3% and 2% respectively, the maximum error in the measurement of density would be

(1996)

(a) 12% (b) 14%
(c) 7% (d) 9%.

15. Percentage errors in the measurement of mass and speed are 2% and 3% respectively. The error in the estimate of kinetic energy obtained by measuring mass and speed will be **(1995)**

(a) 8% (b) 2%
(c) 12% (d) 10%.

16. A certain body weighs 22.42 g and has a measured volume of 4.7cc. The possible error in the measurement of mass and volume are 0.01 g and 0.1cc. Then maximum error in the density will be

(1991)

(a) 22% (b) 2%

(c) 0.2% (d) 0.02%.

Significant Figures

17. The area of a rectangular field (in m^2) of length 55.3 m and breadth 25 m after rounding off the value for correct significant digit is : **(2022)**

(a) 138×10^1 (b) 1382

(c) 1382.5 (d) 14×10^2

18. Taking into account of the significant figures, what is the value of $9.99m - 0.0099m$? **(2020)**

(a) 9.9801 m (b) 9.98 m

(c) 9.980 m (d) 9.9 m

Dimensions of Physical Quantities

19. The dimensions $[MLT^{-2} A^{-2}]$ belong to the : **(2022)**

(a) magnetic flux

(b) self inductance

(c) magnetic permeability

(d) electric permittivity

20. Plane angle and solid angle have **(2022)**

(a) Units but no dimensions

(b) Dimensions but no units

(c) No units and no dimensions

(d) Both units and dimensions

21. If E and G respectively denote energy and gravitational constant, then $\frac{E}{G}$ has the dimensions of **(2021)**

(a) $[M^2][L^{-2}][T^{-1}]$

(b) $[M^2][L^{-1}][T^0]$

(c) $[M][L^{-1}][T^{-1}]$

(d) $[M][L^0][T^0]$

22. Dimensions of stress are **(2020)**

(a) $[MLT^{-2}]$

(b) $[ML^2 T^{-2}]$

(c) $[ML^0 T^{-2}]$

(d) $[ML^{-1} T^{-2}]$

23. The pair of quantities having same dimensions is

(Karnataka NEET 2013)

(a) Impulse and Surface Tension

(b) Angular momentum and Work

(c) Work and Torque

(d) Young's modulus and Energy

24. The dimensions of $(\mu_0 \varepsilon_0)^{-1/2}$ are

(Mains 2012, 2011)

(a) $\left[L^{1/2} T^{-1/2}\right]$ (b) $[L^{-1} T]$

(c) $[LT^{-1}]$ (d) $\left[L^{1/2} T^{1/2}\right]$

25. The dimension of $\frac{1}{2}\varepsilon_0 E^2$, where ε_0 is permittivity of free space and E is electric field, is **(2010)**

(a) $ML^2 T^{-2}$ (b) $ML^{-1} T^{-2}$

(c) $ML^2 T^{-1}$ (d) MLT^{-1}

26. If the dimensions of a physical quantity are given by $M^a L^b T^c$, then the physical quantity will be **(2009)**

(a) velocity if $a = 1, b = 0, c = -1$

(b) acceleration if $a = 1, b = 1, c = -2$

(c) force if $a = 0, b = -1, c = -2$

(d) pressure if $a = 1, b = -1, c = -2$

27. Which two of the following five physical parameters have the same dimensions?

1. energy density
2. refractive index
3. dielectric constant
4. Young's modulus
5. magnetic field

(2008)

(a) 1 and 4 (b) 1 and 5
(c) 2 and 4 (d) 3 and 5

28. Dimensions of resistance in an electrical circuit, in terms of dimension of mass M, of length L, of time T and of current I, would be **(2007)**

(a) $[ML^2T^{-2}]$
(b) $[ML^2T^{-1}I^{-1}]$
(c) $[ML^2T^{-3}I^{-2}]$
(d) $[ML^2T^{-3}I^{-1}]$

29. The ratio of the dimensions of Planck's constant and that of moment of inertia is the dimensions of **(2005)**

(a) time
(b) frequency
(c) angular momentum
(d) velocity.

30. The dimensions of universal gravitational constant are **(2004, 1992)**

(a) $[M^{-1}L^3T^{-2}]$
(b) $[ML^2T^{-1}]$
(c) $[M^{-2}L^3T^{-2}]$
(d) $[M^{-2}L^2T^{-1}]$

31. The dimensions of Planck's constant equals to that of **(2001)**

(a) energy
(b) momentum
(c) angular momentum
(d) power.

32. Which pair do not have equal dimensions? **(2000)**

(a) Energy and torque
(b) Force and impulse
(c) Angular momentum and Planck's constant
(d) Elastic modulus and pressure.

33. The dimensions of impulse are equal to that of **(1996)**

(a) pressure
(b) linear momentum
(c) force
(d) angular momentum

34. Which of the following dimensions will be the same as that of time? **(1996)**

(a) $\frac{L}{R}$ (b) $\frac{C}{L}$
(c) LC (d) $\frac{R}{L}$

35. The dimensions of RC is **(1995)**

(a) square of time
(b) square of inverse time
(c) time
(d) inverse time.

36. Which of the following has the dimensions of pressure ? **(1994, 1990)**

(a) $[MLT^{-2}]$

(b) $[ML^{-1}T^{-2}]$

(c) $[ML^{-2}T^{-2}]$

(d) $[M^{-1}L^{-1}]$

37. Of the following quantities, which one has dimensions different from the remaining three? **(1989)**

(a) Energy per unit volume

(b) Force per unit area

(c) Product of voltage and charge per unit volume

(d) Angular momentum.

Dimensional Formulae and Dimensional Equations

38. The dimensional formula of magnetic flux is **(1999)**

(a) $[M^0L^{-2}T^{-2}A^{-2}]$

(b) $ML^0T^{-2}A^{-2}]$

(c) $[ML^2T^{-2}A^{-1}]$

(d) $[ML^2T^{-1}A^3]$

39. The dimensional formula of permeability of free space μ_0 is **(1991)**

(a) $[MLT^{-2}A^{-2}]$

(b) $[M^0L^1T]$

(c) $[M^0L^2T^{-1}A^2]$

(d) none of these.

40. According to Newton, the viscous force acting between liquid layers of area A and velocity gradient $\Delta v/\Delta Z$ is given by $F = -\eta A\frac{\Delta v}{\Delta Z}$, where η is constant called coefficient of viscosity. The dimensional formula of η is **(1990)**

(a) $[ML^{-2}T^{-2}]$ (b) $[M^0L^0T^0]$

(c) $[ML^2T^{-2}]$ (d) $[ML^{-1}T^{-1}]$.

41. Dimensional formula of self inductance is **(1989)**

(a) $[MLT^{-2}A^{-2}]$

(b) $[ML^2T^{-1}A^{-2}]$

(c) $[ML^2T^{-2}A^{-2}]$

(d) $[ML^2T^{-2}A^{-1}]$

42. The dimensional formula of torque is **(1989)**

(a) $[ML^2T^{-2}]$ (b) $[MLT^{-2}]$

(c) $[ML^{-1}T^{-2}]$ (d) $[ML^{-2}T^{-2}]$.

43. If C and R denote capacitance and resistance, the dimensional formula of CR is **(1988)**

(a) $[M^0L^0T^1]$

(b) $[M^0L^0T^0]$

(c) $[M^0L^0T^{-1}]$

(d) not expressible in terms of MLT.

44. The dimensional formula of angular momentum is **(1988)**

(a) $[ML^2T^{-2}]$

(b) $[ML^{-2}T^{-1}]$

(c) $[MLT^{-1}]$

(d) $[ML^2T^{-1}]$.

45. If force $[F]$, acceleration $[A]$ and time $[T]$ are chosen as the fundamental physical quantities. Find the dimensions of energy. **(2021)**

(a) $[F][A^{-1}][T$

(b) [F][A][T]

(c) $[F][A][T^2]$

(d) $[F][A][T^{-1}]$

46. A physical quantity of the dimensions of length that can be formed out of c, G and $\frac{e^2}{4\pi\varepsilon_0}$ is [c is velocity of light, G is the universal constant of gravitation and e is charge] **(2017)**

(a) $c^2\left[G\frac{e^2}{4\pi\varepsilon_0}\right]^{1/2}$

(b) $\frac{1}{c^2}\left[\frac{e^2}{G4\pi\varepsilon_0}\right]^{1/2}$

(c) $\frac{1}{c}G\frac{e^2}{4\pi\varepsilon_0}$

(d) $\frac{1}{c^2}\left[G\frac{e^2}{4\pi\varepsilon_0}\right]^{1/2}$

47. Planck's constant (h), speed of light in vacuum (c) and Newton's gravitational constant (G) are three fundamental constants. Which of the following combinations of these has the dimension of length? **(NEET-II 2016)**

(a) $\frac{\sqrt{hG}}{c^{3/2}}$ (b) $\frac{\sqrt{hG}}{c^{5/2}}$

(c) $\sqrt{\frac{hc}{G}}$ (d) $\sqrt{\frac{Gc}{h^{3/2}}}$

48. If dimensions of critical velocity v_c of a liquid flowing through a tube are expressed as $[\eta^x \rho^y r^z]$ where η, ρ and r are the coefficient of viscosity of liquid, density of liquid and radius of the tube respectively, then the values of x, y and z are given by **(2015)**

(a) $-1, -1, -1$ (b) 1,1,1

(c) $1, -1, -1$ (d) $-1, -1, 1$

49. If force (F), velocity (V) and time (T) are taken as fundamental units, then the dimensions of mass are **(2014)**

(a) $[FVT^{-1}]$ (b) $[FVT^{-2}]$

(c) $[FV^{-1}T^{-1}]$ (d) $[FV^{-1}T]$

50. The density of a material in CGS system of units is 4 g cm^{-3}. In a system of units in which unit of length is 10 cm and unit of mass is 100 g, the value of density of material will be **(Mains 2011)**

(a) 0.04 (b) 0.4

(c) 40 (d) 400

51. The velocity v of a particle at time t is given by $v = at + \frac{b}{t+c}$, where a, b and c are constants. The dimensions of a, b and c are **(2006)**

(a) [L], [LT] and $[LT^{-2}]$

(b) $[LT^{-2}]$, [L] and [T]

(c) $[L^2]$, [T] and $[LT^{-2}]$

(d) $[LT^{-2}]$, [LT] and [L]

52. An equation is given herc $\left(P + \frac{a}{V^2}\right) = b\frac{\theta}{V}$ where P = Pressure, V = Volume and θ = Absolute temperature. If a and b are constants, the dimensions of a will be **(1996)**

(a) $[ML^{-5}T^{-1}]$ (b) $[ML^5T^1]$

(c) $[ML^5T^{-2}]$ (d) $[M^{-1}L^5T^2]$.

53. Which of the following is a dimensional constant? **(1995)**

(a) Relative density

(b) Gravitational constant

(c) Refractive index

(d) Poisson's ratio.

54. Turpentine oil is flowing through a tube of length l and radius r. The pressure difference between the two ends of the tube is P. The viscosity of oil is given by $\eta = \frac{P(r^2-x^2)}{4vl}$ where v is the velocity of oil at a distance x from the axis of the tube. The dimensions of η are **(1993)**

(a) $[M^0 L^0 T^0]$ (b) $[MLT^{-1}]$

(c) $[ML^2 T^{-2}]$ (d) $[ML^{-1} T^{-1}]$

55. The time dependence of a physical quantity p is given by $p = p_0 \exp(-\alpha t^2)$, where α is a constant and t is the time. The constant α **(1993)**

(a) is dimensionless

(b) has dimensions $[T^{-2}]$

(c) has dimensions $[T^2]$

(d) has dimensions of p

56. P represents radiation pressure, c represents speed of light and S represents radiation energy striking per unit area per sec. The non zero integers x, y, z such that $P^x S^y c^z$ is dimensionless are **(1992)**

(a) $x = 1, y = 1, z = 1$

(b) $x = -1, y = 1, z = 1$

(c) $x = 1, y = -1, z = 1$

(d) $x = 1, y = 1, z = -1$

57. The frequency of vibration f of a mass m suspended from a spring of spring constant k is given by a relation $f = am^x k^y$, where a is a dimensionless constant. The values of x and y are

(a) $x = \frac{1}{2}, y = \frac{1}{2}$

(b) $x = -\frac{1}{2}, y = -\frac{1}{2}$

(c) $x = \frac{1}{2}, y = -\frac{1}{2}$

(d) $x = -\frac{1}{2}, y = \frac{1}{2}$

58. If $x = at + bt^2$, where x is the distance travelled by the body in kilometers while t is the time in seconds, then the units of b is **(1989)**

(a) km/s (b) kms

(c) km/s^2 (d) kms^2

ANSWER KEY

1.	(a)	2.	(c)	3.	(c)	4.	(3)	5.	(2)	6.	(a)
7.	(c)	8.	(c)	9.	(c)	10.	(d)	11.	(c)	12.	(b
13.	(d)	14.	(d)	15.	(a)	16.	(b)	17.	(d)	18.	(b)
19.	(c)	20.	(a)	21.	(b)	22.	(d)	23.	(c)	24.	(c)
25.	(b)	26.	(d)	27.	(a)	28.	(c)	29.	(b)	30.	(a)
31.	(c)	32.	(b)	33.	(b)	34.	(a)	35.	(c)	36.	(b)
37.	(d)	38.	(c)	39.	(a)	40.	(d)	41.	(c)	42.	(a)
43.	(a)	44.	(d)	45.	(c)	46.	(d)	47.	(a)	48.	(c)
49.	(d)	50.	(c)	51.	(b)	52.	(c)	53.	(b)	54.	(d)
55.	(b)	56.	(c)	57.	(d)	58.	(c)				

Hints & Explanations

1. **(a) :** $K = \frac{Qx}{A(T_1-T_2)t}$, where Q is the amount of heat flow, x is the thickness of the slab, A is the area of cross-section, and t is the time taken.

$$K = \frac{\text{Jm}}{\text{m}^2\text{Ks}} = \text{W}\frac{1}{\text{m}}\frac{1}{\text{K}} = \text{Wm}^{-1}\text{ K}^{-1}$$

2. **(c) :** Damping force, $F \propto v$ or $F = kv$

where k is the constant of proportionality

$$\therefore\ k = \frac{F}{v} = \frac{\text{N}}{\text{ms}^{-1}} = \frac{\text{kgms}^{-2}}{\text{ms}^{-1}} = \text{kgs}^{-1}$$

3. **(c) :** Force between two charges

$$F = \frac{1}{4\pi\varepsilon_0}\frac{q^2}{r^2} \Rightarrow \varepsilon_0 = \frac{1}{4\pi}\frac{q^2}{Fr^2} = \text{C}^2/\text{N}-\text{m}^2$$

4. **(3) :** Error arise due to unpredictable fluctuation in temperature and voltage supply are → random errors.

5. **(2) :** $\rho = \frac{M}{V}$

$$\rho = \frac{M}{\pi r^2 \ell}$$

$$\frac{\Delta\rho}{\rho} = \frac{\Delta M}{M} + \frac{2\Delta r}{r} + \frac{\Delta\ell}{\ell}$$

$$\frac{\Delta\rho}{\rho}\% = \left[\frac{0.002}{0.4} + \frac{2(0.001)}{(0.3)} + \frac{0.02}{5}\right]\times 100\%$$

$$= \frac{1}{2}\% + \frac{2}{3}\% + \frac{2}{5}\%$$

$$= 1.6\%$$

6. **(a) :** Given : Pitch = 1 mm, Number of division on circular scale, $N = 100$

Least count, L.C. $= \frac{\text{Pitch}}{N} = \frac{1}{100} = 0.01$ mm
So, diameter, $d =$ main scale reading + (circular scale reading × least count)

$d = 0 + 52 \times 0.01; d = 0.52$ mm;

$d = 0.052$ cm

7. **(c) :** Given : least count = 0.01 mm and number of circular scale divisions = 50.

∴ Pitch = L.C × No. of circular scale division

$$= 0.01 \times 50 = 0.5 \text{ mm.}$$

8. **(c) :** $X = \frac{A^2B^{1/2}}{C^{1/3}D^3}$

Maximum percentage error in X

$= \left(\frac{dX}{X}\right) \times 100$

$= \left(2\frac{dA}{A} + \frac{1}{2}\frac{dB}{B} + \frac{1}{3}\frac{dC}{C} + 3\frac{dD}{D}\right) \times 100$

$= 2 \times 1 + \frac{1}{2} \times 2 + \frac{1}{3} \times 3 + 3 \times 4 = 16\%$

9. **(c) :** If n divisions of vernier scale coincides with $(n-1)$ divisions of main scale.

Therefore, $n\text{VSD} = (n-1)\text{MSD} \Rightarrow$

$1\text{VSD} = \frac{(n-1)}{n}\text{MSD}$

∴ Least count = 1MSD − 1VSD = 1MSD − $\frac{(n-1)}{n}$MSD

$$= 1\text{MSD} - 1\text{MSD} + \frac{1}{n}\text{MSD} = \frac{1}{n}\text{MSD}$$

$$= \frac{1}{n} \times \frac{1}{n} = \frac{1}{n^2} \text{ cm } \left[\because 1\text{MSD} = \frac{1}{n} \text{ cm}\right]$$

10. **(d) :** Diameter of the ball

= MSR + CSR × (Least count) − Zero error

= 5 mm + 25 × 0.001 cm − (−0.004)cm

= 0.5 cm + 25 × 0.001 cm − (−0.004)cm

= 0.529 cm.

11. **(c) :** As $P = \frac{a^3b^2}{cd}$

% error in P is $\frac{\Delta P}{P} \times 100 = \left[3\left(\frac{\Delta a}{a}\right) + 2\left(\frac{\Delta b}{b}\right) + \frac{\Delta c}{c} + \frac{\Delta d}{d}\right] \times 100$

$= [3 \times 1\% + 2 \times 2\% + 3\% + 4\%] = 14\%$

12. **(b) :** From the relation, $h = ut + \frac{1}{2}gt^2$

$$h = \frac{1}{2}gt^2 \Rightarrow g$$

$$= \frac{2h}{t^2} (\text{ body initially at rest })$$

Taking natural logarithm on both sides, we get $\ln g = \ln h - 2\ln t$

Differentiating, $\frac{\Delta g}{g} = \frac{\Delta h}{h} - 2\frac{\Delta t}{t}$

For maximum permissible error,

or $\left(\frac{\Delta g}{g} \times 100\right)_{\max} = \left(\frac{\Delta h}{h} \times 100\right) + 2 \times \left(\frac{\Delta t}{t} \times 100\right)$

According to problem $\frac{\Delta h}{h} \times 100 = e_1$ and $\frac{\Delta t}{t} \times 100 = e_2$

Therefore, $\left(\frac{\Delta g}{g} \times 100\right)_{\max} = e_1 + 2e_2$

13. **(d) :** $V = \frac{4}{3}\pi R^3; \ln V = \ln\left(\frac{4}{3}\pi\right) + \ln R^3$

Differentiating, $\frac{dV}{V} = 3\frac{dR}{R}$

Error in the determination of the volume $= 3 \times 2\% = 6\%$

14. (d) : Maximum error in mass $\left(\frac{\Delta m}{m}\right) =$ $3\% = \frac{3}{100}$ and maximum error in length $\left(\frac{\Delta l}{l}\right) = 2\% = \frac{2}{100}$.

Maximum error in the measurement of density

$$\frac{\Delta \rho}{\rho} = \frac{\Delta m}{m} + \left(3 \times \frac{\Delta l}{l}\right) = \frac{3}{100} + \left(3 \times \frac{2}{100}\right)$$
$$= \frac{3}{100} + \frac{6}{100} = \frac{9}{100}$$
$$= 9\%$$

15. (a) : Percentage error in mass $= 2\% = \frac{2}{100}$ and percentage error in speed $= 3\% = \frac{3}{100}$ $\therefore$ K.E. $= \frac{1}{2}mv^2$

Therefore the error in measurement of kinetic energy

$$\frac{\Delta K.E.}{K.E.} = \frac{\Delta m}{m} + 2 \times \frac{\Delta v}{v} = \frac{2}{100} + 2 \times \frac{3}{100}$$
$$= \frac{8}{100} = 8\%$$

16. (b) : Density $\rho = \frac{\text{mass } m}{\text{volume } V}$

Take logarithm to take base e on the both sides of eqn (i), we get $\ln \rho = \ln m - \ln V$
Differentiate eqn (ii), on both sides, we get $\frac{\Delta \rho}{\rho} = \frac{\Delta m}{m} - \frac{\Delta V}{V}$ Errors are always added.

Error in the density ρ will be

$$= \left[\frac{\Delta m}{m} + \frac{\Delta V}{V}\right] \times 100\%$$
$$= \left[\frac{0.01}{22.42} + \frac{0.1}{4.7}\right] \times 100\%$$
$$= 2\%$$

17. (d) : Given, that, length $(l) = 55.3$ m

Breadth $(b) = 25$ m

The area of rectangular field is, $A = l \times b$

$$= 55.3 \times 25$$
$$= 1382.5 \text{ m}^2 = 1.3825 \times 10^3 \text{ m}^2$$
$$\simeq 1.4 \times 10^3 = 14 \times 10^2$$

18. (b) : Least number of significant figure are 3. Hence, required answer will be 9.98 m.

19. (c) : Dimensions of magnetic flux $= [ML^2 T^{-2} A^{-1}]$

Dimensions of self inductance $= [ML^2 T^{-2} A^{-2}]$

Dimensions of magnetic permeability $= [MLT^{-2} A^{-2}]$

Dimensions of electrical permittivity $= [M^{-1} L^{-3} T^4 A^2]$

So, the correct option is (c)

20. (a) : Plane angle and solid angle have supplementary units. Radian (rad) is the unit of plane angle and steradian (sr) is the unit of solid angle. Plane angle and solid angle are dimensionless quantities.

21. (b) : Dimensions of energy $[E] = [ML^2 T^{-2}]$

Dimensions of gravitational constant $[G] = [M^{-1} L^3 T^{-2}]$

So, the dimensions of $\left[\frac{E}{G}\right] = \frac{[ML^2 T^{-2}]}{[M^{-1} L^3 T^{-2}]}$

$= [M^2 L^{-1} T^0] = [M^2][L^{-1}][T^0]$

22. **(d) :** We know, stress $= \frac{\text{Force}}{\text{Area}}$

Dimensions of force is $[M^1 L^1 T^{-2}]$ and that of area is $[L^2]$.

$\therefore$ Dimensions of stress $= \frac{[M^1 L^1 T^{-2}]}{[L^2]} =$

$[M^1 L^{-1} T^{-2}]$.

23. **(c) :** Impulse = Force × time =

$[MLT^{-2}][T] = [MLT^{-1}]$

Surface tension $= \frac{\text{Force}}{\text{length}} = \frac{[MLT^{-2}]}{[L]} = [ML^0 T^{-2}]$

Angular momentum = Moment of inertia × angular velocity

$= [ML^2][T^{-1}] = [ML^2 T^{-1}]$

Work = Force × distance =

$[MLT^{-2}][L] = [ML^2 T^{-2}]$

Energy $= [ML^2 T^{-2}]$

Torque = Force × distance =

$[MLT^{-2}][L] = [ML^2 T^{-2}]$

Young's modulus $= \frac{\text{Force / Area}}{\text{Change in length / original length}}$

$$= \frac{[MLT^{-2}]/[L^2]}{[L]/[L]} = [ML^{-1} T^{-2}]$$

Hence, among the given pair of physical quantities work and torque have the same dimensions $[ML^2 T^{-2}]$.

24. **(c) :** The speed of the light in vacuum is

$$c = \frac{1}{\sqrt{\mu_0 \varepsilon_0}} = (\mu_0 \varepsilon_0)^{-1/2} \therefore \left[(\mu_0 \varepsilon_0)^{-1/2}\right]$$

$$= [c] = [LT^{-1}]$$

25. **(b) :** Energy density of an electric field E is $u_E = \frac{1}{2}\varepsilon_0 E^2$ where ε_0 is permittivity of free space

$$u_E = \frac{\text{Energy}}{\text{Volume}} = \frac{ML^2 T^{-2}}{L^3} = ML^{-1} T^{-2}$$

Hence, the dimension of $\frac{1}{2}\varepsilon_0 E^2$ is

$ML^{-1} T^{-2}$

26. **(d) :** Pressure, $P = \frac{\text{force}}{\text{area}} =$

$\frac{\text{mass} \times \text{acceleration}}{\text{area}}$

$\therefore [P] = \frac{M^1 LT^{-2}}{L^2} = [M^1 L^{-1} T^{-2}] = M^a L^b T^c$.

$\therefore a = 1, b = -1, c = -2$.

27. **(a) :** [Energy density] $= \left[\frac{\text{Work done}}{\text{Volume}}\right]$

$$= \frac{MLT^{-2} \cdot L}{L^3} = [ML^{-1} T^{-2}]$$

[Young's modulus] $= [Y] = \left[\frac{\text{Force}}{\text{Area}}\right] \times \frac{[l]}{[\Delta l]}$

$$= \frac{MLT^{-2}}{L^2} \cdot \frac{L}{L} = [ML^{-1} T^{-2}]$$

The dimensions of 1 and 4 are the same.

28. **(c) :** According to Ohm's law, $V = RI$ or

$R = \frac{V}{I}$

Dimensions of $V = \frac{W}{q} = \frac{[ML^2 T^{-2}]}{[IT]}$

$$\therefore R = \frac{[ML^2 T^{-2}/IT]}{[I]} = [ML^2 T^{-3} I^{-2}]$$

29. **(b) :** $\frac{h}{I} = \frac{E\lambda}{c \times I} = \frac{[ML^2 T^{-2}][L]}{[LT^{-1}] \times [ML^2]}$

$$\frac{h}{I} = [T^{-1}] = \text{ frequency}$$

30. **(a) :** Gravitational constant

$G = \frac{\text{force} \times (\text{distance})^2}{\text{mass} \times \text{mass}}$

$\therefore$ Dimensions of $G = \frac{[MLT^{-2}][L^2]}{[M][M]} =$

$[M^{-1} L^3 T^{-2}]$

31. **(c) :** Dimensions of Planck's constant

$$h = \frac{\text{Energy}}{\text{Frequency}} = \frac{[ML^2 T^{-2}]}{[T^{-1}]}$$

$$= [ML^2 T^{-1}]$$

Dimensions of angular momentum L

= Moment of inertia (I) × Angular velocity (ω)

$= [ML^2][T^{-1}] = [ML^2 T^{-1}]$

32. **(b) :** Dimensions of force = $[MLT^{-2}]$

Dimensions of impulse = $[MLT^{-1}]$.

33. **(b) :** Impulse = Force × Time.

Therefore dimensional formula of impulse

= Dimensional formula of force × Dimensional formula of time = $[MLT^{-2}][T] = [MLT^{-1}]$ and dimensional formula of linear momentum $[p] = [MLT^{-1}]$.

34. **(a) :** Out of given relation we have to find which relation have dimension as similar with dimension of time so as we know dimension of 'L' inductance = $ML^2Q^{-2} = ML^2I^{-2}T^{-2}$

dimension of 'R' resistance = $ML^2T^{-3}I^{-2}$

dimension of 'C' capacitance = $M^{-1}L^{-2}T^4I^2$

so dimension of $\frac{L}{R} = \frac{ML^2I^{-2}T^{-2}}{ML^2T^{-3}I^{-2}} \Rightarrow T$

hence option (a) is correct.

35. **(c) :** Units of RC = ohm × ohm^{-1} × second = second. Therefore dimensions of RC = time.

36. **(b) :** Pressure = $\frac{\text{Force}}{\text{Area}}$

Therefore dimensions of pressure

$= \frac{\text{Force}}{\text{Area}} = ML^{-1} T^{-2}$.

37. **(d) :** Dimensions of energy E = $[ML^2 T^{-2}]$

Dimensions of volume $v = [L^3]$

Dimensions of force $F = [MLT^{-2}]$

Dimensions of area $A = [L^2]$

Dimensions of voltage $V = [ML^2 T^{-3} A^{-1}]$

Dimensions of charge $q = [AT]$

Dimensions of angular momentum L = $[ML^2 T^{-1}]$

$\therefore$ Dimensions of $\frac{E}{v} = \frac{[ML^2 T^{-2}]}{[L^3]} = [ML^{-1} T^{-2}]$

Dimensions of $\frac{F}{A} = \frac{[MLT^{-2}]}{[L^2]} = [ML^{-1} T^{-2}]$

Dimensions of $\frac{Vq}{v} = \frac{[ML^2 T^{-3} A^{-1}][AT]}{[L^3]} =$ $[ML^{-1} T^{-2}]$

Dimensions of angular momentum is $[ML^2 T^{-1}]$ while other three has dimensions $[ML^{-1} T^{-2}]$

38. **(c) :** Magnetic flux, $\phi = BA = \left(\frac{F}{IL}\right) A$

$= \frac{[MLT^{-2}][L^2]}{[A][L]} = [ML^2\ T^{-2}\ A^{-1}]$.

39. **(a) :** Permeability of free space

$$\mu_0 = \frac{2\pi \times \text{force} \times \text{distance}}{\text{current} \times \text{current} \times \text{length}}$$

Dimensional formula of $\mu_0 = \frac{[MLT^{-2}][L]}{[A][A][L]} =$

$[MLT^{-2}\ A^{-2}]$

40. **(d) :** Dimensions of force F = $[MLT^{-2}]$

Dimensions of velocity gradient

$\frac{\Delta v}{\Delta Z} = \frac{[LT^{-1}]}{[L]} = [T^{-1}]$

Dimensions of area $A = [L^2]$

Given $F = -\eta A \frac{\Delta v}{\Delta Z}$

Dimensional formula for coefficient of viscocity

$$\eta = \frac{F}{(A)\left(\frac{\Delta v}{\Delta Z}\right)} = \frac{[MLT^{-2}]}{[L^2][T^{-1}]} = [ML^{-1}\ T^{-1}]$$

41. **(c) :** Induced emf $|\varepsilon| = L\frac{dI}{dt}$ where L is the self inductance and $\frac{dI}{dt}$ is the rate of change of current.

$\therefore$ Dimensional formula of

$$L = \frac{|\varepsilon|}{\frac{dI}{dt}} = \frac{[ML^2\ T^{-3}\ A^{-1}]}{[AT^{-1}]} = [ML^2\ T^{-2}\ A^{-2}]$$

42. **(a) :** Torque (τ) = Force × distance

Dimensional formula for (τ) =

$[MLT^{-2}][L] = [ML^2\ T^{-2}]$

43. **(a) :** Capacitance $C = \frac{\text{Charge}}{\text{Potential difference}}$

Dimensions of $C = \frac{[AT]}{[ML^2\ T^{-3}\ A^{-1}]} =$

$[M^{-1}\ L^{-2}\ T^4\ A^2]$

Resistance $R = \frac{\text{Potential difference}}{\text{Current}} = \frac{[ML^2\ T^{-3}\ A^{-1}]}{[A]}$

$= [ML^2\ T^{-3}\ A^{-2}]$

Dimensional formula of $CR =$

$[M^{-1}\ L^{-2}\ T^4\ A^2][ML^2\ T^{-3}\ A^{-2}] = [T]$ As the (CR) has dimensions of time and so is called time constant of CR circuit.

44. **(d) :** Angular momentum L

= Moment of inertia I × Angular velocity ω.

$\therefore$ Dimensional formula

$L = [ML^2][T^{-1}] = [ML^2\ T^{-1}]$

45. **(c) :** Let for energy, $[E] = F^\alpha A^\beta T^\gamma$

or $[M^1\ L^2\ T^{-2}] = [MLT^{-2}]^\alpha [LT^{-2}]^\beta [T]^\gamma$

$M^1\ L^2\ T^{-2} = M^\alpha L^{\alpha+\beta} T^{-2\alpha-2\beta+\gamma}$

Comparing from both sides, $\alpha = 1$

$\alpha + \beta = 2 \Rightarrow \beta = 1$

$-2\alpha - 2\beta + \gamma = -2 \Rightarrow \gamma = 2$

$\therefore$ Energy = $[F][A][T^2]$

46. **(d) :** Dimensions of $\frac{e^2}{4\pi\varepsilon_0} = [F \times d^2] =$

$[ML^3\ T^{-2}]$

Dimensions of $G = [M^{-1}\ L^3\ T^{-2}]$,

Dimensions of $c = [LT^{-1}]$

$l \propto \left(\frac{e^2}{4\pi\varepsilon_0}\right)^p G^q c^r \therefore [L^1]$

$= [ML^3\ T^{-2}]^p [M^{-1}\ L^3\ T^{-2}]^q [LT^{-1}]^r$

On comparing both sides and solving, we get

$$p=\frac{1}{2}, q=\frac{1}{2} \text{ and } r=-2 \therefore l \propto \frac{1}{c^2}\left[\frac{Ge^2}{4\pi\varepsilon_0}\right]^{1/2}$$

47. **(a) :** According to question, $l \propto h^p c^q G^r$

$$l = kh^p c^q G^r$$

Writing dimensions of physical quantities on both sides, $[M^0LT^0] = [ML^2\,T^{-1}]^p[LT^{-1}]^q[M^{-1}\,L^3\,T^{-2}]^r$

Applying the principle of homogeneity of dimensions, we get $p-r=0$ ...(ii), $2p+q+3r=1$ .....(iii),$-p-q-2r=0$ .....(iv) Solving eqns. (ii), (iii) and (iv), we get $p=r=\frac{1}{2}, q=-\frac{3}{2}$

From eqn. (i), we get $l = K\frac{\sqrt{hG}}{c^{3/2}}$

48. **(c) :** $[v_c] = [\eta^x \rho^y y^z]$ (given)

Writing the dimensions of various quantities in eqn. (i), we get $[M^0LT^{-1}] = [ML^{-1}\,T^{-1}]^x[ML^{-3}\,T^0]^y[M^0LT^0]^z$

$$= [M^{x+y}\,L^{-x-3y+z}\,T^{-x}]$$

Applying the principle of homogeneity of dimensions, we get $x+y=0; -x-3y+z=1; -x=-1$

On solving, we get $x=1, y=-1, z=-1$

49. **(d) :** Let mass $m \propto F^a V^b T^c$ or

$m = kF^aV^bT^c$ where k is a dimensionless constant and a, b and c are the exponents.

Writing dimensions on both sides, we get

$$\left[ML^0T^0\right]=\left[MLT^{-2}\right]^a\left[LT^{-1}\right]^b[T]^c$$

$$\left[ML^0T^0\right]=\left[M^aL^{a+b}T^{-2a-b+c}\right]$$

Applying the principle of homogeneity of dimensions, we get

a=1 ...(ii), $a+b=0$ ...(iii),

$-2a-b+c=0$

Solving eqns. (ii), (iii) and (iv), we get a = 1, b=-1, c = 1

From eqn. (i), $[m]=\left[FV^{-1}T\right]$

50. **(c) :** As $n_1u_1 = n_2u_2 \Rightarrow 4\frac{g}{cm^3} = n_2\frac{100\text{ g}}{(10\text{ cm})^3}$

$$\Rightarrow n_2 = 40$$

51. **(b) :** $v = at + \frac{b}{t+c}$

As c is added to t, ∴ $[c] = [T]$

$[at] = [LT^{-1}]$ or, $[a] = \frac{[LT^{-1}]}{[T]} = [LT^{-2}]$

$\frac{[b]}{[T]} = [LT^{-1}]$ or, $[b] = [L]$.

52. **(c) :** Equation $\left(P+\frac{a}{V^2}\right) = b\frac{\theta}{V}$. Since $\frac{a}{V^2}$ is added to the pressure, therefore dimensions of $\frac{a}{V^2}$ and pressure (P) will be the same.

And dimensions of $\frac{a}{V^2} = \frac{a}{[L^3]^2} =$

$[ML^{-1}\,T^{-2}]$ or $= [ML^5\,T^{-2}]$.

53. (b) : Relative density, refractive index and Poisson's ratio all the three are ratios, therefore they are dimensionless constants.

54. (d) : Dimensions of $P = [ML^{-1}\,T^{-2}]$

Dimensions of $r = [L]$,

Dimensions of $v = [LT^{-1}]$

Dimensions of $l = [L]$

$\therefore$ Dimensions of $\eta = \frac{[P][r^2 - x^2]}{[4vl]} =$

$\frac{[ML^{-1}\,T^{-2}][L^2]}{[LT^{-1}][L]}$

$= [ML^{-1}\,T^{-1}]$

55. (b) : Given: $p = p_0 e^{-\alpha t^2}$

αt^2 is a dimensionless

$\therefore \alpha = \frac{1}{t^2} = \frac{1}{[T^2]} = [T^{-2}]$

56. (c) : Let $k = P^x S^y c^z$

k is a dimensionless

Dimensions of $k = [M^0\,L^0\,T^0]$

Dimensions of

$$P = \frac{\text{Force}}{\text{Area}} = \frac{[MLT^{-2}]}{[L^2]}$$

$$= [ML^{-1}\,T^{-2}]$$

Dimensions of

$$S = \frac{\text{Energy}}{\text{Area} \times \text{time}} = \frac{[ML^2\,T^{-2}]}{[L^2][T]}$$

$$= [MT^{-3}]$$

Dimensions of $c = [LT^{-1}]$

Substituting these dimensions in eqn (i), we get

$[M^0\,L^0\,T^0]$

$= [ML^{-1}\,T^{-2}]^x[MT^{-3}]^y[LT^{-1}]^z$

Applying the principle of homogeneity of dimensions, we get

$x + y = 0$ ... (.ii), $-x + z = 0$ ... (iii),

$-2x - 3y - z = 0$ ....(iv)

Solving (ii), (iii) and (iv), we get

$x = 1, y = -1, z =$

57. (d) : $f = am^x k^y$

Dimensions of frequency $f =$

$[M^0\,L^0\,T^{-1}]$

Dimensions of constant $a = [M^0\,L^0\,T^0]$

Dimensions of mass $m = [M]$

Dimensions of spring constant $k =$

$[MT^{-2}]$

Putting these value in equation (i), we get $[M^0\,L^0\,T^{-1}] = [M]^x[MT^{-2}]^y$

Applying principle of homogeneity of dimensions, we get $x + y = 0$

$-2y = -1$ or $y = \frac{1}{2}, x = -\frac{1}{2}$

58. (c) : Units of $b = \frac{x}{t^2} = \frac{\text{km}}{\text{s}^2}$

Chapter: 2

MOTION IN A STRAIGHT LINE

Average Velocity and Average Speed

1. A vehicle travels half the distance with speed v and the remaining distance with speed 2v. Its average speed is **(2023)**

(1) $\frac{2v}{3}$ (2) $\frac{4v}{3}$

(3) $\frac{3v}{4}$ (4) $\frac{v}{3}$

2. A particle covers half of its total distance with speed v_1 and the rest half distance with speed v_2. Its average speed during the complete journey is **(Mains 2011)**

(a) $\frac{v_1+v_2}{2}$ (b) $\frac{v_1v_2}{v_1+v_2}$

(c) $\frac{2v_1v_2}{v_1+v_2}$ (d) $\frac{v_1^2v_2^2}{v_1^2+v_2^2}$

3. A car moves from X to Y with a uniform speed v_u and returns to X with a uniform speed v_d. The average speed for this round trip is **(2007)**

(a) $\sqrt{v_u v_d}$ (b) $\frac{v_d v_u}{v_d+v_u}$

(c) $\frac{v_u+v_d}{2}$ (d) $\frac{2v_d v_u}{v_d+v_u}$

4. A car runs at a constant speed on a circular track of radius 100 m, taking 62.8 seconds for every circular lap. The average velocity and average speed for each circular lap respectively is **(2006)**

(a) 10 m/s, 0

(b) 0,0

(c) 0,10 m/s

(d) 10 m/s, 10 m/s.

5. A car moves a distance of 200 m. It covers the first half of the distance at speed 40 km/h and the second half of distance at speed v. The average speed is 48 km/h. The value of v is **(1991)**

(a) 56 km/ (b) 60 km/h

(c) 50 km/h (d) 48 km/h.

6. A bus travelling the first one-third distance at a speed of 10 km/h, the next one-third at 20 km/h and at last one-third at 60 km/h. The average speed of the bus is **(1991)**

(a) 9 km/h (b) 16 km/h

(c) 18 km/h (d) 48 km/h.

7. A car covers the first half of the distance between two places at 40 km/h and another half at 60 km/h. The average speed of the car is **(1990)**

(a) 40 km/h (b) 48 km/h

(c) 50 km/h (d) 60 km/h.

Instantaneous Velocity and Speed

8. The displacement-time graphs of two moving particles make angles of 30° and 45° with the x-axis as shown in the figure. The ratio of their respective velocity is

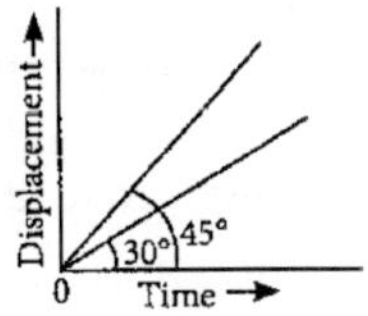

(a) $\sqrt{3}:1$ (b) $1:1$

(c) $1:2$ (d) $1:\sqrt{3}$

9. Two cars P and Q start from a point at the same time in a straight line and their positions are represented by $x_P(t) = (at + bt^2)$ and $x_Q(t) = (ft - t^2)$. At what time do the cars have the same velocity? **(NEET-II 2016)**

(a) $\frac{a-f}{1+b}$ (b) $\frac{a+f}{2(b-1)}$

(c) $\frac{a+f}{2(1+b)}$ (d) $\frac{f-a}{2(1+b)}$

10. If the velocity of a particle is $v = At + Bt^2$, where A and B are constants, then the distance travelled by it between 1 s and 2 s is **(NEET-I 2016)**

(a) $\frac{3}{2}A + \frac{7}{3}B$ (b) $\frac{A}{2} + \frac{B}{3}$

(c) $\frac{3}{2}A + 4B$ (d) $3A + 7B$

11. The displacement ' x ' (in meter) of a particle of mass ' m ' (in kg) moving in one dimension under the action of a force, is related to time ' t ' (in sec) by $t = \sqrt{x} + 3$. The displacement of the particle when its velocity is zero, will be **(Karnataka NEET 2013)**

(a) 4 (b) 0 m (zero)

(c) 6 m (d) 2 m

12. A particle shows distance-time curve as given in this figure. The maximum instantaneous velocity of the particle is around the point **(2008)**

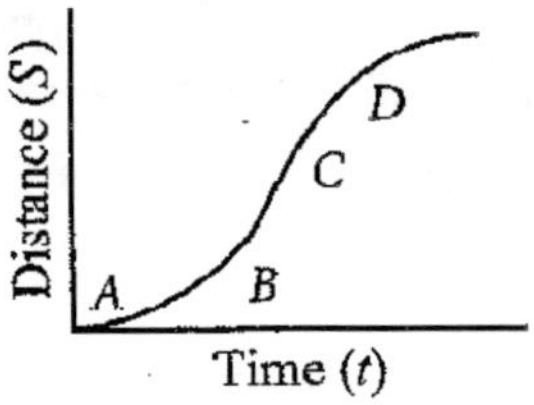

(a) D (b) A

(c) B (d) C

13. The position x of a particle with respect to time t along x-axis is given by $x = 9t^2 - t^3$ where x is in metres and t in seconds. What will be the position of this particle when it achieves maximum speed along the $+x$ direction? **(2007)**

(a) 54 m (b) 81 m

(c) 24 m (d) 32 m

14. A particle moves along a straight line OX. At a time t (in seconds) the distance x (in metres) of the particle from O is given by $x = 40 + 12t - t^3$. How long would the particle travel before coming to rest? **(2006)**

(a) 16 m (b) 24 m

(c) 40 m (d) 56 m

15. The displacement x of a particle varies with time t as $x = ae^{-\alpha t} + be^{\beta t}$, where a, b, α and β are positive constants. The velocity of the particle will **(2005)**

(a) be independent of β

(b) drop to zero when $\alpha = \beta$

(c) go on decreasing with time

(d) go on increasing with time.

16. The displacement-time graph of a moving particle is shown below. The instantaneous velocity of the particle is negative at the point **(1994)**

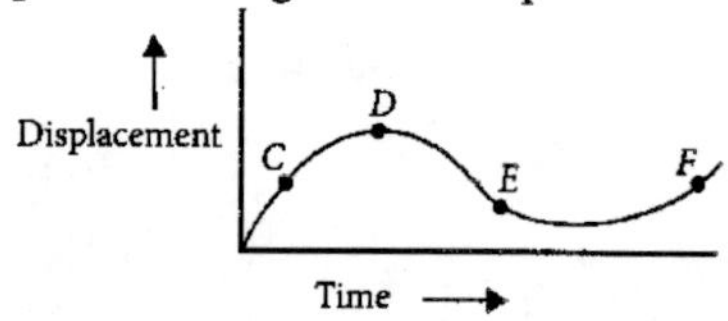

(a) E (b) F

(c) C (d) D

17. Which of the following curve does not represent motion in one dimension? **(1992)**

(a) 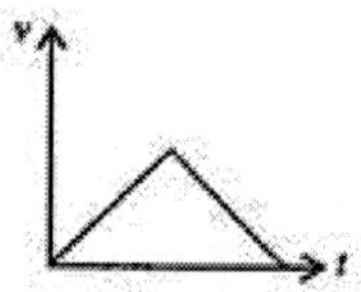

(b) 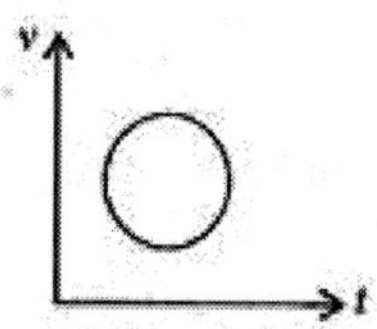

(c) 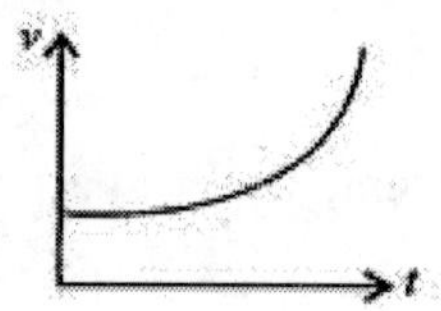

(d) 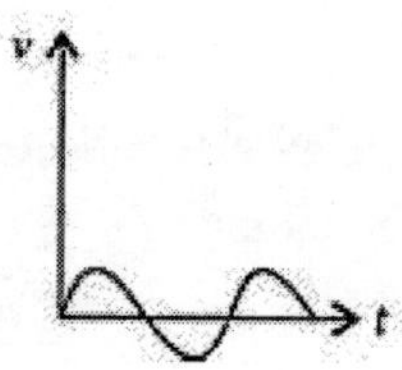

Acceleration

18. A particle of unit mass undergoes one-dimensional motion such that its velocity varies according to $v(x) = \beta x^{-2n}$, where β and n are constants and x is the position of the particle. The acceleration of the particle as a function of x, is given by **(2015 Cancelled)**

(a) $-2\beta^2 x^{-2n+1}$

(b) $-2n\beta^2 e^{-4n+1}$

(c) $-2n\beta^2 x^{-2n-1}$

(d) $-2n\beta^2 x^{-4n-1}$

19. The motion of a particle along a straight line is described by equation $x = 8 + 12t - t^3$ where x is in metre and t in second. The retardation of the particle when its velocity becomes zero is **(2012)**

(a) 24 m s^{-2} (b) zero

(c) 6 m s^{-2} (d) 12 m s^{-2}

20. A particle moves a distance x in time t according to equation $x = (t+5)^{-1}$. The acceleration of particle is proportional to **(2010)**

(a) (velocity) $\frac{3}{2}$

(b) (distance)^2

(c) (distance))$^{-2}$

(d) (velocity))$^{\frac{2}{3}}$

21. A particle moving along x-axis has acceleration f, at time t, given by $f = f_0\left(1 - \frac{t}{T}\right)$, where f_0 and T are constants. The particle at $t = 0$ has zero velocity. In the time interval between $t = 0$ and the instant when $f = 0$, the particle's velocity (v_x) is **(2007)**

(a) $\frac{1}{2} f_0 T^2$ (b) $f_0 T^2$

(c) $\frac{1}{2} f_0 T$ (d) $f_0 T$

22. Motion of a particle is given by equation $s = (3t^3 + 7t^2 + 14t + 8)$m. The value of acceleration of the particle at $t = 1$sec is **(2000)**

(a) 10 m/s^2 (b) 32 m/s^2

(c) 23 m/s^2 (d) 16 m/s^2

23. The position x of a particle varies with time, (t) as $x = at^2 - bt^3$. The acceleration will be zero at time t is equal to **(1997)**

(a) $\frac{a}{3b}$ (b) zero

(c) $\frac{2a}{3b}$ (d) $\frac{a}{b}$

24. The acceleration of a particle is increasing linearly with time t as bt. The particle starts from origin with an initial velocity v_0. The distance travelled by the particle in time t will be **(1995)**

(a) $v_0 t + \frac{1}{3} bt^2$ (b) $v_0 t + \frac{1}{2} bt^2$

(c) $v_0 t + \frac{1}{6} bt^3$ (d) $v_0 t + \frac{1}{3} bt^3$

25. A particle moves along a straight line such that its displacement at any time t is given by $s = (t^3 - 6t^2 + 3t + 4)$ metres. The velocity when the acceleration is zero is **(1994)**

(a) 3 m/s (b) 42 m/s

(c) -9 m/s (d) -15 m/s

Kinematic Equations for Uniformly Accelerated Motion

26. The ratio of the distance travelled by a freely falling body in the $1^{st}, 2^{nd}, 3^{rd}$ and 4th second **(2022)**

(a) $1:2:3:4$ (b) $1:4:9:16$

(c) $1:3:5:7$ (d) $1:1:1:1$

27. A ball is thrown vertically downward with a velocity of 20 m/s from the top of a tower. It hits the ground after some time with a velocity of 80 m/s. The height of the tower is $(g = 10 \text{ m/s}^2)$ **(2020)**

(a) 360 m (b) 340 m

(c) 320 m (d) 300 m

28. A stone falls freely under gravity. It covers distances h_1, h_2 and h_3 in the first 5 seconds, the next 5 seconds and the next 5 seconds respectively. The relation between h_1, h_2 and h_3 is **(2013)**

(a) $h_2 = 3h_1$ and $h_3 = 3h_2$

(b) $h_1 = h_2 = h_3$

(c) $h_1 = 2h_2 = 3h_3$

(d) $h_1 = \frac{h_2}{3} = \frac{h_3}{5}$

29. A boy standing at the top of a tower of 20 m height drops a stone. Assuming $g = 10 \text{ m s}^{-2}$, the velocity with which it hits the ground is **(2011)**

(a) 10.0 m/s (b) 20.0 m/s

(c) 40.0 m/s (d) 5.0 m/s

30. A ball is dropped from a high rise platform at $t = 0$ starting from rest. After 6 seconds another ball is thrown downwards from the same platform with a speed v. The two balls meet at $t = 18$ s. What is the value of v ? (Take $g = 10\ m/s^2$) **(2010)**

(a) $75\ m/s$ (b) $55\ m/s$

(c) $40\ m/s$ (d) $60\ m/s$

31. A particle starts its motion from rest under the action of a constant force. If the distance covered in first 10 seconds is S_1 and that covered in the first 20 seconds is S_2, then **(2009)**

(a) $S_2 = 3S_1$ (b) $S_2 = 4S_1$

(c) $S_2 = S_1$ (d) $S_2 = 2S_1$

32. A particle moves in a straight line with a constant acceleration. It changes its velocity from $10\ m\ s^{-1}$ to $20\ m\ s^{-1}$ while passing through a distance 135 m in t second. The value of t is **(2008)**

(a) 1 (b) 9

(c) 10 (d) 1.8

33. The distance travelled by a particle starting from rest and moving with an acceleration $\frac{4}{3}\ m\ s^{-2}$, in the third second is **(2008)**

(a) $\frac{10}{3}$ m (b) $\frac{19}{3}$ m

(c) 6 m (d) 4 m

34. Two bodies A (of mass 1 kg) and B (of mass 3 kg) are dropped from heights of 16 m and 25 m, respectively. The ratio of the time taken by them to reach the ground is **(2006)**

(a) $4/5$ (b) $5/4$

(c) $12/5$ (d) $5/12$

35. A ball is thrown vertically upward. It has a speed of $10\ m/sec$ when it has reached one half of its maximum height. How high does the ball rise? (Take $g = 10\ m/s^2$) **(2005)**

(a) 10 m (b) 5 m

(c) 15 m (d) 20 m

36. A man throws balls with the same speed vertically upwards one after the other at an interval of 2 seconds. What should be the speed of the throw so that more than two balls are in the sky at any time? (Given $g = 9.8\ m/s^2$) **(2003)**

(a) more than $19.6\ m/s$

(b) at least $9.8\ m/s$

(c) any speed less than $19.6\ m/s$

(d) only with speed $19.6\ m/s$

37. If a ball is thrown vertically upwards with speed u, the distance covered during the last t seconds of its ascent is **(2003)**

(a) ut (b) $\frac{1}{2}gt^2$

(c) $ut - \frac{1}{2}gt^2$ (d) $(u + gt)t$

38. A particle is thrown vertically upward. Its velocity at half of the height is $10\ m/s$, then the maximum height attained by it ($g = 10\ m/s^2$) **(2001)**

(a) 8 (b) 20 m

(c) 10 m (d) 16 m.

39. A car moving with a speed of $40\ km/h$ can be stopped by applying brakes after atleast 2 m. If the same car is moving with a speed of $80\ km/h$, what is the minimum stopping distance? **(1998)**

(a) 4 m (b) 6 m
(c) 8 m (d) 2 m

40. If a car at rest accelerates uniformly to a speed of 144 km/h in 20 s, it covers a distance of **(1997)**

(a) 1440 cm (b) 2980 cm
(c) 20 m (d) 400 m

41. A body dropped from a height h with initial velocity zero, strikes the ground with a velocity 3 m/s. Another body of same mass dropped from the same height h with an initial velocity of 4 m/s. The final velocity of second mass, with which it strikes the ground is **(1996)**

(a) 5 m/s (b) 12 m/s
(c) 3 m/s (d) 4 m/s.

42. The water drop falls at regular intervals from a tap 5 m above the ground. The third drop is leaving the tap at instant the first drop touches the ground. How far above the ground is the second drop at that instant? **(1995)**

(a) 3.75 m (b) 4.00 m
(c) 1.25 m (d) 2.50 m.

43. A car accelerates from rest at a constant rate α for some time after which it decelerates at a constant rate β and comes to rest. If total time elapsed is t, then maximum velocity acquired by car will be

(1994)

(a) $\frac{(\alpha^2-\beta^2)t}{\alpha\beta}$ (b) $\frac{(\alpha^2+\beta^2)t}{\alpha\beta}$
(c) $\frac{(\alpha+\beta)t}{\alpha\beta}$ (d) $\frac{\alpha\beta t}{\alpha+\beta}$

44. The velocity of train increases uniformly from $\frac{20\text{ km}}{\text{h}}$ to $\frac{60\text{ km}}{\text{h}}$ in 4 hours. The distance travelled by the train during this period is

(1994)

(a) 160 km (b) 180 km
(c) 100 km (d) 120 km

45. A body starts from rest, what is the ratio of the distance travelled by the body during the 4th and 3rd second? **(1993)**

(a) $\frac{7}{5}$ (b) $\frac{5}{7}$
(c) $\frac{7}{3}$ (d) $\frac{3}{7}$

46. A body dropped from top of a tower fall through 40 m during the last two seconds of its fall. The height of tow er is ($g = 10\text{ m/s}^2$) **(1992)**

(a) 60 m (b) 45 m
(c) 80 m (d) 50 m

47. What will be the ratio of the distance moved by a freely falling body from rest in 4th and 5th seconds of journey? **(1989)**

(a) 4: 5 (b) 7: 9
(c) 16: 25 (d) 1: 1

48. A car is moving along a straight road with a uniform acceleration. It passes through two points P and Q separated by a distance with velocity 30 km/h and 40 km/h respectively. The velocity of the car midway between P and Q is **(1988)**

(a) 33.3 km/h (b) $20\sqrt{2}$ km/h
(c) $25\sqrt{2}$ km/h (d) 35 km/h

Relative Velocity

49. Preeti reached the metro station and found that the escalator was not working. She walked up the stationary escalator in time t_1. On other days, if she remains stationary on the moving escalator, then the escalator takes her up in time t_2. The time taken by her to walk up on the moving escalator will be **(2017)**

(a) $\frac{t_1 t_2}{t_2 - t_1}$ (b) $\frac{t_1 t_2}{t_2 + t_1}$

(c) $t_1 - t_2$ (d) $\frac{t_1 + t_2}{2}$

50. A bus is moving with a speed of 10 m s^{-1} on a straight road. A scooterist wishes to overtake the bus in 100 s. If the bus is at a distance of 1 km from the scooterist, with what speed should the scooterist chase the bus? **(2009)**

(a) 40 m s^{-1} (b) 25 m s^{-1}

(c) 10 m s^{-1} (d) 20 m s^{-1}

51. A train of 150 metre length is going towards north direction at a speed of 10 m/s. A parrot flies at the speed of 5 m/s towards south direction parallel to the railways track. The time taken by the parrot to cross the train is **(1988)**

(a) 12 s (b) 8 s

(c) 15 s (d) 10 s

ANSWER KEY

1.	(b)	2.	(c)	3.	(d)	4.	(c)	5.	(b)	6.	(c)
7.	(b)	8.	(d)	9.	(d)	10.	(a)	11.	(b)	12.	(d)
13.	(a)	14.	(a)	15.	(d)	16.	(a)	17.	(b)	18.	(d)
19.	(d)	20.	(a)	21.	(c)	22.	(b)	23.	(a)	24.	(c)
25.	(c)	26.	(c)	27.	(d)	28.	(d)	29.	(b)	30.	(a)
31.	(b)	32.	(b)	33.	(a)	34.	(a)	35.	(a)	36.	(a)
37.	(b)	38.	(c)	39.	(c)	40.	(d)	41.	(a)	42.	(a)
43.	(d)	44.	(a)	45.	(a)	46.	(b)	47.	(b)	48.	(c)
49.	(b)	50.	(d)	51.	(d)						

Hints & Explanations

1. **(b) :**

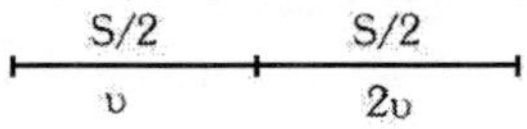

$$V_{avg} = \frac{2v_1v_2}{v_1+v_2} = \frac{2(v)(2v)}{v+2v} = \frac{4v^2}{3v} = \frac{4v}{3}$$

2. **(c) :** Let S be the total distance travelled by the particle. Let t_1 be the time taken by the particle to cover first half of the distance. Then $t_1 = \frac{S/2}{v_1} = \frac{S}{2v_1}$

Let t_2 be the time taken by the particle to cover remaining half of the distance. Then $t_2 = \frac{S/2}{v_2} = \frac{S}{2v_2}$

Average speed, $v_{av} = \frac{\text{Total distance travelled}}{\text{Total time taken}}$

$$= \frac{S}{t_1+t_2} = \frac{S}{\frac{S}{2v_1}+\frac{S}{2v_2}} = \frac{2v_1v_2}{v_1+v_2}$$

3. **(d) :** Average speed =

$\frac{\text{total distance travelled}}{\text{total time taken}}$

$$= \frac{s+s}{t_1+t_2} = \frac{2s}{\frac{s}{v_u}+\frac{s}{v_d}} = \frac{2v_uv_d}{v_d+v_u}.$$

4. **(c) :** Distance travelled in one rotation (lap) = $2\pi r$

∴ Average speed

$$= \frac{\text{distance}}{\text{time}} = \frac{2\pi r}{t} = \frac{2\times 3.14\times 100}{62.8} =$$

10 m s^{-1}

Net displacement in one lap = 0

Average velocity = $\frac{\text{net displacement}}{\text{time}} = \frac{0}{t} = 0.$

5. **(b) :** Total distance travelled = 200 m

Total time taken = $\frac{100}{40} + \frac{100}{v}$

Average speed = $\frac{\text{total distance travelled}}{\text{total time taken}}$

$$48 = \frac{200}{\left(\frac{100}{40}+\frac{100}{v}\right)} \text{ or } 48 = \frac{2}{\left(\frac{1}{40}+\frac{1}{v}\right)}$$

or $\frac{1}{40}+\frac{1}{v} = \frac{1}{24}$ or $\frac{1}{v} = \frac{1}{24} - \frac{1}{40} = \frac{5-3}{120} = \frac{1}{60}$

or $v = 60$ km/h

6. **(c) :** Total distance travelled = s

Total time taken = $\frac{s/3}{10} + \frac{s/3}{20} + \frac{s/3}{60}$

$$= \frac{s}{30} + \frac{s}{60} + \frac{s}{180} = \frac{10s}{180} = \frac{s}{18}$$

Average speed = $\frac{\text{total distance travelled}}{\text{total time taken}}$

$$= \frac{s}{s/18} = 18 \text{ km/h}$$

7. **(b) :** Total distance covered = s

Total time taken = $\frac{s/2}{40} + \frac{s/2}{60} = \frac{5s}{240} = \frac{s}{48}$

∴ Average speed = $\frac{\text{total distance cover}}{\text{total time taken}}$

$$= \frac{s}{\left(\frac{s}{48}\right)} = 48 \text{ km/h}$$

8. **(d) :** The slope of displacement time graph gives velocity so, $v_1 = \tan 30°$

$v_2 = \tan 45°$

so, $\frac{v_1}{v_2} = \frac{\tan 30°}{\tan 45°} = \frac{1}{\sqrt{3}\times 1} = 1:\sqrt{3}$

9. **(d) :** Position of the car P at any time t, is

$x_P(t) = at + bt^2;\ v_P(t) = \frac{dx_P(t)}{dt}$

$= a + 2bt$

Similarly, for car Q,

$x_Q(t) = ft - t^2;\ v_Q(t) = \frac{dx_Q(t)}{dt}$

$= f - 2t$

$\because\ v_P(t) = v_Q(t)$

(Given)

$\therefore\ a + 2bt = f - 2t$ or, $2t(b+1) =$

$f - a \therefore t = \frac{f-a}{2(1+b)}$

10. **(a) :** Velocity of the particle is

$v = At + Bt^2$

$\frac{ds}{dt} = At + Bt^2; \int ds = \int (At + Bt^2)dt$

$\therefore s = \frac{At^2}{2} + B\frac{t^3}{3} + C$

$s(t = 1\text{ s}) = \frac{A}{2} + \frac{B}{3} + C; s(t = 2\text{ s})$

$= 2A + \frac{8}{3}B + C$

Required distance $= s(t = 2\text{ s}) - s(t =$ $1\text{ s})$

$= \left(2A + \frac{8}{3}B + C\right) - \left(\frac{A}{2} + \frac{B}{3} + C\right) = \frac{3}{2}A + \frac{7}{3}B$

11. **(b) :** Given $t = \sqrt{x} + 3$ or $\sqrt{x} = t - 3$

Squaring both sides, we get $x = (t - 3)^2$

Velocity, $v = \frac{dx}{dt} = \frac{d}{dt}(t-3)^2 = 2(t - 3)$

Velocity of the particle becomes zero, when

$2(t - 3) = 0$ or $= 3$ s,

At $t = 3$ s, $x = (3-3)^2 = 0$ m

12. **(d) :**

Because the slope is highest at C, $v = \frac{ds}{dt}$ is maximum

13. **(a) :** Given: $x = 9t^2 - t^3$

Speed $v = \frac{dx}{dt} = \frac{d}{dt}(9t^2 - t^3) = 18t - 3t^2$.

For maximum speed, $\frac{dv}{dt} = 0 \Rightarrow 18 - 6t = 0 \therefore t = 3$ s

$\therefore x_{max} = 81\text{ m} - 27\text{ m} = 54\text{ m}$

14. **(a) :** $x = 40 + 12t - t^3$

$\therefore$ Velocity, $v = \frac{dx}{dt} = 12 - 3t^2$

When particle come to rest, $\frac{dx}{dt} = v = 0$

$\therefore\ 12 - 3t^2 = 0 \Rightarrow 3t^2 = 12 \Rightarrow t =$ 2sec.

Distance travelled by the particle before coming to rest

$\int_0^s ds = \int_0^2 v dt$ or $s = \int_0^2 (12 - 3t^2)dt = 12t - \frac{3t^3}{3}\Big|_0^2$

$s = 12 \times 2 - 8 = 24 - 8 = 16$ m.

15. **(d) :**

$x = ae^{-\alpha t} + be^{\beta t};\ \frac{dx}{dt} = -a\alpha e^{-\alpha t} + b\beta e^{\beta t}$

$v = -a\alpha e^{-\alpha t} + b\beta e^{\beta t}$

Velocity will increases with time

16. **(a) :** The velocity $(v) = \frac{ds}{dt}$

Therefore, instantaneous velocity at point E is negative.

17. **(b) :** In one dimensional motion, the body can have one value of velocity at a time but not two values of velocities at a time.

18. **(d) :** According to question, velocity of unit mass varies as

$v(x) = \beta x^{-2n}$ ... (i), $\frac{dv}{dx} = -2n\beta x^{-2n-1}$

Acceleration of the particle is given by

$$a = \frac{dv}{dt} = \frac{dv}{dx} \times \frac{dx}{dt} = \frac{dv}{dx} \times v$$

Using equation (i) and (ii), we get

$a = (-2n\beta x^{-2n-1}) \times (\beta x^{-2n}) = -2n\beta^2 x^{-4n-1}$

19. **(d) :** Given: $x = 8 + 12t - t^3$

Velocity, $v = \frac{dx}{dt} = 12 - 3t^2$

When $v = \hat{v}, 12 - 3t^2 = 0$ or $t = 2$ s

$$a = \frac{dv}{dt} = -6t$$

$$a|_{t=2\text{ s}} = -12 \text{ m s}^{-2}$$

Retardation = 12 m s^{-2}

20. **(a) :** Distance, $x = (t + 5)^{-1}$

Velocity, $v = \frac{dx}{dt} = \frac{d}{dt}(t + 5)^{-1} = -(t + 5)^{-2}$

Acceleration,

$a = \frac{dv}{dt} = \frac{d}{dt}[-(t + 5)^{-2}] = 2(t + 5)^{-3}$

From equation (ii), we get

$v^{3/2} = -(t + 5)^{-3}$

Substituting this in equation (iii), we get

Acceleration,

$a = -2v^{3/2}$ or $a \propto$ (velocity))$^{3/2}$

From equation (i), we get $x^3 = (t + 5)^{-3}$

Substituting this in equation (iii), we get

Acceleration, $a = 2x^3$ or $a \propto$ (distance))^3

Hence option (a) is correct.

21. **(c) :** Given: At time $t = 0$, velocity, $v = 0$.

Acceleration $f = f_0\left(1 - \frac{t}{T}\right)$

At $f = 0, 0 = f_0\left(1 - \frac{t}{T}\right)$ Since f_0 is a constant,

$\therefore 1 - \frac{t}{T} = 0$ or $t = T$.

Also, acceleration $f = \frac{dv}{dt}$

$\therefore \int_0^{v_x} dv = \int_{t=0}^{t=T} f dt = \int_0^T f_0\left(1 - \frac{t}{T}\right) dt$

$\therefore v_x = \left[f_0 t - \frac{f_0 t^2}{2T}\right]_0^T = f_0 T - \frac{f_0 T^2}{2T} = \frac{1}{2} f_0 T.$

22. **(b) :** $\frac{ds}{dt} = 9t^2 + 14t + 14 \Rightarrow \frac{d^2s}{dt^2} = 18t + 14 = a$ $a_{t=1\text{ s}} = 18 \times 1 + 14 = 32 \text{ m/s}^2$

23. **(a) :** Distance $(x) = at^2 - bt^3$

Therefore velocity

$(v) = \frac{dx}{dt} = \frac{d}{dt}(at^2 - bt^3) = 2at - 3bt^2$

Acceleration

$= \frac{dv}{dt} = \frac{d}{dt}(2at - 3bt^2) = 2a - 6bt = 0$

or $t = \frac{2a}{6b} = \frac{a}{3b}$

24. **(c) :** Acceleration $\propto bt$. i.e., $\frac{d^2x}{dt^2} = a \propto bt$

Integrating, $\frac{dx}{dt} = \frac{bt^2}{2} + C$

Initially, $t = 0, dx/dt = v_0$

Therefore, $\frac{dx}{dt} = \frac{bt^2}{2} + v_0$

Integrating again, $x = \frac{bt^3}{6} + v_0t + C$

When $t = 0, x = 0 \Rightarrow C = 0$.

i.e., distance travelled by the particle

in time $t = v_0t + \frac{bt^3}{6}$.

25. **(c) :**

Displacement $(s) = t^3 - 6t^2 + 3t + 4$ m

Velocity $(v) = \frac{ds}{dt} = 3t^2 - 12t + 3$

Acceleration $(a) = \frac{dv}{dt} = 6t - 12$.

When $a = 0$, we get $t = 2$ seconds.

Therefore velocity when the acceleration is zero is

$v = 3 \times (2)^2 - (12 \times 2) + 3 = -9$ m/s

26. **(c) :** Distance travelled by a body during free fall is given by $S = ut + \frac{1}{2}at^2$

Here, $u = 0$ and $a = g$ $\therefore$

$S \propto t^2$

Here for 1st second, $S_1 = Kt^2 = K$

For 2nd second, $S_2 = K(2)^2 = 4K$

For 3rd second, $S_3 = K(3)^2 = 9K$

For 4th second, $S_4 = K(4)^2 = 16K$

Distance covered in 2 seconds,

$4K - K = 3K$

Distance covered in 3rd seconds,

$9K - 4K = 5K$

Distance covered in 4th seconds,

$16K - 9K = 7K$

$\therefore$ Ratio of distances travelled by the freely falling body will be 1: 3: 5: 7

27. **(d) :** Here, $u = \frac{20\text{ m}}{\text{s}}, v = \frac{80\text{ m}}{\text{s}}, g = \frac{10\text{ m}}{\text{s}^2}, h = ?$ $v^2 = u^2 + 2gh$

$\Rightarrow 80^2 = 20^2 + 2 \times 10 \times h$. Hence, $h = 300$ m

28. **(d) :** Distance covered by the stone in first 5 seconds (i.e. $t = 5$ s) is

$$h_1 = \frac{1}{2}g(5)^2 = \frac{25}{2}g$$

Distance travelled by the stone in next 5 seconds (i.e. $t = 10$ s) is

$$h_1 + h_2 = \frac{1}{2}g(10)^2 = \frac{100}{2}g$$

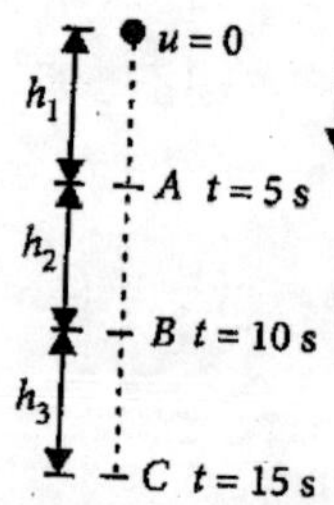

Distance travelled by the stone in next 5 seconds (i.e. $t = 15$ s) is

$$h_1 + h_2 + h_3 = \frac{1}{2}g(15)^2 = \frac{225}{2}g$$

Subtract (i) from (ii), we get

$$(h_1 + h_2) - h_1 = \frac{100}{2}g - \frac{25}{2}g = \frac{75}{2}g$$

$$h_2 = \frac{75}{2}g = 3h_1$$

Subtract (ii) from (iii), we get

$$(h_1 + h_2 + h_3) - (h_2 + h_1) = \frac{225}{2}g - \frac{100}{2}g$$

$$h_3 = \frac{125}{2}g = 5h_1$$

From (i), (iv) and (v), we get $h_1 = \frac{h_2}{3} = \frac{h_3}{5}$

29. **(b) :** Here, $u = 0, g = 10 \text{ m s}^{-2}, h = 20 \text{ m}$

Let v be the velocity with which the stone hits the ground.

$\therefore v^2 = u^2 + 2gh$

or $v = \sqrt{2gh} = \sqrt{2 \times 10 \times 20} = 20 \text{ m/s}$

$[\because u = 0]$

30. **(a) :** Let the two balls meet after ts at distance x from the platform.

For the first ball, $u = 0, t = 18 \text{ s}, g = 10 \text{ m/s}^2$

Using $h = ut + \frac{1}{2}gt^2$

$$\therefore x = \frac{1}{2} \times 10 \times 18^2$$

For the second ball, $u = v, t = 12 \text{ s}, g = 10 \text{ m/s}^2$

Using $h = ut + \frac{1}{2}gt^2$

$$\therefore x = v \times 12 + \frac{1}{2} \times 10 \times 12^2$$

From equations (i) and (ii), we get

$$\frac{1}{2} \times 10 \times 18^2 = 12v + \frac{1}{2} \times 10 \times (12)^2$$

or $12v = \frac{1}{2} \times 10 \times [(18)^2 - (12)^2]$

$12v = \frac{1}{2} \times 10 \times 30 \times 6$ or $v = \frac{1 \times 10 \times 30 \times 6}{2 \times 12} = 75 \text{ m/s}$

31. **(b) :** Given $u = 0$

Distance travelled in 10 s, $S_1 = \frac{1}{2}a \cdot 10^2 = 50a$

Distance travelled in

20 s, $S_2 = \frac{1}{2}a \cdot 20^2 = 200a \therefore S_2 = 4S_1$

32. **(b) :** $v^2 - u^2 = 2as$

Given $v = 20 \text{ m s}^{-1}, u = 10 \text{ m s}^{-1}, s = 135 \text{ m}$

$$\therefore a = \frac{400-100}{2 \times 135} = \frac{300}{270} = \frac{10}{9} \text{ m/s}^2$$

$$v = u + at \Rightarrow t = \frac{v-u}{a} = \frac{10 \text{ m/s}}{\frac{10}{9} \text{ m/s}^2}$$

$$= 9 \text{ s}$$

33. **(a) :** Distance travelled in the 3rd second = Distance travelled in 3 s - distance travelled in 2 s

As, $u = 0, S_{(3^{rd}s)} = \frac{1}{2}a \cdot 3^2 - \frac{1}{2}a \cdot 2^2 = \frac{1}{2} \cdot a \cdot 5$

Given $a = \frac{4}{3} \text{ m s}^{-2}; \therefore S_{(3^{rd})} = \frac{1}{2} \times \frac{4}{3} \times 5 = \frac{10}{3} \text{ m}$

34. **(a) :** Time taken by a body fall from a height h to reach the ground is $t = \sqrt{\frac{2h}{g}}$

$$\therefore \frac{t_A}{t_B} = \frac{\sqrt{\frac{2h_A}{g}}}{\sqrt{\frac{2h_B}{g}}} = \sqrt{\frac{h_A}{h_B}} = \sqrt{\frac{16}{25}} = \frac{4}{5}.$$

35. **(a) :** As, $v^2 = u^2 - 2gh$

After reaching maximum height velocity becomes zero.

$$0 = (10)^2 - 2 \times 10 \times \frac{h}{2} \therefore h = \frac{200}{20}$$

$$= 10 \text{ m}$$

36. **(a) :** Interval of ball thrown = 2 s

If we want that minimum three (more than two) balls remain in air then time of flight of first ball must be greater than 4 s.

$$T > 4\text{sec or } \frac{2u}{g} > 4\text{sec} \Rightarrow u > 19.6 \text{ m/s}$$

37. **(b) :** Let total height = H

Time of ascent = T

So, $H = uT - \frac{1}{2}gT^2$

Distance covered by ball in time $(T - t)$sec.

$$y = u(T - t) - \frac{1}{2}g(T - t)^2$$

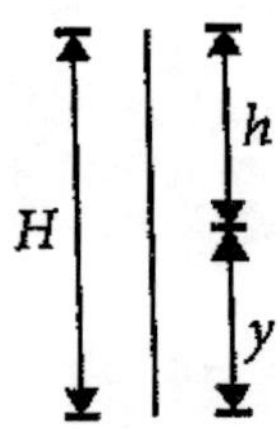

So distance covered by ball in last t sec., $h = H - y$

$$= \left[uT - \frac{1}{2}gT^2\right] - \left[u(T - t) - \frac{1}{2}g(T - t)^2\right]$$

By solving and putting $T = \frac{u}{g}$ we will get $h = \frac{1}{2}gt^2$.

38. **(c) :** For half height,

$$10^2 = u^2 - 2g\frac{h}{2}$$

For total height,

$$0 = u^2 - 2gh$$

From (i) and (ii)

$$\Rightarrow 10^2 = \frac{2gh}{2} \Rightarrow h = 10 \text{ m}$$

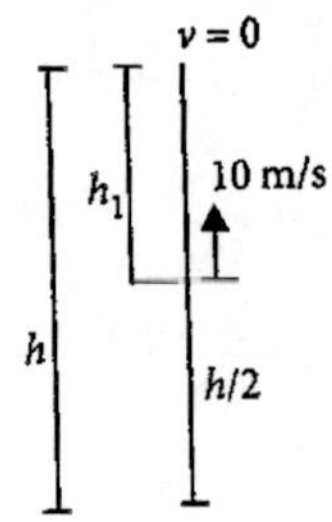

39. **(c) :** 1st case $v^2 - u^2 = 2as$

$$0 - \left(\frac{100}{9}\right)^2 = 2 \times a \times 2$$

$$a = -\frac{10^4}{81 \times 4} \text{ m/s}^2$$

2nd case : $0 - \left(\frac{200}{9}\right)^2 = 2 \times \left(-\frac{10^4}{81 \times 4}\right) \times s$

$[\because 80 \text{ km/h} = 200/9 \text{ m/s}]$

or = 8 m.

40. **(d) :** Initial velocity $u = 0$,

Final velocity = 144 km/h = 40 m/s

and time = 20 s

Using $v = u + at \Rightarrow a = v/t = 2 \text{ m/s}^2$

Again, $= ut + \frac{1}{2}at^2 = \frac{1}{2} \times 2 \times (20)^2 = 400$ m.

41. **(a) :** Initial velocity of first body $(u_1) = 0$; Final velocity $(v_1) = 3$ m/s and initial velocity of second body $(u_2) = 4$ m/s

Height $(h) = \frac{v_1^2}{2g} = \frac{(3)^2}{2\times9.8} = 0.46$ m

Therefore required velocity of the second body,

$v_2 = \sqrt{u_2^2 + 2gh}$

$= \sqrt{(4)^2 + 2\times 9.8\times 0.46} = 5$ m/s

42. **(a) :** Height of tap = 5 m. For the first drop,

$$5 = ut + \frac{1}{2}gt^2 = \frac{1}{2}\times 10t^2 = 5t^2 \text{ or } t = 1 \text{ s}$$

It means that the third drop leaves after one second of the first drop, or each drop leaves after every 0.5 s. Distance covered by the second drop in 0.5 s $= \frac{1}{2}gt^2 = \frac{1}{2}\times 10\times(0.5)^2 = 1.25$ m Therefore distance of the second drop above the ground $= 5 - 1.25 = 3.75$ m

43. **(d) :** Initial velocity $(u) = 0$; acceleration in the first phase $= \alpha$; deceleration in the second phase $= \beta$ and total time $= t$. When car is accelerating then final velocity $(v) = u + \alpha t = 0 + \alpha t_1$ or $t_1 = \frac{v}{\alpha}$ and when car is decelerating, then final velocity $0 = v - \beta t$ or $t_2 = \frac{v}{\beta}$

Therefore total time $(t) = t_1 + t_2 = \frac{v}{\alpha} + \frac{v}{\beta}$

$$t = v\left(\frac{1}{\alpha} + \frac{1}{\beta}\right) = v\left(\frac{\beta+\alpha}{\alpha\beta}\right) \text{ or } v = \frac{\alpha\beta t}{\alpha+\beta}$$

44. **(a) :** Initial velocity $(u) = 20$ km/h; Final velocity $(v) = 60$ km/h and time $(t) = 4$ hours.

velocity $(v) = 60 = u + at = 20 + (a\times 4)$

or, $a = \frac{60-20}{4} = 10$ km/h^2.

Therefore distance travelled in 4 hours is

$$s = ut + \frac{1}{2}at^2 = (20\times 4) + \frac{1}{2}\times 10 \times (4)^2 = 160 \text{ km}$$

45. **(a) :** Distance covered in n^{th} second is given by

$$s_n = u + \frac{a}{2}(2n-1)$$

Here, $u = 0$. $\therefore s_4 = 0 + \frac{a}{2}(2\times 4 - 1) = \frac{7a}{2}$

$$s_3 = 0 + \frac{a}{2}(2\times 3 - 1) = \frac{5a}{2} \quad \therefore \frac{s_4}{s_3} = \frac{7}{5}$$

46. **(b) :** Let h be height of the tower and t is the time taken by the body to reach the ground.

Here, $u = 0, a = g$

$\therefore h = ut + \frac{1}{2}gt^2$ or $h = 0\times t + \frac{1}{2}gt^2$

or $h = \frac{1}{2}gt^2$

Distance covered in last two seconds is

$40 = \frac{1}{2}gt^2 - \frac{1}{2}g(t-2)^2$ or $40 = \frac{1}{2}gt^2 - \frac{1}{2}g(t^2 + 4 - 4t)$

or $40 = (2t-2)g$ or $t = 3$ s

From eqn (i), we get $h = \frac{1}{2}\times 10\times(3)^2$

or $h = 45$ m

47. **(b) :** Distance covered in n^{th} second is given by

$$s_n = u + \frac{a}{2}(2n-1)$$

Given : $u = 0, a = g$

$$\therefore s_4 = \frac{g}{2}(2\times4-1) = \frac{7g}{2}$$

$$s_5 = \frac{g}{2}(2\times5-1) = \frac{9g}{2} \quad \therefore \frac{s_4}{s_5} = \frac{7}{9}$$

48. **(c) :**

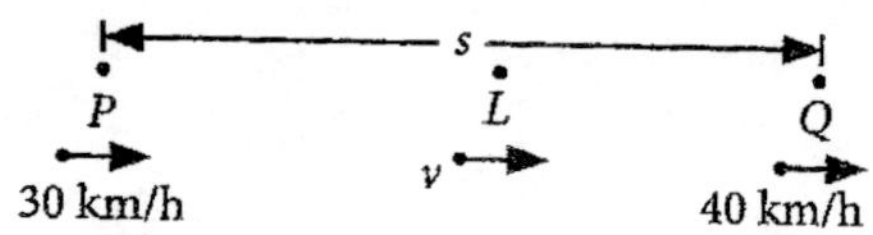

Let $PQ = s$ and L is the midpoint of PQ and v be velocity of the car at point L.

Using third equation of motion, we get $(40)^2 - (30)^2 = 2a\,s$

or $a = \frac{(40)^2-(30)^2}{2s} = \frac{350}{s}$

Also, $v^2 - (30)^2 = 2a\frac{s}{2}$ or $v^2 - (30)^2 = 2\times\frac{350}{s}\times\frac{s}{2}$

or $v = 25\sqrt{2}$ km/h

[Using (i)]

49. **(b) :** Let v_1 is the velocity of Preeti on stationary escalator and d is the distance travelled by her $\therefore v_1 = \frac{d}{t_1}$

Again, let v_2 is the velocity of escalator

$\therefore v_2 = \frac{d}{t_2}$ $\therefore$ Net velocity of Preeti on moving escalator with respect to

$$v = v_1 + v_2 = \frac{d}{t_1} + \frac{d}{t_2} = d\left(\frac{t_1+t_2}{t_1t_2}\right)$$

The time taken by her to walk up on the moving escalator will be

$$t = \frac{d}{v} = \frac{d}{d\left(\frac{t_1+t_2}{t_1t_2}\right)} = \frac{t_1t_2}{t_1+t_2}$$

50. **(d)** : Let v_s be the velocity of the scooter, the distance between the scooter and the bus = 1000 m,

The velocity of the bus = 10 m s^{-1}

Time taken to overtake = 100 s

Relative velocity of the scooter with respect to the bus = $(v_s - 10)$

$\therefore \frac{1000}{(v_s-10)} = 100\text{ s} \Rightarrow v_s = 20\text{ m s}^{-1}$.

51. **(d) :** Choose the positive direction of x-axis to be from south to north. Then

velocity of train $v_T = +10\text{ m s}^{-1}$

velocity of parrot $v_P = -5\text{ m s}^{-1}$

Relative velocity of parrot with respect to train

$$= v_P - v_T = (-5\text{ m s}^{-1}) - (+10\text{ m s}^{-1})$$

$$= -15\text{ m s}^{-1}$$

i.e. parrot appears to move with a speed of 15 m s^{-1} from north to south

$\therefore$ Time taken by parrot to cross the train

$$= \frac{150\text{ m}}{15\text{ m s}^{-1}} = 10\text{ s}$$

Chapter: 3

MOTION IN A PLANE

Scalars and Vectors

1. Identify the vector quantity among the following. **(1997)**

(a) Distance
(b) Angular momentum
(c) Heat (d) Energy

Addition and Subtraction of Vectors- Graphical Method

2. Six vectors, $\vec{a}$ through $\vec{f}$ have the magnitudes and directions indicated in the figure. Which of the following statements is true? **(2010)**

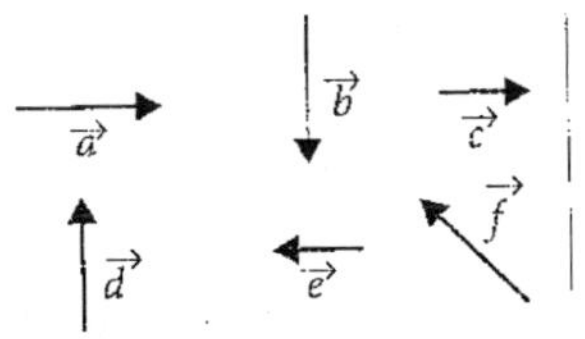

(a) $\vec{b}+\vec{c}=\vec{f}$ (b) $\vec{d}+\vec{c}=\vec{f}$

(c) $\vec{d}+\vec{e}=\vec{f}$ (d) $\vec{b}+\vec{e}=\vec{f}$

Resolution of Vectors

3. If a unit vector is represented by $0.5\hat{\imath}-0.8\hat{\jmath}+c\hat{k}$ then the value of c is **(1999)**

(a) $\sqrt{0.01}$ (b) $\sqrt{0.11}$
(c) 1 (d) $\sqrt{0.39}$

Vector Addition-Analytical Method

4. If the magnitude of sum of two vectors is equal to the magnitude of difference of the two vectors, the angle between these vectors is **(NEET-I 2016)**

(a) 45° (b) 180°

(c) 0° (d) 90°

5. The vectors $\vec{A}$ and $\vec{B}$ are such that $|\vec{A}+\vec{B}|=|\vec{A}-\vec{B}|$. The angle between the two vectors is **(2006,1996,1991)**

(a) 45° (b) 90°

(c) 60° (d) 75°

6. If $|\vec{A}+\vec{B}|=|\vec{A}|+|\vec{B}|$ then angle between A and B will be **(2001)**

(a) 90° (b) 120°

(c) 0° (d) 60°

7. The magnitude of vectors $\vec{A},\vec{B}$ and $\vec{C}$ are 3,4 and 5 units respectively. If $\vec{A}+\vec{B}=\vec{C}$, the angle between $\vec{A}$ and $\vec{B}$ is **(1988)**

(a) $\pi/2$ (b) $\cos^{-1}(0.6)$

(c) $\tan^{-1}(7/5)$ (d) $\pi/4$.

Motion in a Plane

8. The x and y coordinates of the particle at any time are $x=5t-2t^2$ and $y=10t$ respectively, where x and y are in metres and t in seconds. The acceleration of the particle at $t=2$ s is **(2017)**

(a) $5\ \text{m s}^{-2}$ (b) $-4\ \text{m s}^{-2}$

(c) $-8\ \text{m s}^{-2}$ (d) 0

9. The position vector of a particle $\vec{R}$ as a function of time is given by $\vec{R}=4\sin(2\pi t)\hat{\imath}+4\cos(2\pi t)\hat{\jmath}$ where R is in meters, t is in seconds and $\hat{\imath}$ and $\hat{\jmath}$ denote unit vectors along x-and y-directions, respectively. Which one of the following statements is wrong for the motion of particle? **(2015)**

(a) Magnitude of the velocity of particle is 8π meter/second.

(b) Path of the particle is a circle of radius 4 meter.

(c) Acceleration vector is along $-\vec{R}$.

(d) Magnitude of acceleration vector is $\frac{v^2}{R}$, where v is the velocity of particle.

10. A particle is moving such that its position coordinates (x, y) are $(2\text{ m}, 3\text{ m})$ at time $t = 0$, $(6\text{ m}, 7\text{ m})$ at time $t = 2\text{ s}$ and $(13\text{ m}, 14\text{ m})$ at time $= 5\text{ s}$. Average velocity vector $(\vec{v}_{\text{av}})$ from $t = 0$ to $t = 5\text{ s}$ is **(2014)**

(a) $\frac{1}{5}(13\hat{\imath} + 14\hat{\jmath})$ (b) $\frac{7}{3}(\hat{\imath} + \hat{\jmath})$

(c) $2(\hat{\imath} + \hat{\jmath})$ (d) $\frac{11}{5}(\hat{\imath} + \hat{\jmath})$

11. A body is moving with velocity 30 m/s towards east. After 10 seconds its velocity becomes 40 m/s towards north. The average acceleration of the body is **(2011)**

(a) 1 m/s^2 (b) 7 m/s^2

(c) $\sqrt{7}\text{ m/s}^2$ (d) 5 m/s^2

12. A particle moves in $x - y$ plane according to rule $x = a\sin\omega t$ and $y = a\cos\omega t$. The particle follows **(Mains 2010)**

(a) an elliptical path

(b) a circular path

(c) a parabolic path

(d) a straight line path inclined equally to x and y-axes

13. A particle starting from the origin (0,0) moves in a straight line in the (x, y) plane. Its coordinates at a later time are $(\sqrt{3}, 3)$. The path of the particle makes with the x-axis an angle of **(2007)**

(a) 45° (b) 60°

(c) 0° (d) 30°

14. A bus is moving on a straight road towards north with a uniform speed of 50 km/ hour then it turns left through90°. If the speed remains unchanged after turning, the increase in the velocity of bus in the turning process is **(1989)**

(a) 70.7 km/hr along south-west direction

(b) zero

(c) 50 km/hr along west

(d) 70.7 km/hr along north-west direction

Motion in a Plane with Constant Acceleration

15. A car starts from rest and accelerates at 5 m/s^2. At $= 4\text{ s}$, a ball is dropped out of a window by a person sitting in the car. What is the velocity and acceleration of the ball at $t = 6\text{ s}$? (Take $g = 10\text{ m/s}^2$) **(2021)**

(a) $20\sqrt{2}\text{ m/s}, 10\text{ m/s}^2$

(b) $20\text{ m/s}, 5\text{ m/s}^2$

(c) $20\text{ m/s}, 0$

(d) $20\sqrt{2}\text{ m/s}, 0$

16. When an object is shot from the bottom of a long smooth inclined plane kept at an angle 60° with horizontal, it can travel a distance x_1 along the plane. But when the inclination is decreased to 30° and the same object is shot with the same velocity, it can travel x_2 distance. Then $x_1 : x_2$ will be **(2019)**

(a) $1:2\sqrt{3}$ (b) $1:\sqrt{2}$

(c) $\sqrt{2}:1$ (d) $1:\sqrt{3}$

17. A particle has initial velocity $(2\hat{\imath}+3\hat{\jmath})$ and acceleration $(0.3\hat{\imath}+0.2\hat{\jmath})$. The magnitude of velocity after 10 seconds will be **(2012)**

(a) $9\sqrt{2}$ units (b) $5\sqrt{2}$ units

(c) 5 units (d) 9 units

18. A particle has initial velocity $(3\hat{\imath}+4\hat{\jmath})$ and has acceleration $(0.4\hat{\imath}+0.3\hat{\jmath})$. Its speed after 10 s is **(2010)**

(a) 7 units (c) 8.5 units

(b) $7\sqrt{2}$ units (d) 10 units

19. A man is slipping on a frictionless inclined plane and a bag falls down from the same height. Then the velocity of both is related as (v_m = velocity of man and v_B = velocity of bag) **(2000)**

(a) $v_B > v_m$ (b) $v_B < v_m$

(c) $v_B = v_m$ (d) v_B and v_m can't be related.

Relative Velocity in Two Dimensions

20. The speed of a swimmer in still water is 20 m/s. The speed of river water is 10 m/s and is flowing due east. If he is standing on the south bank and wishes to cross the river along the shortest path, the angle at which he should make his strokes w.r.t. north is, given by **(2019)**

(a) 45° west (b) 30° west

(c) 0° (d) 60° west

21. Two boys are standing at the ends A and B of a ground where $AB = a$. The boy at B starts running in a direction perpendicular to AB with velocity v_1. The boy at A starts running simultaneously with velocity v and catches the other in a time t, where t is **(2005)**

(a) $\frac{a}{\sqrt{v^2+v_1^2}}$ (b) $\frac{a}{v+v_1}$

(c) $\frac{a}{v-v_1}$ (d) $\sqrt{\frac{a^2}{v^2-v_1^2}}$

22. The width of river is 1 km. The velocity of boat is 5 km/hr. The boat covered the width of river in shortest time 15 min. Then the velocity of river stream is **(2000, 1998)**

(a) 3 km/hr (b) 4 km/hr

(c) $\sqrt{29}$ km/hr (d) $\sqrt{41}$ km/hr

23. A person aiming to reach exactly opposite point on the bank of a stream is swimming with a speed of 0.5 m/s at an angle of 120° with the direction of flow of water. The speed of water in the stream, is **(1999)**

(a) 0.25 m/s (b) 0.5 m/s

(c) 1.0 m/s (d) 0.433 m/s

24. Two particles A and B are connected by a rigid rod AB. The rod slides along perpendicular rails as shown here. The velocity of A to the left is 10 m/s.

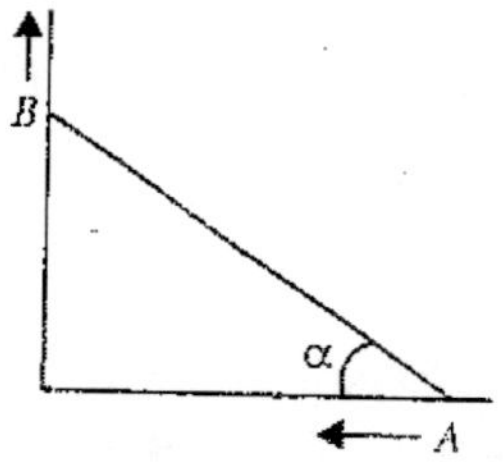

What is the velocity of B when angle = 60°? **(1998)**

(a) 10 m/s (b) 9.8 m/s

(c) 5.8 m/s (d) 17.3 m/s.

25. A boat is sent across a river with a velocity of 8 km h^{-1}. If the resultant velocity of boat is 10 km h^{-1}, then velocity of river is **(1994, 1993)**

(a) 12.8 km h^{-1} (b) 6 km h^{-1}

(c) 8 km h^{-1} (d) 10 km h^{-1}

Projectile Motion

26. A bullet is fired from a gun at the speed of 280 m s–1 in the direction 30° above the horizontal. The maximum height attained by the bullet is (g = 9.8 m s–2, sin 30° = 0.5)

(a) 2000 m (b) 1000 m

(c) 3000 m (d) 2800 m

27. A ball is projected with a velocity, 10 ms^{-1} at an angle of 60° with the vertical direction. Its speed at the highest point of its trajectory will be **(2022)**

(a) zero (b) $5\sqrt{3} \text{ m s}^{-1}$

(c) 5 m s^{-1} (d) 10 m s^{-1}

28. A particle moving in a circle of radius R with a uniform speed taken a time T to complete one revolution. If this particle were projected with the same speed at an angle ' θ ' to the horizontal, the maximum height attained by it equal $4R$. The angle of projection θ, is then given by **(2021)**

(a) $\theta = \sin^{-1}\left(\frac{2gT^2}{\pi^2 R}\right)^{1/2}$

(b) $\theta = \cos^{-1}\left(\frac{gT^2}{\pi^2 R}\right)^{1/2}$

(c) $\theta = \cos^{-1}\left(\frac{\pi^2 R}{gT^2}\right)^{1/2}$

(d) $\theta = \sin^{-1}\left(\frac{\pi^2 R}{gT^2}\right)^{1/2}$

29. A projectile is fired from the surface of the earth with a velocity of 5 m s^{-1} and angle θ with the horizontal. Another projectile fired from another planet with a velocity of 3 m s^{-1} at the same angle follows a trajectory which is identical with the trajectory of the projectile fired from the earth. The value of the acceleration due to gravity on the planet is (in ms^{-2}) is (Given $g = 9.8 \text{ m s}^{-2}$) **(2014)**

(a) 3.5 (b) 5.9

(c) 16.3 (d) 110.8

(2023)

30. The velocity of a projectile at the initial point A is $(2\hat{i} + 3\hat{j})$m/s. Its velocity (in m/s) at point B is **(2013)**

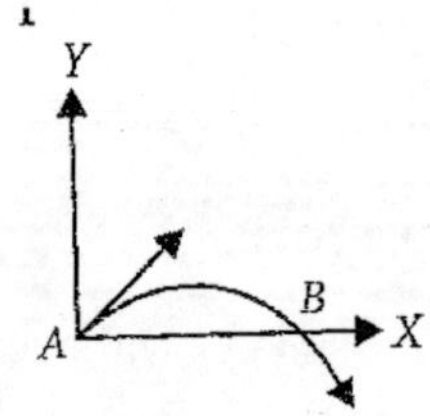

(a) $2\hat{\imath} - 3\hat{\jmath}$ (b) $2\hat{\imath} + 3\hat{\jmath}$

(c) $-2\hat{\imath} - 3\hat{\jmath}$ (d) $-2\hat{\imath} + 3\hat{\jmath}$

31. The horizontal range and the maximum height of a projectile are equal. The angle of projection of the projectile is **(2012)**

(a) $\theta = \tan^{-1}\left(\frac{1}{4}\right)$

(b) $\theta = \tan^{-1}(4)$

(c) $\theta = \tan^{-1}(2)$

(d) $\theta = 45°$

32. A missile is fired for maximum range with an initial velocity of 20 m/s. If $= 10 \text{ m/s}^2$, the range of the missile is **(2011)**

(a) 40 m (b) 50 m

(c) 60 m (d) 20 m

33. A projectile is fired at an angle of 45° with the horizontal. Elevation angle of the projectile at its highest point as seen from the point of projection, is **(Mains 2011)**

(a) 45° (b) 60°

(c) $\tan^{-1}\left(\frac{1}{2}\right)$ (d) $\tan^{-1}\left(\frac{\sqrt{3}}{2}\right)$

34. The speed of a projectile at its maximum height is half of its initial speed. The angle of projection is **(Mains 2010)**

(a) 60° (b) 15°

(c) 30° (d) 45°

35. A particle of mass m is projected with velocity v making an angle of 45° with the horizontal. When the particle lands on the level ground the magnitude of the change in its momentum will be **(2008)**

(a) $mv\sqrt{2}$ (b) zero

(c) $2mv$ (d) $mv/\sqrt{2}$

36. For angles of projection of a projectile at angle $(45° - \theta)$ and $(45° + \theta)$, the horizontal range described by the projectile are in the ratio of **(2006)**

(a) 2: 1 (b) 1: 1

(c) 2: 3 (d) 1: 2

37. A particle A is dropped from a height and another particle B is projected in horizontal direction with speed of 5 m/s from the same height then correct statement is **(2002)**

(a) particle A will reach at ground first with respect to particle B

(b) particle B will reach at ground first with respect to particle A

(c) both particles will reach at ground simultaneously

(d) both particles will reach at ground with same speed.

38. Two projectiles of same mass and with same velocity are thrown at an angle 60° and 30° with the horizontal, then which will remain same **(2000)**

(a) time of flight

(b) rangc of projectile

(c) maximum height acquired

(d) all of them.

39. If a body A of mass M is thrown with velocity v at an angle of 30° to the horizontal and another body B of the same mass is thrown with the same speed at an angle of 60° to the horizontal, the ratio of horizontal range of A to B will be

(1992,1990)

(a) $1:3$ (b) $1:1$

(c) $1:\sqrt{3}$ (d) $\sqrt{3}:1$.

40. The maximum range of a gun of horizontal terrain is 16 km. If $g = 10\ \text{m s}^{-2}$, then muzzle velocity of a shell must be **(1990)**

(a) $160\ \text{m s}^{-1}$ (b) $200\sqrt{2}\ \text{m s}^{-1}$

(c) $400\ \text{m s}^{-1}$ (d) $800\ \text{m s}^{-1}$

Uniform Circular Motion

41. Two particles A and B are moving in uniform circular motion in concentric circles of radii r_A and r_B with speed v_A and v_B respectively. Their time period of rotation is the same. The ratio of angular speed of A to that of B will be **(2019)**

(a) $1:1$ (b) $r_A:r_B$

(c) $v_A:v_B$ (d) $r_B:r_A$

42. A particle starting from rest, moves in a circle of radius 'r'. It attains a velocity of V_0 m/s in the nth round. Its angular acceleration will be

(Odisha NEET 2019)

(a) $\frac{V_0}{n}$ rad/s^2 (b) $\frac{V_0}{2\pi n r^2}$ rad/s^2

(c) $\frac{V_0^2}{4\pi n r^2}$ rad/s^2 (d) $\frac{V_0^2}{4\pi n r}$ rad/s^2

43. In the given figure, $a = 15\ \text{m s}^{-2}$ represents the total acceleration of a particle moving in the clockwise direction in a circle of radius $R = 2.5$ m at a given instant of time. The speed of the particle is

(NEET-II 2016)

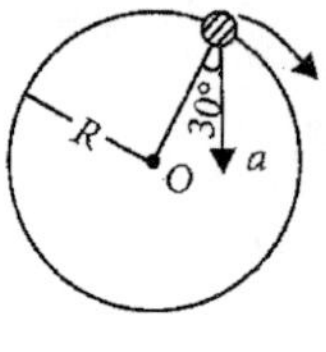

(a) $4.5\ \text{m s}^{-1}$ (b) $5.0\ \text{m s}^{-1}$

(c) $5.7\ \text{m s}^{-1}$ (d) $6.2\ \text{m s}^{-1}$

44. A particle moves in a circle of radius 5 cm with constant speed and time period 0.2πs. The acceleration of the particle is

(2011)

(a) $15\ \text{m/s}^2$ (b) $25\ \text{m/s}^2$

(c) $36\ \text{m/s}^2$ (d) $5\ \text{m/s}^2$

45. A stone tied to the end of a string of 1 m long is whirled in a horizontal circle with a constant speed. If the stone makes 22 revolutions in 44 seconds, what is the magnitude and direction of acceleration of the stone? **(2005)**

(a) $\pi^2\ \text{m s}^{-2}$ and direction along the radius towards the centre

(b) $\pi^2\ \text{m s}^{-2}$ and direction along the radius away from the centre

(c) $\pi^2\ \text{m s}^{-2}$ and direction along the tangent to the circle

(d) $\pi^2/4\ \text{m s}^{-2}$ and direction along the radius towards the centre.

46. A particle moves along a circle of radius $\left(\frac{20}{\pi}\right)$ m with constant tangential acceleration. If the velocity of the particle is 80 m/s at the end of the second revolution after motion has begun, the tangential acceleration is **(2003)**

(a) 40 m/s^2 (b) $640\pi m/s^2$

(c) $160\pi m/s^2$ (d) $40\pi m/s^2$

47. Two particles having mass M and m are moving in a circular path having radius R and r. If their time period are same then the ratio of angular velocity will be **(2001)**

(a) $\frac{r}{R}$ (b) $\frac{R}{r}$

(c) 1 (d) $\sqrt{\frac{R}{r}}$

48. Two racing cars of masses m_1 and m_2 are moving in circles of radii r_1 and r_2 respectively. Their speeds are such that each makes a complete circle in the same time t. The ratio of the angular speeds of the first to the second car is **(1999)**

(a) $r_1 : r_2$ (b) $m_1 : m_2$

(c) 1 : 1 (d) $m_1 m_2 : r_1 r_2$

49. A body is whirled in a horizontal circle of radius 20 cm. It has an angular velocity of 10rad/s. What is its linear velocity at any point on circular path? **(1996)**

(a) 20 m/s (b) $\sqrt{2}$ m/s

(c) 10 m/s (d) 2 m/s

50. The angular speed of a flywheel making 120 revolutions/minute is **(1995)**

(a) 4πrad/s (b) $4\pi^2$rad/s

(c) πrad/s (d) 2πrad/s

51. An electric fan has blades of length 30 cm measured from the axis of rotation. If the fan is rotating at 120rpm, the acceleration of a point on the tip of the blade is **(1990)**

(a) 1600 m s^{-2} (b) 47.4 m s^{-2}

(c) 23.7 m s^{-2} (d) 50.55 m s^{-2}

ANSWER KEY

1.	(b)	2.	(c)	3.	(b)	4.	(d)	5.	(b)	6.	(c)
7.	(a)	8.	(b)	9.	(a)	10.	(d)	11.	(d)	12.	(b)
13.	(b)	14.	(a)	15.	(a)	16.	(d)	17.	(b)	18.	(b)
19.	(c)	20.	(b)	21.	(d)	22.	(a)	23.	(a)	24.	(d)
25.	(b)	26.	(2)	22.	(b)	28.	(a)	29.	(a)	30.	(a)
31.	(b)	32.	(a)	33.	(c)	34.	(a)	35.	(a)	36.	(b)
37.	(c)	38.	(b)	39.	(b)	40.	(c)	41.	(a)	42.	(c)
43.	(c)	44.	(d)	45.	(a)	46.	(a)	47.	(c)	48.	(c)
49.	(d)	50.	(a)	51.	(b)						

Hints & Explanations

1. **(b)** : Since the angular momentum has both magnitude and direction, it is a vector quantity.

2. **(c)** :

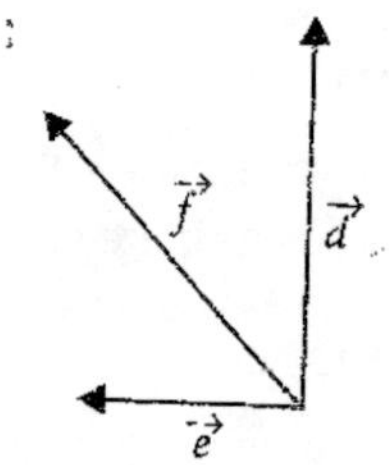

From figure, $\vec{d} + \vec{e} = \vec{f}$

3. **(b)** : For a unit vector $\hat{n}, |\hat{n}| = 1$

$|0.5\hat{\imath} - 0.8\hat{\jmath} + c\hat{k}|^2 = 1^2 \Rightarrow 0.25 + 0.64 + c^2 = 1$ or $c = \sqrt{0.11}$

4. **(d)** : Let the two vectors be $\vec{A}$ and $\vec{B}$.

Then, magnitude of sum of $\vec{A}$ and $\vec{B}$,

$|\vec{A} + \vec{B}| = \sqrt{A^2 + B^2 + 2AB\cos\theta}$

and magnitude of difference of $\vec{A}$ and $\vec{B}$

$|\vec{A} - \vec{B}| = \sqrt{A^2 + B^2 - 2AB\cos\theta}$, $|\vec{A} + \vec{B}| = |\vec{A} - \vec{B}|$ (given) or $\sqrt{A^2 + B^2 + 2AB\cos\theta} = \sqrt{A^2 + B^2 - 2AB\cos\theta}$

$\Rightarrow 4AB\cos\theta = 0 \because 4AB \neq 0, \therefore \cos\theta = 0$ or $\theta = 90°$

5. **(b)** : Let θ be angle between $\vec{A}$ and $\vec{B}$

$|\vec{A} + \vec{B}| = |\vec{A} - \vec{B}|$, then $|\vec{A} + \vec{B}|^2 = |\vec{A} - \vec{B}|^2$

$A^2 + B^2 + 2AB\cos\theta = A^2 + B^2 - 2AB\cos\theta$

or $4AB\cos\theta = 0$ or $\cos\theta = 0$ or $\theta = 90°$

6. **(c)** : $|\vec{A} + \vec{B}| = |\vec{A}| + |\vec{B}|$ if $\vec{A} \parallel \vec{B}. \theta = 0°$ [i.e. $\vec{A}, \vec{B}$ are in same direction]

7. **(a)** : Let θ be angle between $\vec{A}$ and $\vec{B}$.

Given: $A = |\vec{A}| = 3$ units, $B = |\vec{B}| = 4$ units, $C = |\vec{C}| = 5$ units

$|\vec{A} + \vec{B}| = |\vec{C}| \Rightarrow A^2 + 2AB\cos\theta + B^2 = C^2$

$9 + 2AB\cos\theta + 16 = 25$ or $2AB\cos\theta = 0$ or $\cos\theta = 0 \therefore \theta = 90°$.

8. **(b)** : $x = 5t - 2t^2, y = 10t$

$\frac{dx}{dt} = 5 - 4t, \frac{dy}{dt} = 10 \therefore v_x = 5 - 4t, v_y = 10$

$\frac{dv_x}{dt} = -4, \frac{dv_y}{dt} = 0 \therefore a_x = -4, a_y = 0$

Acceleration, $\vec{a} = a_x\hat{\imath} + a_y\hat{\jmath} = -4\hat{\imath}$

$\therefore$ The acceleration of the particle at $t = 2$ s is -4 m s^{-2}.

9. **(a)** : Here, $\vec{R} = 4\sin(2\pi t)\hat{\imath} + 4\cos(2\pi t)\hat{\jmath}$

The velocity of the particle is

$$\vec{v} = \frac{d\vec{R}}{dt} = \frac{d}{dt}[4\sin(2\pi t)\hat{\imath} + 4\cos(2\pi t)\hat{\jmath}]$$
$$= 8\pi\cos(2\pi t)\hat{\imath} - 8\pi\sin(2\pi t)\hat{\jmath}$$

Its magnitude is

$|\vec{v}| = \sqrt{(8\pi\cos(2\pi t))^2 + (-8\pi\sin(2\pi t))^2}$

$= \sqrt{64\pi^2\cos^2(2\pi t) + 64\pi^2\sin^2(2\pi t)}$
$= \sqrt{64\pi^2[\cos^2(2\pi t) + \sin^2(2\pi t)]}$
$= \sqrt{64\pi^2}$ (As $\sin^2\theta + \cos^2\theta = 1$)
$= 8\pi$m/s

10. **(d)** : At time $t = 0$, the position vector of the particle is $\vec{r}_1 = 2\hat{\imath} + 3\hat{\jmath}$.

At time $= 5$ s, the position vector of the particle is $\vec{r}_2 = 13\hat{\imath} + 14\hat{\jmath}$.

Displacement from $\vec{r}_1$ to $\vec{r}_2$ is

$\Delta\vec{r} = \vec{r}_2 - \vec{r}_1 = (13\hat{\imath} + 14\hat{\jmath}) - (2\hat{\imath} + 3\hat{\jmath})$
$= 11\hat{\imath} + 11\hat{\jmath}$

$\therefore$ Average velocity,

$\vec{v}_{av} = \frac{\Delta\vec{r}}{\Delta t} = \frac{11\hat{\imath}+11\hat{\jmath}}{5-0} = \frac{11}{5}(\hat{\imath} + \hat{\jmath})$

11. **(d)** :

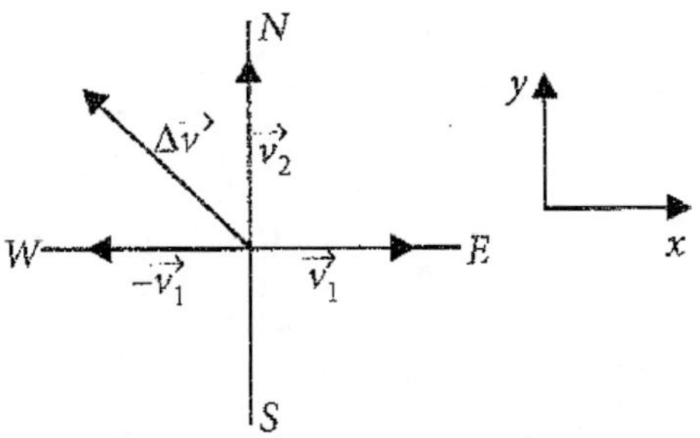

Velocity towards east direction, $\vec{v}_1 = 30\hat{\imath}$ m/s

Velocity towards north direction, $\vec{v}_2 = 40\hat{\jmath}$ m/s

Change in velocity, $\Delta\vec{v} = \vec{v}_2 - \vec{v}_1 = (40\hat{\jmath} - 30\hat{\imath})$

$\therefore |\Delta\vec{v}| = |40\hat{\jmath} - 30\hat{\imath}| = 50$ m/s

Average acceleration, $\vec{a}_{av} = \frac{\text{Change in velocity}}{\text{Time interval}}$

$$\vec{a}_{av} = \frac{\vec{v}_2 - \vec{v}_1}{\Delta t} = \frac{\Delta\vec{v}}{\Delta t}; |\vec{a}_{av}| = \frac{|\Delta\vec{v}|}{\Delta t}$$
$$= \frac{50 \text{ m/s}}{10 \text{ s}} = 5 \text{ m/s}^2$$

12. **(b)** : $x = a\sin\omega t$ or $\frac{x}{a} = \sin\omega t$

$y = a\cos\omega t$ or $\frac{y}{a} = \cos\omega t$

Squaring and adding, we get

$\frac{x^2}{a^2} + \frac{y^2}{a^2} = 1$ ($\because \cos^2\omega t + \sin^2\omega t = 1$)

or $x^2 + y^2 = a^2$

This is the equation of a circle. Hence particle follows a circular path.

13. **(b)** : Let θ be the angle which the particle makes with an x-axis.

From figure,

$\tan\theta = \frac{3}{\sqrt{3}} = \sqrt{3}$

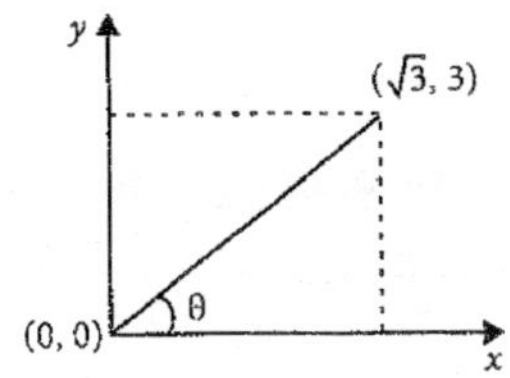

or, $\theta = \tan^{-1}(\sqrt{3}) = 60°$

14. **(a)** : $\vec{v}_1 = 50$ km/hr due north $\vec{v}_2 = 50$ km/hr due west $-\vec{v}_1 = 50$ km/hr due south

Magnitude of change in velocity

$= |\vec{v}_2 - \vec{v}_1| = |\vec{v}_2 + (-\vec{v}_1)|$

$= \sqrt{(50)^2 + (50)^2} = 70.7\ \text{km/hr}$

$= \sqrt{v_2^2 + (-v_1)^2}$

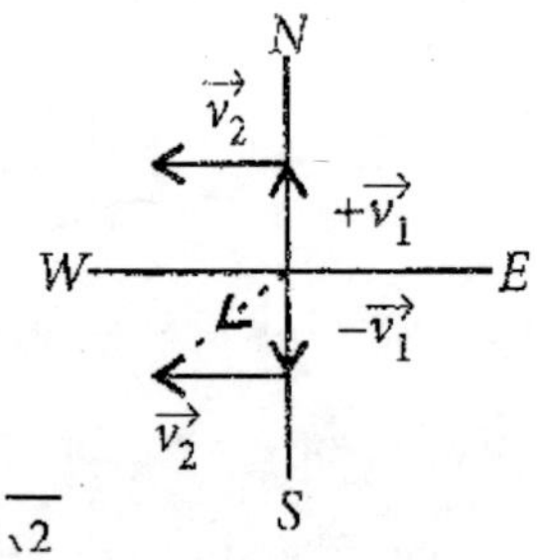

$\vec{v} = 70.7\ \text{km/hr}$ along south-west direction

15. **(a) :** Given : $u_x = 0, a_x = 5\ \text{m/s}^2$

At $t = 4$ s ball is dropped $a_y = g = 10\ \text{m/s}^2$

Let v_x is the velocity of ball at the time $= 4$ s.

$v_x = u_x + a_x t = 0 + 5 \times 4 = 20\ \text{m/s}$

v_y is the velocity of ball after leaving at $t = 6$ s

$v_y = u_y + a_y t' = 0 + g \times 2 = 20\ \text{m/s}$

Resultant velocity of ball at $t = 6$ s

$$v = \sqrt{v_x^2 + v_y^2} = \sqrt{20^2 + 20^2} \Rightarrow v$$

$$= 20\sqrt{2}\ \text{m/s}$$

Acceleration of the ball will be due to gravity i.e., $= 10\ \text{m/s}^2$.

16. **(d) :** $v^2 - u^2 = 2ax$

For case $I: v^2 = u^2 - 2(g\sin\theta_1)x_1$

$[\because a = -g\sin\theta]$

$$x_1 = \frac{u^2}{2g\sin\theta_1}$$

$[\because v = 0]$

For case II :

$v^2 = u^2 - (2g\sin\theta_2)x_2$

$$x_2 = \frac{u^2}{2g\sin\theta_2}$$

$$\therefore \frac{x_1}{x_2} = \frac{\sin\theta_2}{\sin\theta_1} = \frac{\sin 30^\circ}{\sin 60^\circ} = \frac{1}{\sqrt{3}}$$

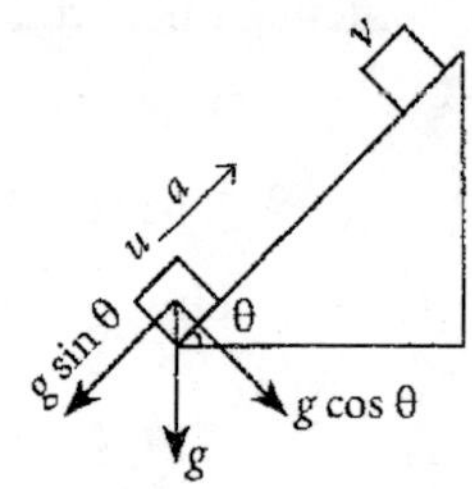

17. **(b) :** Here, $\vec{u} = 2\hat{i} + 3\hat{j}, \vec{a} = 0.3\hat{i} + 0.2\hat{j}, t = 10$ s

As $\vec{v} = \vec{u} + \vec{a}t$

$\therefore\ \vec{v} = (2\hat{i} + 3\hat{j}) + (0.3\hat{i} + 0.2\hat{j})(10)$

$= 2\hat{i} + 3\hat{j} + 3\hat{i} + 2\hat{j}$

$= 5\hat{i} + 5\hat{j}$

$|\vec{v}| = \sqrt{(5)^2 + (5)^2} = 5\sqrt{2}$ units

18. **(b) :** Here, Initial velocity, $\vec{u} = 3\hat{i} + 4\hat{j}$

Acceleration, $\vec{a} = 0.4\hat{i} + 0.3\hat{j}$; time, $t = 10$ s

Let $\vec{v}$ be velocity of a particle after 10 s.

Using, $\vec{v} = \vec{u} + \vec{a}t \therefore \vec{v} = (3\hat{i} + 4\hat{j}) + (0.4\hat{i} + 0.3\hat{j})(10)$

$= 3\hat{i} + 4\hat{j} + 4\hat{i} + 3\hat{j} = 7\hat{i} + 7\hat{j}$

Speed of the particle after 10 s = $|\vec{v}| = \sqrt{(7)^2 + (7)^2} = 7\sqrt{2}$ units

19. **(c)** : Vertical acceleration in both the cases is g, whereas horizontal velocity is constant.

20. **(b)** :

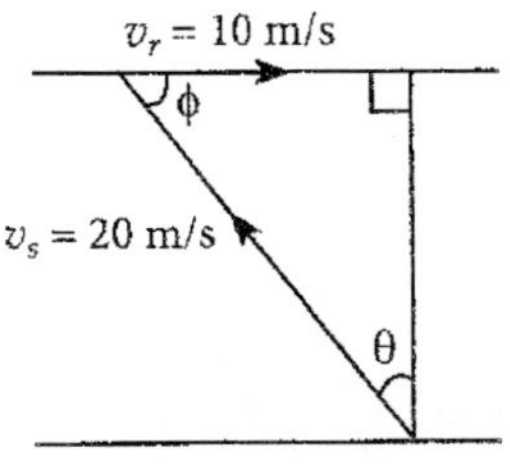

$$\cos\phi = \frac{10}{20} = \frac{1}{2} \text{ or } \phi = 60^\circ \Rightarrow \theta = 180^\circ - (90^\circ + 60^\circ) = 30^\circ$$

21. **(d)** : $t = \frac{a}{v'} = \frac{a}{\sqrt{v^2 - v_1^2}}$

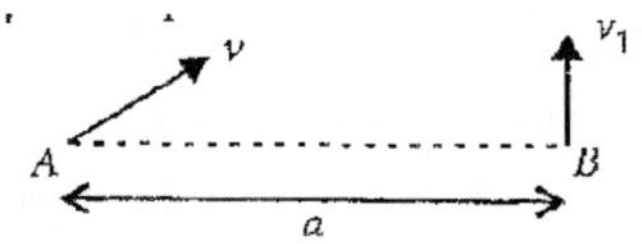

22. **(a)** : $v_{\text{Resultant}} = \frac{1 \text{ km}}{1/4\text{hr}} = 4$ km/hr

$\therefore v_{\text{River}} = \sqrt{5^2 - 4^2} = 3$ km/hr

23. **(a)** : Let v be the velocity of river water. As shown in figure,

$$\sin 30^\circ = \frac{v}{0.5}$$

or, $v = 0.5 \sin 30^\circ$

$= 0.5 \times (1/2) = 0.25$ m/s

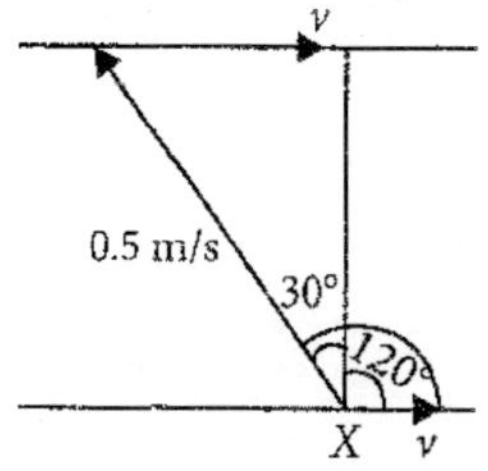

24. **(d)** : Let particle B move upwards with velocity v, then $\tan 60^\circ = \frac{v}{10}$; $v = \sqrt{3} \times 10 = 17.3$ m/s.

25. **(b)** : Let the velocity of river be v_R and velocity of boat is v_B.

$\therefore$ Resultant velocity

$= \sqrt{v_B^2 + v_R^2 + 2v_Bv_R\cos\theta}$

$(10) = \sqrt{v_B^2 + v_R^2 + 2v_Bv_R\cos 90^\circ}$

$(10) = \sqrt{(8)^2 + v_R^2}$ or $(10)^2 = (8)^2 + v_R^2$

$v_R^2 = 100 - 64$ or $v_R = 6$ km/hr

26. **(b)** : $H_{\max} = \frac{u^2 \sin^2\theta}{2g}$

$$= \frac{(280)^2 (\sin 30^\circ)^2}{2(9.8)}$$

=1000 m

27. **(b)** : : Ball is projected with a velocity, $u = 10$ m/s

Angle of projection, $\theta = 90^\circ - 60^\circ = 30^\circ$

The velocity of a projectile at the highest point will be

$v = u\cos\theta = 10 \times \cos 30°$

$= 10 \times \frac{\sqrt{3}}{2} = 5\sqrt{3}$ m/s

28. **(a)** : We know, $T = \frac{2\pi R}{u} \Rightarrow u = \frac{2\pi R}{T}$

Here : $H_{max} = 4R$

$H_{max} = \frac{u^2\sin^2\theta}{2g}$

Putting the value of u and H_{max} in equation (i), we get

$4R = \left(\frac{2\pi R}{T}\right)^2 \times \frac{\sin^2\theta}{2g} \Rightarrow \theta$

$= \sin^{-1}\left(\frac{2gT^2}{\pi^2 R}\right)^{1/2}$

29. **(a)** : The equation of trajectory is

$y = x\tan\theta - \frac{gx^2}{2u^2\cos^2\theta}$

where θ is the angle of projection and u is the velocity with which projectile is projected.

For equal trajectories and for same angles of projection,

$\frac{g}{u^2} =$ constant

As per question, $\frac{9.8}{5^2} = \frac{g'}{3^2}$

where g' is acceleration due to gravity on the planet.

$g' = \frac{9.8 \times 9}{25} = 3.5$ m s^{-2}

30. **(a)** : At point B, X component of velocity remains unchanged while Y component reverses its direction.

$\therefore$ The velocity of the projectile at point B is $2\hat{i} - 3\hat{j}$ m/s.

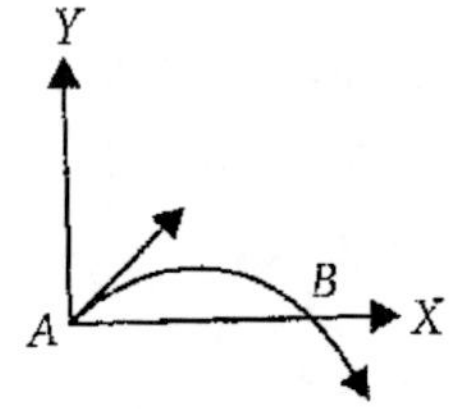

31. **(b)** : Horizontal range, $R = \frac{u^2\sin 2\theta}{g}$

where u is the velocity of projection and θ is the angle of projection.

Maximum height, $H = \frac{u^2\sin^2\theta}{2g}$

According to question $R = H$

$\therefore \frac{u^2\sin 2\theta}{g} = \frac{u^2\sin^2\theta}{2g}$ or, $\frac{2u^2\sin\theta\cos\theta}{g} = \frac{u^2\sin^2\theta}{2g}$

$\tan\theta = 4$ or $\theta = \tan^{-1}(4)$

32. **(a)** :

Sol. Here, $u = 20$ m/s, $g = 10$ m/s^2

For maximum range, angle of projection is $\theta = 45°$

$\therefore R_{max} = \frac{u^2\sin 90°}{g} = \frac{u^2}{g}$

$\left(\because R = \frac{u^2\sin 2\theta}{g}\right)$

$= \frac{(20\text{ m/s})^2}{(10\text{ m/s}^2)} = 40$ m

33. **(c)** : Let ϕ be elevation angle of the projectile at its highest point as seen from the point of projection O and θ

be angle of projection with the horizontal.

From figure, $\tan\phi = \frac{H}{R/2}$

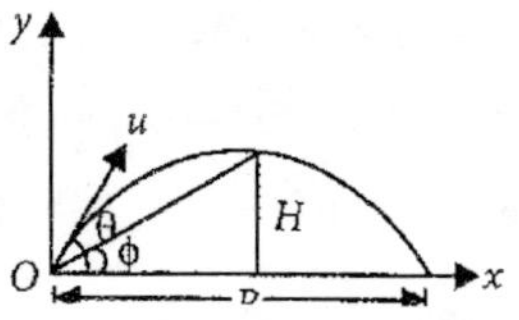

In case of projectile motion

Maximum height, $H = \frac{u^2\sin^2\theta}{2g}$

Horizontal range, $R = \frac{u^2\sin 2\theta}{g}$

Substituting these values of H and R in (i), we get

$$\tan\phi = \frac{\frac{u^2\sin^2\theta}{2g}}{\frac{u^2\sin 2\theta}{2g}} = \frac{\sin^2\theta}{\sin 2\theta} = \frac{\sin^2\theta}{2\sin\theta\cos\theta} =$$

$\frac{1}{2}\tan\theta$

Here, $\theta = 45^\circ$ $\therefore$ $\tan\phi = \frac{1}{2}\tan 45^\circ = \frac{1}{2}$ $(\because \tan 45^\circ = 1)$

$\phi = \tan^{-1}\left(\frac{1}{2}\right)$

34. **(a)** : Let v be velocity of a projectile at maximum height H. $v = u\cos\theta$

According to given problem,

$v = \frac{u}{2}$

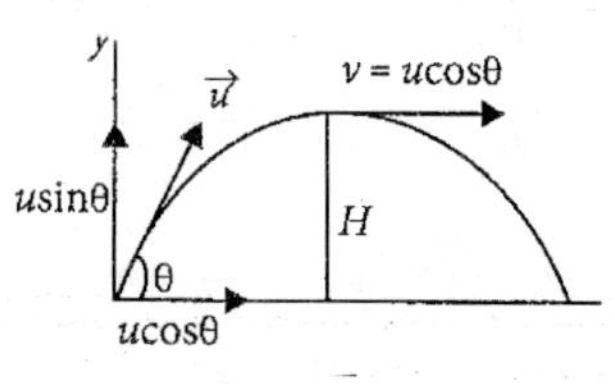

$\therefore \frac{u}{2} = u\cos\theta \Rightarrow \cos\theta = \frac{1}{2} \Rightarrow \theta = 60^\circ$

35. **(a)** :

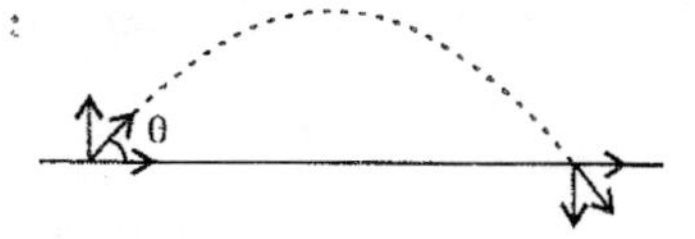

Motion in a Plane

The horizontal momentum does not change. The change in vertical momentum is

$$mv\sin\theta - (-mv\sin\theta) = 2mv\frac{1}{\sqrt{2}}$$

$$= \sqrt{2}mv$$

36. **(b)** : Horizontal range, $R = \frac{u^2\sin 2\theta}{g}$

For angle of projection $(45^\circ - \theta)$, the horizontal range is

$$\therefore R_1 = \frac{u^2\sin[2(45^\circ - \theta)]}{g}$$

$$= \frac{u^2\sin(90^\circ - 2\theta)}{g}$$

$$= \frac{u^2\cos 2\theta}{g}$$

For angle of projection $(45^\circ + \theta)$, the horizontal range is

$$R_2 = \frac{u^2\sin[2(45^\circ + \theta)]}{g}$$

$$= \frac{u^2\sin(90^\circ + 2\theta)}{g} = \frac{u^2\cos 2\theta}{g}$$

$$\therefore \frac{R_1}{R_2} = \frac{u^2\cos 2\theta/g}{u^2\cos 2\theta/g} = \frac{1}{1}.$$

37. **(c)** : Time required to reach the ground is dependent on the vertical motion of the particle. Vertical motion of both the particles A and B are exactly same. Although particle B has an initial velocity, but that is in horizontal direction and it has no component in vertical (component of a vector at a direction of $90° = 0$) direction. Hence they will reach the ground simultaneously.

38. **(b)** : As $\theta_2 = (90 - \theta_1)$,

So range of projectile, $R_1 = \frac{v_0^2 \sin 2\theta}{g} = \frac{v_0^2 2\sin\theta\cos\theta}{g}$

$$R_2 = \frac{v_0^2 2\sin(90-\theta_1)\cos(90-\theta_1)}{g}$$

$$R_2 = \frac{v_0^2 2\cos\theta_1 \sin\theta_1}{g} = R_1$$

39. **(b)** : For the given velocity of projection u, the horizontal range is the same for the angle of projection θ and $90° - \theta$.

Horizontal range, $R = \frac{u^2 \sin 2\theta}{g}$

$\therefore$ For body $A, R_A = \frac{u^2 \sin(2\times 30°)}{g} = \frac{u^2 \sin 60°}{g}$

For body $B, R_B = \frac{u^2 \sin(2\times 60°)}{g}$

$$R_B = \frac{u^2 \sin 120°}{g} = \frac{u^2 \sin(180° - 60°)}{g}$$

$$= \frac{u^2 \sin 60°}{g}$$

The range is the same whether the angle is θ or $90° - \theta$

$\therefore$ The ratio of ranges is 1: 1.

40. **(c)** : Horizontal range, $R = \frac{u^2 \sin 2\theta}{g}$

For maximum horizontal range, $\theta = 45°$

$R_m = \frac{u^2}{g}$ where u be muzzle velocity of a shell.

$\therefore$ $(1600\text{ m}) = \frac{u^2}{(10\text{ m s}^{-2})^2}$ or $u = 400\text{ m s}^{-1}$.

41. **(a)** : Time period, $T = \frac{2\pi}{\omega}$

As $T_A = T_B$. So, $\frac{2\pi}{\omega_A} = \frac{2\pi}{\omega_B}$ or $\omega_A : \omega_B = 1:1$

42. **(c)** : Distance travelled in n^{th} rounds $= (2\pi r)n$

Using $v^2 = u^2 + 2as$ or, $V_0^2 = 0 + 2a(2\pi r)n \Rightarrow a = \frac{V_0^2}{4\pi n r}$

Angular acceleration, $\alpha = \frac{a}{r} = \frac{V_0^2}{4\pi n r^2}\text{ rad/s}^2$

43. **(c)** : Here, $a = 15\text{ m s}^{-2}, R = 2.5\text{ m}$

From figure, $a_c = a\cos 30° = 15 \times \frac{\sqrt{3}}{2}\text{ m s}^{-2}$

As we know, $a_c = \frac{v^2}{R} \Rightarrow v = \sqrt{a_c R}$

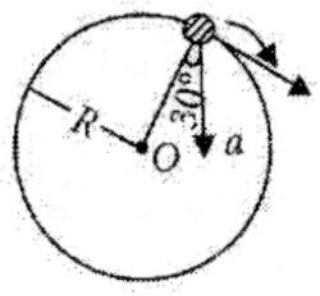

$\therefore\ v = \sqrt{15 \times \frac{\sqrt{3}}{2} \times 2.5} = 5.69 \simeq 5.7 \text{ m s}^{-1}$

44. **(d)** : Here, radius, $R = 5 \text{ cm} = 5 \times 10^{-2} \text{ m}$

Time period, $T = 0.2\pi s$

Centripetal acceleration

$$a_c = \omega^2 R = \left(\frac{2\pi}{T}\right)^2 R = \left(\frac{2\pi}{0.2\pi}\right)^2 (5 \times 10^{-2})$$
$$= 5 \text{ m/s}^2$$

As particle moves with constant speed, therefore its tangential acceleration is zero. So, $a_t = 0$

The acceleration of the particle is $a = \sqrt{a_c^2 + a_t^2} = 5 \text{ m/s}^2$ It acts towards the centre of the circle.

45. **(a)** : $a = r\omega^2; \omega = 2\pi v$

42 revolution = 44 s ⇒ 1 revolution = $44/22 = 2 \text{ s}$ $v = 1/2 \text{ Hz}$

$a = r\omega^2 = 1 \times \frac{4\pi^2}{4} = \pi^2 \text{ m/s}^2.$

It is the centripetal acceleration towards the center.

46. **(a)** : Radius of circle $= \frac{20}{\pi}$

In two resolution it covers 4π angular displacement or $4\pi r$ distance linearly

After two resolutions if velocity become = 80 m/s

So $v^2 = v^2 + 2as$

a = tangential acceleration

s = linear displacement

U = 0

$$(80)^2 = 2 \times a \times 4\pi \times \frac{20}{\pi}$$

$$\frac{80}{2} = a$$

$$a = 40 m/s^2$$

47. **(c)** : $\omega = \frac{2\pi}{t}$; As t is same $\therefore \frac{\omega_1}{\omega_2} = 1$

48. **(c)** : $t = \frac{2\pi}{\omega_1} = \frac{2\pi}{\omega_2} \Rightarrow \frac{\omega_1}{\omega_2} = \frac{1}{1}$

49. **(d)** : Radius of circle $(r) = 20 \text{ cm} = 0.2 \text{ m}$ and angular velocity $(\omega) = 10 \text{rad/s}$

Linear velocity $(v) = r\omega = 0.2 \times 10 = 2 \text{ m/s}$.

50. **(a)** : Number of revolutions per minute $(n) = 120$.

Therefore angular speed $(\omega) = \frac{2\pi n}{60} = \frac{2\pi \times 120}{60} = 4\pi \text{rad/s}$

51. **(b)** : Frequency of rotation $v = 120\text{rpm} = 2\text{rps}$

length of blade $r = 30 \text{ cm} = 0.3 \text{ m}$

Centripetal acceleration $a = \omega^2 r = (2\pi v)^2 r$

$= 4\pi^2 v^2 r = 4\pi^2 (2)^2 (0.3) = 47.4 \text{ m s}^{-2}$

Chapter: 4

LOW OF MOTION

Newton's First Law of Motion

1. Physical independence of force is a consequence of **(1991)**
   (a) third law of motion
   (b) second law of motion
   (c) first law of motion
   (d) all of these laws

Newton's Second Law of Motion

2. A ball of mass 0.15 kg is dropped from a height 10 m, strikes the ground and rebounds to the same height. The magnitude of impulse imparted to the ball is ($g = 10\ \mathrm{m/s^2}$) nearly **(2021)**
   (a) 1.4 kg m/s (b) 0 kg m/s
   (c) 4.2 kg m/s (d) 2.1 kg m/s

3. The force F acting on a particle of mass m is indicated by the force-time graph as shown. The change in momentum of the particle over the time interval from zero to 8 s is] **(2014)**

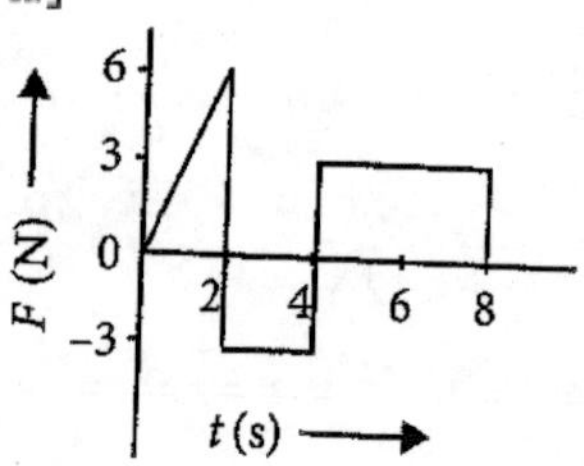

   (a) 24 N s (b) 20 N s
   (c) 12 N s (d) 6 N s

4. A stone is dropped from a height h. It hits the ground with a certain momentum P. If the same stone is dropped from a height 100% more than the previous height, the momentum when it hits the ground will change by **(Mains 2012)**
   (a) 68% (b) 41%
   (c) 200% (d) 100%

5. A body, under the action of a force $\vec{F} = 6\hat{\imath} - 8\hat{\jmath} + 10\hat{k}$, acquires an acceleration of $1\ \mathrm{m/s^2}$. The mass of this body must be **(2009)**
   (a) 10 kg (b) 20 kg
   (c) $10\sqrt{2}$ kg (d) $2\sqrt{10}$ kg

6. Sand is being dropped on a conveyer belt at the rate of Mkg/s. The force necessary to keep the belt moving with a constant velocity of v m/s will be **(2008)**
   (a) $\frac{Mv}{2}$ newton (b) zero
   (c) Mv newton (d) $2Mv$ newton

7. An object of mass 3 kg is at rest. Now a force of $\vec{F} = 6t^2\hat{\imath} + 4t\hat{\jmath}$ is applied on the object then velocity of object at $t = 3$ s is **(2002)**
   (a) $18\hat{\imath} + 3\hat{\jmath}$ (b) $18\hat{\imath} + 6\hat{\jmath}$
   (c) $3\hat{\imath} + 18\hat{\jmath}$ (d) $18\hat{\imath} + 4\hat{\jmath}$

8. A cricketer catches a ball of mass 150gm in 0.1sec moving with speed 20 m/s, then he experiences force of **(2001)**
   (a) 300 N (b) 30 N
   (c) 3 N (d) 0.3 N

9. If the force on a rocket, moving with a velocity of 300 m/s is 210 N, then the rate of combustion of the fuel is **(1999)**

(a) 0.07 kg/s (b) 1.4 kg/s

(c) 0.7 kg/s (d) 10.7 kg/s

10. A bullet is fired from a gun. The force on the bullet is given by $F = 600 - 2 \times 10^5 t$ where, F is in newton and t in seconds. The force on the bullet becomes zero as soon as it leaves the barrel. What is the average impulse imparted to the bullet? **(1998)**

(a) 9Ns (b) zero

(c) 1.8Ns (d) 0.9Ns

11. A 5000 kg rocket is set for vertical firing. The exhaust speed is 800 m s^{-1}. To give an initial upward acceleration of 20 m s^{-2}, the amount of gas ejected per second to supply the needed thrust will be ($g = 10$ m s^{-2}) **(1998)**

(a) 185.5 kg s^{-1} (b) 187.5 kg s^{-1}

(c) 127.5 kg s^{-1} (d) 137.5 kg s^{-1}

12. A force of 6 N acts on a body at rest and of mass 1 kg. During this time, the body attains a velocity of 30 m/s. The time for which the force acts on the body is **(1997)**

(a) 7 seconds (b) 5 seconds

(c) 10 seconds (d) 8 seconds

13. A 10 N force is applied on a body produce in it an acceleration of 1 m/s^2. The mass of the body is

(a) 15 kg (b) 20 kg

(c) 10 kg (d) 5 kg

14. A force vector applied on a mass is represented as $\vec{F} = 6\hat{i} - 8\hat{j} + 10\hat{k}$ and accelerates with 1 m/s^2. What will be the mass of the body? **(1996)**

(a) 10 kg (b) 20 kg

(c) $10\sqrt{2}$ kg (d) $2\sqrt{10}$ kg

15. In a rocket, fuel burns at the rate of 1 kg/s. This fuel is ejected from the rocket with a velocity of 60 km/s. This exerts a force on the rocket equal to **(1994)**

(a) 6000 N (b) 60000 N

(c) 60 N (d) 600 N

16. A satellite in force free space sweeps stationary interplanetary dust at a rate of $dM/dt = \alpha v$, where M is mass and v is the speed of satellite and α is a constant. The acceleration of satellite is **(1994)**

(a) $\frac{-\alpha v^2}{2M}$ (b) $-\alpha v^2$

(c) $\frac{-2\alpha v^2}{M}$ (d) $\frac{-\alpha v^2}{M}$

17. A particle of mass m is moving with a uniform velocity v_1. It is given an impulse such that its velocity becomes v_2. The impulse is equal to **(1990)**

(a) $m[|v_2| - |v_1|]$ (b) $\frac{1}{2}m[v_2^2 - v_1^2]$

(c) $m[v_1 + v_2]$ (d) $m[v_2 - v_1]$

18. A 600 kg rocket is set for a vertical firing. If the exhaust speed is 1000 m s^{-1}, the mass of the gas ejected per second to supply the thrust needed to overcome the weight of rocket is **(1996)** **(1990)**

(a) 117.6 kg s^{-1} (b) 58.6 kg s^{-1}

(c) 6 kg s^{-1} (d) 76.4 kg s^{-1}

Newton's Third Law of Motion

19. A rigid ball of mass m strikes a rigid wall at 60° and gets reflected without loss of speed as shown in the figure. The value of impulse imparted by the wall on the ball will be **(NEET-II 2016)**

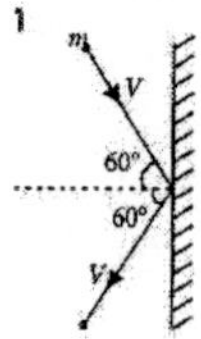

(a) mV (b) 2mV

(c) $\frac{mV}{2}$ (d) $\frac{mV}{3}$

20. A body of mass M hits normally a rigid wall with velocity V and bounces back with the same velocity. The impulse experienced by the body is **(2011)**

(a) MV (b) 1.5MV

(c) $2MV$ (d) zero

21. A 0.5 kg ball moving with a speed of 12 m/s strikes a hard wall at an angle of 30° with the wall. It is reflected with the same speed at the same angle. If the ball is in contact with the wall for 0.25 seconds, the average force acting on the wall is **(2006)**

(a) 96 N (b) 48 N

(c) 24 N (d) 12 N

22. A body of mass 3 kg hits a wall at an angle of 60° and returns at the same angle. The impact time was 0.2 s. The force exerted on the wall **(2000)**

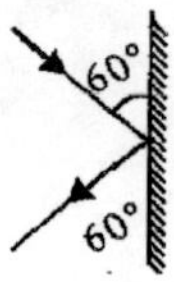

(a) $150\sqrt{3}$ N (b) $50\sqrt{3}$ N

(c) 100 N (d) $75\sqrt{3}$ N

Conservation of Momentum

23. A shell of mass m is at rest initially. It explodes into three fragments having mass in the ratio 2:2:1. If the fragments having equal mass fly off along mutually perpendicular directions with speed v, the speed of the third (lighter) fragment is

(a) v (b) $\sqrt{2}v$

(c) $2\sqrt{2}v$ (d) $3\sqrt{2}v$

24. An object flying in air with velocity $(20\hat{i} + 25\hat{j} - 12\hat{k})$ suddenly breaks in two pieces whose masses are in the ratio 1:5. The smaller mass flies off with a velocity $(100\hat{i} + 35\hat{j} + 8\hat{k})$.
The velocity of the larger piece will be **(Odisha NEET 2019)**

(a) $4\hat{i} + 23\hat{j} - 16\hat{k}$

(b) $-100\hat{i} - 35\hat{j} - 8\hat{k}$

(c) $20\hat{i} + 15\hat{j} - 80\hat{k}$

(d) $-20\hat{i} - 15\hat{j} - 80\hat{k}$.

25. An explosion breaks a rock into three parts in a horizontal plane. Two of them go off at right angles to each other. The first part of mass 1 kg moves with a speed of 12 m s^{-1} and the second part of mass 2 kg moves with 8 m s^{-1} speed. If the third part flies off with 4 m s^{-1} speed, then its mass is **(2013)**

(a) 7 kg (b) 17 kg

(c) 3 kg (d) 5 kg

26. A person holding a rifle (mass of person and rifle together is 100 kg) stands on a smooth surface and fires 10 shots horizontally, in 5 s. Each bullet has a mass of 10 g with a muzzle velocity of $800 \mathrm{~m} \mathrm{~s}^{-1}$. The final velocity acquired by the person and the average force exerted on the person are **(Karnataka NEET 2013)**

(a) $-0.08 \mathrm{~m} \mathrm{~s}^{-1}, 16 \mathrm{~N}$

(b) $-0.8 \mathrm{~m} \mathrm{~s}^{-1}, 16 \mathrm{~N}$

(c) $-1.6 \mathrm{~m} \mathrm{~s}^{-1}, 16 \mathrm{~N}$

(d) $-1.6 \mathrm{~m} \mathrm{~s}^{-1}, 8 \mathrm{~N}$

27. An explosion blows a rock into three parts. Two parts go off at right angles to each other. These two are, 1 kg first part moving with a velocity of $12 \mathrm{~m} \mathrm{~s}^{-1}$ and 2 kg second part moving with a velocity $8 \mathrm{~m} \mathrm{~s}^{-1}$. If the third part flies off with a velocity of $4 \mathrm{~m} \mathrm{~s}^{-1}$, its mass would be **(2009)**

(a) 7 kg (b) 17 kg

(c) 3 kg (d) 5 kg

28. A 1 kg stationary bomb is exploded in three parts having mass 1:1:3 respectively. Parts having same mass move in perpendicular direction with velocity 30 m/s, then the velocity of bigger part will be **(2001)**

(a) $10\sqrt{2}$ m/s (b) $\frac{10}{\sqrt{2}}$ m/s

(c) $15\sqrt{2}$ m/s (d) $\frac{15}{\sqrt{2}}$ m/s

29. A mass of 1 kg is thrown up with a velocity of 100 m/s. After 5 seconds, it explodes into two parts. One part of mass 400 g comes down with a velocity 25 m/s. The velocity of other part is (Take $g = 10 \mathrm{~m} \mathrm{~s}^{-2}$)

(a) 40 m/s (b) 80 m/s

(c) 100 m/s (d) 60 m/s

30. A shell, in flight, explodes into four unequal parts. Which of the following is conserved? **(1998)**

(a) Potential energy (b) Momentum

(c) Kinetic energy (d) Both (a) and (c).

31. A man fires a bullet of mass 200 g at a speed of 5 m/s. The gun is of one kg mass. By what velocity the gun rebounds backward? **(1996)**

(a) 1 m/s (b) 0.01 m/s

(c) 0.1 m/s (d) 10 m/s.

32. A body of mass 5 kg explodes at rest into three fragments with masses in the ratio 1:1:3. The fragments with equal masses fly in mutually perpendicular directions with speeds of 21 m/s. The velocity of heaviest fragment in m/s will be **(1989)**

(a) $7\sqrt{2}$ (b) $5\sqrt{2}$

(c) $3\sqrt{2}$ (d) $\sqrt{2}$

Equilibrium of a Particle

33. A particle moving with velocity $\vec{v}$ is acted by three forces shown by the vector triangle PQR. The velocity of the particle will **(2019)**

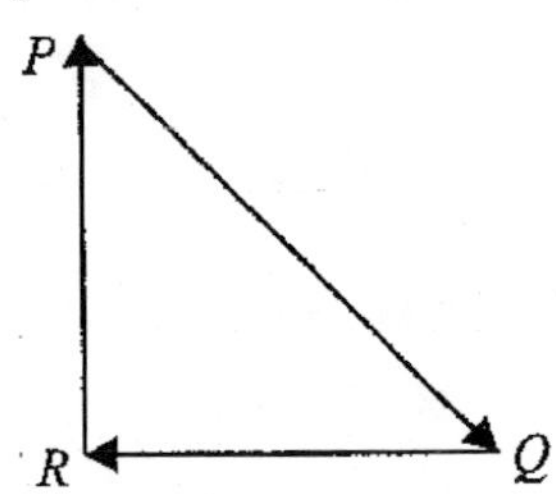

(a) change according to the smallest force $\overrightarrow{QR}$

(b) increase

(c) decrease

(d) remain constant

34. Three forces acting on a body are shown in the figure. To have the resultant force only along the y-direction, the magnitude of the minimum additional force needed is

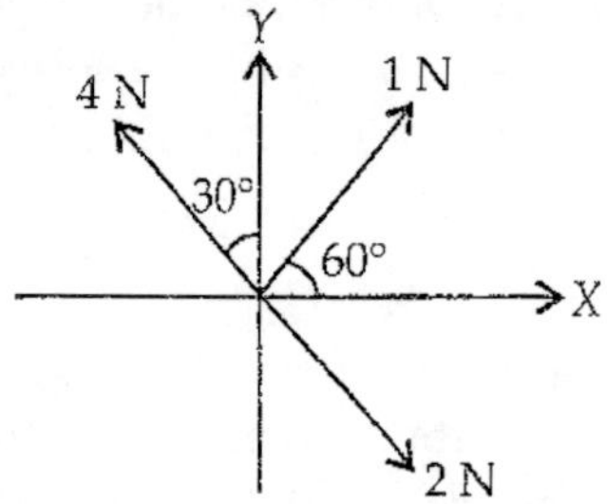

(a) $\frac{\sqrt{3}}{4}$ N (b) $\sqrt{3}$ N

(c) 0.5 N (d) 1.5 N

Common Forces in Mechanics

35. Calculate the maximum acceleration of a moving car so that a body lying on the floor of the car remains stationary. The coefficient of static friction between the body and the floor is 0.15 ($g = 10\ m\ s^{-2}$).

(2023)

(a) 150 $m\ s^{-2}$ (b) 1.5 $m\ s^{-2}$

(c) 50 $m\ s^{-2}$ (d) 1.2 $m\ s^{-2}$

36. Which one of the following statements is incorrect? **(2018)**

(a) Rolling friction is smaller than sliding friction.

(b) Limiting value of static friction is directly proportional to normal reaction.

(c) Frictional force opposes the relative motion.

(d) Coefficient of sliding friction has dimensions of length.

37. A plank with a box on it at one end is gradually raised about the other end. As the angle of inclination with the horizontal reaches 30°, the box starts to slip and slides 4.0 m down the plank in 4.0 s. The coefficients of static and kinetic friction between the box and the plank will be, respectively

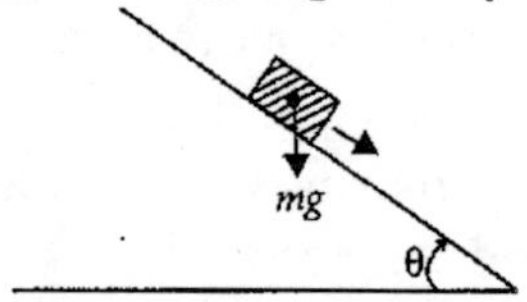

(a) 0.5 and 0.6 (b) 0.4 and 0.3

(c) 0.6 and 0.6 (d) 0.6 and 0.5

38. A block A of mass m_1 rests on a horizontal table. A light string connected to it passes over a frictionless pulley at the edge of table and from its other end another block B of mass m_2 is suspended. The coefficient of kinetic friction between the block and the table is μ_k. When the block A is sliding on the table, the tension in the string is

(2015 Cancelled)

(a) $\frac{m_1 m_2 (1+\mu_k) g}{(m_1+m_2)}$ (b) $\frac{m_1 m_2 (1-\mu_k) g}{(m_1+m_2)}$

(c) $\frac{(m_2+\mu_k m_1) g}{(m_1+m_2)}$ (d) $\frac{(m_2-\mu_k m_1) g}{(m_1+m_2)}$

39. A system consists of three masses m_1, m_2 and m_3 connected by a string passing over a pulley P. The mass m_1 hangs freely and m_2 and m_3 are on a rough horizontal table (the coefficient of friction $= \mu$). The pulley is frictionless and of negligible mass. The downward acceleration of mass m_1 is (Assume $m_1 = m_2 = m_3 = m$) **(2014)**

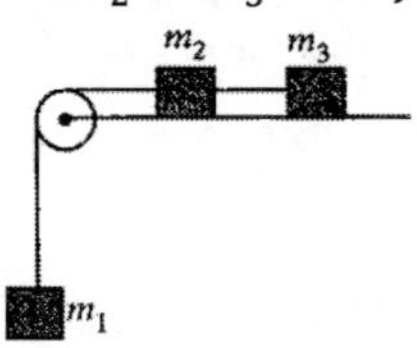

(a) $\frac{g(1-g\mu)}{9}$ (b) $\frac{2g\mu}{3}$

(c) $\frac{g(1-2\mu)}{3}$ (d) $\frac{g(1-2\mu)}{2}$

40. The upper half of an inclined plane of inclination θ is perfectly smooth while lower half is rough. A block starting from rest at the top of the plane will again come to rest at the bottom, if the coefficient of friction between the block and lower half of the plane is given by **(2013)**

(a) $\mu = 2\tan\theta$ (b) $\mu = \tan\theta$

(c) $\mu = \frac{1}{\tan\theta}$ (d) $\mu = \frac{2}{\tan\theta}$

41. A conveyor belt is moving at a constant speed of 2 m s^{-1}. A box is gently dropped on it. The coefficient of friction between them is $\mu = 0.5$. The distance that the box will move relative to belt before coming to rest on it, taking $g = 10 \text{ m s}^{-2}$, is **(Mains 2011)**

(a) 0.4 m (b) 1.2 m

(c) 0.6 m (d) zero

42. A block of mass m is in contact with the cart C as shown in the figure. The coefficient of static friction between the block and the cart is μ. The acceleration α of the cart that will prevent the block from falling satisfies **(2010)**

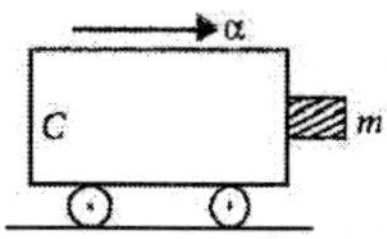

(a) $\alpha > \frac{mg}{\mu}$ (b) $\alpha > \frac{g}{\mu m}$

(c) $\alpha \geq \frac{g}{\mu}$ (d) $\alpha < \frac{g}{\mu}$

43. A block B is pushed momentarily along a horizontal surface with an initial velocity V. If μ is the coefficient of sliding friction between B and the surface, block B will come to rest after a time **(2007)**

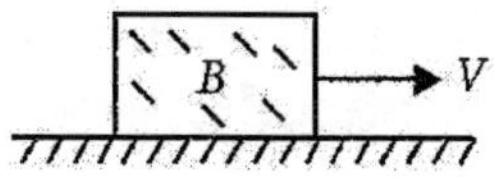

(a) $g\mu/V$ (b) g/V

(c) V/g (d) $V/(g\mu)$

44. The coefficient of static friction, μ_s, between block A of mass 2 kg and the table as shown in the figure is 0.2 . What would be the maximum mass value of block B so that the two blocks do not move? The string and the pulley are assumed to be smooth and massless. ($g = 10 \text{ m/s}^2$)]

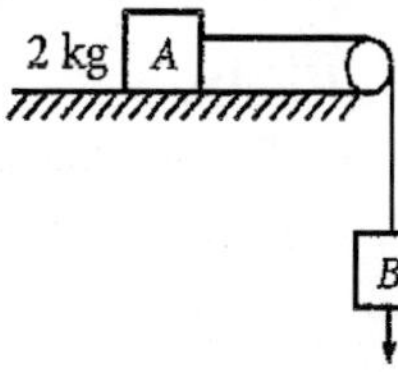

(a) 2.0 kg (b) 4.0 kg
(c) 0.2 kg (d) 0.4 kg

45. A block of mass 10 kg placed on rough horizontal surface having coefficient of friction $\mu = 0.5$, if a horizontal force of 100 N acting on it then acceleration of the block will be **(2002)**
(a) $10\ m/s^2$ (b) $5\ m/s^2$
(c) $15\ m/s^2$ (d) $0.5\ m/s^2$

46. On the horizontal surface of a truck a block of mass 1 kg is placed ($\mu = 0.6$) and truck is moving with acceleration $5\ m/s^2$ then the frictional force on the block will be **(2001)**
(a) 5 N (b) 6 N
(c) 5.88 N (d) 8 N

47. A block has been placed on a inclined plane with the slope angle θ, block slides down the plane at constant speed. The coefficient of kinetic friction is equal to **(1993)**
(a) $\sin\theta$ (b) $\cos\theta$
(c) g (d) $\tan\theta$

48. Consider a car moving along a straight horizontal road with a speed of 72 km/h. If the coefficient of static friction between the tyres and the road is 0.5 , the shortest distance in which the car can be stopped is (taking $g = 10\ m/s^2$) **(1992)**
(a) 30 m (b) 40 m
(c) 72 m (d) 20 m

49. A heavy uniform chain lies on horizontal table top. If the coefficient of friction between the chain and the table surface is 0.25 , then the maximum fraction of the length of the chain that can hang over one edge of the table is **(1991)**
(a) 20% (b) 25%
(c) 35% (d) 15%

50. Starting from rest, a body slides down a 45° inclined plane in twice the time it takes to slide down the same distance in the absence of friction. The coefficient of friction between the body and the inclined plane is
(a) 0.80 (b) 0.75
(c) 0.25 (d) 0.33

Circular Motion

51. A block of mass 10 kg is in contact against the inner wall of a hollow cylindrical drum of radius 1 m. The coefficient of friction between the block and the inner wall of the cylinder is 0.1 . The minimum angular velocity needed for the cylinder to keep the block stationary when the cylinder is vertical and rotating about its axis, will be ($g = 10\ m/s^2$)
(a) 10π rad/s (b) $\sqrt{10}$ rad/s
(c) $\frac{10}{2\pi}$ rad/s (d) 10 rad/s

52. One end of string of length l is connected to a particle of mass m and the other end is connected to a small peg on a smooth horizontal table. If the particle moves in circle with speed v, the net force on the particle (directed towards centre) will be (T represents the tension in the string) **(2017)**
(a) $T + \frac{mv^2}{l}$ (b) $T - \frac{mv^2}{l}$
(c) zero (d) T

53. A car is negotiating a curved road of radius R. The road is banked at an angle θ. The coefficient of friction between the tyres of the car and the road is μ_s. The maximum safe velocity on this road is **(NEET-I 2016)**

(a) $\sqrt{\frac{g}{R}\frac{\mu_s+\tan\theta}{1-\mu_s\tan\theta}}$ (b) $\sqrt{\frac{g}{R^2}\frac{\mu_s+\tan\theta}{1-\mu_s\tan\theta}}$

(c) $\sqrt{gR^2\frac{\mu_s+\tan\theta}{1-\mu_s\tan\theta}}$ (d) $\sqrt{gR\frac{\mu_s+\tan\theta}{1-\mu_s\tan\theta}}$

54. Two stones of masses m and $2m$ are whirled in horizontal circles, the heavier one in a radius $r/2$ and the lighter one in radius r. The tangential speed of lighter stone is n times that of the value of heavier stone when they experience same centripetal forces. The value of n is **(2015)**

(a) 4 (b) 1

(c) 2 (d) 3

55. A car is moving in a circular horizontal track of radius 10 m with a constant speed of 10 m/s. A bob is suspended from the roof of the car by a light wire of length 1.0 m. The angle made by the wire with the vertical is

(Karnataka NEET 2013)

(a) $\pi/3$ (b) $\pi/6$

(c) $\pi/4$ (d) $0°$

56. A car of mass 1000 kg negotiates a banked curve of radius 90 m on a frictionless road. If the banking angle is 45°, the speed of the car is **(2012)**

(a) $20\ \text{m s}^{-1}$ (b) $30\ \text{m s}^{-1}$

(c) $5\ \text{m s}^{-1}$ (d) $10\ \text{m s}^{-1}$

57. A car of mass m is moving on a level circular track of radius R. If μ_s represents the static friction between the road and tyres of the car, the maximum speed of the car in circular motion is given by **(Mains 2012)**

(a) $\sqrt{\mu_s mRg}$ (b) $\sqrt{\frac{Rg}{\mu_s}}$

(c) $\sqrt{\frac{mRg}{\mu_s}}$ (d) $\sqrt{\mu_s Rg}$

58. A gramophone record is revolving with an angular velocity ω. A coin is placed at a distance r from the centre of the record. The static coefficient of friction is μ. The coin will revolve with the record if **(2010)**

(a) $r = \mu g\omega^2$ (b) $r < \frac{\omega^2}{\mu g}$

(c) $r \leq \frac{\mu g}{\omega^2}$ (d) $r \geq \frac{\mu g}{\omega^2}$

59. A roller coaster is designed such that riders experience "weightlessness" as they go round the top of a hill whose radius of curvature is 20 m. The speed of the car at the top of the hill is between **(2008)**

(a) 16 m/s and 17 m/s

(b) 13 m/s and 14 m/s

(c) 14 m/s and 15 m/s

(d) 15 m/s and 16 m/s

60. A tube of length L is filled completely with an incompressible liquid of mass M and closed at both the ends. The tube is then rotated in a horizontal plane about one of its ends with a uniform angular velocity ω. The force exerted by the liquid at the other end is **(2006)**

(a) $\frac{ML^2\omega^2}{2}$ (b) $\frac{ML\omega^2}{2}$

(c) $\frac{ML^2\omega}{2}$ (d) $ML\omega^2$

61. A 500 kg car takes a round turn of radius 50 m with a velocity of 36 km/hr. The centripetal force is

(a) 1000 N (b) 750 N

(c) 250 N (d) 1200 N

62. A ball of mass 0.25 kg attached to the end of a string of length 1.96 m is moving in a horizontal circle. The string will break if the tension is more than 25 N. What is the maximum speed with which the ball can be moved? **(1998)**

(a) 5 m/s (b) 3 m/s

(c) 14 m/s (d) 3.92 m/s.

63. When milk is churned, cream gets separated due to **(1991)**

(a) centripetal force

(b) centrifugal force

(c) fricitional force

(d) gravitational force

Solving Problems in Mechanics

64. A small block slides down on a smooth inclined plane, starting from rest at time $t = 0$. Let S_n be the distance travelled by the block in the interval $t = n - 1$ to $t = n$. Then, the ratio $\frac{S_n}{S_{n+1}}$ is **(2021)**

(a) $\frac{2n}{2n-1}$ (b) $\frac{2n-1}{2n}$

(c) $\frac{2n-1}{2n+1}$ (d) $\frac{2n+1}{2n-1}$

65. Two bodies of mass 4 kg and 6 kg are tied to the ends of a massless string. The string passes over a pulley which is frictionless (see figure). The acceleration of the system in terms of acceleration due to gravity (g) is **(2020)**

(1999

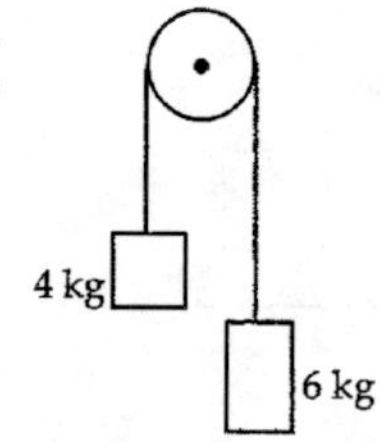

(a) g (b) $g/2$

(c) $g/5$ (d) $g/10$

66. A block of mass m is placed on a smooth inclined wedge ABC of inclination θ as shown in the figure.

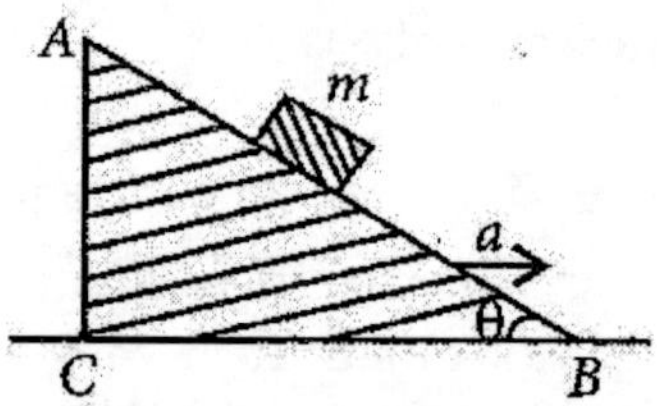

The wedge is given an acceleration a towards the right. The relation between a and θ for the block to remain stationary on the wedge is

(a) $a = \frac{g}{\operatorname{cosec}\theta}$ (b) $a = \frac{g}{\sin\theta}$

(c) $a = g\cos\theta$ (d) $a = g\tan\theta$

67. Two blocks A and B of masses $3m$ and m respectively are connected by a massless and inextensible string. The whole system is suspended by a massless spring as shown in figure. The magnitudes of acceleration of A and B immediately after the string is cut, are respectively **(2017)**

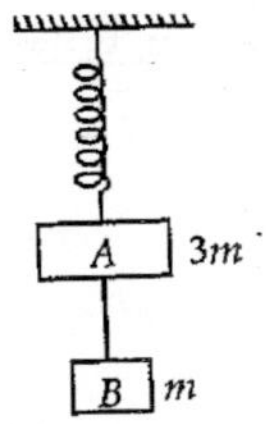

(a) $\frac{g}{3}, g$ (b) g, g

(c) $\frac{g}{3}, \frac{g}{3}$ (d) $g, \frac{g}{3}$

68. A balloon with mass m is descending down with an acceleration a (where $< g$). How much mass should be removed from it so that it starts moving up with an acceleration? **(2014)**

(a) $\frac{2ma}{g+a}$ (b) $\frac{2ma}{g-a}$

(c) $\frac{ma}{g+a}$ (d) $\frac{ma}{g-a}$

69. Three blocks with masses $m, 2m$ and $3m$ are connected by strings, as shown in the figure. After an upward force F is applied on block m, the masses move upward at constant speed v.

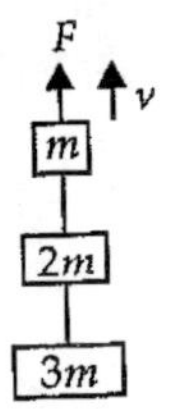

What is the net force on the block of mass $2m$? (is the acceleration due to gravity) **(2013)**

(a) $3mg$ (b) $6mg$

(c) zero (d) $2mg$

70. A person of mass 60 kg is inside a lift of mass 940 kg and presses the button on control panel. The lift starts moving upwards with an acceleration 1.0 m/s^2. If $g = 10 \text{ m s}^{-2}$, the tension in the supporting cable is **(2011)**

(a) 8600 N (b) 9680 N

(c) 11000 N (d) 1200 N

71. The mass of a lift is 2000 kg. When the tension in the supporting cable is 28000 N, then its acceleration is **(2009)**

(a) 4 m s^{-2} upwards

(b) 4 m s^{-2} downwards

(c) 14 m s^{-2} upwards

(d) 30 m s^{-2} downwards

72. A block of mass m is placed on a smooth wedge of inclination θ. The whole system is accelerated horizontally so that the block does not slip on the wedge. The force exerted by the wedge on the block will be (g is acceleration due to gravity) **(2004)**

(a) $mg\cos\theta$ (b) $mg\sin\theta$

(c) mg (d) $mg/\cos\theta$

73. A man weighs 80 kg. He stands on a weighing scale in a lift which is moving upwards with a uniform acceleration of 5 m/s^2. What would be the reading on the scale? ($g = 10 \text{ m/s}^2$) **(2003)**

(a) zero (b) 400 N

(c) 800 N (d) 1200 N

74. A monkey of mass 20 kg is holding a vertical rope. The rope will not break when a mass of 25 kg is suspended from it but will break if the mass exceeds 25 kg. What is the maximum acceleration with which the monkey can climb up along the rope? ($g = 10\ m/s^2$) **(2003)**

(a) $5\ m/s^2$ (b) $10\ m/s^2$

(c) $25\ m/s^2$ (d) $2.5\ m/s^2$

75. A lift of mass 1000 kg which is moving with acceleration of $1\ m/s^2$ in upward direction, then the tension developed in string which is connected to lift is

(a) 9800 N (b) 10,800 N

(c) 11,000 N (d) 10,000 N

76. Two masses as shown in the figure are suspended from a massless pulley. The acceleration of the system when masses are left free is **(2000)**

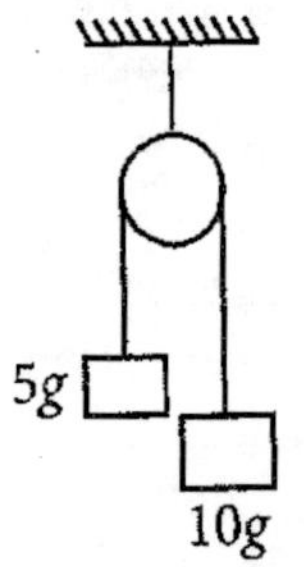

(a) $\frac{2g}{3}$ (b) $\frac{g}{3}$

(c) $\frac{g}{9}$ (d) $\frac{g}{7}$

77. A mass of 1 kg is suspended by a thread. It is

(i) lifted up with an acceleration $4.9\ m/s^2$,

(ii) lowered with an acceleration $4.9\ m/s^2$.

The ratio of the tensions is **(1998)**

(a) 1:3 (b) 1:2

(c) 3:1 (d) 2:1

78. A mass M is placed on a very smooth wedge resting on a surface without friction. Once the mass is released, the acceleration to be given to the wedge so that M remains at

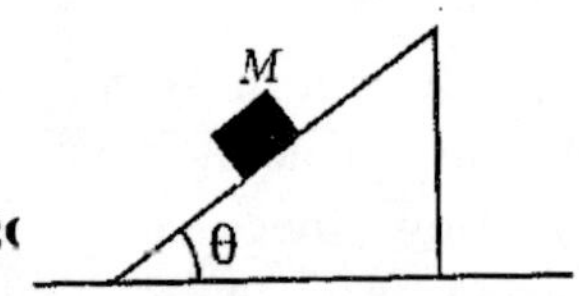

rest is a where **(1998)**

(a) a is applied to the left and $a = g\tan\theta$

(b) a is applied to the right and $a = g\tan\theta$

(c) a is applied to the left and $a = g\sin\theta$

(d) a is applied to the left and $a = g\cos\theta$

79. A monkey is decending from the branch of a tree with constant acceleration. If the breaking strength of branch is 75% of the weight of the monkey, the minimum acceleration with which monkey can slide down without breaking the branch is

(a) (b) $3g/4$

(c) $g/4$ (d) $g/2$

ANSWER KEY

1.	(c)	2.	(c)	3.	(c)	4.	(b)	5.	(c)	6.	(c)
7.	(b)	8.	(b)	9.	(c)	10.	(d)	11.	(b)	12.	(b)
13.	(c)	14.	(c)	15.	(b)	16.	(d)	17.	(d)	18.	(c)
19.	(a)	20.	(c)	21.	(c)	22.	(a)	23.	(c)	24.	(a)
25.	(d)	26.	(*)	27.	(d)	28.	(a)	29.	(c)	30.	(b)
31.	(a)	32.	(a)	33.	(d)	34.	(c)	35.	(b)	36.	(d)
37.	(d)	38.	(a)	39.	(c)	40.	(a)	41.	(a)	42.	(c)
43.	(d)	44.	(d)	45.	(b)	46.	(a)	47.	(d)	48.	(b)
49.	(a)	50.	(b)	51.	(d)	52.	(d)	53.	(d)	54.	(c)
55.	(c)	56.	(b)	57.	(d)	58.	(c)	59.	(c)	60.	(b)
61.	(a)	62.	(c)	63.	(b)	64.	(c)	65.	(c)	66.	(d)
67.	(a)	68.	(a)	69.	(c)	70.	(c)	71.	(a)	72.	(d)
73.	(d)	74.	(d)	75.	(b)	76.	(b)	77.	(c)	78.	(a)
79.	(c)										

Hints & Explanations

1. **(c) :** Newton's first law of motion is related to physical independence of force.

2. **(c) :** Mass, $m = 0.15$ kg; $h_1 = 10$ m, $h_2 = 10$ m; $g = 10 \text{ m/s}^2$ The velocity at the time of strike when going downwards.

$v = -\sqrt{2gh_1}$

and when move up $v' = \sqrt{2gh_2}$

Impulse = change in momentum

$mv' - mv = 2mv$ (As $h_1 = h_2$) $= 2 \times 0.15 \times \sqrt{2 \times 10 \times 10} = 4.2$ kg m/s

3. **(c) :**

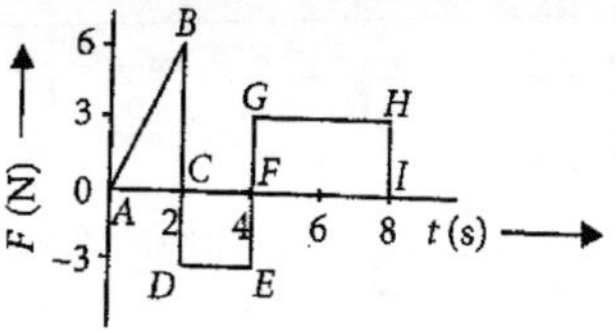

Change in momentum = Area under F - t graph in that interval

= Area of $\triangle ABC$ − Area of rectangle $CDEF$+ Area of rectangle FGHI

$= \frac{1}{2} \times 2 \times 6 - 3 \times 2 + 4 \times 3 = 12 \text{ N s}^{+}$

4. **(b) :** When a stone is dropped from a height h, it hits the ground with a momentum

$P = m\sqrt{2gh}$ ...(i)

where m is the mass of the stone

When the same stone is dropped from a height $2h$ (i.e. 100% of initial), then its momentum with which it hits the ground becomes $P' = m\sqrt{2g(2h)} = \sqrt{2}P$ (Using (i)) ...(ii)

% change in momentum $= \frac{P'-P}{P} \times 100\%$

$$= \frac{\sqrt{2}P - P}{P} \times 100\% = 41\%$$

5. **(c)** : $\vec{F} = 6\hat{\imath} - 8\hat{\jmath} + 10\hat{k}$

$|\vec{F}| = \sqrt{36+64+100} = \sqrt{200}$ N

$= 10\sqrt{2}$ N.

Acceleration, $a = 1 \text{ m s}^{-2}$

$\therefore$ Mass, $= \frac{10\sqrt{2}}{1} = 10\sqrt{2}$ kg.

6. **(c)** : $F = \frac{d}{dt}(Mv) = v\frac{dM}{dt} + M\frac{dv}{dt}$

As v is a constant, $F = v\frac{dM}{dt}$. But $\frac{dM}{dt} = M$ kg/s

$\therefore$ To keep the conveyer belt moving at m/s, force needed $= vM$ newton.

7. **(b)** : Mass, = 3 kg, force, $F = 6t^2\hat{\imath} + 4t\hat{\jmath}$

$\therefore$ acceleration, $a = \frac{F}{m} = \frac{6t^2\hat{\imath}+4t\hat{\jmath}}{3} = 2t^2\hat{\imath} + \frac{4}{3}t\hat{\jmath}$

Now, $a = \frac{dv}{dt} = 2t^2\hat{\imath} + \frac{4}{3}t\hat{\jmath}$

$\therefore dv = \left(2t^2\hat{\imath} + \frac{4}{3}t\hat{\jmath}\right)dt \;\therefore v$

$$= \int_0^3 \left(2t^2\hat{\imath} + \frac{4}{3}t\hat{\jmath}\right)dt$$

$$= \frac{2}{3}t^3\hat{\imath} + \frac{4}{6}t^2\hat{\jmath}\Big|_0^3 = 18\hat{\imath} + 6\hat{\jmath}.$$

8. **(b)** : Impulse = Change in momentum

$F \cdot \Delta t = m \cdot v; F = \frac{m \cdot v}{\Delta t} = \frac{150\times10^{-3}\times20}{0.1} =$ 30 N.

9. **(c)** : Force $= \frac{d}{dt}$(momentum)

$$= \frac{d}{dt}(mv) = v\left(\frac{dm}{dt}\right) \Rightarrow 210$$

$$= 300\left(\frac{dm}{dt}\right)$$

$\frac{dm}{dt}$ = rate of combustion $= \frac{210}{300} =$ 0.7 kg/s

10. **(d)** : When $F = 0, 600 - 2\times10^5 t = 0$

$$\therefore t = \frac{600}{2\times10^5} = 3\times10^{-3} \text{ s}$$

Now, impulse, $I = \int_0^t F dt =$

$\int_0^t (600 - 2\times10^5 t)dt$

$600t - 2\times10^5\frac{t^2}{2}$

$= 600\times3\times10^{-3} - 10^5\times(3\times10^{-3})^2$

or, $I = 1.8 - 0.9 = 0.9$ N s.

11. **(b)** : Thrust $= M(g+a) = u\frac{dm}{dt}$

$$\frac{dm}{dt} = \frac{M(g+a)}{u} = \frac{5000(10+20)}{800}$$

$= 187.5$ kg/s

12. **(b)** : Force $(F) = 6$ N; Initial velocity $(u) = 0$;

Mass $(m) = 1$ kg and final velocity $(v) = 30$ m/s.

Therefore acceleration $(a) = \frac{F}{m} = \frac{6}{1} = 6 \text{ m/s}^2$ and final velocity $(v) = 30 = u + at = 0 + 6\times t$ or $t = 5$ seconds.

13. **(c)** : Force $(F) = 10$ N and acceleration $(a) = 1$ m/s^2.

Mass $(m) = \frac{F}{a} = \frac{10}{1} = 10$ kg.

14. **(c)** : $\vec{F} = 6\hat{\imath} - 8\hat{\jmath} + 10\hat{k}$

$|\vec{F}| = \sqrt{6^2 + 8^2 + (10)^2} = \sqrt{36 + 64 + 100}$

$= 10\sqrt{2}$ M

a = 1m/s

F = ma

$10\sqrt{2} = M \times 1$

$M = 10\sqrt{2}$ kg

15. **(b)** : Rate of burning of fuel $\left(\frac{dm}{dt}\right) =$ 1 kg/s and velocity of ejected fuel $(v) = 60$ km/s $= 60 \times 10^3$ m/s

Force = Rate of change of momentum

$$= \frac{dp}{dt} = \frac{d(mv)}{dt} = v\frac{dm}{dt}$$

$$= (60 \times 10^3) \times 1$$

$$= 60000 \text{ N}$$

16. **(d)** : Rate of change of mass $= \frac{dM}{dt} = \alpha v$.

Retarding force = Rate of change of momentum

= Velocity × Rate of change in mass = $-v \times \frac{dM}{dt}$

$= -v \times \alpha v = -\alpha v^2$. (Minus sign of v due to deceleration)

Therefore, acceleration $= -\frac{\alpha v^2}{M}$.

17. **(d)** : Impulse is a vector quantity and is equal to change in momentum of the body thus, (same as $F \times t$ where t is short) Impulse $= mv_2 - mv_1 = m(v_2 - v_1)$

18. **(c)** : Thrust is the force with which the rocket moves upward given by $F = u\frac{dm}{dt}$

Thus mass of the gas ejected per second to supply the thrust needed to overcome the weight of the rocket is

$\frac{dm}{dt} = \frac{F}{u} = \frac{m \times a}{u}$ or $\frac{dm}{dt} = \frac{600 \times 10}{1000} = 6$ kg s^{-1}

19. **(a)** : Given, $p_i = p_f = mV$

Change in momentum of the ball =

$\vec{p}_f - \vec{p}_i$

$= -(p_{fx}\hat{\imath} - p_{fy}\hat{\jmath}) - (p_{ix}\hat{\imath} - p_{iy}\hat{\jmath})$

$= -\hat{\imath}(p_{fx} + p_{ix}) - \hat{\jmath}(p_{fy} - p_{iy})$

$= -2p_{ix}\hat{\imath} - 0\hat{\jmath} = -mV\hat{\imath}$

Here, $p_{ix} = p_{fx} = p_i \cos 60° = \frac{mV}{2}$

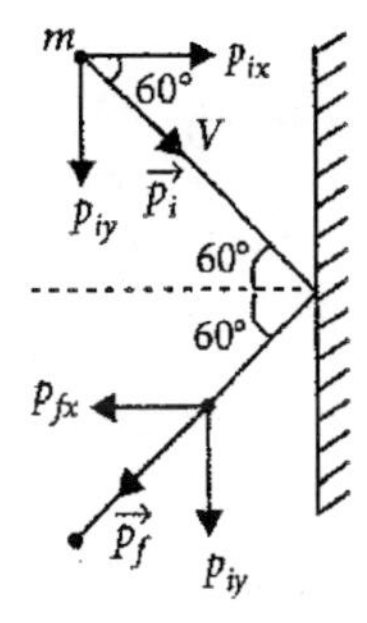

∵ Impulse imparted by the wall = change in the momentum of the ball = mV.

20. **(c) :** Impulse = Change in linear momentum

$= MV - (-MV) = 2MV$

21. **(c) :** Components of momentum parallel to the wall are in the same direction and components of momentum perpendicular to the wall are opposite to each other. Therefore change of momentum = $2mv\sin\theta$.

$F \times t$ = change in momentum = $2mv\sin\theta$

$\therefore F = \frac{2mv\sin\theta}{t} = \frac{2\times0.5\times12\times\sin30^\circ}{0.25} = 48 \times \frac{1}{2} = 24$ N.

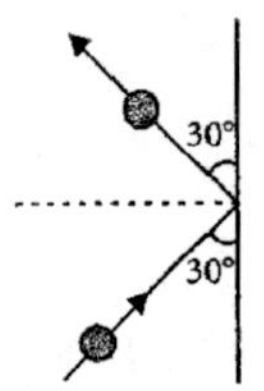

22. **(a) :**

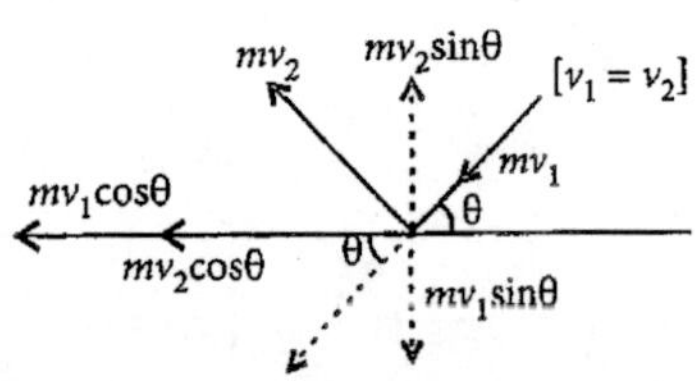

Change in momentum = $mv_2\sin\theta - (mv_1\sin\theta) = 2mv\sin\theta$

$= 2 \times 3 \times 10 \times \sin 60^\circ = 60 \times \frac{\sqrt{3}}{2}$

Force = Change in momentum / Impact time

$= \frac{30\sqrt{3}}{0.2} = 150\sqrt{3}$ N

23. **(c) :** Masses Ratio = 2 : 2 : 1

Initial mass = m

$M_1 = \frac{2m}{5}\ M_2 = \frac{2m}{5}\ M_3 = \frac{m}{5}$

Appling momentum conservation [same mass have velocity 'v' in perpendicular direction]

$m_1v_1 + m_2v_2 + m_3v_3 \qquad V_i = V_y = V$

$\frac{2m}{5}Vi + \frac{2m}{5}Vj + \frac{m}{5}\vec{V}_3 = 0$

$\vec{V}_3 = -(2V_i + 2V_j)$

$|\vec{V}_3| = \sqrt{(-2v)^2 + (-2v)^2} = \sqrt{8v^2} = 2\sqrt{2v}$

24. **(a) :** From the law of conservation of linear momentum $m\vec{v} = m_1\vec{v}_1 + m_2\vec{v}_2$

$\Rightarrow 6k(20\hat{\imath} + 25\hat{\jmath} - 12\hat{k})$

$= k(100\hat{\imath} + 35\hat{\jmath} + 8\hat{k}) + 5k\vec{v}_2$

$\Rightarrow 5\vec{v}_2 = (120 - 100)\hat{\imath} + (150 - 35)\hat{\jmath} + (-72 - 8)\hat{k}$

$\Rightarrow 5\vec{v}_2 = 20\hat{\imath} + 115\hat{\jmath} - 80\hat{k}$

$\Rightarrow \vec{v}_2 = 4\hat{\imath} + 23\hat{\jmath} - 16\hat{k}$

25. **(d) :** The situation is as shown in the figure.

According to law of conservation of linear momentum

$\vec{p}_1 + \vec{p}_2 + \vec{p}_3 = 0$

$\therefore \vec{p}_3 = -(\vec{p}_1 + \vec{p}_2)$

Here, $\vec{p}_1 = (1\text{ kg})(12\text{ m s}^{-1})\hat{\imath} =$ $12\hat{\imath}\text{ kg m s}^{-1}$

$\vec{p}_2 = (2\text{ kg})(8\text{ m s}^{-1})\hat{\jmath} = 16\hat{\jmath}\text{ kg m s}^{-1}$

$\therefore \vec{p}_3 = -(12\hat{\imath} + 16\hat{\jmath})\text{kgms}^{-1}$

The magnitude of p_3 is

$$p_3 = \sqrt{(12)^2 + (16)^2} = 20\text{ kg m s}^{-1}$$

$$\therefore m_3 = \frac{p_3}{v_3} = \frac{20\text{ kg m s}^{-1}}{4\text{ m s}^{-1}} = 5\text{ kg}$$

26. **(*)** : None of the given options is correct.

100 Kg = mass of man + rifle

99.9 Kg = left after 10 shot being fired

Momentum of 10 shot = 0.1×800=80 Ns

Momentum of (men + rifle) = mv = 80

= 99.9×V = 80

$$V = \frac{80}{99.9} \Rightarrow 0.8 m/s$$

Force Exerted by 10 bullet =

$$\frac{\text{Change in momentum}}{\Delta t}$$

$$= \frac{10\times0.01\times800}{55} = 16\text{N}$$

27. **(d)**

$\vec{P}_1+\vec{P}_2+\vec{P}_3=0$ $\quad P_1 = 1\times12 = 12$ N-S (along x-axis)

$\vec{P}_3=-(\vec{P}_1+\vec{P}_2)$ $\quad P_2 = 2\times8 = 16$ N–S (along y-axis)

$\vec{P}_3 = -(12\hat{i}+16\hat{j})$

$$|\vec{P}_3| = \sqrt{(-12)^2+(-16)^2} = \sqrt{400} = 20\text{ N-S}$$

Mass of third part = $\frac{P_3}{V} = \frac{20}{4} = 5kg$

28. **(a)** : Apply conservation of linear momentum.

Total momentum before explosion

= total momentum after explosion

$$0 = \frac{m}{5}v_1\hat{\imath} + \frac{m}{5}v_2\hat{\jmath} + \frac{3m}{5}\vec{v}_3$$

$$\Rightarrow \frac{3m}{5}\vec{v}_3 = -\frac{m}{5}[v_1\hat{\imath} + v_2\hat{\jmath}]$$

$$\vec{v}_3 = \frac{-v_1}{3}\hat{\imath} - \frac{v_2}{3}\hat{\jmath}$$

$$\therefore v_1 = v_2 = 30\text{ m/s}$$

$$\vec{v}_3 = -10\hat{\imath} - 10\hat{\jmath};\ v_3 = 10\sqrt{2}\text{ m/s}$$

29. **(c)** : Velocity after $5\text{ s}, v = u - gt = 100 - 10\times5 = 50\text{ m/s}$ By conservation of momentum $1\times50 = 0.4\times(-25) + 0.6\times v'$

$$60 = 0.6\times v' \Rightarrow v' = 100\text{ m/s}$$

upwards

30. **(b)** : In absence of External force momentum is conserved

31. **(a)** : Mass of bullet $(m_1) = 200\text{ g} = 0.2\text{ kg}$; speed of bullet $(v_1) = 5\text{ m/s}$ and mass of gun $(m_2) = 1\text{ kg}$. Before firing, total momentum is zero. After firing total momentum is $m_1v_1 + m_2v_2$.

From the law of conservation of momentum

$m_1v_1 + m_2v_2 = 0$ or

$$v_2 = \frac{-m_1v_1}{m_2} = \frac{-0.2\times5}{1} = -1\text{ m/s}$$

32. **(a) :** Since 5 kg body explodes into three fragments with masses in the ratio 1: 1: 3 thus, masses of fragments will be 1 kg, 1 kg and 3 kg respectively. The magnitude of resultant momentum of two fragments each of mass 1 kg, moving with velocity 21 m/s, in perpendicular directions is

$\sqrt{(m_1v_1)^2+(m_2v_2)^2} = \sqrt{(21)^2+(21)^2}$

$= 21\sqrt{2}$ kg m/s

According to law of conservation of linear momentum

$m_3v_3 = 21\sqrt{2}$ or $3v_3$

$= 21\sqrt{2}$ or $v_3 = 7\sqrt{2}$ m/s

33. **(d) :** As per triangle law, $\vec{F}_1+\vec{F}_2+\vec{F}_3=0$ i.e., net force on the particle is zero. So, acceleration is also zero. Hence velocity of the particle will remain constant.

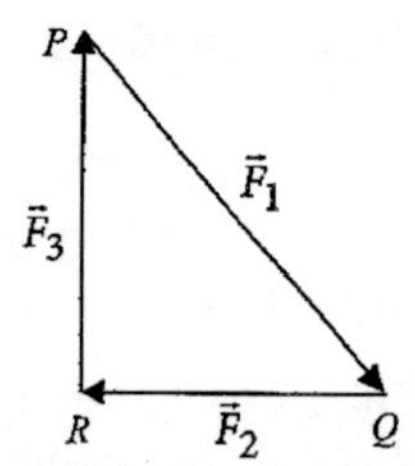

34. **(c) :** Taking x-components, the total should be zero.

$1\times\cos 60^\circ + 2\cos 60^\circ + x - 4\cos 60^\circ$

$= 0$

$\therefore\ x = 0.5$ N

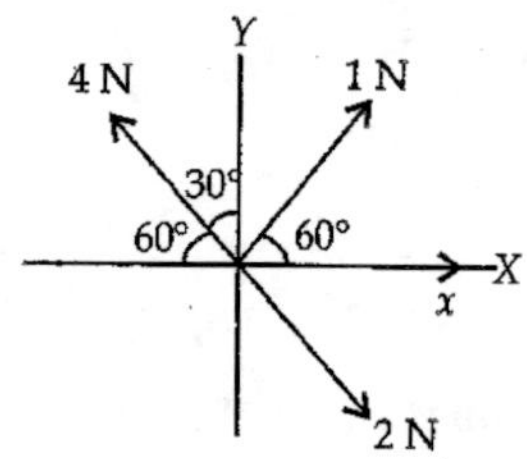

35. **(b) :** $F_S = ma$

$f_L = ma_{\max}$

$\mu mg = ma_{\max}$

$a_{\max} = \mu g$

$= 0.15(10)$

$= 1.5 m/s^2$

36. **(d) :** Coefficient of sliding friction has no dimension.

$f = \mu_s N \Rightarrow \mu_s = \frac{f}{N}$

37. **(d) :** Let μ_s and μ_k be the coefficients of static and kinetic friction between the box and the plank respectively. When the angle of inclination θ reaches 30°, the block just slides,

$\therefore\ \mu_s = \tan\theta = \tan 30^\circ = \frac{1}{\sqrt{3}} = 0.6$

If a is the acceleration produced in the block, then $ma = mg\sin\theta - f_k$ (where f_k is force of kinetic friction) $=$

$mg\sin\theta - \mu_k N$ (as $f_k = \mu_k N$)

$= mg\sin\theta - \mu_k mg\cos\theta$

$a = g(\sin\theta - \mu_k\cos\theta)$

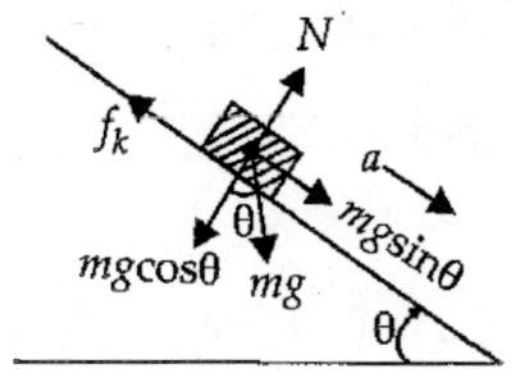

As $g = 10\text{ m s}^{-2}$ and $\theta = 30^\circ$

$\therefore\ a = (10\text{ m s}^{-2})(\sin 30^\circ - \mu_k \cos 30^\circ)$

If s is the distance travelled by the block in time t, then

$$s = \frac{1}{2}at^2(\text{ as } u = 0) \text{ or } a = \frac{2s}{t^2}$$

But $s = 4.0$ m and $t = 4.0$ s (given)

$$\therefore\ a = \frac{2(4.0\text{ m})}{(4.0\text{ s})^2} = \frac{1}{2}\text{ m s}^{-2}$$

Substituting this value of a in eqn. (i), we get

$$\frac{1}{2}\text{ m s}^{-2} = (10\text{ m s}^{-2})\left(\frac{1}{2} - \mu_k\frac{\sqrt{3}}{2}\right)$$

$\frac{1}{10} = 1 - \sqrt{3}\mu_k$ or

$\sqrt{3}\mu_k = 1 - \frac{1}{10} = \frac{9}{10} = 0.9$

or $\mu_k = \frac{0.9}{\sqrt{3}} = 0.5$

38. **(a) :**

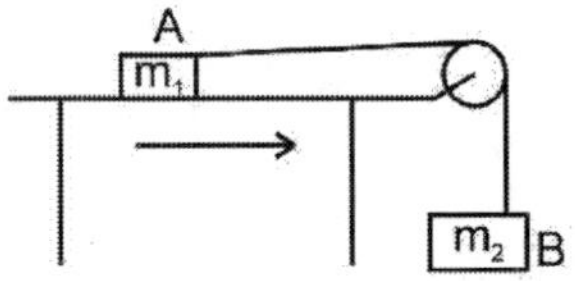

Kinetic friction = μ_k

Block 'A' is sliding toward right due to tension, Net acceleration is also toward right

FBD of A Block

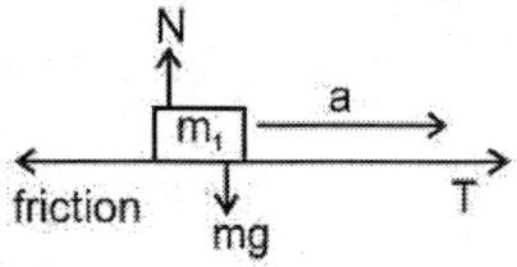

$T - \mu_k N = m_1 a$ .....(i)

$N = m_1 g$

FBD of 'B' Block

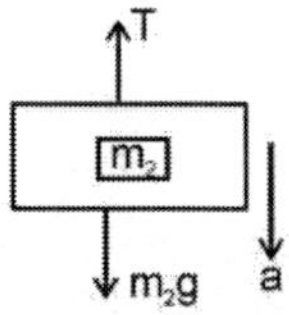

$m_2 g - T = m_2 a$ ....(ii)

adding eq (i) & (ii)

$m2g - \mu_k N = m_1 a + m_2 a$

$m_2 g - m_1 g \mu_k = (m_1 + m_2)a$

$$\frac{g(m_2 - m_1\mu_k)}{(m_1 + m_2)} = a$$

So Tension will be

$T = m_1 a + \mu_k N$

$$T = m_1\left[\frac{g(m_2 - m_1\mu_k)}{m_1 + m_2}\right] + \mu_k m_1 g$$

$$T = m_1 g\left[\frac{m_2 - m_1\mu_k}{m_1 + m_2} + \mu_k\right]$$

$$T = m_1 g\left[\frac{m_2 - m_1\mu_k + m_1\mu_k + m_2\mu_k}{m_1 + m_2}\right]$$

$$T = m_1 g\left[\frac{m_2(1 + \mu_k)}{m_1 + m_2}\right]$$

$$T = m_1 m_2 g\left[\frac{1 + \mu_k}{m_1 + m_2}\right]$$

39. **(c)** : Force of friction on mass $m_2 = \mu m_2 g$ Force of friction on mass $m_3 = \mu m_3 g$ Let a be common acceleration of the system.

$$\therefore a = \frac{m_1 g - \mu m_2 g - \mu m_3 g}{m_1 + m_2 + m_3}$$

Here, $m_1 = m_2 = m_3 = m$

$$\therefore a = \frac{mg - \mu mg - \mu mg}{m + m + m}$$

$$= \frac{mg - 2\mu mg}{3m} = \frac{g(1-2\mu)}{3}$$

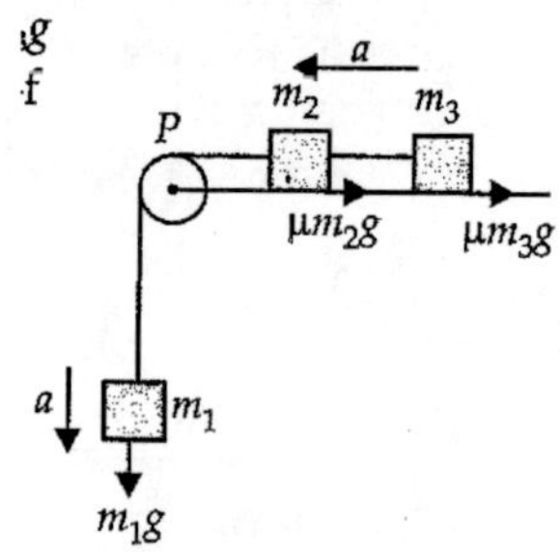

Hence, the downward acceleration of mass m_1 is $\frac{g(1-2\mu)}{3}$.

40. **(a) :**

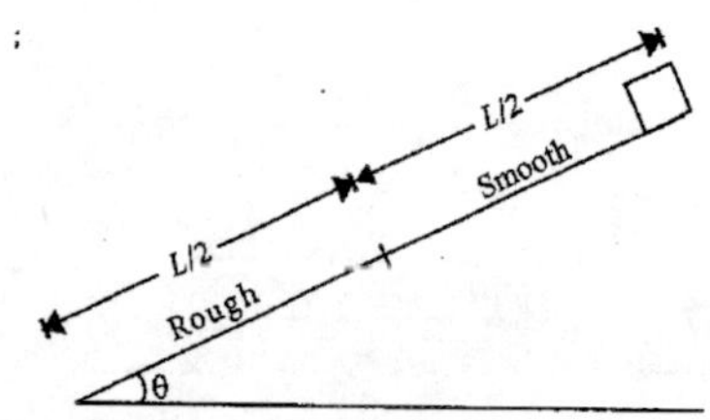

For upper half smooth plane

Acceleration of the block, $a = g\sin\theta$

Here, $u = 0$ (block starts from rest)

$a = g\sin\theta, s = \frac{L}{2}$

Using, $v^2 - u^2 = 2as$, we have $v^2 - 0 = 2 \times g\sin\theta \times \frac{L}{2}$

$v = \sqrt{gL\sin\theta}$

$v = \sqrt{gL\sin\theta}$

For lower half rough plane

Acceleration of the block, $a' = g\sin\theta - \mu g\cos\theta$

where μ is the coefficient of friction between the block and lower half of the plane

Here, $u = v = \sqrt{gL\sin\theta}$

$v = 0$ (block comes to rest)

$a = a' = g\sin\theta - \mu g\cos\theta, s = \frac{L}{2}$

Again, using $v^2 - u^2 = 2as$, we have

$$0 - (\sqrt{gL\sin\theta})^2 = 2 \times (g\sin\theta - \mu g\cos\theta) \times \frac{L}{2}$$

$$-gL\sin\theta = (g\sin\theta - \mu g\cos\theta)L - \sin\theta = \sin\theta - \mu\cos\theta$$

$\mu\cos\theta = 2\sin\theta$ or $\mu = 2\tan\theta$

41. **(a) :** Force of friction, $f = \mu mg$

$$\therefore a = \frac{f}{m} = \frac{\mu mg}{m} = \mu g = 0.5 \times 10 = 5 \text{ m s}^{-2}$$

Using $v^2 - u^2 = 2aS, 0^2 - 2^2 = 2(-5) \times S \Rightarrow S = 0.4$ m

42. **(c)** : Pseudo force or fictitious force, $F_{\text{fic}} = m\alpha$

Force of friction, $f = \mu N = \mu m\alpha$

The block of mass m will not fall as long as

$f \geq mg; \mu m\alpha \geq mg$

$\alpha \geq \frac{g}{\mu}$

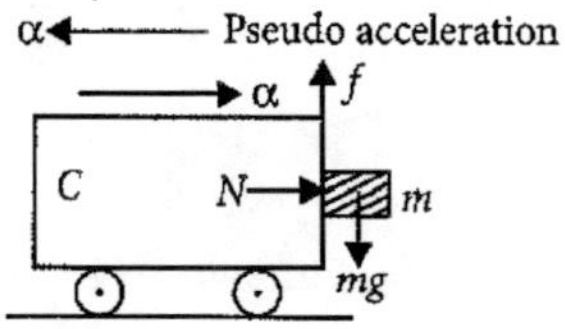

43. **(d)** : Given $u = V$, final velocity = 0.

Using $v = u + at$ $\therefore 0 = V - at$ or,

$-a = \frac{0-V}{t} = -\frac{V}{t}$

Force of friction, $f = \mu R = \mu mg$

Retardation, $a = \mu g$ $\therefore t = \frac{V}{a} = \frac{V}{\mu g}$.

44. **(d):**

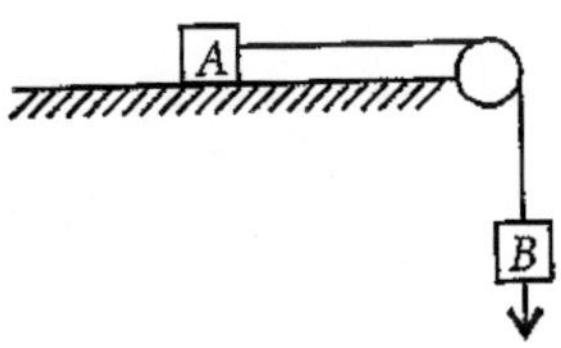

Free body diagram of two masses is

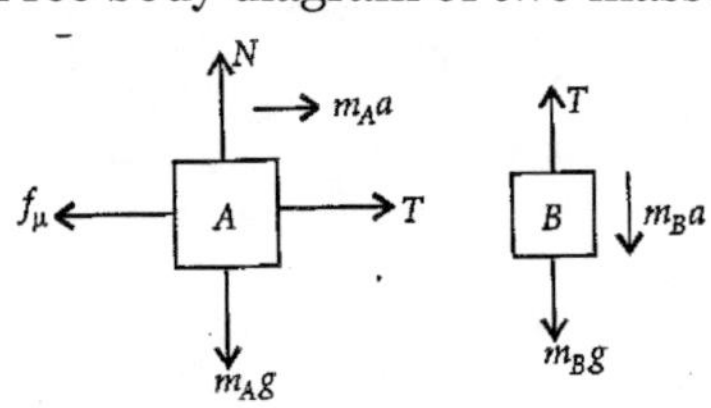

We get equations

$T + m_A a = f$ or $T = \mu N_A$ (for $a = 0$)

and $T = m_B a + m_B g$ or $T = m_B g$ (for $a = 0$)

$\therefore \mu N_A = m_B g \Rightarrow m_B = \mu m_A = 0.2 \times 2 = 0.4$ kg

45. **(b)** :

$m = 10$ kg, $R = mg$

$\therefore$ Frictional force = f_k

$= \mu_k R = \mu_k mg = 0.5 \times 10 \times 10 = 50$ N

$\therefore$ Net force acting on the body,

$F = P - f_k = 100 - 50 = 50$ N

$\therefore$ Acceleration of the block, $a = F/m = 50/10 = 5$ m/s^2

46. **(a) :**

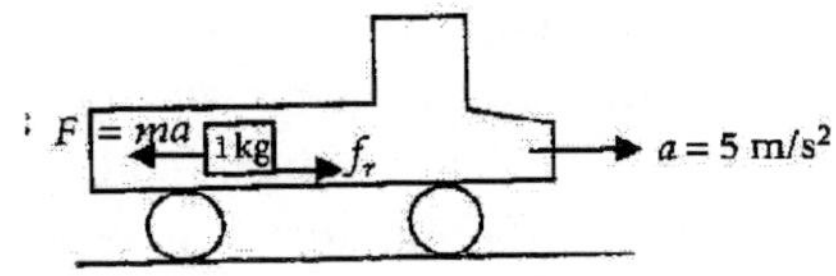

$f_{rL} = \mu_s N = \mu_s \times mg = 0.6 \times 1 \times 10$

$= 6$N

f_{rL} is the force of limiting friction.

where f_{rL} is the force of limiting frict

Pseudo force = $ma = 1 \times 5; F = 5$ N

If $F < f_{rL}$ block does not move. So static friction is present.

Static friction = applied force. $\therefore f_r = 5$ N

47. **(d)** : The acceleration is nullified by force of kinetic friction on the block.

$mg\sin\theta$ is force downwards.

μ_k is the coefficient of kinetic friction.

$\mu_k mg\cos\theta$ is friction force acting upwards.

$\therefore mg\sin\theta - \mu_k mg\cos\theta$ = mass × acceleration

acceleration = 0 as v is constant $\therefore \mu_k = \tan\theta$

48. **(b)** : Car initial speed = 72 km/h =

$72 \times \frac{5}{18} = 20 m/s$

Retardation due to friction b/w type an Road = $\mu g = 5$ m/s^2

Applying 3rd eq of motion.

$V^2 = v^2 + 2aS$

$0 = (20)^2 - 2 \times 5 \times 5$

$\frac{400}{10} = S$

$S = 40$ m

49. **(a)** : Let M is the mass of the chain of length L. If y is the maximum length of chain which can hang outside the table without sliding, then for equilibrium of the chain, the weight of hanging part must be balanced by the force of friction on the portion of the table.

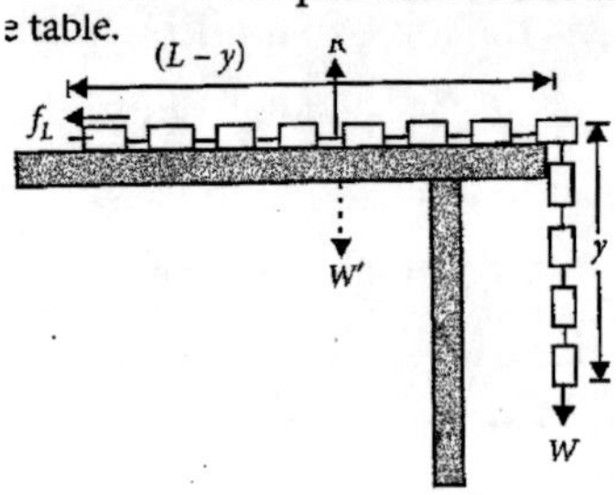

$W = f_L$ ...(i)

But from figure

$W = \frac{M}{L} yg$ and $R = W' = \frac{M}{L}(L - y)g$

So that $f_L = \mu R = \mu \frac{M}{L}(L - y)g$

Substituting these values of W and f_L in eqn.(i), we get

$\mu \frac{M}{L}(L - y)g = \frac{M}{L} yg$

or $\mu(L - y) = y$

or $y = \frac{\mu L}{\mu+1} = \frac{0.25L}{1.25} = \frac{L}{5}$

or $\frac{y}{L} = \frac{1}{5} = \frac{1}{5} \times 100\% = 20\%$

50. **(b)** : The various forces acting on the body have been shown in the figure. The force on the body down the inclined plane in presence of friction is

$F = mg\sin\theta - f = mg\sin\theta - \mu N$

$= ma$

or $a = g\sin\theta - \mu g\cos\theta$.

Since block is at rest thus initial velocity $u = 0$

∴ Time taken to slide down the plane

$t_1 = \sqrt{\frac{2s}{a}} = \sqrt{\frac{2s}{g\sin\theta - \mu g\cos\theta}}$

In absence of friction time taken will be

$t_2 = \sqrt{\frac{2s}{g\sin\theta}}$

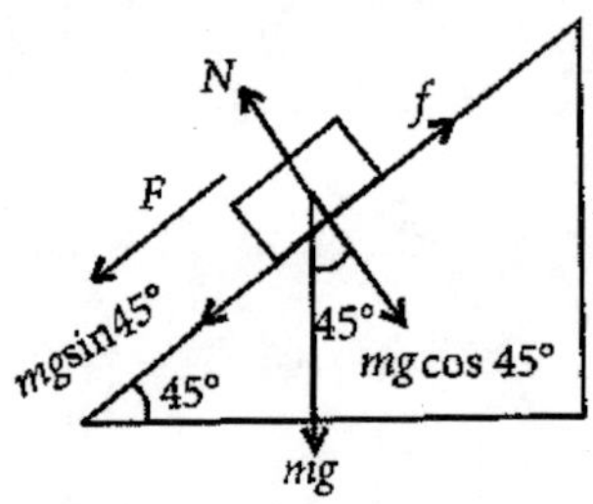

Given : $t_1 = 2t_2$

$\therefore t_1^2 - 4t_2^2$ or $\frac{2s}{g(\sin\theta - \mu\cos\theta)} = \frac{2s \times 4}{g(\sin\theta)}$

or $\sin\theta = 4\sin\theta - 4\mu\cos\theta$

or $\mu = \frac{3}{4}\tan\theta = 0.75$

51. **(d)** : To keep the block stationary,

Frictional force ≥ Weight $\mu N \geq Mg$

Here, $N = M\omega^2 r$

$r = 1$ m, $\mu = 0.1$

For minimum ω, $\mu M\omega^2 r = Mg$

$$\omega = \sqrt{\frac{g}{\mu r}} = \sqrt{\frac{10}{0.1 \times 1}} = 10\text{rads}^{-1}$$

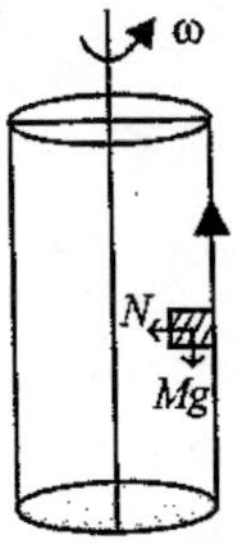

52. **(d)** : Centripetal force $\left(\frac{mv^2}{l}\right)$ is provided by tension so net force on the particle will be equal to tension T.

53. **(d)** :

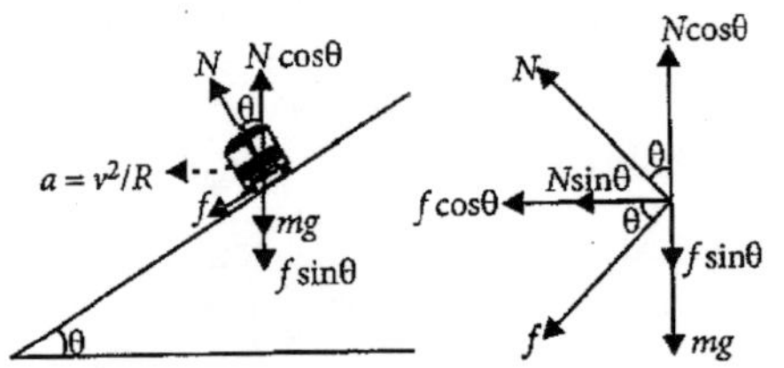

For vertical equilibrium on the road,

$N\cos\theta = mg + f\sin\theta \Rightarrow mg =$

$N\cos\theta - f\sin\theta$ ...(i)

Centripetal force for safe turning,

$N\sin\theta + f\cos\theta = \frac{mv^2}{R}$ ...(ii)

From eqns. (i) and (ii), we get

$$\frac{v^2}{Rg} = \frac{N\sin\theta + f\cos\theta}{N\cos\theta - f\sin\theta} \Rightarrow \frac{v^2_{\max}}{Rg} = \frac{N\sin\theta + \mu_s N\cos\theta}{N\cos\theta - \mu_s N\sin\theta}$$

$$v_{\max} = \sqrt{Rg\left(\frac{\mu_s + \tan\theta}{1 - \mu_s\tan\theta}\right)}$$

54. **(c)** : Let v be tangential speed of heavier stone. Then, centripetal force experienced by lighter stone is

$$(F_c)_{\text{lighter}} = \frac{m(nv)^2}{r}$$

and that of heavier stone is $(F_c)_{\text{heavier}} = \frac{2mv^2}{(r/2)}$

But $(F_c)_{\text{lighter}} = (F_c)_{\text{heavier}}$

$\therefore \frac{m(nv)^2}{r} = \frac{2mv^2}{(r/2)}$ or, $n^2\left(\frac{mv^2}{r}\right) = 4\left(\frac{mv^2}{r}\right)$

$n^2 = 4$ or $n = 2$

55. **(c)** : Let θ is the angle made by the wire with the vertical.

$$\therefore \tan\theta = \frac{v^2}{rg}$$

Here, $v = 10$ m/s, $r = 10$ m, $g = 10$ m/s^2

$$\therefore \tan\theta = \frac{(10\text{ m/s})^2}{10\text{ m}(10\text{ m/s}^2)} = 1$$

$$\theta = \tan^{-1}(1) = \frac{\pi}{4}$$

56. **(b)** : Here, $m = 1000$ kg, $R = 90$ m, $\theta = 45°$

For banking, $\tan\theta = \frac{v^2}{Rg}$

or $v = \sqrt{Rg\tan\theta} = \sqrt{90 \times 10 \times \tan 45°}$

$= 30\text{ m s}^{-1}$

57. **(d)**: Force of friction provides the necessary centripetal force.

$\frac{mv^2}{R} \le \mu_s N;\ v^2 \le \frac{\mu_s RN}{m}$

$v^2 \le \mu_s Rg$

or $v \le \sqrt{\mu_s Rg}$

$[\because N = mg]$

$\therefore$ The maximum speed of the car in circular motion is $v_{\max} = \sqrt{\mu_s Rg}$

58. **(c)** : The coin will revolve with the record, if Force of friction ≥ centripetal force

$\mu mg \geq mr\omega^2$ or $r \leq \frac{\mu g}{\omega^2}$

59. **(c)** : $mg = \frac{mv^2}{R} \Rightarrow v = \sqrt{Rg}$

$v = \sqrt{20 \times 10} = \sqrt{200} = 14.1 \text{ m/s}$

i.e., Between 14 and 15 m/s.

60. **(b)** : The center of the tube will be at length $L/2$.

So radius $r = L/2$.

The force exerted by the liquid at the other end

= centrifugal force

Centrifugal force = $Mr\omega^2 =$

$M\left(\frac{L}{2}\right)\omega^2 = \frac{ML\omega^2}{2}$

61. **(a)** : $F_{\text{centripetal}} = \frac{mv^2}{R}$; $v = \left(36 \times \frac{5}{18}\right) \text{m/s}$

$F_{\text{centripetal}} = \frac{500 \times \left(36 \times \frac{5}{18}\right)^2}{50} = 1000 \text{ N}$

62. **(c)** : $\frac{mv^2}{r} = 25$; $v = \sqrt{\frac{25 \times 1.96}{0.25}} = 14 \text{ m/s}$.

63. **(b)** : When milk is churned, cream gets separated due to centrifugal force.

64. **(c)**: The acceleration is $a = g\sin\theta$

Initial velocity, $u = 0$

Distance travelled in n^{th} second $S_{n^{\text{th}}} = u + \frac{1}{2}a(2n-1)$

$S_{n^{\text{th}}} = \frac{1}{2}a(2n-1)$ ...(i)

$S_{(n+1)^{\text{th}}} = \frac{1}{2}a[2(n+1)-1]$ ...(ii)

On dividing eqn (i) by (ii), we get

$\therefore \frac{S_{n^{\text{th}}}}{S_{(n+1)^{\text{th}}}} = \frac{(2n-1)}{(2n+1)}$

65. **(c)** : Given : $m_1 = 4$ kg, $m_2 = 6$ kg

From the diagram,

$T - m_1 g = m_1 a$ ...(i)

$m_2 g - T = m_2 a$ ...(ii)

Solving equation (i) and (ii)

$a = \frac{(m_2 - m_1)g}{m_2 + m_1} = \frac{(6-4)g}{10} = \frac{2}{10}g$

$= \frac{g}{5}$

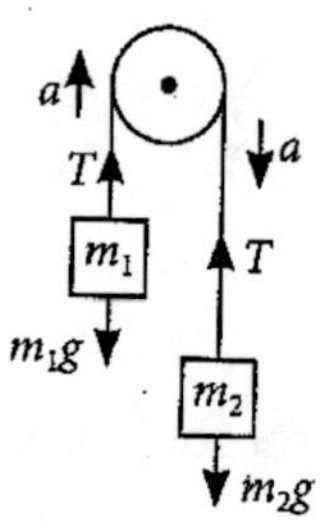

66. **(d)** : In non-inertial frame,

$N\sin\theta = ma$ ...(i)

$N\cos\theta = mg$ ...(ii)

From (i) and (ii),

$\tan\theta = \frac{a}{g}$

$\Rightarrow a = g\tan\theta$

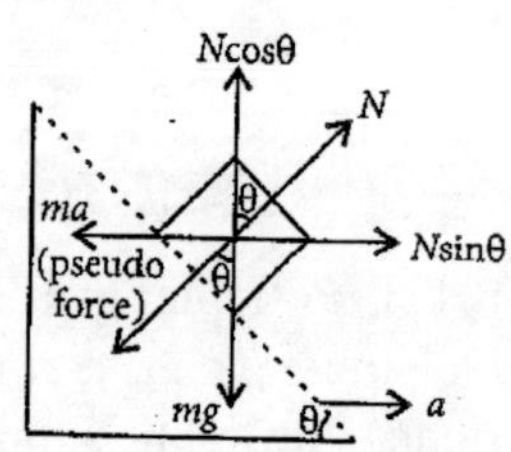

67. **(a) :** Before the string is cut

$kx = T + 3mg$ ...(i)

$T = mg$ ...(ii)

From eqns. (i) and (ii)

$kx = 4mg$

Just after the string is cut

$T = 0$

$a_A = \frac{kx-3mg}{3m}$

$a_A = \frac{4mg-3mg}{3m} = \frac{mg}{3m} = \frac{g}{3}$

and $a_B = g$.

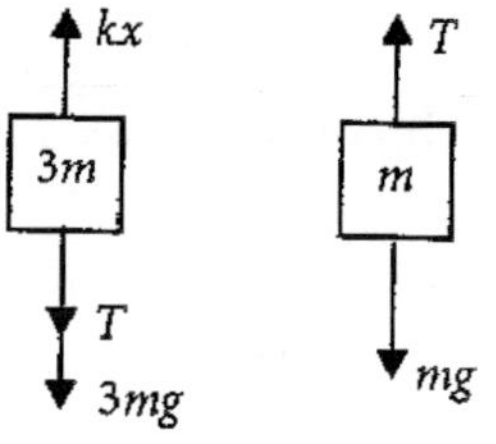

Before the string is cut

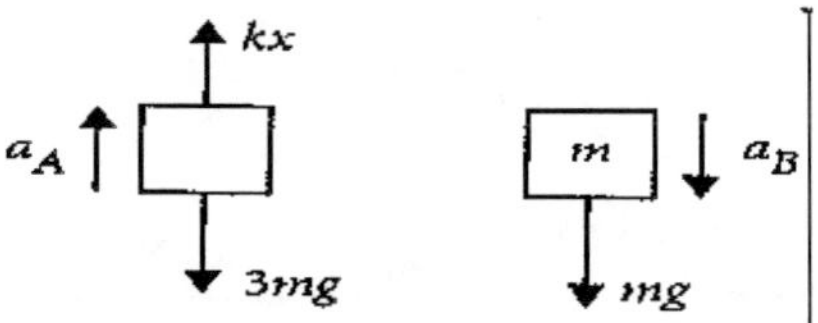

After the string is cut

68. **(a) :** Let F be the upthrust of the air. As the balloon is descending down with an acceleration a

$\therefore$ mg – F = ma ...(i)

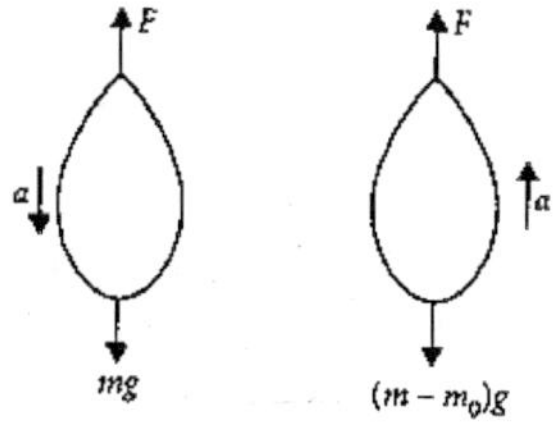

Let mass m_0 be removed from the balloon so that it starts moving up with an acceleration a. Then,

$F - (m - m_0)g = (m - m_0)a$

$F - mg + m_0g = ma - m_0a$

...(ii)

Adding eqn. (i) and eqn. (ii), we get

$m_0g = 2ma - m_0a; m_0g + m_0a = 2ma$

$m_0(g + a) = 2ma$

$$m_0 = \frac{2ma}{a+g}$$

69. **(c) :** As all blocks are moving with constant speed, therefore, acceleration is zero. So net force on each block is zero.

70. **(c) :** Here, Mass of a person, $m =$ 60 kg

Mass of lift, = 940 kg,

$a = 1 \text{ m/s}^2, g = 10 \text{ m/s}^2$

Let T be the tension in the supporting cable.

$\therefore T - (M + m)g = (M + m)a$

$T = (M + m)(a + g)$

$= (940 + 60)(1 + 10)$

$= 11000$ N

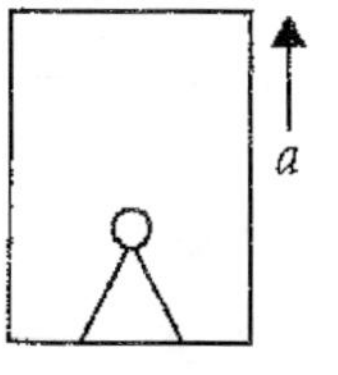

71. **(a) :** $F - Mg = Ma$

$8000 = 2000a$

$\therefore$ Acceleration is

4 m s^{-2} upwards.

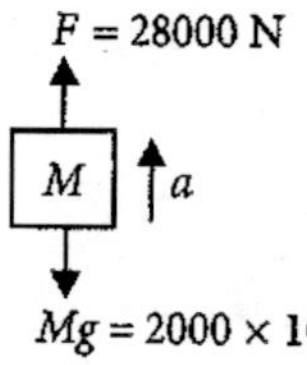

72. **(d)** : The wedge is given an acceleration to the left.

∴ The block has a pseudo acceleration to the right, pressing against the wedge because of which the block is not moving.

∴ $mg\sin\theta = ma\cos\theta$

or $a = \frac{g\sin\theta}{\cos\theta}$

Total reaction of the wedge on the block is $N = mg\cos\theta + ma\sin\theta$

or $N = mg\cos\theta + \frac{mg\sin\theta \cdot \sin\theta}{\cos\theta}$

or $N = \frac{mg(\cos^2\theta + \sin^2\theta)}{\cos\theta} = \frac{mg}{\cos\theta}$.

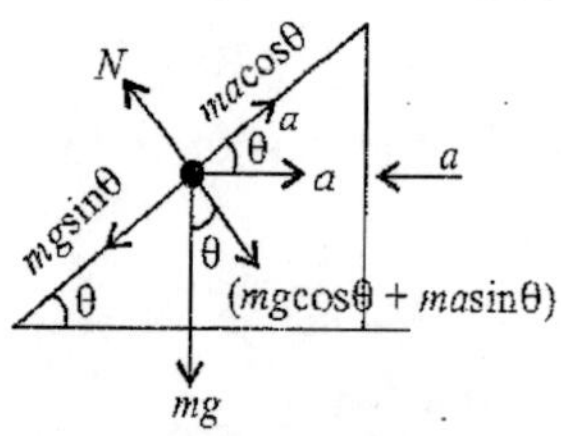

73. **(d)** : When the lift is accelerating upwards with acceleration a, then reading on the scale

$R = m(g + a) = 80(10 + 5)\text{N}$

$= 1200 \text{ N}$

74. **(d)** : Let T be the tension in the rope when monkey climbs up with an acceleration a. Then,

$T - mg = ma$

$$25g - 20g = 20a \Rightarrow a = \frac{5 \times 10}{20}$$

$$= 2.5 \text{ m/s}^2$$

75. **(b)** : For a lift which is moving in upward direction with an acceleration a, the tension T developed in the string connected to the lift is given by $T = m(g + a)$.

Here $m = 1000$ kg, $a = 1 \text{ m/s}^2, g = 9.8 \text{ m/s}^2$

∴ $T = 1000(9.8 + 1) = 10{,}800$ N

76. **(b)** : The force equations are

$T - 5g = 5a$

$10g - T = 10a$

Adding, $10g - 5g = 15a$

or $a = \frac{5g}{15} = \frac{g}{3}$.

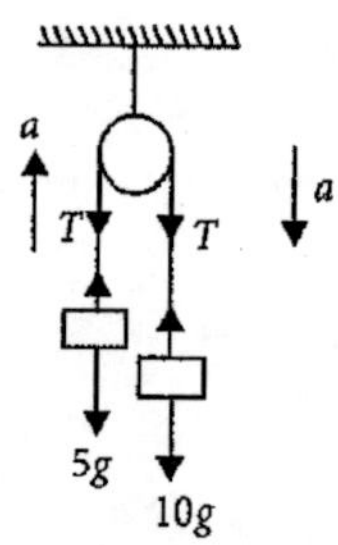

77. **(c)** : Upward acceleration, $ma = T_1 - mg$

$T_1 = m(g + a)$

Downward acceleration, $ma = mg - T_2$

or, $T_2 = m(g - a)$

$$\frac{T_1}{T_2} = \frac{g + a}{g - a} = \frac{9.8 + 4.9}{9.8 - 4.9} = \frac{3}{1}$$

78. **(a)** : The pseudo acceleration for the body $a' = a$

If the pseudo force $Ma\cos\theta = Mg\sin\theta$, then the body will be at rest, $a =$

$g\tan\theta$ This horizontal acceleration should be applied to the wedge to the left.

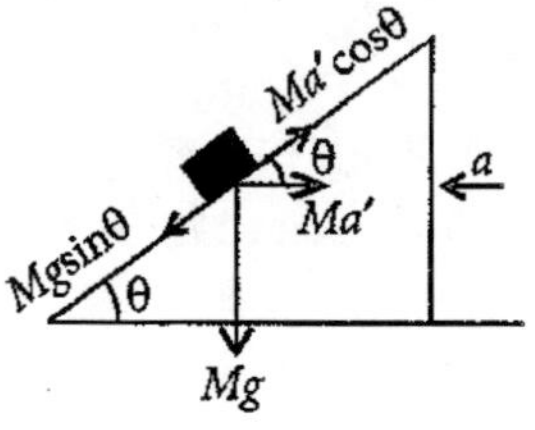

79. **(c) :** Let T be the tension in the branch of a tree when monkey is decending with acceleration a

Thus, $mg - T = ma$

also, $T = 75\%$ of weight of monkey

$T = \left(\frac{75}{100}\right)mg = \frac{3}{4}mg$

$\therefore ma = mg - \left(\frac{3}{4}\right)mg = \frac{1}{4}mg$ or $a = \frac{g}{4}$

Chapter: 5

WORK, ENERGY AND POWER

Introduction

1. A particle moves so that its position vector is given by $\vec{r} = \cos\omega t\hat{x} + \sin\omega t\hat{y}$, where ω is a constant. Which of the following is true? **(NEET-I 2016)**
   (a) Velocity is perpendicular to $\vec{r}$ and acceleration is directed towards the origin.
   (b) Velocity is perpendicular to $\vec{r}$ and acceleration is directed away from the origin.
   (c) Velocity and acceleration both are perpendicular to $\vec{r}$.
   (d) Velocity and acceleration both are parallel to $\vec{r}$.

2. If vectors $\vec{A} = \cos\omega t\hat{\imath} + \sin\omega t\hat{\jmath}$ and $\vec{B} = \cos\frac{\omega t}{2}\hat{\imath} + \sin\frac{\omega t}{2}\hat{\jmath}$ are functions of time, then the value of t at which they are orthogonal to each other is **(2015)**
   (a) $t = \frac{\pi}{\omega}$ (b) $t = 0$
   (c) $t = \frac{\pi}{4\omega}$ (d) $t = \frac{\pi}{2\omega}$

3. If a vector $2\hat{\imath} + 3\hat{\jmath} + 8\hat{k}$ is perpendicular to the vector $4\hat{\jmath} - 4\hat{\imath} + \alpha\hat{k}$, then the value of α is **(2005)**
   (a) ½ (b) $-1/2$
   (c) 1 (d) -1

4. The vector sum of two forces is perpendicular to their vector differences. In that case, the forces **(2003)**
   (a) are equal to each other
   (b) are equal to each other in magnitude
   (c) are not equal to each other in magnitude
   (d) cannot be predicted.

5. The position vector of a particle is $\vec{r} = (a\cos\omega t)\hat{\imath} + (a\sin\omega t)\hat{\jmath}$. The velocity of the particle is **(1995)**
   (a) directed towards the origin
   (b) directed away from the origin
   (c) parallel to the position vector
   (d) perpendicular to the position vector.

6. The angle between the two vectors $\vec{A} = 3\hat{\imath} + 4\hat{\jmath} + 5\hat{k}$ and $\vec{B} = 3\hat{\imath} + 4\hat{\jmath} - 5\hat{k}$ will be **(1994)**
   (a) 90° (b) 180°
   (c) zero (d) 45°

Notions of Work and Kinetic Energy: The Work-Energy Theorem

7. Consider a drop of rain water having mass 1 g falling from a height of 1 km. It hits the ground with a speed of $50\ \text{m s}^{-1}$. Take g constant with a value $10\ \text{m s}^{-2}$. The work done by the (i)

gravitational force and the (ii) resistive force of air is **(2017)**

(a) (i) 1.25 J (ii) −8.25 J

(b) (i) 100 J (ii) 8.75 J

(c) (i) 10 J (ii) −8.75 J

(d) (i) −10 J (ii) −8.25 J

8. A particle of mass 10 g moves along a circle of radius 6.4 cm with a constant tangential acceleration. What is the magnitude of this acceleration if the kinetic energy of the particle becomes equal to 8×10^{-4} J by the end of the second revolution after the beginning of the motion? **(NEET-I 2016)**

(a) $0.18\ m/s^2$ (b) $0.2\ m/s^2$

(c) $0.1\ m/s^2$ (d) $0.15\ m/s^2$

9. A bullet of mass 10 g leaves a rifle at an initial velocity of 1000 m/s and strikes the earth at the same level with a velocity of 500 m/s. The work done in joule for overcoming the resistance of air will be **(1989)**

(a) 375 (b) 3750

(c) 5000 (d) 500

10. A particle moves from a point $(-2\hat{i} + 5\hat{j})$ to $(4\hat{j} + 3\hat{k})$ when a force of $(4\hat{i} + 3\hat{j})$N is applied. How much work has been done by the force?

(NEET-II 2016)

(a) 8 J (b) 11 J (c) 5 J (d) 2 J

11. A uniform force of $(3\hat{i} + \hat{j})$ newton acts on a particle of mass 2 kg. Hence the particle is displaced from position $(2\hat{i} + \hat{k})$ metre to position $(4\hat{i} + 3\hat{j} - \hat{k})$ metre. The work done by the force on the particle is **(2013)**

(a) 13 J (b) 15 J

(c) 9 J (d) 6 J

12. A body moves a distance of 10 m along a straight line under the action of a 5 N force. If the work done is 25 J, then angle between the force and direction of motion of the body is **(1997)**

(a) 60° (b) 75°

(c) 30° (d) 45°

13. A body, constrained to move in *y*-direction, is subjected to a force given by $\vec{F} = (-2\hat{i} + 15\hat{j} + 6\hat{k})$N. The work done by this force in moving the body through a distance of $10\hat{j}$ m along *y*-axis, is **(1994)**

(a) 150 J (b) 20 J

(c) 190 J (d) 160 J

14. When a body moves with a constant speed along a circle **(1994)**

(a) no work is done on it

(b) no acceleration is produced in it

(c) its velocity remains constant

(d) no force acts on it.

Kinetic Energy

15. A particle of mass 5 m at rest suddenly breaks on its own into three fragments. Two fragments of mass *m* each move along mutually perpendicular direction with speed *v* each. The energy released during the process is **(Odisha NEET 2019)**

(a) $\frac{3}{5}mv^2$ (b) $\frac{5}{3}mv^2$

(c) $\frac{3}{2}mv^2$ (d) $\frac{4}{3}mv^2$

16. A body of mass $(4m)$ is lying in $x-y$ plane at rest. It suddenly explodes into three pieces. Two pieces, each of mass (m) move perpendicular to each other with equal speeds (v). The total kinetic energy generated due to explosion is **(2014)**

(a) mv^2 (b) $\frac{3}{2}mv^2$

(c) $2mv^2$ (d) $4mv^2$

17. An engine pumps water continuously through a hose. Water leaves the hose with a velocity v and m is the mass per unit length of the water jet. What is the rate at which kinetic energy is imparted to water? **(2009)**

(a) mv^3 (b) $\frac{1}{2}mv^2$

(c) $\frac{1}{2}m^2v^2$ (d) $\frac{1}{2}mv^3$

18. A shell of mass 200gm is ejected from a gun of mass 4 kg by an explosion that generates 1.05 kJ of energy. The initial velocity of the shell is **(2008)**

(a) $40\ m\ s^{-1}$ (b) $120\ m\ s^{-1}$

(c) $100\ m\ s^{-1}$ (d) $80\ m\ s^{-1}$

19. A bomb of mass 30 kg at rest explodes into two pieces of masses 18 kg and 12 kg. The velocity of 18 kg mass is $6\ m\ s^{-1}$. The kinetic energy of the other mass is **(2005)**

(a) 324 J (b) 486 J

(c) 256 J (d) 524 J

20. A particle of mass m_1 is moving with a velocity v_1 and another particle of mass m_2 is moving with a velocity v_2. Both of them have the same momentum but their different kinetic energies are E_1 and E_2 respectively. If $m_1 > m_2$ then **(2004)**

(a) $E_1 < E_2$ (b) $\frac{E_1}{E_2} = \frac{m_1}{m_2}$

(c) $E_1 > -E_2$ (d) $E_1 = E_2$

21. A ball of mass 2 kg and another of mass 4 kg are dropped together from a 60 feet tall building. After a fall of 30 feet each towards earth, their respective kinetic energies will be in the ratio of **(2004)**

(a) $\sqrt{2}:1$ (b) $1:4$

(c) $1:2$ (d) $1:\sqrt{2}$

22. A stationary particle explodes into two particles of masses m_1 and m_2 which move in opposite directions with velocities v_1 and v_2. The ratio of their kinetic energies E_1/E_2 is **(2003)**

(a) m_2/m_1 (b) m_1/m_2

(c) 1 (d) m_1v_2/m_2v_1

23. If kinetic energy of a body is increased by 300% then percentage change in momentum will be **(2002)**

(a) 100% (b) 150%

(c) 265% (d) 73.2%.

24. A particle is projected making an angle of 45° with horizontal having kinetic energy K. The kinetic energy at highest point will be **(2001, 1997)**

(a) $\frac{K}{\sqrt{2}}$ (b) $\frac{K}{2}$

(c) $2K$ (d) K

25. Two bodies with kinetic energies in the ratio of $4:1$ are moving with equal linear momentum. The ratio of their masses is **(1999)**

(a) $4:1$ (b) $1:1$

(c) $1:2$ (d) $1:4$.

26. Two bodies of masses m and $4m$ are moving with equal kinetic energies. The ratio of their linear momenta is **(1998,1997,1989)**

(a) $1:2$ (b) $1:4$

(c) $4:1$ (d) $1:1$

27. The kinetic energy acquired by a mass m in travelling distance d, starting from rest, under the action of a constant force is directly proportional to **(1994)**

(a) m (b) m^0

(c) $\sqrt{m}$ (d) $1/\sqrt{m}$

28. Two masses of 1 g and 9 g are moving with equal kinetic energies. The ratio of the magnitudes of their respective linear momenta is **(1993)**

(a) $1:9$ (b) $9:1$

(c) $1:3$ (d) $3:1$

29. A particle of mass M is moving in a horizontal circle of radius R with uniform speed v. When it moves from one point to a diametrically opposite point, its **(1992)**

(a) kinetic energy change by $Mv^2/4$

(b) momentum does not change

(c) momentum change by $2Mv$

(d) kinetic energy changes by Mv^2

Work done by a Variable Force

30. A force $F = 20 + 10y$ acts on a particle in y-direction where F is in newton and y in meter. Work done by this force to move the particle from $y = 0$ to $y = 1$ m is **(2019)**

(a) 20 J (b) 30 J

(c) 5 J (d) 25 J

31. Force F on a particle moving in a straight line varies with distance d as shown in figure. The work done on the particle during its displacement of 12 m is **(2011)**

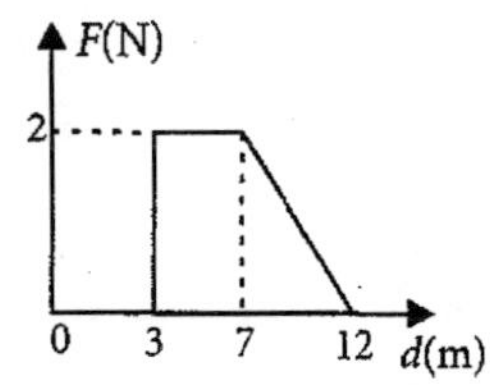

(a) 18 J (b) 21 J

(c) 26 J (d) 13 J

32. A body of mass 3 kg is under a constant force which causes a displacement s in metres in it, given by the relation $s = \frac{1}{3}t^2$, where t is in seconds. Work done by the force in 2 seconds is **(2006)**

(a) $\frac{19}{5}$ J (b) $\frac{5}{19}$ J

(c) $\frac{3}{8}$ J (d) $\frac{8}{3}$ J

33. A force F acting on an object varies with distance x as shown here. The force is in N and x in m. The work done by the force in moving the object from $x = 0$ to $x = 6$ m is **(2005)**

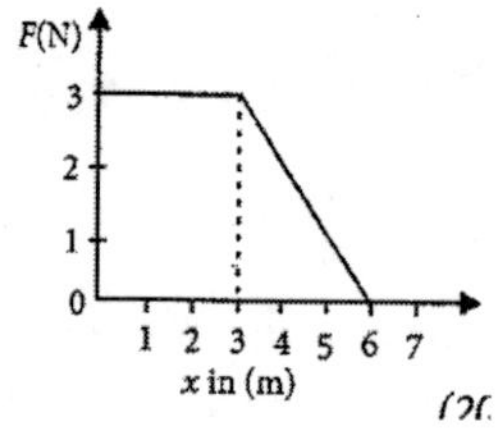

(a) 18.0 J (b) 13.5 J
(c) 9.0 J (d) 4.5 J.

34. A force acts on a 3 g particle in such a way that the position of the particle as a function of time is given by $x = 3t - 4t^2 + t^3$, where x is in metres and t is in seconds. The work done during the first 4 second is **(1998)**

(a) 490 mJ (b) 450 mJ
(c) 240 mJ (d) 530 mJ

35. A position dependent force, $F = (7 - 2x + 3x^2)$N acts on a small body of mass 2 kg and displaces it from $x = 0$ to $x = 5$ m. The work done in joule is **(1994,1992)**

(a) 135 (b) 270
(c) 35 (d) 70

The Concept of Potential Energy

36. The potential energy of a particle in a force field is $U = \frac{A}{r^2} - \frac{B}{r}$ where A and B are positive constants and r is the distance of the particle from the centre of the field. For stable equilibrium, the distance of the particle is **(2012)**

(a) $\frac{B}{2A}$ (b) $\frac{2A}{B}$
(c) $\frac{A}{B}$ (d) $\frac{B}{A}$

37. The potential energy of a system increases if work is done **(2011)**

(a) upon the system by a nonconservative force
(b) by the system against a conservative force
(c) by the system against a nonconservative force
(d) upon the system by a conservative force.

38. The potential energy between two atoms, in a molecule, is given by $U(x) = \frac{a}{x^{12}} - \frac{b}{x^6}$ where a and b are positive constants and x is the distance between the atoms. The atom is in stable equilibrium, when **(1995)**

(a) $x = \left(\frac{2a}{b}\right)^{1/6}$ (b) $x = \left(\frac{11a}{5b}\right)^{1/6}$
(c) $x = 0$ (d) $x = \left(\frac{a}{2b}\right)^{1/6}$

The Conservation of Mechanical Energy

39. A particle is released from height S from the surface of the Earth. At a certain height its kinetic energy is three times its potential energy. The height from the surface of earth and the speed of the particle at that instant are respectively **(2021)**

(a) $\frac{S}{4}, \sqrt{\frac{3gS}{2}}$ (b) $\frac{S}{4}, \frac{3gS}{2}$

(c) $\frac{S}{4}, \frac{\sqrt{3gS}}{2}$ (d) $\frac{S}{2}, \frac{\sqrt{3gS}}{2}$

40. A mass m is attached to a thin wire and whirled in a vertical circle. The wire is most likely to break when **(2019)**

(a) inclined at an angle of 60° from vertical

(b) the mass is at the highest point

(c) the wire is horizontal

(d) the mass is at the lowest point

41. A body initially at rest and sliding along a frictionless track from a height h (as shown in the figure) just completes a vertical circle of

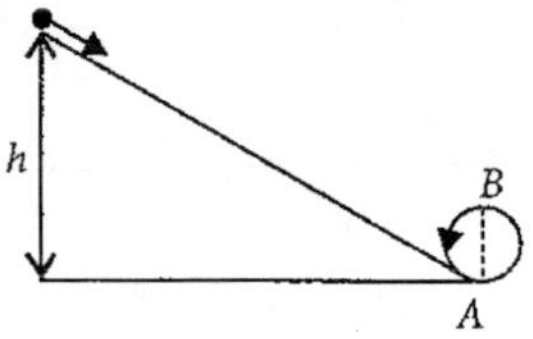

diameter $AB = D$. The height h is equal to **(2018)**

(a) $\frac{3}{2}D$ (b) D

(c) $\frac{7}{5}D$ (d) $\frac{5}{4}D$

42. What is the minimum velocity with which a body of mass m must enter a vertical loop of radius R so that it can complete the loop? **(NEET-I 2016)**

(a) $\sqrt{3gR}$ (b) $\sqrt{5gR}$

(c) $\sqrt{gR}$ (d) $\sqrt{2gR}$

43. A particle with total energy E is moving in a potential energy region $U(x)$. Motion of the particle is restricted to the region when

(Karnataka NEET 2013)

(a) $U(x) < E$ (b) $U(x) = 0$

(c) $U(x) \le E$ (d) $U(x) > E$

44. A stone is tied to a string of length l and is whirled in a vertical circle with the other end of the string as the centre. At a certain instant of time, the stone is at its lowest position and has a speed u. The magnitude of the change in velocity as it reaches a position where the string is horizontal (g being acceleration due to gravity) is **(2003)**

(a) $\sqrt{2(u^2 - gl)}$ (b) $\sqrt{u^2 - gl}$

(c) $u - \sqrt{u^2 - 2gl}$ (d) $\sqrt{2gl}$

45. A child is sitting on a swing. Its minimum and maximum heights from the ground 0.75 m and 2 m respectively, its maximum speed will be **(2001)**

(a) 10 m/s (b) 5 m/s

(c) 8 m/s (d) 15 m/s

46. As shown in the figure, a mass is performing vertical circular motion. The average velocity of the particle is increased, then at which point will the string break? **(2000)**

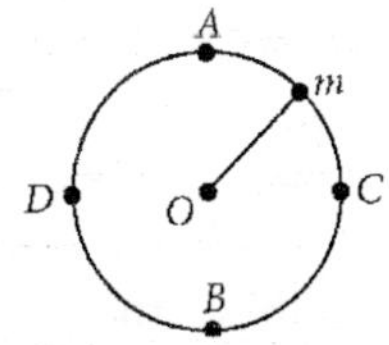

(a) A (b) B

(c) C (d) D

The Potential Energy of a Spring

47. The potential energy of a long spring when stretched by 2 cm is U. If the spring is stretched by 8 cm, potential energy stored in it will be **(2023)**

(a) 4 U (b) 8 U

(c) 16 U (d) 2 U

48. Two similar springs P and Q have spring constants K_P and K_Q, such that $K_P > K_Q$. They are stretched first by the same amount (case a), then by the same force (case b). The work done by the springs W_P and W_Q are related as, in case (a) and case (b) respectively **(2015 Cancelled)**

(a) $W_P > W_Q; W_Q > W_P$

(b) $W_P < W_Q; W_Q < W_P$

(c) $W_P = W_Q; W_P > W_Q$

(d) $W_P = W_Q; W_P = W_Q$

49. A block of mass M is attached to the lower end of a vertical spring. The spring is hung from a ceiling and has force constant value k. The mass is released from rest with the spring initially unstretched. The maximum extension produced in the length of the spring will be **(2009)**

(a) $2Mg/k$ (b) $4Mg/k$

(c) $Mg/2k$ (d) Mg/k

50. A vertical spring with force constant k is fixed on a table. A ball of mass m at a height h above the free upper end of the spring falls vertically on the spring so that the spring is compressed by a distance d. The net work done in the process is **(2007)**

(a) $mg(h+d) - \frac{1}{2}kd^2$

(b) $mg(h-d) - \frac{1}{2}kd^2$

(c) $mg(h-d) + \frac{1}{2}kd^2$

(d) $mg(h+d) + \frac{1}{2}kd^2$

51. The potential energy of a long spring when stretched by 2 cm is U. If the spring is stretched by 8 cm the potential energy stored in it is **(2006)**

(a) $U/4$ (b) $4U$

(c) $8U$ (d) $16U$

52. A mass of 0.5 kg moving with a speed of 1.5 m/s on a horizontal smooth surface, collides with a nearly weightless spring of force constant = 50 N/m. The maximum compression of the spring would be **(2004)**

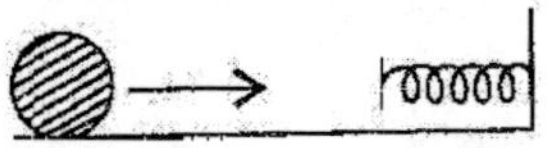

(a) 0.15 m (b) 0.12 m

(c) 1.5 m (d) 0.5 m

53. When a long spring is stretched by 2 cm, its potential energy is U. If the spring is stretched by 10 cm, the potential energy stored in it will be **(2003)**

(a) $\frac{U}{5}$ (b) $5U$

(c) $10U$ (d) 25U

54. Two springs A and B having spring constant K_A and $K_B (K_A = 2K_B)$ are stretched by applying force of equal magnitude. If energy stored in spring A is E_A then energy stored in B will be **(2001)**

(a) $2E_A$ (b) $\frac{E_A}{4}$

(c) $E_A/2$ (d) $4E_A$

Various Forms of Energy: The Law of Conservation of Energy

55. A body of mass 1 kg is thrown upwards with a velocity 20 m/s. It momentarily comes to rest after attaining a height of 18 m. How much energy is lost due to air friction? ($g = 10\ m/s^2$) **(2009)**

(a) 30 J (b) 40 J

(c) 10 J (d) 20 J

56. 300 J of work is done in sliding a 2 kg block up an inclined plane of height 10 m. Work done against friction is (Take $g = 10\ m/s^2$) **(2006)**

(a) 1000 J (b) 200 J

(c) 100 J (d) zero.

Power

57. An electric lift with a maximum load of 2000 kg (lift + passengers) is moving up with a constant speed of $1.5\ m\ s^{-1}$. The frictional force opposing the motion is 3000 N. The minimum power delivered by the motor to the lift in watts is ($g = 10\ m\ s^{-2}$) **(2022)**

(a) 23000 (b) 20000

(c) 34500 (d) 23500

58. Water falls from a height of 60 m at the rate of 15 kg/s to operate a turbine. The losses due to frictional force are 10% of the input energy. How much power is generated by the turbine? ($g = 10\ m/s^2$) **(2021)**

(a) 7.0 kW (b) 10.2 kW

(c) 8.1 kW (d) 12.3 kW

59. A body of mass 1 kg begins to move under the action of a time dependent force $\vec{F} = (2t\hat{\imath} + 3t^2\hat{\jmath})N$, where $\hat{\imath}$ and $\hat{\jmath}$ are unit vectors along x and y axis. What power will be developed by the force at the time ? **(NEET-I 2016)**

(a) $(2t^3 + 3t^4)W$

(b) $(2t^3 + 3t^5)W$

(c) $(2t^2 + 3t^3)W$

(d) $(2t^2 + 4t^4)W$

60. The heart of a man pumps 5 litres of blood through the arteries per minute at a pressure of 150 mm of mercury. If the density of mercury be $13.6 \times 10^3\ kg/m^3$ and $g = 10\ m/s^2$ then the power (in watt) is **(2015)**

(a) 3.0 (b) 1.50

(c) 1.70 (d) 2.35

61. A particle of mass m is driven by a machine that delivers a constant power k watts. If the particle starts from rest, the force on the particle at time t is **(2015 Cancelled)**

(a) $\sqrt{2mk}t^{-1/2}$ (b) $\frac{1}{2}\sqrt{mk}t^{-1/2}$

(c) $\sqrt{\frac{mk}{2}}t^{-1/2}$ (d) $\sqrt{mk}t^{-1/2}$

62. One coolie takes 1 minute to raise a suitcase through a height of 2 m but the second coolie takes 30 s to raise the same suitcase to the same height.

The powers of two coolies are in the ratio **(Karnataka NEET 2013)**

(a) 1: 3 (b) 2: 1

(c) 3: 1 (d) 1: 2

63. A car of mass m starts from rest and accelerates so that the instantaneous power delivered to the car has a constant magnitude P_0. The instantaneous velocity of this car is proportional to **(Mains 2012)**

(a) t^2P_0 (b) $t^{\frac{1}{2}}$

(c) $t^{-1/2}$ (d) $\frac{t}{\sqrt{m}}$

64. A body projected vertically from the earth reaches a height equal to earth's radius before returning to the earth. The power exerted by the gravitational force is greatest **(2011)**

(a) at the highest position of the body

(b) at the instant just before the body hits the earth

(c) it remains constant all through

(d) at the instant just after the body is projected

65. An engine pumps water through a hose pipe. Water passes through the pipe and leaves it with a velocity of 2 m/s. The mass per unit length of water in the pipe is 100 kg/m. What is the power of the engine? **(2010)**

(a) 400 W (b) 200 W

(c) 100 W (d) 800 W

66. A particle of mass M, starting from rest, undergoes uniform acceleration. If the speed acquired in time T is V, the power delivered to the particle is **(Mains 2010)**

(a) $\frac{MV^2}{T}$ (b) $\frac{1}{2}\frac{MV^2}{T^2}$

(c) $\frac{MV^2}{T^2}$ (d) $\frac{1}{2}\frac{MV^2}{T}$

67. Water falls from a height of 60 m at the rate of 15 kg/s to operate a turbine. The losses due to frictional forces are 10% of energy. How much power is generated by the turbine ? ($g = 10\ \text{m/s}^2$) **(2008)**

(a) 12.3 kW (b) 7.0 kW

(c) 8.1 kW (d) 10.2 kW

68. If $\vec{F} = (60\hat{\imath} + 15\hat{\jmath} - 3\hat{k})\text{N}$ and $\vec{v} = (2\hat{\imath} - 4\hat{\jmath} + 5\hat{k})\text{m/s}$, then instantaneous power is **(2000)**

(a) 195 watt (b) 45 watt

(c) 75 watt (d) 100 watt

69. How much water a pump of 2 kW can raise in one minute to a height of 10 m? (take $g = 10\ \text{m/s}^2$) **(1990)**

(a) 1000 liters (b) 1200 liters

(c) 100 liters (d) 2000 liters

Collisions

70. Body A of mass $4m$ moving with speed u collides with another body B of mass $2m$, at rest. The collision is head on and elastic in nature. After the collision the fraction of energy lost by the colliding body A is **(2019)**

(a) 5/9 (b) 1/9

(c) 8/9 (d) 4/9

71. A moving block having mass m, collides with another stationary block having mass 4 m. The lighter block comes to rest after collision. When the initial velocity of the lighter block is v, then the value of coefficient of restitution (e) will be **(2018)**

(a) 0.5 (b) 0.25

(c) 0.8 (d) 0.4

72. A bullet of mass 10 g moving horizontally with a velocity of 400 m s^{-1} strikes a wooden block of mass 2 kg which is suspended by light inextensible string of length 5 m. As a result, the centre of gravity of the block is found to rise a vertical distance of 10 cm. The speed of the bullet after it emerges out horizontally from the block will be **(NEET-II 2016)**

(a) 100 m s^{-1} (b) 80 m s^{-1}

(c) 120 m s^{-1} (d) 160 m s^{-1}

73. Two identical balls A and B having velocities of 0.5 m s^{-1} and -0.3 m s^{-1} respectively collide elastically in one dimension. The velocities of B and A after the collision respectively will be **(NEET-II 2016, 1994, 1991)**

(a) -0.5 m s^{-1} and 0.3 m s^{-1}

(b) 0.5 m s^{-1} and -0.3 m s^{-1}

(c) -0.3 m s^{-1} and 0.5 m s^{-1}

(d) 0.3 m s^{-1} and 0.5 m s^{-1}

74. Two particles A and B, move with constant velocities $\vec{v}_1$ and $\vec{v}_2$. At the initial moment their position vectors are $\vec{r}_1$ and $\vec{r}_2$ respectively. The condition for particles A and B for their collision is **(2015)**

(a) $\vec{r}_1 \times \vec{v}_1 = \vec{r}_2 \times \vec{v}_2$

(b) $\vec{r}_1 - \vec{r}_2 = \vec{v}_1 - \vec{v}_2$

(c) $\frac{\vec{r}_1-\vec{r}_2}{|\vec{r}_1-\vec{r}_2|} = \frac{\vec{v}_2-\vec{v}_1}{|\vec{v}_2-\vec{v}_1|}$

(d) $\vec{r}_1 \cdot \vec{v}_1 = \vec{r}_2 \cdot \vec{v}_2$

75. A ball is thrown vertically downwards from a height of 20 m with an initial velocity v_0. It collides with the ground, loses 50 percent of its energy in collision and rebounds to the same height. The initial velocity v_0 is (Take $g = 10 \text{ m s}^{-2}$) **(2015)**

(a) 28 m s^{-1} (b) 10 m s^{-1}

(c) 14 m s^{-1} (d) 20 m s^{-1}

76. On a frictionless surface, a block of mass M moving at speed v collides elastically with another block of same mass M which is initially at rest. After collision the first block moves at an angle θ to its initial direction and has a speed $v/3$. The second block's speed after the collision is **(2015)**

(a) $\frac{3}{\sqrt{2}}v$ (b) $\frac{\sqrt{3}}{2}v$

(c) $\frac{2\sqrt{2}}{3}v$ (d) $\frac{3}{4}v$

77. Two particles of masses m_1, m_2 move with initial velocities u_1 and u_2. On collision, one of the particles get excited to higher level, after absorbing energy ε. If final velocities of particles be v_1 and v_2 then we must have **(2015 Cancelled)**

(a) $\frac{1}{2}m_1u_1^2 + \frac{1}{2}m_2u_2^2 - \varepsilon = \frac{1}{2}m_1v_1^2 + \frac{1}{2}m_2v_2^2$

(b) $\frac{1}{2}m_1^2u_1^2 + \frac{1}{2}m_2^2u_2^2 + \varepsilon = \frac{1}{2}m_1^2v_1^2 + \frac{1}{2}m_2^2v_2^2$

(c) $m_1^2u_1 + m_2^2u_2 - \varepsilon = m_1^2v_1 + m_2^2v_2$

(d) $\frac{1}{2}m_1u_1^2 + \frac{1}{2}m_2u_2^2 = \frac{1}{2}m_1v_1^2 + \frac{1}{2}m_2v_2^2 - \varepsilon$

78. Two spheres A and B of masses m_1 and m_2 respectively collide. A is at rest initially and B is moving with velocity v along x-axis. After collision B has a velocity $\frac{v}{2}$ in a direction perpendicular to the original direction. The mass A moves after collision in the direction **(2012)**

(a) same as that of B

(b) opposite to that of B

(c) $\theta = \tan^{-1}\left(\frac{1}{2}\right)$ to the x-axis

(d) $\theta = \tan^{-1}\left(-\frac{1}{2}\right)$ to the x-axis

79. A mass m moving horizontally (along the x-axis) with velocity v collides and sticks to a mass of $3m$ moving vertically upward (along the y-axis) with velocity $2v$. The final velocity of the combination is **(Mains 2011)**

(a) $\frac{3}{2}v\hat{i} + \frac{1}{4}v\hat{j}$ (b) $\frac{1}{4}v\hat{i} + \frac{3}{2}v\hat{j}$

(c) $\frac{1}{3}v\hat{i} + \frac{2}{3}v\hat{j}$ (d) $\frac{2}{3}v\hat{i} + \frac{1}{3}v\hat{j}$

80. A ball moving with velocity 2 m/s collides head on with another stationary ball of double the mass. If the coefficient of restitution is 0.5 , then their velocities (in m/s) after collision will be **(2010)**

(a) 0,1 (b) 1,1

(c) 1,0.5 (d) 0,2

81. Two equal masses m_1 and m_2 moving along the same straight line with velocities +3 m/s and −5 m/s respectively collide elastically. Their velocities after the collision will be respectively **(1998)**

(a) −4 m/s and +4 m/s

(b) +4 m/s for both

(c) −3 m/s and +5 m/s

(d) −5 m/s and +3 m/s.

82. A rubber ball is dropped from a height of 5 m on a plane. On bouncing it rises to 1.8 m. The ball loses its velocity on bouncing by a factor of **(1998)**

(a) $\frac{3}{5}$ (b) $\frac{2}{5}$

(c) $\frac{16}{25}$ (d) $\frac{9}{25}$

83. A metal ball of mass 2 kg moving with speed of 36 km/h has a head on collision with a stationary ball of mass 3 kg. If after collision, both the balls move as a single mass, then the loss in K.E. due to collision is **(1997)**

(a) 100 J (b) 140 J

(c) 40*J* (d) 60 J.

84. A moving body of mass m and velocity 3 km/ hour collides with a body at rest of mass $2m$ and sticks to it. Now the combined mass starts to move. What will be the combined velocity? **(1996)**

(a) 3 km/ hour (b) 4 km/ hour

(c) 1 km/ hour (d) 2 km/ hour

85. The coefficient of restitution e for a perfectly elastic collision is **(1988)**

(a) 1 (b) 0

(c) ∞ (d) -1

ANSWER KEY

1.	(a)	2.	(a)	3.	(b)	4.	(b)	5.	(d)	6.	(a)
7.	(c)	8.	(c)	9.	(b)	10.	(c)	11.	(c)	12.	(a)
13.	(a)	14.	(a)	15.	(d)	16.	(b)	17.	(d)	18.	(c)
19.	(b)	20.	(a)	21.	(c)	22.	(a)	23.	(a)	24.	(b)
25.	(d)	26.	(a)	27.	(b)	28.	(c)	29.	(c)	30.	(d)
31.	(d)	32.	(d)	33.	(b)	34.	(d)	35.	(a)	36.	(b)
37.	(b)	38.	(a)	39.	(a)	40.	(d)	41.	(d)	42.	(b)
43.	(c)	44.	(a)	45.	(b)	46.	(b)	47.	(c)	48.	(a)
49.	(a)	50.	(a)	51.	(d)	52.	(a)	53.	(d)	54.	(a)
55.	(d)	56.	(c)	57.	(c)	58.	(c)	59.	(b)	60.	(c)
61.	(c)	62.	(d)	63.	(b)	64.	(b)	65.	(d)	66.	(d)
67.	(c)	68.	(b)	69.	(b)	70.	(c)	71.	(b)	72.	(c)
73.	(b)	74.	(c)	75.	(d)	76.	(c)	77.	(a)	78.	(d)
79.	(b)	80.	(a)	81.	(d)	82.	(a)	83.	(d)	84.	(c)
85.	(a)										

Hints & Explanations

1. **(a) :** Given, $\vec{r} = \cos\omega t\hat{x} + \sin\omega t\hat{y}$

$$\therefore\ \vec{v} = \frac{d\vec{r}}{dt} = -\omega\sin\omega t\hat{x} + \omega\cos\omega t\hat{y}$$

$$\vec{a} = \frac{d\vec{v}}{dt} = -\omega^2\cos\omega t\hat{x} - \omega^2\sin\omega t\hat{y}$$

$$= -\omega^2\vec{r}$$

Since position vector $(\vec{r})$ is directed away from the origin, so, acceleration $(-\omega^2\vec{r})$ is directed towards the origin.

Also,

$$\vec{r}\cdot\vec{v} = (\cos\omega t\hat{x} + \sin\omega t\hat{y})\cdot(-\omega\sin\omega t\hat{x} + \omega\cos\omega t\hat{y})$$

$$= -\omega\sin\omega t\cos\omega t + \omega\sin\omega t\cos\omega t = 0$$

$$\Rightarrow \vec{r}\perp\vec{v}$$

2. **(a) :** Two vectors $\vec{A}$ and $\vec{B}$ are orthogonal to each other, if their scalar product is zero i.e. $\vec{A}\cdot\vec{B} = 0$

Here, $\vec{A} = \cos\omega t\hat{\imath} + \sin\omega t\hat{\jmath}$

and $\vec{B} = \cos\frac{\omega t}{2}\hat{\imath} + \sin\frac{\omega t}{2}\hat{\jmath}$

$$\therefore\ \vec{A}\cdot\vec{B} = (\cos\omega t\hat{\imath} + \sin\omega t\hat{\jmath})\cdot\left(\cos\frac{\omega t}{2}\hat{\imath} + \sin\frac{\omega t}{2}\hat{\jmath}\right)$$

$$= \cos\omega t\cos\frac{\omega t}{2} + \sin\omega t\sin\frac{\omega t}{2}$$

$$= \cos\left(\omega t - \frac{\omega t}{2}\right)$$

But $\vec{A}\cdot\vec{B} = 0$ (as $\vec{A}$ and $\vec{B}$ are orthogonal to each other)

$\therefore \cos\left(\omega t - \frac{\omega t}{2}\right) = 0$

$\cos\left(\omega t - \frac{\omega t}{2}\right) = \cos\frac{\pi}{2}$ or $\omega t - \frac{\omega t}{2} = \frac{\pi}{2}$

$\frac{\omega t}{2} = \frac{\pi}{2}$ or $t = \frac{\pi}{\omega}$

3. **(b)** : $\vec{a} = 2\hat{\imath} + 3\hat{\jmath} + 8\hat{k}, \vec{b} = 4\hat{\jmath} - 4\hat{\imath} + \alpha\hat{k}$

$\vec{a}\cdot\vec{b} = 0$ if $\vec{a} \perp \vec{b}$

$(2\hat{\imath} + 3\hat{\jmath} + 8\hat{k})\cdot(-4\hat{\imath} + 4\hat{\jmath} + \alpha\hat{k}) = 0$

or, $-8 + 12 + 8\alpha = 0 \Rightarrow 4 + 8\alpha = 0$

$\Rightarrow \alpha = -1/2$.

4. **(b)** : Given: $(\vec{F}_1 + \vec{F}_2) \perp (\vec{F}_1 - \vec{F}_2)$

$\therefore (\vec{F}_1 + \vec{F}_2)\cdot(\vec{F}_1 - \vec{F}_2) = 0$

$F_1^2 - F_2^2 - \vec{F}_1\cdot\vec{F}_2 + \vec{F}_2\cdot\vec{F}_1 = 0 \Rightarrow F_1^2 = F_2^2$

i.e. F_1, F_2 are equal to each other in magnitude.

5. **(d)** : Position vector of the particle

$\vec{r} = (a\cos\omega t)\hat{\imath} + (a\sin\omega t)\hat{\jmath}$

velocity vector

$$\vec{v} = \frac{d\vec{r}}{dt} = (-a\omega\sin\omega t)\hat{\imath} + (a\omega\cos\omega t)\hat{\jmath}$$

$= \omega[(-a\sin\omega t)\hat{\imath} + (a\cos\omega t)\hat{\jmath}]$

$\vec{v}\cdot\vec{r} = \omega a[-\sin\omega t\hat{\imath} + \cos\omega t\hat{\jmath})]$

$\cdot\, [a\cos\omega t\hat{\imath} + a\sin\omega t\hat{\jmath}]$

$= \omega[-a^2\sin\omega t\cos\omega t + a^2\cos\omega t\sin\omega t]$

$= 0$

Therefore velocity vector is perpendicular to the position vector.

6. **(a)** : $\vec{A} = 3\hat{\imath} + 4\hat{\jmath} + 5\hat{k}$ and $\vec{B} = 3\hat{\imath} + 4\hat{\jmath} - 5\hat{k}$

$$\cos\theta = \frac{\vec{A}\cdot\vec{B}}{|\vec{A}||\vec{B}|}$$

$$= \frac{(3\hat{\imath} + 4\hat{\jmath} + 5\hat{k})\cdot(3\hat{\imath} + 4\hat{\jmath} - 5\hat{k})}{\left[\sqrt{(3)^2 + (4)^2 + (5)^2}\right]\times\left[\sqrt{(3)^2 + (4)^2 + (5)^2}\right]}$$

$$= \frac{9 + 16 - 25}{50} = 0 \text{ or } \theta = 90°.$$

7. **(c)** : Here, $m = 1\text{ g} = 10^{-3}\text{ kg}$, $h = 1\text{ km} = 1000\text{ m}, v = 50\text{ m s}^{-1}, g = 10\text{ m s}^{-2}$.

(i) The work done by the gravitational force

$= mgh = 10^{-3} \times 10 \times 1000 = 10\text{ J}$

(ii) The total work done by gravitational force and the resistive force of air is equal to change in kinetic energy of rain drop.

$\therefore \quad W_g + W_r = \frac{1}{2}mv^2 - 0$

$10 + W_r = \frac{1}{2} \times 10^{-3} \times 50 \times 50$

or $\quad W_r = -8.75\text{ J}$

8. **(c)** : Here, $m = 10\text{ g} = 10^{-2}\text{ kg}, R = 6.4\text{ cm} = 6.4 \times 10^{-2}\text{ m}$ $\quad K_f = 8 \times 10^{-4}\text{ J}, K_i = 0, a_t = ?$

Using work energy theorem,

Work done by all the forces = Change in KE

$$W_{\text{tangential force}} + W_{\text{centripetal force}} = K_f - K_i$$

$$\Rightarrow a_t = \frac{K_f}{4\pi Rm} = \frac{8 \times 10^{-4}}{4 \times \frac{22}{7} \times 6.4 \times 10^{-2} \times 10^{-2}}$$

$= 0.099 \approx 0.1 \text{ m s}^{-2}$

9. **(b) :** Work done = change in kinetic energy of the body $W = \frac{1}{2} \times 0.01[(1000)^2 - (500)^2] = 3750$ joule

10. **(c) :** Here $\vec{r}_1 = (-2\hat{\imath} + 5\hat{\jmath})\text{m}, \vec{r}_2 = (4\hat{\jmath} + 3\hat{k})\text{m}$

$\vec{F} = (4\hat{\imath} + 3\hat{\jmath})\text{N}, W = ?$

Work done by force F in moving from $\vec{r}_1$ to $\vec{r}_2$,

$W = \vec{F} \cdot (\vec{r}_2 - \vec{r}_1) \Rightarrow W$

$= (4\hat{\imath} + 3\hat{\jmath}) \cdot (4\hat{\jmath} + 3\hat{k} + 2\hat{\imath} - 5\hat{\jmath})$

$= (4\hat{\imath} + 3\hat{\jmath}) \cdot (2\hat{\imath} - \hat{\jmath} + 3\hat{k}) = 8 + (-3)$

$= 5 \text{ J}$

11. **(c) :** Here, $\vec{F} = (3\hat{\imath} + \hat{\jmath})\text{N}$

Initial position, $\vec{r}_1 = (2\hat{\imath} + \hat{k})\text{m}$

Final position, $\vec{r}_2 = (4\hat{\imath} + 3\hat{\jmath} - \hat{k})\text{m}$

Displacement, $\vec{r} = \vec{r}_2 - \vec{r}_1$

$\vec{r} = (4\hat{\imath} + 3\hat{\jmath} - \hat{k})\text{m} - (2\hat{\imath} + \hat{k})\text{m}$

$= 2\hat{\imath} + 3\hat{\jmath} - 2\hat{k} \text{ m}$

Work done, $W = \vec{F} \cdot \vec{r} = (3\hat{\imath} + \hat{\jmath}) \cdot (2\hat{\imath} + 3\hat{\jmath} - 2\hat{k})$

$= 6 + 3 = 9 \text{ J}$

12. **(a) :** Distance $(s) = 10$ m; Force $(F) = 5$ N and work done $(W) = 25$ J

Work done $(W) = Fs\cos\theta$

$\therefore 25 = 5 \times 10\cos\theta = 50\cos\theta$

or $\cos\theta = 25/50 = 0.5$ or $\theta = 60°$

13. **(a) :** Force $\vec{F} = (-2\hat{\imath} + 15\hat{\jmath} + 6\hat{k})\text{N}$, and distance,

$d = 10\hat{\jmath}$ m

Work done, $W = \vec{F} \cdot \vec{d} = (-2\hat{\imath} + 15\hat{\jmath} + 6\hat{k}) \cdot (10\hat{\jmath})$

$= 150\text{Nm} = 150 \text{ J}$

14. **(a) :** Every resolution give zero displacement

15. **(d) :** Let the speed of the third fragment of mass $3m$ be v'.

From law of conservation of linear momentum,

$3mv' = \sqrt{2}mv \Rightarrow v' = \frac{\sqrt{2}v}{3}$ ...(i)

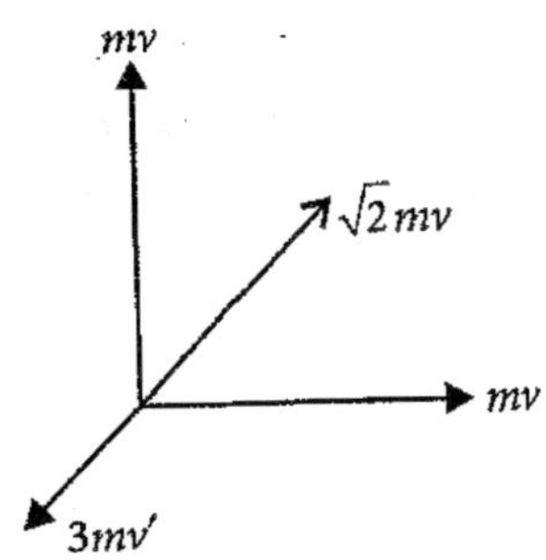

$\therefore$ Energy released during the process is,

$$K.E. = 2\left(\frac{1}{2}mv^2\right) + \frac{1}{2}(3m)v^2$$

$$= mv^2 + \frac{1}{2}(3m)\frac{2v^2}{9}$$

(Using eqn. (i))

$= mv^2 + \frac{mv^2}{3} = \frac{4}{3}mv^2.$

16. **(b) :**

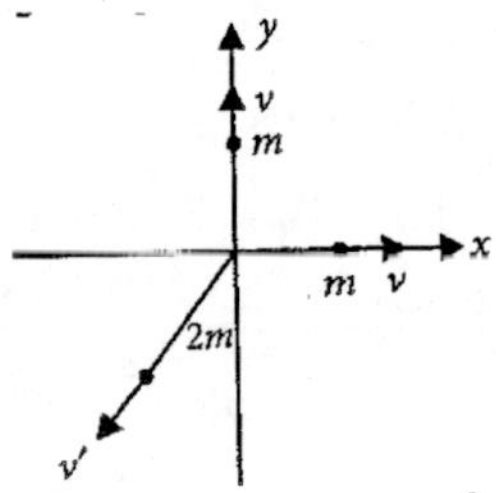

Let $\vec{v}'$ be velocity of third piece of mass 2 m.

Initial momentum, $\vec{p}_i = 0$ (As the body is at rest)

Final momentum, $\vec{p}_f = mv\hat{\imath} + mv\hat{\jmath} + 2m\vec{v}'$

According to law of conservation of momentum

$$\vec{p}_i = \vec{p}_f \text{ or, } 0 = mv\hat{\imath} + mv\hat{\jmath} + 2m\vec{v}' \text{ or, } \vec{v}' = -\frac{v}{2}\hat{\imath} - \frac{v}{2}\hat{\jmath}$$

The magnitude of v' is

$$v' = \sqrt{\left(-\frac{v}{2}\right)^2 + \left(-\frac{v}{2}\right)^2} = \frac{v}{\sqrt{2}}$$

Total kinetic energy generated due to explosion

$$= \frac{1}{2}mv^2 + \frac{1}{2}mv^2 + \frac{1}{2}(2m)v'^2$$

$$= \frac{1}{2}mv^2 + \frac{1}{2}mv^2 + \frac{1}{2}(2m)\left(\frac{v}{\sqrt{2}}\right)^2$$

$$= mv^2 + \frac{mv^2}{2} = \frac{3}{2}mv^2$$

17. **(d) :** Velocity of water is v, mass flowing per unit length is m.

$\therefore$ Mass flowing per second $= mv$

$\therefore$ Rate of kinetic energy or K.E. per second $= \frac{1}{2}(mv)v^2 = \frac{1}{2}mv^3.$

18. **(c) :** $mv = Mv' \Rightarrow v' = \left(\frac{m}{M}\right)v$

Total K.E. of the bullet and gun = $\frac{1}{2}mv^2 + \frac{1}{2}Mv'^2$

Total K.E. $= \frac{1}{2}mv^2 + \frac{1}{2}M \cdot \frac{m^2}{M^2}v^2$

Total K.E. $= \frac{1}{2}mv^2\left\{1 + \frac{m}{M}\right\}$

or $= \left\{\frac{1}{2} \times 0.2\right\}\left\{1 + \frac{0.2}{4}\right\}v^2 = 1.05 \times 1000$ J

$$\Rightarrow v^2 = \frac{4 \times 1.05 \times 1000}{0.1 \times 4.2} = 100^2 \therefore v = 100 \text{ m s}^{-1}$$

19. **(b) :** According to law of conservation of linear momentum,

$30 \times 0 = 18 \times 6 + 12 \times v$

$\Rightarrow -108 = 12v \Rightarrow v = -9$ m/s.

Negative sign indicates that both fragments move in opposite directions.

K.E. of 12 kg $= \frac{1}{2}mv^2 = \frac{1}{2} \times 12 \times 81 =$ 486 J

20. **(a) :** Kinetic energy $= \frac{p^2}{2m}$

$$\therefore \frac{E_1}{E_2} = \frac{p_1^2/2m_1}{p_2^2/2m_2} \Rightarrow \frac{E_1}{E_2} = \frac{m_2}{m_1}$$

or $E_1 < E_2$

[as $m_1 > m_2$]

21. **(c) :** Ratio of their kinetic energy is given as

$$\frac{KE_1}{KE_2} = \frac{(1/2)m_1v_1^2}{(1/2)m_2v_2^2}$$

$v^2 = 2gs$ (zero initial velocity)

which is same for both

$$\therefore \frac{KE_1}{KE_2} = \frac{m_1}{m_2} = \frac{2}{4} = \frac{1}{2}.$$

22. **(a) :** $m_1v_1 = m_2v_2$

$$\frac{E_1}{E_2} = \frac{(1/2)m_1v_1^2}{(1/2)m_2v_2^2} = \frac{m_1^2v_1^2}{m_2^2v_2^2} \cdot \frac{m_2}{m_1} = \frac{m_2}{m_1}$$

23. **(a) :** Let m be the mass of the body and v_1 and v_2 be the initial and final velocities of the body respectively.

$\therefore$ Initial kinetic energy $= \frac{1}{2}mv_1^2$

Final kinetic energy $= \frac{1}{2}mv_2^2$

Initial kinetic energy is increased 300% to get the final kinetic energy.

$$\therefore \frac{1}{2}mv_2^2 = \frac{1}{2}\left(1 + \frac{300}{100}\right)mv_1^2$$

$\Rightarrow v_2 = 2v_1$ or $v_2/v_1 = 2$

Initial momentum $= p_1 = mv_1$

Final momentum $= p_2 = mv_2$

$\therefore \frac{p_2}{p_1} = \frac{mv_2}{mv_1} = \frac{v_2}{v_1} = 2$ or $\therefore p_2 = 2p_1 = \left(1 + \frac{100}{100}\right)p_1$

So momentum has increased 100%.

24. **(b) :** Kinetic energy of the ball $= K$ and angle of projection $(\theta) = 45°$.

Velocity of the ball at the highest point

$= v\cos\theta$

$= v\cos 45° = \frac{v}{\sqrt{2}}$

Therefore kinetic energy of the ball

$$= \frac{1}{2}m \times \left(\frac{v}{\sqrt{2}}\right)^2 = \frac{1}{4}mv^2 = \frac{K}{2}$$

25. **(d) :** K.E. $= \frac{p^2}{2m} \Rightarrow \frac{K.E_1}{K.E_2} = \frac{m_2}{m_1} = \frac{4}{1}$

or $\frac{m_1}{m_2} = \frac{1}{4}$

26. **(a) :** Mass of first body $= m$;

Mass of second body $= 4m$ and $KE_1 = KE_2$.

Linear momentum of a body

$p = \sqrt{2mE} \propto \sqrt{m}$

Therefore $\frac{p_1}{p_2} = \sqrt{\frac{m_1}{m_2}} = \sqrt{\frac{m}{4m}} = \sqrt{\frac{1}{4}} = \frac{1}{2}$

or $p_1 : p_2 = 1 : 2$.

27. **(b) :** $v^2 = u^2 + 2as$ or $v^2 - u^2 = 2as$

or $v^2 - (0)^2 = 2 \times \frac{F}{m} \times s$ or $v^2 = \frac{2Fs}{m}$

and $K.E. = \frac{1}{2}mv^2 = \frac{1}{2}m \times \frac{2Fs}{m} = Fs$.

Thus K.E. is independent of m or directly proportional to m^0.

28. **(c) :** $\frac{K_1}{K_2} = \frac{p_1^2}{p_2^2} \times \frac{M_2^2}{M_1^2}$

Here $K_1 = K_2$

$\therefore \frac{p_1}{p_2} = \sqrt{\frac{M_1}{M_2}} = \sqrt{\frac{1}{9}} = \frac{1}{3}$ or, $p_1 : p_2 = 1:3$

29. **(c)** : On the diametrically opposite points, the velocities have same magnitude but opposite directions. Therefore change in momentum is

$$Mv - (-Mv) = 2Mv$$

30. **(d)** : Given: $F = 20 + 10y$

work done, $W = \int F.dy$

$$= \int_0^1 (20 + 10y)dy = \left[20y + \frac{10}{2}y^2\right]_0^1$$

$$= 20 + \frac{10}{2} = 25 \text{ J}$$

31. **(d)** :

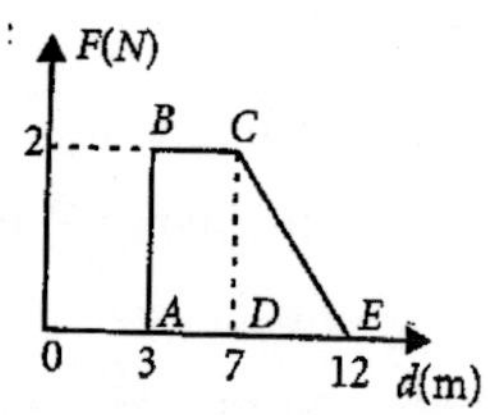

Work done = Area under $(F - d)$ graph

= Area of rectangle $ABCD$ + Area of triangle DCE

$$= 2 \times (7 - 3) + \frac{1}{2} \times 2 \times (12 - 7)$$

$$= 8 + 5 = 13 \text{ J}$$

32. **(d)** : $s = \frac{t^2}{3}; \frac{ds}{dt} = \frac{2t}{3}; \frac{d^2s}{dt^2} = \frac{2}{3}$ m/s^2

Work done, $W = \int Fds = \int m\frac{d^2s}{dt^2}ds$

$$= \int m\frac{d^2s}{dt^2}\frac{ds}{dt}dt = \int_0^2 3 \times \frac{2}{3} \times \frac{2t}{3}dt = \frac{4}{3}\int_0^2 tdt$$

$$= \frac{4}{3}\left|\frac{t^2}{2}\right|_0^2 = \frac{4}{3} \times 2 = \frac{8}{3} \text{ J.}$$

33. **(b)** : Work done = area under $F - x$ curve

= area of trapezium

$$= \frac{1}{2} \times (6 + 3) \times 3 = \frac{9 \times 3}{2} = 13.5 \text{ J}$$

34. **(d)** : $x = 3t - 4t^2 + t^3$

$$V = \frac{dx}{dt} = 3 - 8t + 3t^2$$

$$V_0 = 3 - 8 \times 0 + 3 \times 0^2 = 3 \text{ m/s}$$

$$V_4 = 3 - 8 \times 4 + 3 \times 16 = 19 \text{ m/s}$$

$$W = \frac{1}{2}m(V_4^2 - V_0^2)$$

$$= \frac{1}{2} \times 3 \times 10^{-3}(19^2 - 3^2)$$

$$= 528 \times 10^{-3} \text{ J} \approx 530 \text{ mJ}$$

35. **(a)** : Force $(F) = 7 - 2x + 3x^2$;

Mass $(m) = 2$ kg and displacement $(d) = 5$ m. Therefore work done

$$(W) = \int Fdx = \int_0^5 (7 - 2x + 3x^2)dx$$

$$= [7x - x^2 + x^3]_0^5$$

$$= (7 \times 5) - (5)^2 + (5)^3$$

$$= 35 - 25 + 125$$

$$= 135 \text{ J}$$

36. **(b)** : Here, $U = \frac{A}{r^2} - \frac{B}{r}$

For equilibrium, $\frac{dU}{dr} = 0$

$\therefore\ -\frac{2A}{r^3}+\frac{B}{r^2}=0$ or $\frac{2A}{r^3}=\frac{B}{r^2}$ or $r=\frac{2A}{B}$ 37. (b) (a): $U(x)=\frac{a}{x^{12}}-\frac{b}{x^6}$ or

$-\frac{12a}{x^{13}}-\frac{-6b}{x^7}=0$

or $x^6=\frac{2a}{b}$. Therefore $x=\left(\frac{2a}{b}\right)^{1/6}$

37. **(b) :** Potential energy increases as work done against conservative field

38. **(a) :** $U(x) = \frac{a}{x^{12}}-\frac{b}{x^6}$ or $-\frac{12a}{x^{13}}-\frac{-6b}{x^7}=0$

or $x^6=\frac{2a}{b}$ Therefore $x=\left(\frac{2a}{b}\right)^{1/6}$

39. **(a) :** Let the point is P where K.E. is three times of P.E. Let the height fall is x and speed at P is v.

$KE_p = 3PE_p = 3mg(S-x)$ ...(i)

Use conservation of energy

PE at top $= PE$ at $P + KE$ at P

$mgS = mg(S-x)+KE_p$

$KE_p = mgS - mg(S-x)$ ...(ii)

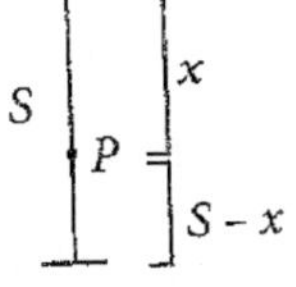

From (i) and (ii)

$3mg(S-x) = mgS - mg(S-x)$

$4mg(S-x) = mgS$

$4S-4x=S \Rightarrow x=\frac{3S}{4}$

So, $S-x=S-\frac{3S}{4}=\frac{S}{4}$

Now, $KE_p=\frac{1}{2}mv^2=3mg(S-x)$

$\frac{v^2}{2}=3g\left(S-\frac{3S}{4}\right)$

$\Rightarrow \frac{v^2}{2}=3g\times\frac{S}{4}$

$\Rightarrow v=\sqrt{\frac{3gS}{2}}$

40. **(d) :** In vertical circular motion, tension in the wire is maximum at the lowermost point, so the wire is most likely to break when the mass is at the lowermost point.

41. **(d) :** As body is at rest initially, i.e., speed = 0.

At point A, speed $= v$.

As track is frictionless, so total mechanical energy will remain constant.

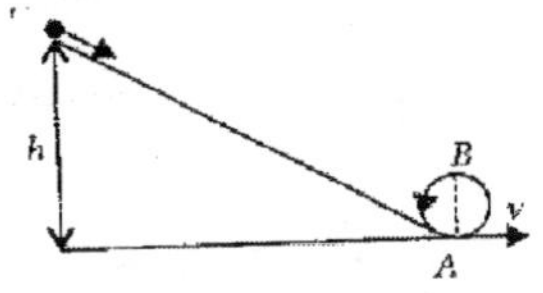

$\therefore$ (T.M.E)$_i$ = (T.M.E)$_f$

$0+mgh=\frac{1}{2}mv^2+0$ or $h=\frac{v^2}{2g}$

For completing the vertical circle, $v \geq \sqrt{5gR}$

$\therefore h = \frac{5gR}{2g} = \frac{5}{2}R = \frac{5}{4}D$

42. **(b) :** Standard Result.

43. **(c) :** conceptual

44. **(a) :** The total energy at A = the total energy at B

$\Rightarrow \frac{1}{2}mu^2 = \frac{1}{2}mv^2 + mgl$

$\Rightarrow v = \sqrt{u^2 - 2gl}$

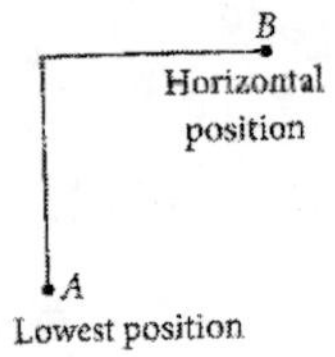

The change in magnitude of velocity = $\sqrt{u^2 + v^2}$

$= \sqrt{2(u^2 - gl)}$

45. **(b) :** Maximum drop in P.E. = maximum gain in K.E.

$mg(2 - 0.75) = \frac{1}{2}mv^2 \Rightarrow v$

$= \sqrt{2g(1.25)} = 5 \text{ m/s}$

46. **(b) :** When a mass is moving in a vertical circle, it string experiences the maximum force when it is at the lowest point B. Therefore, tension at B is maximum

$= \text{Weight} + \frac{mv^2}{R}$

So, the string breaks at point B.

47. **(c)**

$U = \frac{1}{2}kx^2$

for $x = 2$

$U = \frac{1}{2}k(2)^2$

$U' = \frac{1}{2}k(8)^2$

Eq. (2)/eq. (1)

$\Rightarrow \frac{U'}{U} = \left(\frac{8}{2}\right)^2$

$\Rightarrow U' = 16U$

48. **(a) :** Here, $K_P > K_Q$

Case (a): Elongation (x) in each spring is same.

$W_P = \frac{1}{2}K_P x^2, W_Q = \frac{1}{2}K_Q x^2 \therefore W_P > W_Q$

Case (b) : Force of elongation is same.

So, $x_1 = \frac{F}{K_P}$ and $x_2 = \frac{F}{K_Q}$

$W_P = \frac{1}{2}K_P x_1^2 = \frac{1}{2}\frac{F^2}{K_P}$

$W_Q = \frac{1}{2}K_Q x_2^2 = \frac{1}{2}\frac{F^2}{K_Q} \quad \therefore W_P < W_Q$

49. **(a) :** When the mass attached to a spring fixed at the other end is allowed to fall suddenly, it extends the spring by x. Potential energy lost by the mass is gained by the spring.

$Mgx = \frac{1}{2}kx^2 \Rightarrow x = \frac{2Mg}{k}$.

50. **(a) :** Net work done = $W_{mg} + W_{spring}$

$= mg(h+d) - \frac{1}{2}kd^2$

51. **(d) :** Potential energy of a spring

$= \frac{1}{2} \times$ force constant $\times$ (extension $)^2$

$\therefore$ Potential energy $\propto$ (extension $)^2$

or, $\frac{U_1}{U_2} = \left(\frac{x_1}{x_2}\right)^2$ or, $\frac{U_1}{U_2} = \left(\frac{2}{8}\right)^2$

or, $\frac{U_1}{U_2} = \frac{1}{16}$ or, $U_2 = 16U_1 = 16U$

$(\because U_1 = U)$

52. **(a) :** The kinetic energy of mass is converted into energy required to compress a spring which is given by

$\frac{1}{2}mv^2 = \frac{1}{2}kx^2$

$\Rightarrow x = \sqrt{\frac{mv^2}{k}} = \sqrt{\frac{0.5 \times (1.5)^2}{50}} = 0.15$ m.

53. **(d) :** $U = -kx^2, k =$ Spring constant

$\frac{U_1}{U_2} = \frac{x_1^2}{x_2^2} = \frac{4}{100} \Rightarrow U_2 = 25U_1$

54. **(a) :** Energy $= \frac{1}{2}Kx^2 = \frac{1}{2}\frac{F^2}{K}$

$\because \frac{K_A}{K_B} = 2; \therefore \frac{E_A}{E_B} = \frac{1}{2}$ or $E_B = 2E_A$

55. **(d) :** Initial velocity $u = 20$ m/s; $m =$ 1 kg

Kinetic energy = maximum potential energy

Initial kinetic energy $= \frac{1}{2} \times 1 \times 20^2 =$ 200 J

$Mgh(\text{max}) = 200$ J

$\therefore h = 20$ m.

The height travelled by the body, $h' =$ 18 m

$\therefore$ Loss of energy due to air friction

$= mgh - mgh'$

$\Rightarrow$ Energy lost $= 200 \text{ J} - 1 \times 10 \times 18 \text{ J} = 20 \text{ J}$

56. **(c) :** Gain in potential energy $= mgh$

$= 2 \times 10 \times 10 = 200$ J

Gain in potential energy + work done against friction

$\therefore$ Work done against friction $= 300 - 200 = 100$ J

= work done = 300 J

57. **(c) :** Given that,

Mass of lift + passengers, $m = 2000$ kg

Speed, $v = 1.5$ m/s

Frictional force, $F = 3000$ N

Power delivered, $P =$ Force $\times$ velocity ...(i)

Force acting

$F = mg + f$

$F = 2000 \times 10 + 3000$

$F = 23000$ N

Using value of ' F ' in equation (i),

$P = 23000 \times 1.5 = 34500$ W

58. **(c) :** Given, $h = 60$ m

Now, water falls at the rate of 15 kg is

i.e., $\frac{m}{t} = 15$ kg/s

$g = 10$ m/s^2

As loss due to friction is 10%,

therefore only 90% of input energy is used to generate power.

$\therefore P = gh\frac{m}{t}\times\frac{90}{100}$

$P = 10\times 60\times 15\times\frac{90}{100} = 8100\text{ W} \Rightarrow P = 8.1\text{ kW}$

59. **(b)** : Here, $\vec{F} = (2t\hat{\imath} + 3t^2\hat{\jmath})\text{N}, m = 1\text{ kg}$

Acceleration of the body, $\vec{a} = \frac{\vec{F}}{m} = \frac{(2t\hat{\imath}+3t^2\hat{\jmath})\text{N}}{1\text{ kg}}$

Velocity of the body at time t,

$$\vec{v} = \int \vec{a}dt = \int (2t\hat{\imath} + 3t^2\hat{\jmath})dt$$

$$= t^2\hat{\imath} + t^3\hat{\jmath}\text{ m s}^{-1}$$

$\therefore$ Power developed by the force at time t,

$$P = \vec{F}\cdot\vec{v} = (2t\hat{\imath} + 3t^2\hat{\jmath})\cdot(t^2\hat{\imath} + t^3\hat{\jmath})\text{W}$$

$$= (2t^3 + 3t^5)\text{W}$$

60. **(c)** : Here, Volume of blood pumped by man's heart,

$V = 5\text{ litres} = 5\times 10^{-3}\text{ m}^3$

($\because$ 1 litre $= 10^{-3}\text{ m}^3$)

Time in which this volume of blood pumps, $t = 1\text{ min} = 60\text{ s}$

Pressure at which the blood pumps,

$P = 150$ mm of Hg $= 0.15$ m of Hg

$= (0.15\text{ m})(13.6\times 10^3\text{ kg/m}^3)(10\text{ m/s}^2)$

$= 20.4\times 10^3\text{ N/m}^2$

$\therefore$ Power of the heart $= \frac{PV}{t}$

$$= \frac{(20.4\times 10^3\text{ N/m}^2)(5\times 10^{-3}\text{ m}^3)}{60\text{ s}}$$

$$= 1.70\text{ W}$$

61. **(c)** : Constant power acting on the particle of mass m is k watt.

or $P = k; \frac{dW}{dt} = k; dW = kdt$

Integrating both sides, $\int_0^W dW = \int_0^t kdt$

$\Rightarrow W = kt$ ...(i)

Using work energy theorem,

$$W = \frac{1}{2}mv^2 - \frac{1}{2}m(0)^2 \Rightarrow kt = \frac{1}{2}mv^2$$

$$v = \sqrt{\frac{2kt}{m}}$$

Acceleration of the particle, $a = \frac{dv}{dt}$

$$a = \frac{1}{2}\sqrt{\frac{2k}{m}}\frac{1}{\sqrt{t}} = \sqrt{\frac{k}{2mt}}$$

Force on the particle, $F = ma = \sqrt{\frac{mk}{2t}} = \sqrt{\frac{mk}{2}}t^{-1/2}$

62. **(d)** : Power, $P = \frac{\text{Work done}}{\text{Time taken}}$

Here work done ($= mgh$) is same in both cases

$$\therefore \frac{P_1}{P_2} = \frac{t_2}{t_1} = \frac{30\text{ s}}{1\text{ min}} = \frac{30\text{ s}}{60\text{ s}} = \frac{1}{2}$$

63. **(b)** : $P_0 = Fv$

$\because\ F = ma = m\dfrac{dv}{dt}$

$\therefore\ P_0 = mv\frac{dv}{dt}$ or $P_0dt = mvdv$

Integrating both sides, we get

$\int_0^t P_0dt = m\int_0^v vdv\ P_0t = \frac{mv^2}{2}$

$v = \left(\dfrac{2P_0t}{m}\right)^{1/2}$ or $v \propto \sqrt{t}$

64. **(b) :** Power, $\vec{F}\cdot\vec{v} = Fv\cos\theta$

Just before hitting the earth $\theta = 0°$. Hence, the power exerted by the gravitational force is greatest at the instant just before the body hits the earth.

65. **(d) :** Here,

Mass per unit length of water, $\mu = 100$ kg/m

Velocity of water, $v = 2$ m/s

Power of the engine, $P = \mu v^3$

$= (100\text{ kg/m})(2\text{ m/s})^3 = 800$ W

66. **(d) :** Power delivered in time T is $P = F\cdot V = MaV$

or $P = MV\frac{dV}{dT} \Rightarrow PdT = MVdV$

$\Rightarrow\ PT = \frac{MV^2}{2}$ or $P = \frac{1}{2}\frac{MV^2}{T}$

67. **(c) :** Mass of water falling /second = 15 kg/s

$h = 60$ m, $g = 10\text{ m/s}^2$, loss = 10%

i.e., 90% is used.

Power generated = 15 × 10 × 60 × 0.9 = 8100 W = 8.1 kW

68. **(b) :** $P = \vec{F}\cdot\vec{y} = (60\hat{\imath} + 15\hat{\jmath} - 3\hat{k})\cdot(2\hat{\imath} - 4\hat{\jmath} + 5\hat{k})$

$= 120 - 60 - 15 = 45$ watts

69. **(b) :** Power $= \frac{\text{work done}}{\text{time taken}} = \frac{W}{t}$

$\therefore P = \dfrac{M\times g\times h}{t}$

$\Rightarrow\ M = \dfrac{P\times t}{g\times h} = \dfrac{2000\times 60}{10\times 10} = 1200$ kg

i.e., 1200 liters as one liter has a mass of 1 kg.

70. **(c) :** According to conservation of momentum,

$4mu_1 = 4mv_1 + 2mv_2 \Rightarrow 2(u_1 - v_1) = v_2$ ...(i)

From conservation of energy,

$\frac{1}{2}(4m)u_1^2 = \frac{1}{2}(4m)v_1^2 + \frac{1}{2}(2m)v_2^2$

$\Rightarrow 2(u_1^2 - v_1^2) = v_2^2$ ...(ii)

From (i) and (ii), $2(u_1^2 - v_1^2) = 4(u_1 - v_1)^2$

$3v_1 = u_1$ ...(iii)

Now, fraction of loss in kinetic energy for mass $4m$,

$$\frac{\Delta K}{K_i} = \frac{K_i - K_f}{K_i} = \frac{\frac{1}{2}(4m)u_1^2 - \frac{1}{2}(4m)v_1^2}{\frac{1}{2}(4m)u_1^2}$$

Substituting (iii) in (iv), we get $\frac{\Delta K}{K_i} = \frac{8}{9}$

71. **(b) :** Let final velocity of the block of mass, $4m = v'$ Initial velocity of block of mass $4m = 0$

Final velocity of block of mass $m = 0$

According to law of conservation of linear momentum,

$mv + 4m \times 0 = 4mv' + 0 \Rightarrow v' = v/4$

Coefficient of restitution,

$$e = \frac{\text{Relative velocity of separation}}{\text{Relative velocity of approach}}$$

$$= \frac{v/4}{v} = 0.25$$

72. **(c)** : Mass of bullet, $m = 10\text{ g} = 0.01\text{ kg}$

Initial speed of bullet, $u = 400\text{ m s}^{-1}$

Mass of block, $M = 2\text{ kg}$

Length of string, $l = 5\text{ m}$

Speed of the block after collision $= v_1$

Speed of the bullet on emerging from block, = ?

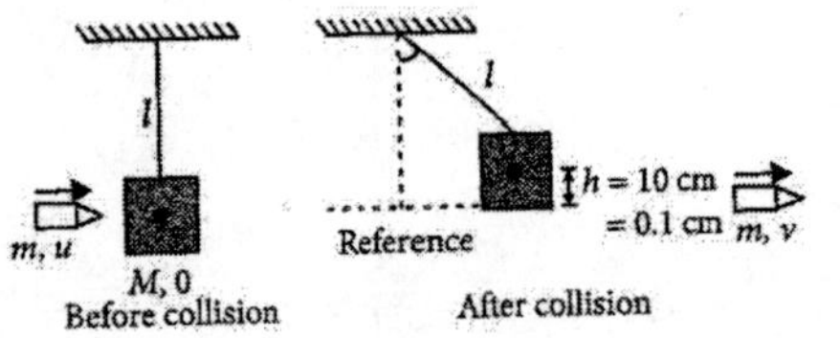

After collision

Using energy conservation principle for the block,

$(\text{KE} + \text{PE})_{\text{Reference}} = (\text{KE} + \text{PE})_h$

$\Rightarrow \frac{1}{2}Mv_1^2 = Mgh$ or, $v_1 = \sqrt{2gh}$

$v_1 = \sqrt{2 \times 10 \times 0.1} = \sqrt{2}\text{ m s}^{-1}$.

Using momentum conservation principle for block and bullet system,

$(M \times 0 + mu)_{\text{Before collision}}$

$= (M \times v_1 + mv)_{\text{After collision}}$

$\Rightarrow 0.01 \times 400 = 2\sqrt{2} + 0.01 \times v$

$\Rightarrow v = \frac{4 - 2\sqrt{2}}{0.01} = 117.15\text{ m s}^{-1}$

$\approx 120\text{ m s}^{-1}$

73. **(b)** : Masses of the balls are same and collision is elastic, so their velocity will be interchanged after collision.

74. **(c)** : Let the particles A and B collide at time t. For their collision, the position vectors of both particles should be same at time t, i.e.,

$\vec{r}_1 + \vec{v}_1 t = \vec{r}_2 + \vec{v}_2 t; \vec{r}_1 - \vec{r}_2 = \vec{v}_2 t - \vec{v}_1 t = (\vec{v}_2 - \vec{v}_1)t$ ...(i)

Also, $|\vec{r}_1 - \vec{r}_2| = |\vec{v}_2 - \vec{v}_1| t$ or $t = \frac{|\vec{r}_1 - \vec{r}_2|}{|\vec{v}_2 - \vec{v}_1|}$

Substituting this value of t in eqn. (i), we get

$$\vec{r}_1 - \vec{r}_2 = (\vec{v}_2 - \vec{v}_1)\frac{|\vec{r}_1 - \vec{r}_2|}{|\vec{v}_2 - \vec{v}_1|}$$

or $\frac{\vec{r}_1 - \vec{r}_2}{|\vec{r}_1 - \vec{r}_2|} = \frac{(\vec{v}_2 - \vec{v}_1)}{|\vec{v}_2 - \vec{v}_1|}$

75. **(d)** : The situation is shown in the figure.

Let v be the velocity of the ball with which it collides with ground. Then according to the law of conservation

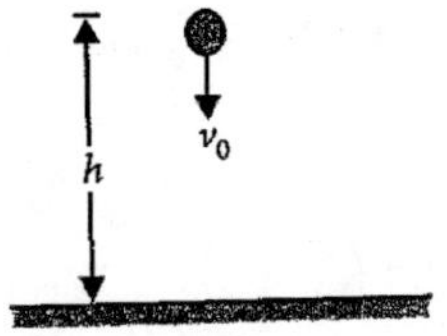

of energy,

Gain in kinetic energy = loss in potential energy

i.e. $\frac{1}{2}mv^2 - \frac{1}{2}mv_0^2 = mgh$ (where m is the mass of the ball)

or $v^2 - v_0^2 = 2gh$ ...(i)

Now, when the ball collides with the ground, 50% of its energy is lost and it rebounds to the same height h.

$$\therefore \frac{50}{100}\left(\frac{1}{2}mv^2\right) = mgh$$

$$\frac{1}{4}v^2 = gh \text{ or } v^2 = 4gh$$

Substituting this value of v^2 in eqn. (i), we get

$$4gh - v_0^2 = 2gh$$

or $v_0^2 = 4gh - 2gh = 2gh$ or $v_0 = \sqrt{2gh}$

Here, $g = 10 \text{ m s}^{-2}$ and $h = 20$ m

$\therefore v_0 = \sqrt{2(10 \text{ m s}^{-2})(20 \text{ m})} = 20 \text{ m s}^{-1}$

76. **(c)** : The situation is shown in the figure.

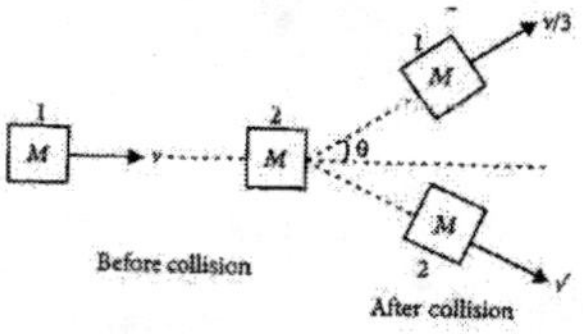

Let v' be speed of second block after the collision.

As the collision is elastic, so kinetic energy is conserved.

According to conservation of kinetic energy,

$$\frac{1}{2}Mv^2 + 0 = \frac{1}{2}M\left(\frac{v}{3}\right)^2 + \frac{1}{2}Mv'^2$$

$$v^2 = \frac{v^2}{9} + v'^2 \text{ or } v'^2 = v^2 - \frac{v^2}{9} = \frac{9v^2 - v^2}{9} = \frac{8}{9}v^2$$

$$v' = \sqrt{\frac{8}{9}v^2} = \frac{\sqrt{8}}{3}v = \frac{2\sqrt{2}}{3}v$$

77. **(a)** : Total initial energy of two particles

$$= \frac{1}{2}m_1u_1^2 + \frac{1}{2}m_2u_2^2$$

Total final energy of two particles

$$= \frac{1}{2}m_2v_2^2 + \frac{1}{2}m_1v_1^2 + \varepsilon$$

Using energy conservation principle,

$$\frac{1}{2}m_1u_1^2 + \frac{1}{2}m_2u_2^2 = \frac{1}{2}m_1v_1^2 + \frac{1}{2}m_2v_2^2 + \varepsilon$$

$$\therefore \frac{1}{2}m_1u_1^2 + \frac{1}{2}m_2u_2^2 - \varepsilon = \frac{1}{2}m_1v_1^2 + \frac{1}{2}m_2v_2^2$$

78. **(d)** :

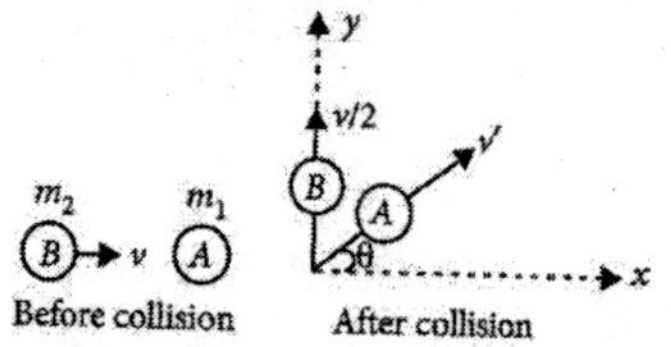

According to law of conservation of linear momentum along x-axis, we get

$m_1 \times 0 + m_2 \times v = m_1 v' \cos\theta$

$m_2 v = m_1 v' \cos\theta$

or $\cos\theta = \frac{m_2 v}{m_1 v'}$ ...(i)

According to law of conservation of linear momentum along y-axis, we get

$m_1 \times 0 + m_2 \times 0 = m_1 v' \sin\theta + m_2 \frac{v}{2}$

$\Rightarrow -m_2 \frac{v}{2} = m_1 v' \sin\theta$

$\sin\theta = -\frac{m_2 v}{2 m_1 v'}$ ...(ii)

Divide (ii) by (i), we get

$\tan\theta = -\frac{1}{2}$ or $\theta = \tan^{-1}\left(-\frac{1}{2}\right)$ to the x-axis

79. **(b) :** $\overleftrightarrow{m} \longrightarrow v$

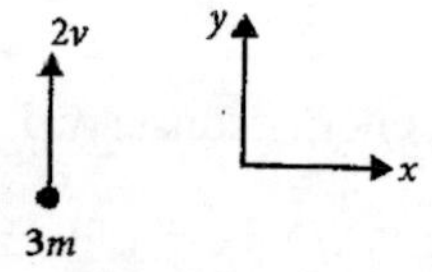

According to conservation of momentum, we get

$$mv\hat{\imath} + (3m)2v\hat{\jmath} = (m + 3m)\overrightarrow{v'}$$

where $\overrightarrow{v'}$ is the final velocity after collision

$$\overrightarrow{v'} = \frac{1}{4}v\hat{\imath} + \frac{6}{4}v\hat{\jmath} = \frac{1}{4}v\hat{\imath} + \frac{3}{2}v\hat{\jmath}$$

80. **(a) :** Here, $m_1 = m, m_2 = 2m$

$u_1 = 2$ m/s, $u_2 = 0$

Coefficient of restitution, $e = 0.5$

Let v_1 and v_2 be their respective velocities after collision.

Applying the law of conservation of linear momentum, we get $m_1 u_1 + m_2 u_2 = m_1 v_1 + m_2 v_2$

$\therefore\ m \times 2 + 2m \times 0 = m \times v_1 + 2m \times v_2$

or $2m = mv_1 + 2mv_2$ or $2 = (v_1 + 2v_2)$ ...(i)

By definition of coefficient of restitution,

$e = \frac{v_2 - v_1}{u_1 - u_2}$

or $e(u_1 - u_2) = v_2 - v_1$

$\Rightarrow 0.5(2 - 0) = v_2 - v_1$ ...(ii)

Solving equations (i) and (ii), we get

$$v_1 = 0 \text{ m/s}, v_2 = 1 \text{ m/s}$$

81. **(d) :** Equal masses after elastic collision interchange their velocities. -5 m/s and $+3$ m/s.

82. **(a) :** Initial energy equation

$mgh = \frac{1}{2}mv^2$ i.e. $10 \times 5 = \frac{1}{2}v_1^2 \Rightarrow v_1 = 10$

After one bounce,

$10 \times 1.8 = \frac{1}{2}v_2^2 \Rightarrow v_2 = 6$

Loss in velocity on bouncing $\frac{6}{10} = \frac{3}{5}$ a factor.

83. **(d) :** Mass of metal ball = 2 kg;
Speed of metal ball $(v_1) = 36$ km/h = 10 m/s and mass of stationary ball = 3 kg

Applying law of conservation of momentum,

$$m_1v_1 + m_2v_2 = (m_1 + m_2)v$$

or, $v = \frac{m_1v_1+m_2v_2}{m_1+m_2} = \frac{(2\times10)+(3\times0)}{2+3} = \frac{20}{5} =$ 4 m/s

Therefore loss of energy

$$= \left[\frac{1}{2}m_1v_1^2 + \frac{1}{2}m_2v_2^2\right] - \frac{1}{2} \times (m_1 + m_2)v^2$$

$$= \left[\frac{1}{2} \times 2 \times (10)^2 + \frac{1}{2} \times 3(0)^2\right] - \frac{1}{2} \times (2 + 3) \times (4)^2$$

$$= 100 - 40 = 60 \text{ J}$$

84. **(c) :** Mass of body $(m_1) = m$; Velocity of first body $(u_1) = 3$ km/ hour; Mass of second body at rest $(m_2) = 2m$ and velocity of second body $(u_2) = 0$.

After combination, mass of the body

$$M = m + 2m = 3m$$

From the law of conservation of momentum, we get $Mv = m_1u_1 + m_2u_2$

or $3mv = (m \times 3) + (2m \times 0) = 3m$ or $v = 1$ km/ hour.

85. **(a) :** For a perfectly elastic collision, $e = 1$ and for a perfectly inelastic collision,

$e = 0$.

Chapter: 6 SYSTEMS OF PARTICLES AND ROTATIONAL MOTION

Centre of Mass

1. Two objects of mass 10 kg and 20 kg respectively are connected to the two ends of a rigid rod of length 10 m with negligible mass. The distance of the center of mass of the system from the 10 kg mass is **(2022)**

(a) $\frac{10}{3}$ m (b) $\frac{20}{3}$ m

(c) 10 m (d) 5 m

2. Two particles of mass 5 kg and 10 kg respectively are attached to the two ends of a rigid rod of length 1 m with negligible mass. The centre of mass of the system from the 5 kg particle is nearly at a distance of **(2020)**

(a) 33 cm (b) 50 cm

(c) 67 cm (d) 80 cm

3. Three masses are placed on the x-axis : 300 g at origin, 500 g at $x = 40$ cm and 400 g at $x = 70$ cm. The distance of the centre of mass from the origin is **(Mains 2012)**

(a) 40 cm (b) 45 cm

(c) 50 cm (d) 30 cm

4. Two bodies of mass 1 kg and 3 kg have position vectors $\hat{\imath} + 2\hat{\jmath} + \hat{k}$ and $-3\hat{\imath} - 2\hat{\jmath} + \hat{k}$, respectively. The centre of mass of this system has a position vector **(2009)**

(a) $-2\hat{\imath} - \hat{\jmath} + \hat{k}$ (b) $2\hat{\imath} - \hat{\jmath} - 2\hat{k}$

(c) $-\hat{\imath} + \hat{\jmath} + \hat{k}$ (d) $-2\hat{\imath} + 2\hat{k}$

5. Consider a system of two particles having masses m_1 and m_2. If the particle of mass m_1 is pushed towards the centre of mass of the particles through a distance d, by what distance would be particle of mass m_2 move so as to keep the centre of mass of the particles at the original position? **(2004)**

(a) $\frac{m_1}{m_1+m_2}d$ (b) $\frac{m_1}{m_2}d$

(c) d (d) $\frac{m_2}{m_1}d$

6. Three identical metal balls, each of radius r are placed touching each other on a horizontal surface such that an equilateral triangle is formed when centres of three balls are joined. The centre of the mass of the system is located at **(1999)**

(a) line joining centres of any two balls

(b) centre of one of the balls

(c) horizontal surface

(d) point of intersection of the medians.

7. The centre of mass of system of particles does not depend on **(1997)**

(a) position of the particles

(b) relative distances between the particles

(c) masses of the particles

(d) forces acting on the particle.

Motion of Centre of Mass

8. Two persons of masses 55 kg and 65 kg respectively, are at the opposite ends of a boat. The length of the boat is 3.0 m and weighs 100 kg. The 55 kg man walks up to the 65 kg man and sits with him. If the boat is in still water the center of mass of the system shifts by **(2012)**

(a) 3.0 m (b) 2.3 m

(c) zero (d) 0.75 m

9. Two particles which are initially at rest, move towards each other under the action of their internal attraction. If their speeds are v and $2v$ at any instant, then the speed of centre of mass of the system will be **(2010)**

(a) $2v$ (b) zero

(c) 1.5v (d) v

10. A man of 50 kg mass is standing in a gravity free space at a height of 10 m above the floor. He throws a stone of 0.5 kg mass downwards with a speed 2 m/s. When the stone reaches the floor, the distance of the man above the floor will be **(2010)**

(a) 9.9 m (b) 10.1 m

(c) 10 m (d) 20 m

Vector Product of Two Vectors

11. Vectors, $\vec{A}, \vec{B}$ and $\vec{C}$ are such that $\vec{A}\cdot\vec{B} = 0$ and $\vec{A}\cdot\vec{C} = 0$. Then the vector parallel to $\vec{A}$ is **(Karnataka NEET 2013)**

(a) $\vec{A}\times\vec{B}$ (b) $\vec{B}+\vec{C}$

(c) $\vec{B}\times\vec{C}$ (d) $\vec{B}$ and $\vec{C}$

12. $\vec{A}$ and $\vec{B}$ are two vectors and θ is the angle between them, if $|\vec{A}\times\vec{B}| = \sqrt{3}(\vec{A}\cdot\vec{B})$, the value of θ is **(2007)**

(a) 45° (b) 30°

(c) 90° (d) 60°

13. If the angle between the vectors $\vec{A}$ and $\vec{B}$ is θ, the value of the product $(\vec{B}\times\vec{A})\cdot\vec{A}$ is equal to **(2005, 1989)**

(a) $BA^2\sin\theta$ (b) $BA^2\cos\theta$

(c) $BA^2\sin\theta\cos\theta$ (d) zero.

14. If $|\vec{A}\times\vec{B}| = \sqrt{3}\vec{A}\cdot\vec{B}$ then the value of $|\vec{A}+\vec{B}|$ is **(2004)**

(a) $(A^2+B^2+AB)^{1/2}$

(b) $\left(A^2+B^2+\frac{AB}{\sqrt{3}}\right)^{1/2}$

(c) $A+B$

(d) $\left(A^2+B^2+\sqrt{3}AB\right)^{1/2}$

15. The resultant of $\vec{A}\times 0$ will be equal to **(1992)**

(a) zero (b) A

(c) zero vector (d) unit vector.

Angular Velocity and its Relation with Linear Velocity

16. What is the value of linear velocity, if $\vec{r} = 3\hat{\imath} - 4\hat{\jmath} + \hat{k}$ and $\vec{\omega} = 5\hat{\imath} - 6\hat{\jmath} + 6\hat{k}$? **(1999)**

(a) $4\hat{\imath} - 13\hat{\jmath} + 6\hat{k}$

(b) $18\hat{\imath} + 13\hat{\jmath} - 2\hat{k}$

(c) $6\hat{\imath} + 2\hat{\jmath} - 3\hat{k}$

(d) $6\hat{\imath} - 2\hat{\jmath} + 8\hat{k}$

Torque and Angular Momentum

17. Find the torque about the origin when a force of $3\hat{j}$ N acts on a particle whose position vector is $2\hat{k}$ m. **(2020)**
(a) $6\hat{\imath}$Nm (b) $6\hat{\jmath}$Nm
(c) $-6\hat{\imath}$Nm (d) $6\hat{k}$Nm

18. The moment of the force, $\vec{F} = 4\hat{\imath} + 5\hat{\jmath} - 6\hat{k}$ at $(2,0,-3)$, about the point $(2,-2,-2)$, is given by **(2018)**
(a) $-8\hat{\imath} - 4\hat{\jmath} - 7\hat{k}$
(b) $-4\hat{\imath} - \hat{\jmath} - 8\hat{k}$
(c) $-7\hat{\imath} - 8\hat{\jmath} - 4\hat{k}$
(d) $-7\hat{\imath} - 4\hat{\jmath} - 8\hat{k}$

19. A force $\vec{F} = \alpha\hat{\imath} + 3\hat{\jmath} + 6\hat{k}$ is acting at a point $\vec{r} = 2\hat{\imath} - 6\hat{\jmath} - 12\hat{k}$. The value of α for which angular momentum about origin is conserved is **(2015)**
(a) zero (b) 1
(c) -1 (d) 2

20. A mass m moves in a circle on a smooth horizontal plane with velocity v_0 at a radius R_0. The mass is attached to a string which passes through a smooth hole in the plane as shown. The tension in the string is increased gradually and finally m moves in a circle of radius $\frac{R_0}{2}$. The final value of the kinetic energy is **(2015 Cancelled)**

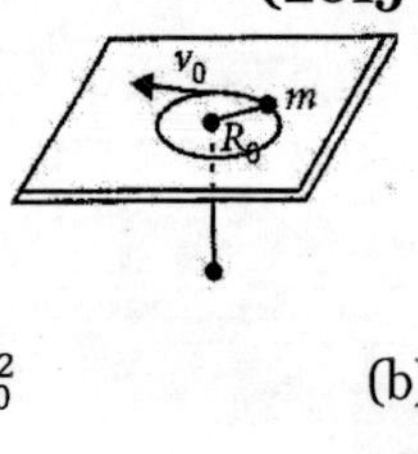

(a) $2mv_0^2$ (b) $\frac{1}{2}mv_0^2$
(c) mv_0^2 (d) $\frac{1}{4}mv_0^2$

21. When a mass is rotating in a plane about a fixed point, its angular momentum is directed along] **(2012)**
(a) a line perpendicular to the plane of rotation
(b) the line making an angle of 45° to the plane of rotation
(c) the radius
(d) the tangent to the orbit.

22. A small mass attached to a string rotates on a frictionless table top as shown. If the tension in the string is increased by pulling the string causing the radius of the circular motion to decrease by a factor of 2 , the kinetic energy of the mass will **(Mains 2011)**

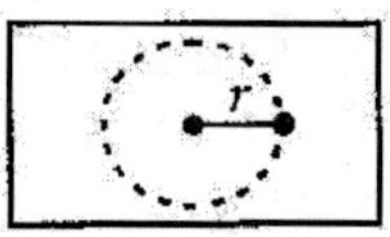

(a) decrease by a factor of 2
(b) remain constant
(c) increase by a factor of 2
(d) increase by a factor of 4

23. If $\vec{F}$ is the force acting on a particle having position vector $\vec{r}$ and $\vec{\tau}$ be the torque of this force about the origin, then **(2009)**
(a) $\vec{r}\cdot\vec{\tau} > 0$ and $\vec{F}\cdot\vec{\tau} < 0$
(b) $\vec{r}\cdot\vec{\tau} = 0$ and $\vec{F}\cdot\vec{\tau} = 0$
(c) $\vec{r}\cdot\vec{\tau} = 0$ and $\vec{F}\cdot\vec{\tau} \neq 0$
(d) $\vec{r}\cdot\vec{\tau} \neq 0$ and $\vec{F}\cdot\vec{\tau} = 0$

24. A particle of mass m moves in the XY plane with a velocity v along the straight line AB. If the angular

momentum of the particle with respect to origin O is L_A when it is at A and L_B when it is at B, then **(2007)**
(a) $L_A = L_B$
(b) the relationship between L_A and L_B depends upon the slope of the line AB
(c) $L_A < L_B$
(d) $L_A > L_B$

25. Find the torque of a force $\vec{F} = -3\hat{\imath} + \hat{\jmath} + 5\hat{k}$ acting at the point $\vec{r} = 7\hat{\imath} + 3\hat{\jmath} + \hat{k}$. **(1997)**
(a) $-21\hat{\imath} + 4\hat{\jmath} + 4\hat{k}$
(b) $-14\hat{\imath} + 34\hat{\jmath} - 16\hat{k}$
(c) $14\hat{\imath} - 38\hat{\jmath} + 16\hat{k}$
(d) $4\hat{\imath} + 4\hat{\jmath} + 6\hat{k}$

26. What is the torque of the force $\vec{F} = 2\hat{\imath} - 3\hat{\jmath} + 4\hat{k}$ N acting at the point $\vec{r} = 3\hat{\imath} + 2\hat{\jmath} + 3\hat{k}$ m about origin? **(1995)**
(a) $-6\hat{\imath} + 6\hat{\jmath} - 12\hat{k}$
(b) $-17\hat{\imath} + 6\hat{\jmath} + 13\hat{k}$
(c) $6\hat{\imath} - 6\hat{\jmath} + 12\hat{k}$
(d) $17\hat{\imath} - 6\hat{\jmath} - 13\hat{k}$

27. A particle of mass $m = 5$ is moving with a uniform speed $v = 3\sqrt{2}$ in the XOY plane along the line $y = x + 4$. The magnitude of the angular momentum of the particle about the origin is **(1991)**
(a) 60 units (b) $40\sqrt{2}$ units
(c) zero (d) 7.5 units

Equilibrium of a Rigid Body

28. A uniform rod of length 200 cm and mass 500 g is balanced on a wedge placed at 40 cm mark. A mass of 2 kg is suspended from the rod at 20 cm and another unknown mass ' m ' is suspended from the rod at 160 cm mark as shown in the figure. Find the value of ' m ' such that the rod is in equilibrium. ($g = 10\ \text{m/s}^2$) **(2021)**

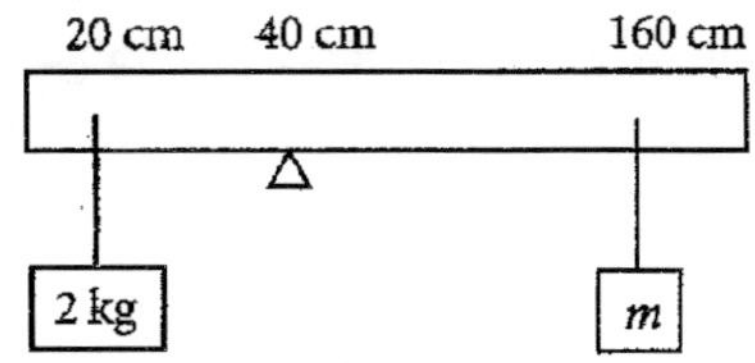

(a) $\frac{1}{12}$ kg (b) $\frac{1}{2}$ kg
(c) $\frac{1}{3}$ kg (d) $\frac{1}{6}$ kg

29. Which of the following statements are correct?
(1) Centre of mass of a body always coincides with the centre of gravity of the body.
(2) Centre of mass of a body is the point at which the total gravitational torque on the body is zero.
(3) A couple on a body produces both translational and rotational motion in a body.
(4) Mechanical advantage greater than one means that small effort can be used to lift a large load. **(2017)**
(a) (1) and (2) (b) (2) and (3)
(c) (3) and (4) (d) (2) and (4)

30. A rod of weight W is supported by two parallel knife edges A and B and is in equilibrium in a horizontal position. The knives are at a distance d from each other. The centre of mass of the rod is at distance x from A. The normal reaction on A is **(2015 celled)**

(a) $\frac{W(d-x)}{x}$ (b) $\frac{W(d-x)}{d}$

(c) $\frac{Wx}{d}$ (d) $\frac{Wd}{x}$

31. ABC is an equilateral triangle with O as its centre. $\vec{F}_1, \vec{F}_2$ and $\vec{F}_3$ represent three forces acting along the sides AB, BC and AC respectively. If the total torque about O is zero then the magnitude of $\vec{F}_3$ is **(2012, 1998)**

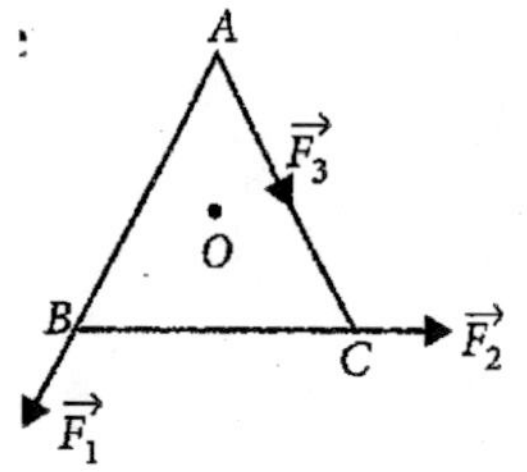

(a) $F_1 + F_2$ (b) $F_1 - F_2$

(c) $\frac{F_1+F_2}{2}$ (d) $2(F_1 + F_2)$

32. (1) Centre of gravity (C.G.) of a body is the point at which the weight of the body acts.

(2) Centre of mass coincides with the centre of gravity if the earth is assumed to have infinitely large radius.

(3) To evaluate the gravitational field intensity due to any body at an external point, the entire mass of the body can be considered to be concentrated at its C.G.

(4) The radius of gyration of any body rotating about an axis is the length of the perpendicular drawn from the C.G. of the body to the axis.

Which one of the following pairs of statements is correct? **(Mains 2010)**

(a) (4) and (1) (b) (1) and (2)

(c) (2) and (3) (d) (3) and (4)

33. A rod of length 3 m and its mass per unit length is directly proportional to distance x from one of its end then its centre of gravity from that end will be at **(2002)**

(a) 1.5 m (b) 2 m

(c) 2.5 m (d) 3.0 m

34. 250 N force is required to raise 75 kg mass from a pulley. If rope is pulled 12 m then the load is lifted to 3 m, the efficiency of pulley system will be **(2001)**

(a) 25% (b) 33.3%

(c) 75% (d) 90%.

35. A couple produces **(1997)**

(a) linear and rotational motion

(b) no motion

(c) purely linear motion

(d) purely rotational motion.

Moment of Inertia

36. The ratio of radius of gyration of a solid sphere of mass M and radius R about its own axis to the radius of gyration of the thin hollow sphere of same mass and radius about its axis is **(2023)**

(a) 5 : 3 (b) 2 : 5

(c) 5 : 2 (d) 3 : 5

37. A solid sphere of mass m and radius R is rotating about its diameter. A solid cylinder of the same mass and same radius is also rotating about its geometrical axis with an angular speed twice that of the sphere. The ratio of their kinetic energies of rotation $(E_{sphere}/E_{cylinder})$ will be

(NEET-II 2016)

(a) 2: 3 (b) 1: 5

(c) 1: 4 (d) 3: 1

38. A light rod of length l has two masses m_1 and m_2 attached to its two ends. The moment of inertia of the system about an axis perpendicular to the rod and passing through the centre of mass is **(NEET-II 2016)**

(a) $\frac{m_1 m_2}{m_1+m_2} l^2$ (b) $\frac{m_1+m_2}{m_1 m_2} l^2$

(c) $(m_1+m_2)l^2$ (d) $\sqrt{m_1 m_2} l^2$

39. From a circular disc of radius R and mass $9M$, a small disc of mass M and radius $R/3$ is removed concentrically. The moment of inertia of the remaining disc about an axis perpendicular to the plane of the disc and passing through its centre is **(Mains 2010)**

(a) $\frac{40}{9} MR^2$ (b) MR^2

(c) $4MR^2$ (d) $\frac{4}{9} MR^2$

40. The ratio of the radii of gyration of a circular disc to that of a circular ring, each of same mass and radius, around their respective axes is **(2008)**

(a) $\sqrt{2}: 1$ (b) $\sqrt{2}: \sqrt{3}$

(c) $\sqrt{3}: \sqrt{2}$ (d) $1: \sqrt{2}$

41. Two bodies have their moments of inertia I and $2I$ respectively about their axis of rotation. If their kinetic energies of rotation are equal, their angular velocity will be in the ratio **(2005)**

(a) 2: 1 (b) 1: 2

(c) $\sqrt{2}: 1$ (d) $1: \sqrt{2}$

42. Three particles, each of mass m gram, are situated at the vertices of an equilateral triangle ABC of side l cm (as shown in the figure). The moment of inertia of the system about a line AX perpendicular to AB and in the plane of ABC, in gram- cm^2 units will be **(2004)**

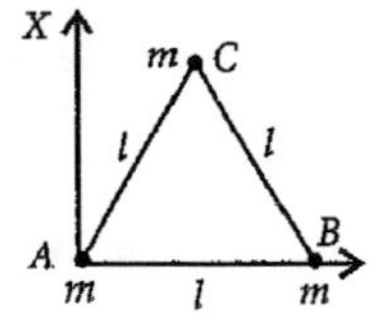

(a) $\frac{3}{4} ml^2$ (b) $2ml^2$

(c) $\frac{5}{4} ml^2$ (d) $\frac{3}{2} ml^2$

43. A circular disc is to be made by using iron and aluminium so that it acquires maximum moment of inertia about geometrical axis. It is possible with **(2002)**

(a) aluminium at interior and iron surrounding it

(b) iron at interior and aluminium surrounding it

(c) using iron and aluminium layers in alternate order

(d) sheet of iron is used at both external surface and aluminium sheet as internal layers.

44. For the adjoining diagram,the correct relation between I_1, I_2, and I_3 is, (I- moment of inertia) **(2000)**

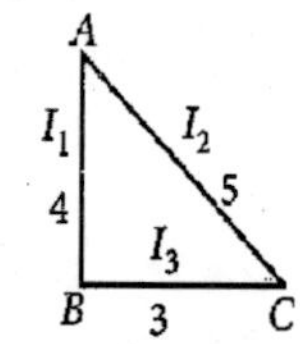

(a) $I_1 > I_2$ (b) $I_2 > I_1$

(c) $I_3 > I_1$ (d) $I_3 > I_2$

45. The ABC is a triangular plate of uniform thickness. The sides are in the ratio shown in the figure. I_{AB}, I_{BC} and I_{CA} are the moments of inertia of the plate about AB,

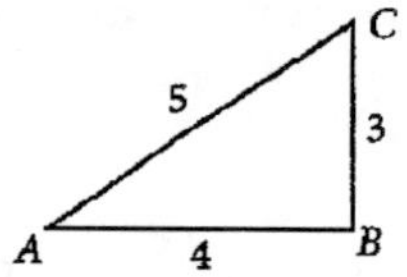

BC and CA respectively. Which one of the following relations is correct? **(1995)**

(a) $I_{AB} + I_{BC} = I_{CA}$

(b) I_{CA} is maximum

(c) $I_{AB} > I_{BC}$

(d) $I_{BC} > I_{AB}$

46. In a rectangle $ABCD(BC = 2AB)$. The moment of inertia is minimum along axis through **(1993)**

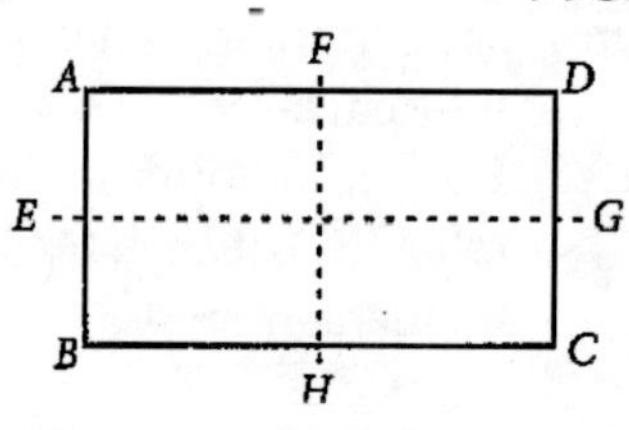

(a) BC (b) BD

(c) HF (d) EG

47. A fly wheel rotating about fixed axis has a kinetic energy of 360 joule when its angular speed is 30radian/sec. The moment of inertia of the wheel about the axis of rotation is **(1990)**

(a) 0.6 kg m^2 (b) 0.15 kg m^2

(c) 0.8 kg m^2 (d) 0.75 kg m^2

48. A ring of mass m and radius r rotates about an axis passing through its centre and perpendicular to its plane with angular velocity ω. Its kinetic energy is **(1988)**

(a) $\frac{1}{2}mr^2\omega^2$ (b) $mr\omega^2$

(c) $mr^2\omega^2$ (d) $\frac{1}{2}mr\omega^2$

Theorems of Perpendicular and Parallel Axes

49. The ratio of the radius of gyration of a thin uniform disc about an axis passing through its centre and normal to its plane to the radius of gyration of the disc about its diameter is **(2022)**

(a) 2: 1 (b) $\sqrt{2}$: 1

(c) 4: 1 (d) 1: $\sqrt{2}$

50. From a circular of mass ' M ' and radius ' R ' an arc corresponding to a 90° sector is removed. The moment of inertia of the remaining part of the ring about an axis passing through the centre of the ring and perpendicular to the plane of the ring is ' K ' times ' MR^2. Then the value of ' K ' is **(2021)**

(a) $\frac{1}{8}$ (b) $\frac{3}{4}$

(c) $\frac{7}{8}$ (d) $\frac{1}{4}$

51. From a disc of radius R and mass M, a circular hole of diameter R, whose rim passes through the centre is cut. What is the moment of inertia of the remaining part of the disc about a perpendicular axis, passing through the centre? **(NEET-I 2016)**

(a) $11MR^2/32$ (b) $9MR^2/32$

(c) $15MR^2/32$ (d) $13MR^2/32$

52. Three identical spherical shells, each of mass m and radius r are placed as shown in figure. Consider an axis XX' which is touching the two shells and passing through the diameter of the third shell. Moment of inertia of the system consisting of these three spherical shells about XX' axis is **(2015 Cancelled)**

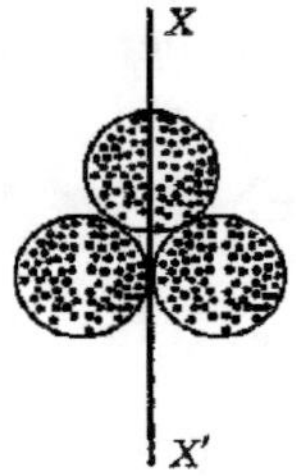

(a) $\frac{16}{5}mr^2$ (b) $4mr^2$

(c) $\frac{11}{5}mr^2$ (d) $3mr^2$

53. The moment of inertia of a uniform circular disc is maximum about an axis perpendicular to the disc and passing through **(Mains 2012)**

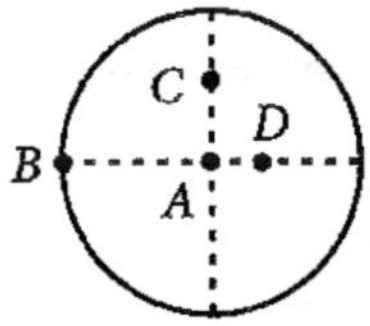

(a) B (b) C

(c) D (d) A

54. The moment of inertia of a thin uniform rod of mass M and length L about an axis passing through its midpoint and perpendicular to its length is I_0. Its moment of inertia about an axis passing through one of its ends and perpendicular to its length is **(2011)**

(a) $I_0 + ML^2/2$ (b) $I_0 + ML^2/4$

(c) $I_0 + 2ML^2$ (d) $I_0 + ML^2$

55. Four identical thin rods each of mass M and length$l$, form a square frame. Moment of inertia of this frame about an axis through the centre of the square and perpendicular to its plane is **(2009)**

(a) $\frac{2}{3}Ml^2$ (b) $\frac{13}{3}Ml^2$

(c) $\frac{1}{3}Ml^2$ (d) $\frac{4}{3}Ml^2$

56. A thin rod of length L and mass M is bent at its midpoint into two halves so that the angle between them is 90°. The moment of inertia of the bent rod about an axis passing through the bending point and perpendicular to the plane defined by the two halves of the rod is **(2008)**

(a) $\frac{ML^2}{6}$ (b) $\frac{\sqrt{2}ML^2}{24}$

(c) $\frac{ML^2}{24}$ (d) $\frac{ML^2}{12}$

57. The moment of inertia of a uniform circular disc of radius R and mass M about an axis touching the disc at its diameter and normal to the disc **(2006)**

(a) $\frac{1}{2}MR^2$ (b) MR^2

(c) $\frac{2}{5}MR^2$ (d) $\frac{3}{2}MR^2$

58. The ratio of the radii of gyration of a circular disc about a tangential axis in the plane of the disc and of a circular ring of the same radius and mass about a tangential axis in the plane of the ring is **(2004)**

(a) 2: 3 (b)2: 1

(c) $\sqrt{5}:\sqrt{6}$ (d) $1:\sqrt{2}$

59. The moment of inertia of a disc of mass M and radius R about an axis, which is tangential to the circumference of the disc and parallel to its diameter is **(1999)**

(a) $\frac{5}{4}MR^2$ (b) $\frac{2}{3}MR^2$

(c) $\frac{3}{2}MR^2$ (d) $\frac{4}{5}MR^2$

60. Moment of inertia of a uniform circular disc about a diameter is I. Its moment of inertia about an axis perpendicular to its plane and passing through a point on its rim will be **(1990)**

(a) $5I$ (b) $3I$

(c) $6I$ (d) $4I$

Kinematics of Rotational Motion about a Fixed Axis

61. The angular speed of a fly wheel moving with uniform angular acceleration changes from 1200rpm to 3120rpm in 16 seconds. The angular acceleration in rad/s^2 is **(2022)**

(a) 2π (b) 4π

(c) 12π (d) 104π

62. A wheel has angular acceleration of 3.0rad/sec^2 and an initial angular speed of 2.00rad/sec. In a time of 2sec it has rotated through an angle (in radians) of **(2007)**

(a) 10 (b) 12

(c) 4 (d) 6

Dynamics of Rotational Motion about a Fixed Axis

63. A solid cylinder of mass 2 kg and radius 4 cm is rotating about its axis at the rate of 3rpm. The torque required to stop it after 2π revolutions is **(2019)**

(a) 2×10^6 N m

(b) 2×10^{-6} N m

(c) 2×10^{-3} N m

(d) 12×10^{-4} N m

64. Three objects, A : (a solid sphere), B : (a thin circular disk) and C : (a circular ring), each have the same mass M and radius R. They all spin with the same angular speed ω about their own symmetry axes. The amounts of work (W) required to bring them to rest, would satisfy the relation **(2018)**

(a) $W_C > W_B > W_A$

(b) $W_A > W_B > W_C$

(c) $W_B > W_A > W_C$

(d) $W_A > W_C > W_B$

65. A rope is wound around a hollow cylinder of mass 3 kg and radius 40 cm. What is the angular acceleration of the cylinder if the rope is pulled with a force of 30 N ? **(2017)**

(a) 0.25rads^{-2} (b) 25rads^{-2}

(c) 5 m s^{-2} (d) 25 m s^{-2}

66. A uniform circular disc of radius 50 cm at rest is free to turn about an axis which is perpendicular to its plane and passes through its centre. It is subjected to a torque which produces a constant angular acceleration of 2.0rads^{-2}. Its net acceleration in ms^{-2} at the end of 2.0 s is approximately **(NEET-I 2016)**

(a) 6.0 (b) 3.0

(c) 8.0 (d) 7.0

67. Point masses m_1 and m_2 are placed at the opposite ends of a rigid rod of length L, and negligible mass. The rod is to be set rotating about an axis perpendicular to it.

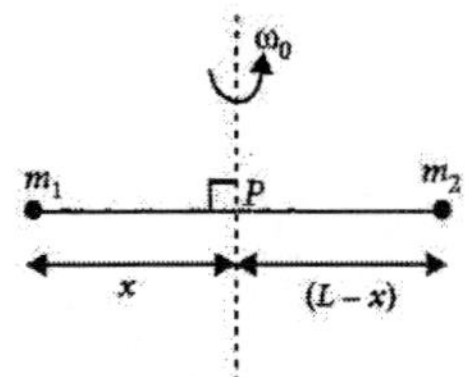

The position of point P on this rod through which the axis should pass so that the work required to set the rod rotating with angular velocity ω_0 is minimum, is given by **(2015)**

(a) $x = \frac{m_2}{m_1} L$ (b) $x = \frac{m_2 L}{m_1+m_2}$

(c) $x = \frac{m_1 L}{m_1+m_2}$ (d) $x = \frac{m_1}{m_2} L$

68. An automobile moves on a road with a speed of 54 km h^{-1}. The radius of its wheels is 0.45 m and the moment of inertia of the wheel about its axis of rotation is 3 kg m^2. If the vehicle is brought to rest in 15 s, the magnitude of average torque transmitted by its brakes to the wheel is **(2015)**

(a) 10.86 kg m^2 s^{-2}

(b) 2.86 kg m^2 s^{-2}

(c) 6.66 kg m^2 s^{-2}

(d) 8.58 kg m^2 s^{-2}

69. A solid cylinder of mass 50 kg and radius 0.5 m is free to rotate about the horizontal axis. A massless string is wound round the cylinder with one end attached to it and other hanging freely. Tension in the string required to produce an angular acceleration of 2 revolutions s^{-2} is **(2014)**

(a) 25 N (b) 50 N

(c) 78.5 N (d) 157 N

70. A rod PQ of mass M and length L is hinged at end P. The rod is kept horizontal by a massless string tied to point Q as shown in figure. When string is cut, the

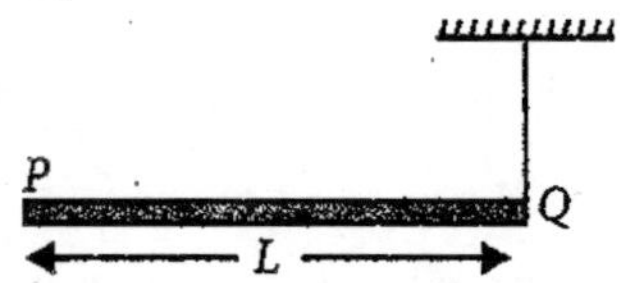

initial angular acceleration of the rod is **(2013)**

(a) $\frac{2g}{L}$ (b) $\frac{2g}{2L}$ (c) $\frac{3g}{2L}$ (d) $\frac{g}{L}$

71. The instantaneous angular position of a point on a rotating wheel is given by the equation $\theta(t) = 2t^3 - 6t^2$. The torque on the wheel becomes zero at **(2011)**

(a) $t = 1$ s (b) $t = 0.5$ s

(c) $t = 0.25$ s (d) $t = 2$ s

72. A uniform rod AB of length l and mass m is free to rotate about point A. The rod is released from rest in the horizontal position. Given that the moment of inertia of the rod about A is $ml^2/3$, the initial angular acceleration of the rod will be **(2007,2006)**

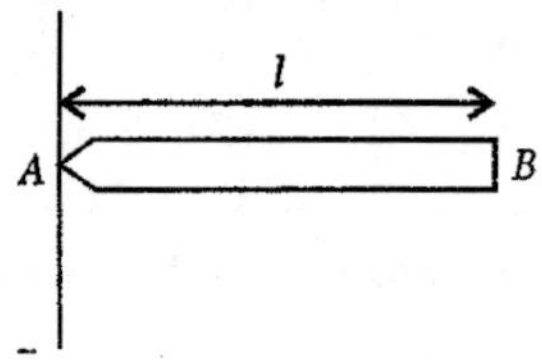

(a) $\frac{mgl}{2}$ (b) $\frac{3}{2}gl$

(c) $\frac{3g}{2l}$ (d) $\frac{2g}{3l}$

73. A wheel having moment of inertia 2 kg m^2 about its vertical axis, rotates at the rate of 60rpm about this axis. The torque which can stop the wheel's rotation in one minute would be **(2004)**

(a) $\frac{2\pi}{15}$ Nm (b) $\frac{\pi}{12}$ N m

(c) $\frac{\pi}{15}$ N m (d) $\frac{\pi}{18}$ N m

74. The moment of inertia of a body about a given axis is 1.2 kg m^2. Initially, the body is at rest. In order to produce a rotational kinetic energy of 1500 joule, an angular acceleration of 25radian/ $\sec^2$ must be applied about that axis for a duration of (1990)

(a) 4 s (b) 2 s

(c) 8 s (d) 10 s

Angular Momentum in case of Rotation about a Fixed Axis

75. A solid sphere is rotating freely about its symmetry axis in free space. The radius of the sphere is increased keeping its mass same. Which of the following physical quantities would remain constant for the sphere? **(2018)**

(a) Angular velocity.

(b) Moment of inertia.

(c) Rotational kinetic energy.

(d) Angular momentum.

76. Two discs of same moment of inertia rotating about their regular axis passing through centre and perpendicular to the plane of disc has angular velocities ω_1 and ω_2. They are brought into contact face to face coinciding the axis of rotation. The expression for loss of energy during this process is **(2017)**

(a) $\frac{1}{4}I(\omega_1 - \omega_2)^2$

(b) $I(\omega_1 - \omega_2)^2$

(c) $\frac{1}{8}I(\omega_1 - \omega_2)^2$

(d) $\frac{1}{2}I(\omega_1 + \omega_2)^2$

77. Two rotating bodies A and B of masses m and $2m$ with moments of inertia I_A and $I_B(I_B > I_A)$ have equal kinetic energy of rotation. If L_A and L_B be their angular momenta respectively, then **(NEET-II 2016)**

(a) $L_A = \frac{L_B}{2}$ (b) $L_A = 2L_B$

(c) $L_B > L_A$ (d) $L_A > L_B$

78. Two discs are rotating about their axes, normal to the discs and passing through the centres of the discs. Disc D_1 has 2 kg mass and 0.2 m radius and initial angular velocity of 50rads^{-1}. Disc D_2 has 4 kg mass, 0.1 m radius and initial angular velocity of 200rads^{-1}. The two discs are brought in contact face to face, with their axes of rotation coincident. The final angular velocity (in rads^{-1}) of the system is **(Karnataka NEET 2013)**

(a) 60 (b) 100
(c) 120 (d) 40

79. A circular platform is mounted on a frictionless vertical axle. Its radius $R = 2$ m and its moment of inertia about the axle is 200 kg m^2. It is initially at rest. A 50 kg man stands on the edge of the platform and begins to walk along the edge at the speed of 1 m s^{-1} relative to the ground. Time taken by the man to complete one revolution is

(Mains 2012)

(a) πs (b) $3\pi/2$ s
(c) 2πs (d) $\pi/2$ s

80. A circular disk of moment of inertia I_t is rotating in a horizontal plane, about its symmetry axis, with a constant angular speed ω_i. Another disk of moment of inertia I_b is dropped coaxially onto the rotating disk. Initially the second disk has zero angular speed. Eventually both the disks rotate with a constant angular speed ω_f. The energy lost by the initially rotating disc to friction is

(2010)

(a) $\frac{1}{2}\frac{I_b^2}{(I_t+I_b)}\omega_i^2$ (b) $\frac{1}{2}\frac{I_t^2}{(I_t+I_b)}\omega_i^2$

(c) $\frac{I_b-I_t}{(I_t+I_b)}\omega_i^2$ (d) $\frac{1}{2}\frac{I_bI_t}{(I_t+I_b)}\omega_i^2$

81. A thin circular ring of mass M and radius r is rotating about its axis with constant angular velocity ω. Two objects each of mass m are attached gently to the opposite ends of a diameter of the ring. The ring now rotates with angular velocity given by

(Mains 2010, 1998)

(a) $\frac{(M+2m)\omega}{2m}$ (b) $\frac{2M\omega}{M+2m}$

(c) $\frac{(M+2m)\omega}{M}$ (d) $\frac{M\omega}{M+2m}$

82. A round disc of moment of inertia I_2 about its axis perpendicular to its plane and passing through its centre is placed over another disc of moment of inertia I_1 rotating with an angular velocity ω about the same axis. The final angular velocity of the combination of discs is

(2004)

(a) $\frac{I_2\omega}{I_1+I_2}$ (b) ω

(c) $\frac{I_1\omega}{I_1+I_2}$ (d) $\frac{(I_1+I_2)\omega}{I_1}$

83. A thin circular ring of mass M and radius r is rotating about its axis with a constant angular velocity ω. Four objects each of mass m, are kept gently to the opposite ends of two perpendicular diameters of the ring. The angular velocity of the ring will be

(2003)

(a) $\frac{M\omega}{4m}$ (b) $\frac{M\omega}{M+4m}$

(c) $\frac{(M+4m)\omega}{M}$ (d) $\frac{(M-4m)\omega}{M+4m}$

84. A disc is rotating with angular speed ω. If a child sits on it, what is conserved?

(2002)

(a) linear momentum.

(b) angular momentum.

(c) kinetic energy.

(d) potential energy.

Rolling Motion

85. A disc of radius 2 m and mass 100 kg rolls on a horizontal floor. Its centre of mass has speed of 20 cm/s. How much work is needed to stop it ? **(2019)**

(a) 1 J (b) 3 J

(c) 30 kJ (d) 2 J

86. A solid cylinder of mass 2 kg and radius 50 cm rolls up an inclined plane of angle inclination 30°. The centre of mass of cylinder has speed of 4 m/s. The distance travelled by the cylinder on the incline surface will be (Take $g = 10\ m/s^2$) **(Odisha NEET 2019)**

(a) 2.2 m (b) 1.6 m

(c) 1.2 m (d) 2.4 m

87. A solid sphere is in rolling motion. In rolling motion a body possesses translational kinetic energy (K_t) as well as rotational kinetic energy (K_r) simultaneously. The ratio $K_t : (K_t + K_r)$ for the sphere is **(2018, 1991)**

(a) 7: 10 (b) 5: 7

(c) 10: 7 (d) 2: 5

88. A disc and a sphere of same radius but different masses roll off on two inclined planes of the same altitude and length. Which one of the two objects gets to the bottom of the plane first? **(NEET-I 2016)**

(a) Both reach at the same time

(b) Depends on their masses

(c) Disc

(d) Sphere

89. The ratio of the accelerations for a solid sphere (mass m and radius R) rolling down an incline of angle θ without slipping and slipping down the incline without rolling is **(2014)**

(a) 5: 7 (b) 2: 3

(c) 2: 5 (d) 7: 5

90. A small object of uniform density rolls up a curved surface with an initial velocity ' v '. It reaches upto a maximum height of $\frac{3v^2}{4g}$ with respect to the initial position. The object is **(2013)**

(a) hollow sphere (b) disc

(c) ring (d) solid sphere.

91. A solid cylinder of mass 3 kg is rolling on a horizontal surface with velocity $4\ m\ s^{-1}$. It collides with a horizontal spring of force constant $200\ N\ m^{-1}$. The maximum compression produced in the spring will be **(2012)**

(a) 0.5 m (b) 0.6 m

(c) 0.7 m (d) 0.2 m

92. A solid cylinder and a hollow cylinder, both of the same mass and same external diameter are released from the same height at the same time on an inclined plane. Both roll down without slipping. Which one will reach the bottom first? **(Mains 2010)**

(a) Both together only when angle of inclination of plane is 45°.

(b) Both together.

(c) Hollow cylinder.

(d) Solid cylinder

93. A drum of radius R and mass M, rolls down without slipping along an inclined plane of angle θ. The frictional force **(2005)**

(a) dissipates energy as heat

(b) decreases the rotational motion

(c) decreases the rotational and translational motion

(d) converts translational energy to rotational energy.

94. A ball rolls without slipping. The radius of gyration of the ball about an axis passing through its centre of mass is K. If radius of the ball be R, then the fraction of total energy associated with its rotational energy will be **(2003)**

(a) $\frac{K^2+R^2}{R^2}$ (b) $\frac{K^2}{R^2}$

(c) $\frac{K^2}{K^2+R^2}$ (d) $\frac{R^2}{K^2+R^2}$

95. A solid cylinder of mass M and radius R rolls without slipping down an inclined plane of length L and height h. What is the speed of its centre of mass when the cylinder reaches its bottom? **(2003,1989)**

(a) $\sqrt{2gh}$ (b) $\sqrt{\frac{3}{4}gh}$

(c) $\sqrt{\frac{4}{3}gh}$ (d) $\sqrt{4gh}$

96. Consider a contact point P of a wheel on ground which rolls on ground without slipping. Then value of displacement of point P when wheel completes half of rotation (If radius of wheel is 1 m) **(2002)**

(a) 2 m (b) $\sqrt{\pi^2+4}$ m

(c) πm (d) $\sqrt{\pi^2+2}$ m

97. A solid sphere of radius R is placed on a smooth horizontal surface. A horizontal force F is applied at height h from the lowest point. For the maximum acceleration of centre of mass, which is correct? **(2002)**

(a) $h = R$

(b) $h = 2R$

(c) $h = 0$

(d) no relation between h and R.

98. A disc is rolling, the velocity of its centre of mass is v_{cm}. Which one will be correct? **(2001)**

(a) The velocity of highest point is $2v_{cm}$ and at point of contact is zero.

(b) The velocity of highest point is v_{cm} and at point of contact is v_{cm}.

(c) The velocity of highest point is $2v_{cm}$ and point of contact is v_{cm}.

(d) The velocity of highest point is $2v_{cm}$ and point of contact is $2v_{cm}$.

99. A solid spherical ball rolls on a table. Ratio of its rotational kinetic energy to total kinetic energy is **(1994)**

(a) ½ (b) 1/6

(c) 7/10 (d) 2/7

100. A solid sphere, disc and solid cylinder all of the same mass and radius are allowed to roll down (from rest) on the inclined plane, then **(1993)**

(a) solid sphere reaches the bottom first

(b) solid sphere reaches the bottom last

(c) disc will reach the bottom first

(d) all reach the bottom at the same time.

101. The speed of a homogenous solid sphere after rolling down an inclined plane of vertical height h from rest without sliding is **(1992)**

(a) $\sqrt{\frac{10}{7}gh}$ (b) $\sqrt{gh}$

(c) $\sqrt{\frac{6}{5}gh}$ (d) $\sqrt{\frac{4}{3}gh}$

102. A solid homogenous sphere of mass M and radius is moving on a rough horizontal surface, partly rolling and partly sliding. During this kind of motion of the sphere **(1988)**

(a) total kinetic energy is conserved

(b) the angular momentum of the sphere about the point of contact with the plane is conserved

(c) only the rotational kinetic energy about the centre of mass is conserved

(d) angular momentum about the centre of mass is conserved.

ANSWER KEY

1.	**(b)**	**2.**	**(c)**	**3.**	**(a)**	**4.**	**(a)**	**5.**	**(b)**	**6.**	**(d)**
7.	**(d)**	**8.**	**(c)**	**9.**	**(b)**	**10.**	**(b)**	**11.**	**(c)**	**12.**	**(d)**
13.	**(d)**	**14.**	**(a)**	**15.**	**(c)**	**16.**	**(b)**	**17.**	**(c)**	**18.**	**(d)**
19.	**(c)**	**20.**	**(a)**	**21.**	**(a)**	**22.**	**(d)**	**23.**	**(b)**	**24.**	**(a)**
25.	**(c)**	**26.**	**(d)**	**27.**	**(a)**	**28.**	**(a)**	**29.**	**(*)**	**30.**	**(b)**
31.	**(a)**	**32.**	**(a)**	**33.**	**(b)**	**34.**	**(c)**	**35.**	**(d)**	**36.**	**(*)**
37.	**(b)**	**38.**	**(a)**	**39.**	**(a)**	**40.**	**(d)**	**41.**	**(c)**	**42.**	**(c)**
43.	**(a)**	**44.**	**(b)**	**45.**	**(d)**	**46.**	**(d)**	**47.**	**(c)**	**48.**	**(a)**
49.	**(b)**	**50.**	**(b)**	**51.**	**(d)**	**52.**	**(b)**	**53.**	**(a)**	**54.**	**(b)**
55.	**(d)**	**56.**	**(d)**	**57.**	**(d)**	**58.**	**(c)**	**59.**	**(a)**	**60.**	**(c)**
61.	**(b)**	**62.**	**(a)**	**63.**	**(b)**	**64.**	**(a)**	**65.**	**(b)**	**66.**	**(c)**
67.	**(b)**	**68.**	**(c)**	**69.**	**(d)**	**70.**	**(c)**	**71.**	**(a)**	**72.**	**(c)**
73.	**(c)**	**74.**	**(b)**	**75.**	**(d)**	**76.**	**(a)**	**77.**	**(c)**	**78.**	**(b)**
79.	**(c)**	**80.**	**(d)**	**81.**	**(d)**	**82.**	**(c)**	**83.**	**(b)**	**84.**	**(b)**
85.	**(b)**	**86.**	**(d)**	**87.**	**(b)**	**88.**	**(d)**	**89.**	**(a)**	**90.**	**(b)**
91.	**(b)**	**92.**	**(d)**	**93.**	**(d)**	**94.**	**(c)**	**95.**	**(c)**	**96.**	**(b)**
97.	**(b)**	**98.**	**(a)**	**99.**	**(d)**	**100.**	**(a)**	**101.**	**(a)**	**102.**	**(b)**

Hints & Explanations

1. **(b) :**

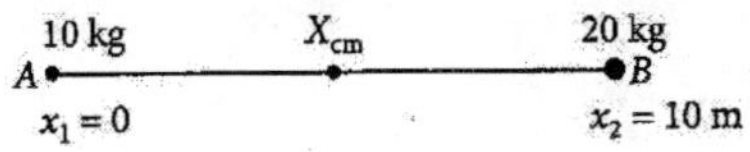

Masses, $m_1 = 10$ kg and $m_2 = 20$ kg

Let the distance between the two masses is = 10 m.

Now, centre of masses for two particle system is written as,

$$X_{COM} = \frac{m_1x_1 + m_2x_2}{m_1 + m_2}$$

Considering point A as origin, so $B = (d, 0)$

$$X_{COM} = \left(\frac{m_1 \times 0 + m_2 d}{m_1 + m_2}\right) = \frac{m_2 d}{m_1 + m_2}$$

$$X_{COM} = \frac{20 \text{ kg} \times 10 \text{ m}}{10 \text{ kg} + 20 \text{ kg}} = \frac{20}{3} \text{ m}$$

2. **(c) :** Given: $m_1 = 5$ kg, $m_2 = 10$ kg and $L = 1$ m

Here center of mass, $X_{cm} = \frac{m_1x_1+m_2x_2}{m_1+m_2}$

$$= \frac{5 \times 0 + 10 \times 1}{15} = \frac{10}{15} = \frac{2}{3}$$

$$= 0.666 \text{ m}; 0.67 \text{ m}$$

$$= 67 \text{ cm}$$

3. **(a) :**

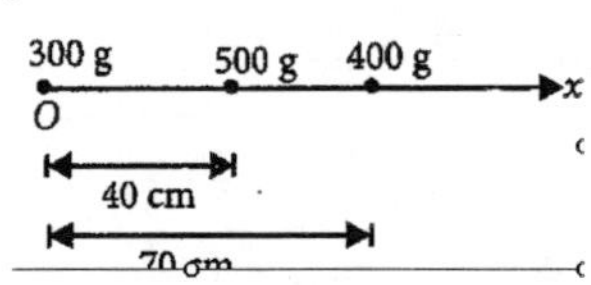

The distance of the centre of mass of the system of three masses from the origin O is

$$X_{CM} = \frac{m_1x_1 + m_2x_2 + m_3x_3}{m_1 + m_2 + m_3}$$

$$= \frac{300 \times 0 + 500 \times 40 + 400 \times 70}{300 + 500 + 400}$$

$$= \frac{500 \times 40 + 400 \times 70}{1200} = \frac{400[50 + 70]}{1200}$$

$$= \frac{50 + 70}{3} = \frac{120}{3} = 40 \text{ cm}$$

4. **(a) :** $\vec{r}_1 = \hat{\imath} + 2\hat{\jmath} + \hat{k}$ for $M_1 = 1$ kg

$\vec{r}_2 = -3\hat{\imath} - 2\hat{\jmath} + \hat{k}$ for $M_2 = 3$ kg

$$r_{C.M.} = \frac{\sum m_i r_i}{\sum m_i}$$

$\Rightarrow r_{C.M.}$

$$= \frac{(1\hat{\imath} + 2\hat{\jmath} + 1\hat{k}) \times 1 + (-3\hat{\imath} - 2\hat{\jmath} + \hat{k}) \times 3}{4}$$

$$\Rightarrow r_{C.M.} = \frac{-8\hat{\imath} - 4\hat{\jmath} + 4\hat{k}}{4} = -2\hat{\imath} - \hat{\jmath} + \hat{k}.$$

5. **(b) :** C.M. $= \frac{m_1x_1+m_2x_2}{m_1+m_2}$

After changing position of m_1 and to keep the position of C.M. same

$$\text{C.M.} = \frac{m_1(x_1 - d) + m_2(x_2 + d_2)}{m_1 + m_2}$$

$0 = \frac{-m_1d+m_2d_2}{m_1+m_2}$ [Substituting value of C.M. from (i)]

$$\Rightarrow d_2 = \frac{m_1}{m_2} d$$

6. **(d)** : Centre of mass of each ball lies on the centre.

⇒ centre of mass of combined body will be at the centroid of equilateral triangle.

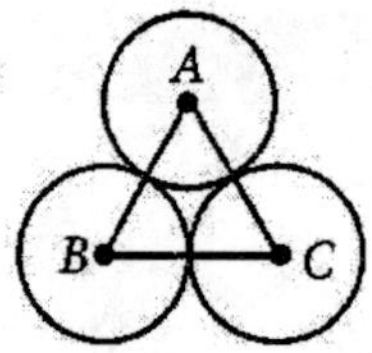

7. **(d)** : The resultant of all forces, on any system of particles, is zero. Therefore their centre of mass does not depend upon the forces acting on the particles.

8. **(c)** : As no external force acts on the system, therefore centre of mass will not shift.

9. **(b)** : As no external force is acting on the system, the centre of mass must be at rest i.e. $v_{CM} = 0$.

10. **(b)** : Since the man is in gravity free space, force on man + stone system is zero.

Therefore centre of mass of the system remains at rest. Let the man goes x m above when the stone reaches the floor, then

$$M_{man} \times x = M_{stone} \times 10$$

$$x = \frac{0.5}{50} \times 10 \text{ or } x = 0.1 \text{ m}$$

Therefore final height of man above floor

$= 10 + x$

$= 10 + 0.1 = 10.1$ m

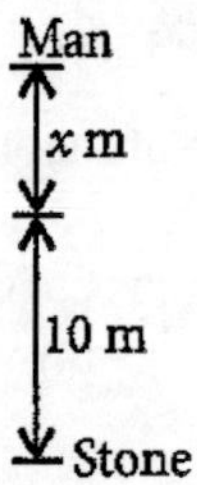

11. **(c)** : given $\vec{A}\cdot\vec{B}=0$

$\Rightarrow \vec{A} \perp \vec{B} \quad \theta = 90^\circ$ [angle Between A and

$\vec{A}\cdot\vec{C}=0$

$\vec{A} \perp \vec{C} \quad \phi = 90^\circ$ [angle Between A and C]

i.e. A in perpendicular to Both B and C

$\vec{B}\times\vec{C} \rightarrow$ gives a vector which perpendicular to both $\vec{B}$

So $\vec{A}$ will be parallel to $\vec{B}\times\vec{C}$

12. **(d)**: $|\vec{A}\times\vec{B}| = \sqrt{3}(\vec{A}\cdot\vec{B})$

$\therefore AB\sin\theta = \sqrt{3}AB\cos\theta$

or, $\tan\theta = \sqrt{3}$ or, $\theta = \tan^{-1}\sqrt{3} = 60°$.

13. **(d)** : Let $\vec{A}\times\vec{B} = \vec{C}$

The cross product of $\vec{B}$ and $\vec{A}$ is perpendicular to the plane containing $\vec{A}$ and $\vec{B}$ i.e. perpendicular to $\vec{A}$.

Therefore product of $(\vec{B}\times\vec{A})\cdot\vec{A} = 0$.

14. **(a)** : $|\vec{A}\times\vec{B}| = \sqrt{3}\vec{A}\cdot\vec{B}$

$|\vec{A}||\vec{B}|\sin\theta = \sqrt{3}|\vec{A}||\vec{B}|\cos\theta$

$\tan\theta = \sqrt{3} \Rightarrow \theta = 60°$

$|\vec{A}+\vec{B}| = \sqrt{|\vec{A}|^2 + |\vec{B}|^2 + 2|\vec{A}||\vec{B}|\cos\theta}$

$= (A^2 + B^2 + AB)^{1/2}$

15. **(c)** : $\vec{A}\times 0$ is a zero vector.

16. **(b)** :

$$\vec{v} = \vec{\omega} \times \vec{r} = \begin{vmatrix} \hat{\imath} & \hat{\jmath} & \hat{k} \\ 5 & -6 & 6 \\ 3 & -4 & 1 \end{vmatrix} = 18\hat{\imath} + 13\hat{\jmath} - 2\hat{k}$$

17. **(c) :** Here, $\vec{F} = 3\hat{\jmath}$ N, $\vec{r} = 2\hat{k}$ m

Torque, $\vec{\tau} = \vec{r} \times \vec{F} = 2\hat{k} \times 3\hat{\jmath} = -6\hat{\imath}$ N m

18. **(d) :** Moment of the force is,

$\vec{\tau} = (\vec{r} - \vec{r}_0) \times \vec{F}$

Here, $\vec{r}_0 = 2\hat{\imath} - 2\hat{\jmath} - 2\hat{k}$

and $\vec{r} = 2\hat{\imath} + 0\hat{\jmath} - 3\hat{k}$

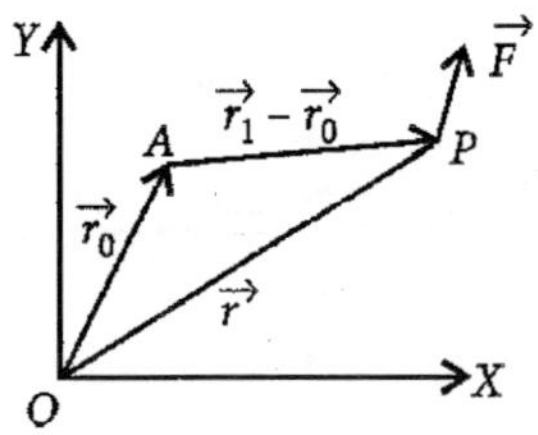

$\therefore \vec{r} - \vec{r}_0 = (2\hat{\imath} + 0\hat{\jmath} - 3\hat{k}) - (2\hat{\imath} - 2\hat{\jmath} - 2\hat{k}) = 0\hat{\imath} + 2\hat{\jmath} - \hat{k}$

$$\therefore \vec{\tau} = \begin{vmatrix} \hat{\imath} & \hat{\jmath} & \hat{k} \\ 0 & 2 & -1 \\ 4 & 5 & -6 \end{vmatrix} = -7\hat{\imath} - 4\hat{\jmath} - 8\hat{k}$$

19. **(c) :** For the conservation of angular momentum about origin, the torque $\vec{\tau}$ acting on the particle will be zero.

By definition, $\vec{\tau} = \vec{r} \times \vec{F}$

Here, $\vec{r} = 2\hat{\imath} - 6\hat{\jmath} - 12\hat{k}$ and $\vec{F} = \alpha\hat{\imath} + 3\hat{\jmath} + 6\hat{k}$

$$\therefore \vec{\tau} = \begin{vmatrix} \hat{\imath} & \hat{\jmath} & \hat{k} \\ 2 & -6 & -12 \\ \alpha & 3 & 6 \end{vmatrix}$$

$= \hat{\imath}(-36 + 36) - \hat{\jmath}(12 + 12\alpha) + \hat{k}(6 + 6\alpha)$

$= -\hat{\jmath}(12 + 12\alpha) + \hat{k}(6 + 6\alpha)$

But $\vec{\tau} = 0$

$\therefore 12 + 12\alpha = 0$ or $\alpha = -1$

and $6 + 6\alpha = 0$ or $\alpha = -1$

20. **(a) :** According to law of conservation of angular momentum

$mvr = mv'r'$

$v_0 R_0 = v\left(\frac{R_0}{2}\right); v = 2v_0$

$\therefore \frac{K_0}{K} = \frac{\frac{1}{2}mv_0^2}{\frac{1}{2}mv^2} = \left(\frac{v_0}{v}\right)^2$

or $\frac{K}{K_0} = \left(\frac{v}{v_0}\right)^2 = (2)^2$

$K = 4K_0 = 2mv_0^2$

21. **(a) :** When a mass is rotating in a plane about a fixed point its angular momentum is directed along a line perpendicular to the plane of rotation.

22. **(d)**

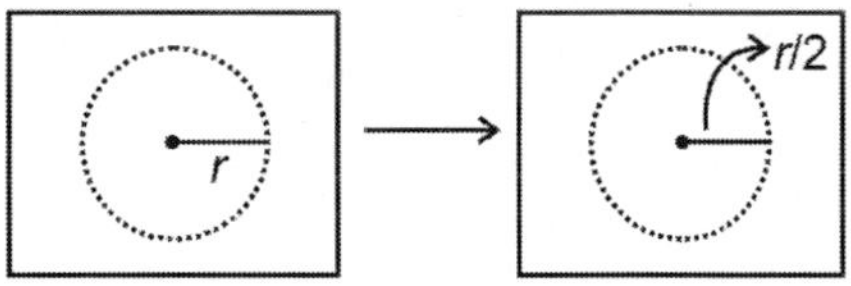

Let initial angular momentum = m v r

final angular momentum $= mv'\frac{r}{2}$

No External force/Torque angular momentum in conserved.

$mvr = mv'\frac{r}{2}$

$\boxed{v' = 2v}$

K.E. initial $= \frac{1}{2}mv^2$

$k_1 = \frac{1}{2}mv^2$

K.E final $= \frac{1}{2}mv'^2$

$$K_2 \Rightarrow \frac{1}{2} m \times (2v)^2 \Rightarrow 4 \times \frac{1}{2} mv^2$$

$$\boxed{K_2 = 4k_1}$$

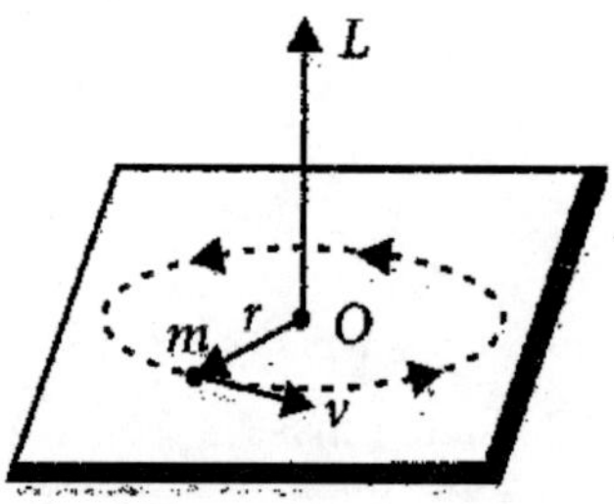

23. **(b) :** Torque is always perpendicular to $\vec{F}$ as well as $\vec{r}$. $\vec{r} \cdot \vec{\tau} = 0$ as well as $\vec{F} \cdot \vec{\tau} = 0$.

24. **(a)**

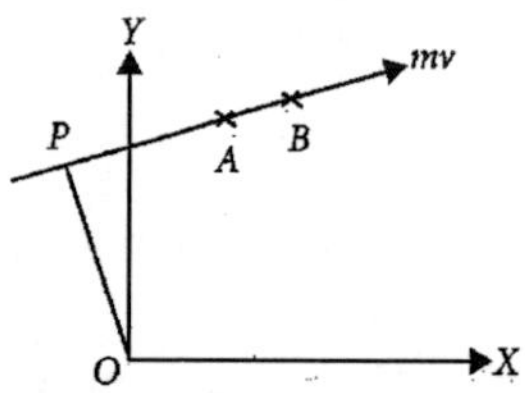

Moment of linear momentum is angular momentum. OP is the same whether the mass is at A or B.

$\therefore L_A = L_B$.

25. **(c)**

26. **(d) :** Force $(\vec{F}) = -3\hat{\imath} + \hat{\jmath} + 5\hat{k}$ and distance of the point $(\vec{r}) = 7\hat{\imath} + 3\hat{\jmath} + \hat{k}$

Torque $\vec{\tau} = \vec{r} \times \vec{F} = \begin{vmatrix} \hat{\imath} & \hat{\jmath} & \hat{k} \\ 7 & 3 & 1 \\ -3 & 1 & 5 \end{vmatrix} = 14\hat{\imath} - 38\hat{\jmath} + 16\hat{k}$

27. **(a) :** $\vec{L} = \vec{r} \times \vec{p}$

$y = x + 4$ line has been shown in the figure.

When $x = 0$,

$y = 4$, So $OP = 4$.

The slope of the line can be obtained by comparing with the equation of line

$$y = mx + c$$

$$m = \tan\theta = 1 \Rightarrow \theta = 45°$$

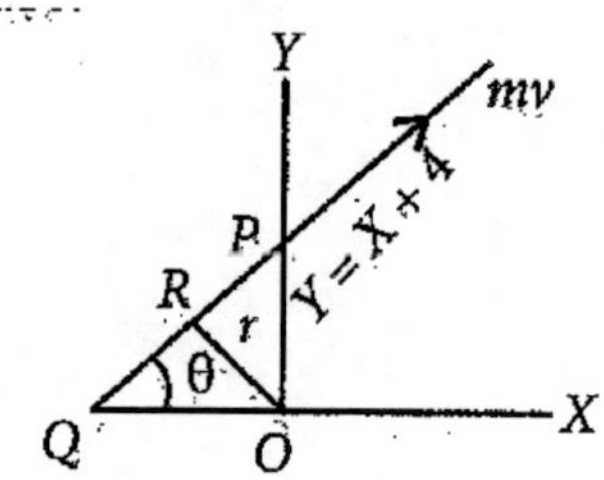

$\angle OQP = \angle OPQ = 45°$

If we draw a line perpendicular to this line.

Length of the perpendicular $= OR$

$$\Rightarrow OR = OP\sin 45° = 4\frac{1}{\sqrt{2}} = \frac{4}{\sqrt{2}} = 2\sqrt{2}$$

Angular momentum of particle going along this line

$$= r \times mv = 2\sqrt{2} \times 5 \times 3\sqrt{2} = 60 \text{ units}$$

28. **(a) :** Here, $AD = 20$ cm

$AE = 160$ cm

$g = 10 \text{ m/s}^2$

Take moments about C

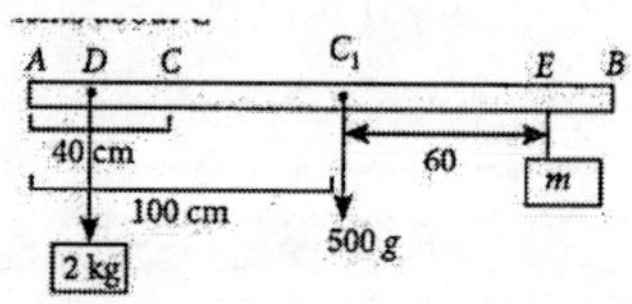

Clockwise moment = Anticlockwise moment

$$2 \times g \times DC = 0.50 \times g \times CC_1 + m \times g \times CE$$

or $2 \times (40 - 20) = 0.500(100 - 40) + m \times (60 + 60)$

or $40 - 30 = 120$ m

or $m = \frac{1}{12}$ kg

29. **(*)** : Centre of gravity of a body is the point at which the total gravitational torque on body is zero. Centre of mass and centre of gravity coincides only for symmetrical bodies.

Hence statements (1) and (2) are incorrect.

A couple of a body produces rotational motion only. Hence statement (3) is incorrect.

Mechanical advantage is greater than one means that the system will require a force that is less than the load in order to move it. Hence statement (4) is correct.

30. **(b)** : Given situation is shown in figure.

N_1 = Normal reaction on A

N_2 = Normal reaction on B

W = Weight of the rod

In vertical equilibrium,

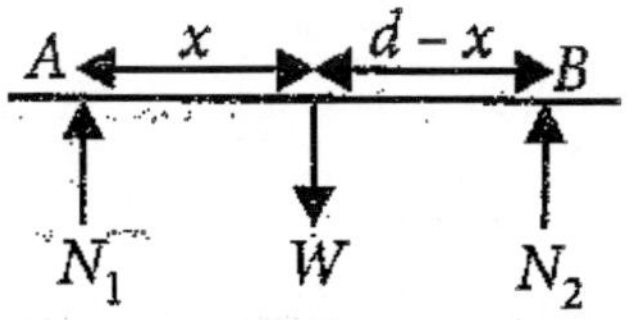

$$N_1 + N_2 = W$$

Torque balance about centre of mass of the rod,

$$N_1 x = N_2(d - x)$$

Putting value of N_2 from equation (i)

$$N_1 x = (W - N_1)(d - x) \Rightarrow N_1 x = Wd - Wx - N_1 d + N_1 x$$

$$\Rightarrow N_1 d = W(d - x); \therefore N_1 = \frac{W(d - x)}{d}$$

31. **(a)** : Let x be the perpendicular distance of centre O of equilateral triangle from each side.

Total torque about $O = 0$

$\Rightarrow F_1 x + F_2 x - F_3 x = 0$ or $F_3 = F_1 + F_2$

32. **(a)** : Conceptual

33. **(b)** : Let us consider an elementary length dx at a distance x from one end.

Its mass $= k \cdot x \cdot dx$

[k = proportionality constant]

Then centre of gravity of the rod x_c is given by

$$x_c = \frac{\int_0^3 kxdx \cdot x}{\int_0^3 kxdx} = \frac{\int_0^3 x^2 dx}{\int_0^3 xdx} = \frac{\left.\frac{x^3}{3}\right|_0^3}{\left.\frac{x^2}{2}\right|_0^3}$$

or $x_c = \frac{27/3}{9/2} = 2.$

$\therefore$ Centre of gravity of the rod will be at distance of 2 m from one end.

34. **(c)** : Load $W = Mg = 75 \times 10 = 750$ N

Effort $P = 250$ N

$\therefore$ Mechanical advantage

$$= \frac{\text{load}}{\text{effort}} = \frac{W}{P} = \frac{750}{250} = 3$$

Velocity ratio

$$= \frac{\text{distance travelled by effort}}{\text{distance travelled by load}} = \frac{12}{3} = 4$$

Efficiency, $\eta = \frac{\text{Mechanical advantage}}{\text{Velocity ratio}} =$ $(3/4) \times 100 = 75\%$.

35. **(d)** : Couple produces rotational motion

36. **(*)** :

Radius of gyration : $K = \sqrt{\frac{I}{m}}$

$$\frac{k_{\text{solid sphere}}}{k_{\text{hollow sphere}}} = \sqrt{\frac{2mR^2/5m}{2mR^2/3m}} = \sqrt{3}:\sqrt{5}$$

37. **(b)** : $\frac{E_{\text{Sphere}}}{E_{\text{Cylinder}}} = \frac{\frac{1}{2}I_s\omega_s^2}{\frac{1}{2}I_c\omega_c^2} = \frac{I_s\omega_s^2}{I_c\omega_c^2}$

Here, $I_s = \frac{2}{5}MR^2, I_c = \frac{1}{2}MR^2, \omega_c = 2\omega_s$

$$\frac{E_{\text{Sphere}}}{E_{\text{Cylinder}}} = \frac{\frac{2}{5}mR^2 \times \omega_s^2}{\frac{1}{2}mR^2 \times (2\omega_s)^2} = \frac{4}{5} \times \frac{1}{4} = \frac{1}{5}$$

38. **(a)** : Here, $l_1 + l_2 = l$

Centre of mass of the system,

$$l_1 = \frac{m_1 \times 0 + m_2 \times l}{m_1 + m_2} = \frac{m_2 l}{m_1 + m_2}$$

$$= l_2 = l - l_1 = \frac{m_1 l}{m_1 + m_2}$$

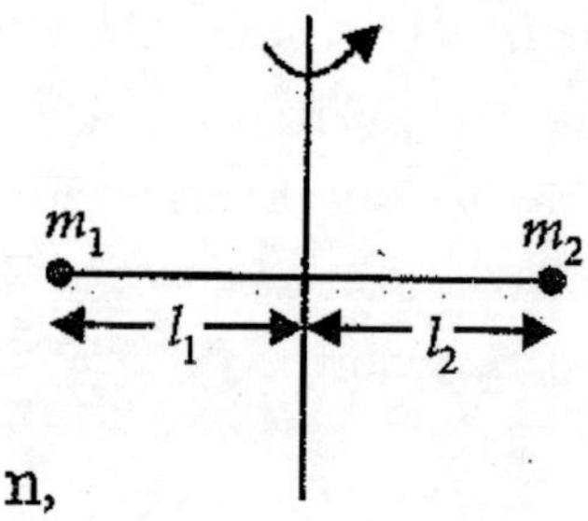

n,

Required moment of inertia of the system,

$$I = m_1 l_1^2 + m_2 l_2^2$$

$$= (m_1 m_2^2 + m_2 m_1^2)\frac{l^2}{(m_1 + m_2)^2}$$

$$= \frac{m_1 m_2 (m_1 + m_2) l^2}{(m_1 + m_2)^2} = \frac{m_1 m_2}{m_1 + m_2} l^2$$

39. **(a)** : Mass of the disc $= 9M$ Mass of removed portion of disc $= M$

The moment of inertia of the complete disc about an axis passing through its centre O and perpendicular to its plane is $I_1 = \frac{9}{2}MR^2$

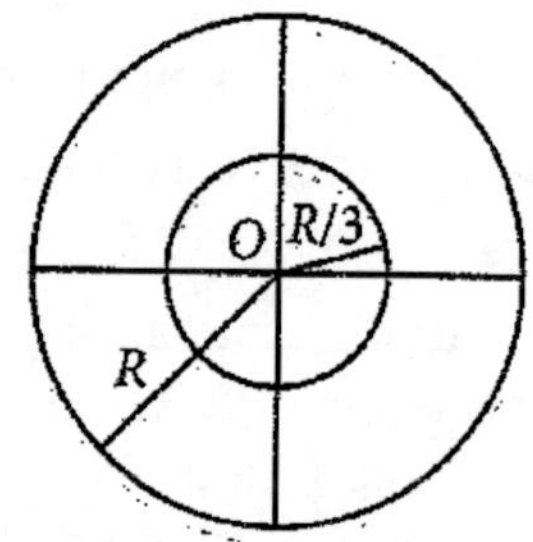

Now, the moment of inertia of the removed portion of the disc

$$I_2 = \frac{1}{2}M\left(\frac{R}{3}\right)^2 = \frac{1}{18}MR^2$$

Therefore, moment of inertia of the remaining portion of disc about O is

$$I = I_1 - I_2 = 9\frac{MR^2}{2} - \frac{MR^2}{18} = \frac{40MR^2}{9}$$

40. **(d)** : M.I. of a circular disc, $Mk^2 = \frac{M \cdot R^2}{2}$

M.I. of a circular ring $= MR^2$.

$\therefore$ Ratio of their radius of gyration $=$ $\frac{1}{\sqrt{2}} : 1 = 1 : \sqrt{2}$

41. **(c)** : K.E. $= \frac{1}{2}I\omega^2$

$\therefore \frac{1}{2}I\omega_1^2 = \frac{1}{2}\cdot 2I\omega_2^2; \frac{\omega_1^2}{\omega_2^2} = \frac{2}{1} \Rightarrow \frac{\omega_1}{\omega_2} = \frac{\sqrt{2}}{1}.$

42. **(c)** : The moment of inertia of the system

$= m_A r_A^2 + m_B r_B^2 + m_C r_C^2$

$= m_A(0)^2 + m(l)^2 + m(l\sin 30°)^2$

$= ml^2 + ml^2 \times (1/4) = (5/4)ml^2$

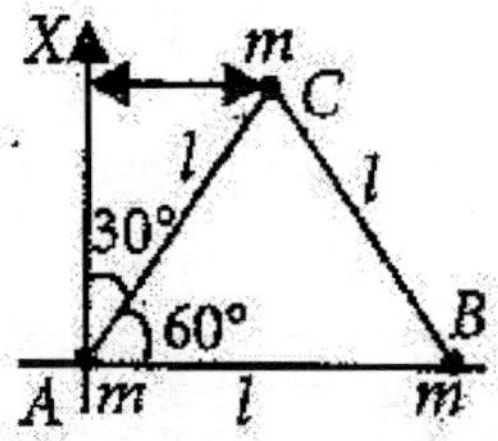

43. **(a)** : A circular disc may be divided into a large number of circular rings. Moment of inertia of the disc will be the summation of the moments of inertia of these rings about the geometrical axis. Now, moment of inertia of a circular ring about its geometrical axis is MR^2, where M is the mass and R is the radius of the ring.
Since the density (mass per unit volume) for iron is more than that of aluminium, the proposed rings made of iron should be placed at a higher radius to get more value of MR^2. Hence to get maximum moment of inertia for the circular disc, aluminium should be placed at interior and iron at the exterior position.

44. **(b)** : As effective distance of mass from BC is greater than the effective distance of mass from AB, therefore $I_2 > I_1$.

45. **(d)** : The intersection of medians is the centre of mass of the triangle. Since the distances of centre of mass from the sides is related as $x_{BC} < x_{AB} < x_{AC}$. Therefore $I_{BC} > I_{AB} > I_{AC}$ or $I_{BC} > I_{AB}$.

46. **(d)** : The moment of inertia is minimum about EG because mass distribution is at minimum distance from EG.

47. **(C)** :

$$\text{K.E.} = \frac{1}{2}I\omega^2$$

$$I = \frac{2\text{ K.E.}}{\omega^2} = \frac{2 \times 360}{30 \times 30} = 0.8 \text{ kg m}^2$$

48. **(a)** : Kinetic energy $= \frac{1}{2}I\omega^2$, and for ring $I = mr^2$.

Hence KE $= \frac{1}{2}mr^2\omega^2$

49. **(b)** : The radius of gyration of thin uniform disc about an axis passing through it centre and normal to its plane is,

$$k = \frac{R}{\sqrt{2}}$$

Radius of gyration of disc about its diametre is $k' = \frac{R}{2}$

Then, $\frac{k}{k'} = \frac{R}{\sqrt{2}} / \frac{R}{2} = \sqrt{2}:1$

50. **(b)** : Here: M is the mass and R is the radius of the ring. Moment of inertia of a ring, $I = MR^2$
If 90° sector is removed, the moment of inertia of the remaining part of ihe ring is

$$I = MR^2 - \frac{MR^2}{4}$$

$$\Rightarrow KMR^2 = \frac{3}{4}MR^2$$

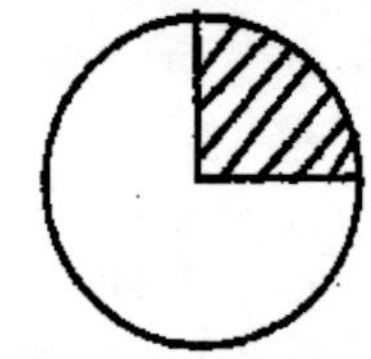

Here $K = \frac{3}{4}$

51. **(d) :** Mass per unit area of disc $= \frac{M}{\pi R^2}$
Mass of removed portion of disc,

$$M' = \frac{M}{\pi R^2} \times \pi \left(\frac{R}{2}\right)^2 = \frac{M}{4}$$

Moment of inertia of removed portion about an axis passing through centre of disc O and perpendicular to the plane of disc,

$$I'_O = I_{O'} + M'd^2$$
$$= \frac{1}{2} \times \frac{M}{4} \times \left(\frac{R}{2}\right)^2 + \frac{M}{4} \times \left(\frac{R}{2}\right)^2$$
$$= \frac{MR^2}{32} + \frac{MR^2}{16} = \frac{3MR^2}{32}$$

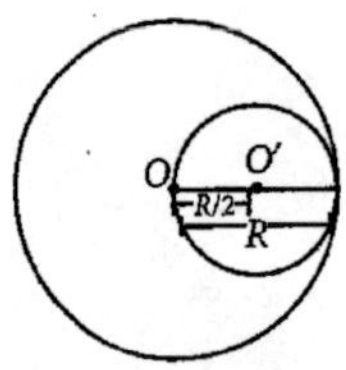

The moment of inertia of complete disc about centre O before removing the portion of the disc

$$I_O = \frac{1}{2} MR^2$$

So, moment of inertia of the disc with removed portion is

$$I = I_O - I'_O = \frac{1}{2} MR^2 - \frac{3MR^2}{32} = \frac{13MR^2}{32}$$

52. **(b) :** Net moment of inertia of the system,

$$I = I_1 + I_2 + I_3.$$

The moment of inertia of a shell about its diameter,

$$I_1 = \frac{2}{3} mr^2$$

The moment of inertia of a shell about its tangent is given by

$$I_2 = I_3 = I_1 + mr^2 = \frac{2}{3} mr^2 + mr^2$$
$$= \frac{5}{3} mr^2$$
$$\therefore I = 2 \times \frac{5}{3} mr^2 + \frac{2}{3} mr^2 = \frac{12mr^2}{3}$$
$$= 4mr^2$$

53. **(a) :** According to the theorem of parallel axes, $I = I_{CM} + Ma^2$
As a is maximum for point B. Therefore I is maximum about B.

54. **(b) :** According to the theorem of parallel axes, the moment of inertia of the thin rod of mass M and length L about an axis passing through one of the ends is

$$I = I_{CM} + Md^2$$

where I_{CM} is the moment of inertia of the given rod about an axis passing through its centre of mass and perpendicular to its length and d is the distance between two parallel axes.
Here, $I_{CM} = I_0, d = \frac{L}{2}$

$$\therefore I = I_0 + M\left(\frac{L}{2}\right)^2 = I_0 + \frac{ML^2}{4}$$

55. **(d) :** Moment of inertia for the rod AB rotating about an axis through the mid-point of AB perpendicular to the plane of the paper is $\frac{Ml^2}{12}$.

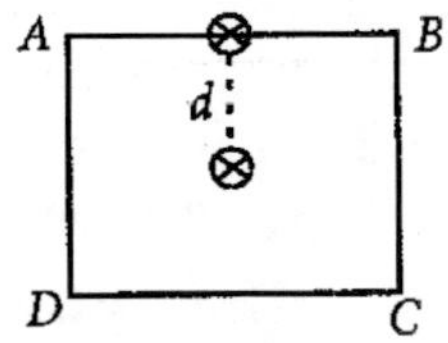

$\therefore$ Moment of inertia about the axis through the centre of the square and parallel to this axis,

$$I = I_0 + Md^2 = M\left(\frac{l^2}{12} + \frac{l^2}{4}\right) = \frac{Ml^2}{3}$$

For all the four rods, $I = \frac{4}{3}Ml^2$.

56. **(d)**

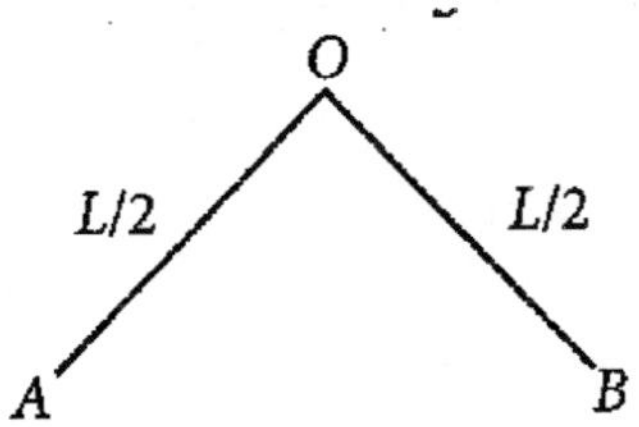

Total mass $= M$, total length $= L$
Moment of inertia of OA about O = Moment of inertia of OB about O

$\Rightarrow$ M.I. $_{\text{total}} = 2 \times \left(\frac{M}{2}\right)\left(\frac{L}{2}\right)^2 \cdot \frac{1}{3} = \frac{ML^2}{12}$

57. **(d)** : Moment of inertia of a uniform circular disc about an axis through its centre and perpendicular to its plane is $I_C = \frac{1}{2}MR^2$

$\therefore$ Moment of inertia of a uniform circular disc about an axis touching the disc at its diameter and normal to the disc is I. By the theorem of parallel axes,

$$I = I_C + Mh^2 = \frac{1}{2}MR^2 + MR^2 = \frac{3}{2}MR^2$$

58. **(c)** : Radius of gyration of disc about a tangential axis in the plane of disc is $\frac{\sqrt{5}}{2}R = K_1$, radius of gyration of circular ring of same radius about a tangential axis in the plane of circular ring is

$$K_2 = \sqrt{\frac{3}{2}}R \;\therefore \frac{K_1}{K_2} = \frac{\sqrt{5}}{\sqrt{6}}$$

59. **(a)** : Moment of inertia of a disc about its diameter $= \frac{1}{4}MR^2$
Using theorem of parallel axes, $I = \frac{1}{4}MR^2 + MR^2 = \frac{5}{4}MR^2$.

60. **(c)** : Moment of inertia of uniform circular disc about diameter $= I$
According to theorem of perpendicular axes.
Moment of inertia of disc about axis

$$= 2I = \frac{1}{2}mr^2$$

Using theorem of parallel axes,
Moment of inertia of disc about the given axis

$$= 2I + mr^2 = 2I + 4I = 6I$$

61. **(b)** : Initial angular speed,

$$\omega_0 = \frac{2\pi \times 1200}{60}\text{rads}^{-1} = 40\pi\text{rads}^{-1}$$

Final angular speed,

$$\omega = \frac{2\pi \times 3120}{60}\text{rads}^{-1} = 104\pi\text{rads}^{-1}$$

$\therefore$ Angular acceleration,

$$\alpha = \frac{\omega - \omega_0}{t} = \frac{104\pi - 40\pi}{16} = 4\pi\text{rads}^{-2}$$

62. **(a)** : Given: Angular acceleration, $\alpha = 3\text{rad/s}^2$

Initial angular velocity $\omega_i = 2\text{rad/s}$
Time $t = 2$ s

Using, $\theta = \omega_i t + \frac{1}{2}\alpha t^2$

$\therefore \theta = 2 \times 2 + \frac{1}{2} \times 3 \times 4 = 4 + 6 = 10$

radians

63. (b) : Given: Mass = 2 kg, Radius $R =$ 4 cm

Initial angular speed

$\omega_0 = 3\text{rpm} = 3 \times \frac{2\pi}{60}\text{rad/s} = \frac{\pi}{10}\text{rad/s}$

We know that, $\omega^2 = \omega_0{}^2 + 2\alpha\theta$

$\Rightarrow 0 = \left(\frac{\pi}{10}\right)^2 + 2 \times \alpha \times 2\pi \times 2\pi \Rightarrow \alpha$

$= \frac{-1}{800}\text{rad/s}^2$

Moment of inertia of a solid cylinder,

$I = \frac{MR^2}{2} = \frac{2 \times \left(\frac{4}{100}\right)^2}{2} = \frac{16}{10^4}$

Torque $\tau = I\alpha = \left(\frac{16}{10^4}\right) \times \left(-\frac{1}{800}\right) = -2 \times 10^{-6}\text{Nm}$

64. (a) : Work done required to bring a object to rest

$\Delta W = \Delta KE$

$\Delta W = \frac{1}{2}I\omega^2$; where $I =$ moment of inertia

For same $\omega, \Delta W \propto I$

For a solid sphere, $I_A = \frac{2}{5}MR^2$

For a thin circular disk, $I_B = \frac{1}{2}MR^2$

For a circular ring, $I_C = MR^2$

$\therefore I_C > I_B > I_A \therefore W_C > W_B > W_A$

65. (b) : Here, $m = 3$ kg, $r = 40$ cm $= 40 \times 10^{-2}$ m, $F = 30$ N Moment of inertia of hollow cylinder about its axis

$= mr^2 = 3\text{ kg} \times (0.4)^2\text{ m}^2 = 0.48\text{ kg m}^2$

The torque is given by, $\tau = I\alpha$

where $I =$ moment of inertia, $\alpha =$ angular acceleration In the given case, $\tau = rF$, as the force is acting perpendicularly to the radial vector.

$\therefore \alpha = \frac{\tau}{I} = \frac{Fr}{mr^2} = \frac{F}{mr} = \frac{30}{3 \times 40 \times 10^{-2}}$

$= \frac{30 \times 100}{3 \times 40}$

$\alpha = 25\text{rads}^{-2}$

66. (c) : Given, $r = 50$ cm $= 0.5$ m, $\alpha = 2.0\text{rads}^{-2}, \omega_0 = 0$

At the end of 2 s,

tangential acceleration, $a_t = r\alpha = 0.5 \times 2 = 1\text{ m s}^{-2}$

radial acceleration, $a_r = \omega^2 r = (\omega_0 + \alpha t)^2 r$

$= (0 + 2 \times 2)^2 \times 0.5 = 8\text{ m s}^{-2}$

$\therefore$ Net acceleration,

$a = \sqrt{a_t^2 + a_r^2} = \sqrt{1^2 + 8^2} = \sqrt{65}$

$\approx 8\text{ m s}^{-2}$

67. (b) : Moment of inertia of the system about the axis of rotation (through point) is

$I = m_1 x^2 + m_2(L - x)^2$

By work energy theorem,

Work done to set the rod rotating with angular velocity $\omega_0 =$ Increase in rotational kinetic energy

$$W=\frac{1}{2}I\omega_0^2=\frac{1}{2}[m_1x^2+m_2(L-x)^2]\omega_0^2$$

For W to be minimum, $\frac{dW}{dx}=0$

i.e. $\frac{1}{2}[2m_1x+2m_2(L-x)(-1)]\omega_0^2=0$

or $m_1x-m_2(L-x)=0$ ($\because \omega_0\neq 0$)

or $(m_1+m_2)x=m_2L$ or $x=\frac{m_2L}{m_1+m_2}$

68. **(c) :** Here, speed of the automobile,

$$v=54\text{ km h}^{-1}=54\times\frac{5}{18}\text{ m s}^{-1}$$
$$=15\text{ m s}^{-1}$$

Radius of the wheel of the automobile, $R=0.45$ m

Moment of inertia of the wheel about its axis of rotation,

$I=3\text{ kg m}^2$

Time in which the vehicle brought to rest, $t=15$ s

The initial angular speed of the wheel is

$$\omega_i=\frac{v}{R}=\frac{15\text{ m s}^{-1}}{0.45\text{ m}}=\frac{1500}{45}\text{rads}^{-1}$$
$$=\frac{100}{3}\text{rads}^{-1}$$

and its final angular speed is

$\omega_f=0$ (as the vehicle comes to rest)

$\therefore$ The angular retardation of the wheel is

$$\alpha=\frac{\omega_f-\omega_i}{t}=\frac{0-\frac{100}{3}}{15\text{ s}}=-\frac{100}{45}\text{rads}^{-2}$$

The magnitude of required torque is

$$\tau=I|\alpha|=(3\text{ kg m}^2)\left(\frac{100}{45}\text{rads}^{-2}\right)$$
$$=\frac{20}{3}\text{ kg m}^2\text{ s}^{-2}=6.66\text{ kg m}^2\text{ s}^{-2}$$

69. **(d) :** Here, mass of the cylinder, $M=50$ kg

Radius of the cylinder, $R=0.5$ m

Angular acceleration, $\alpha=2\text{ rev s}^{-2}$

$=2\times2\pi\text{rads}^{-2}=4\pi\text{rads}^{-2}$

Torque, $\tau=TR$

Moment of inertia of the solid cylinder about its axis, $I=\frac{1}{2}MR^2$

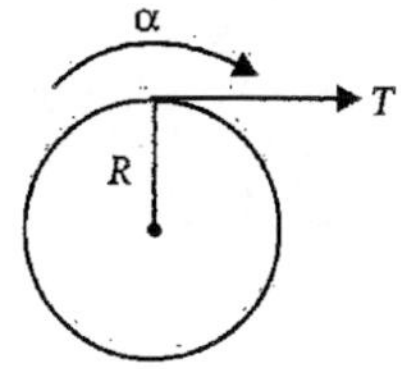

$\therefore$ Angular acceleration of the cylinder,

$$\alpha=\frac{\tau}{I}=\frac{TR}{\frac{1}{2}MR^2}$$

$$T=\frac{MR\alpha}{2}=\frac{50\times0.5\times4\pi}{2}=157\text{ N}$$

70. **(c)**

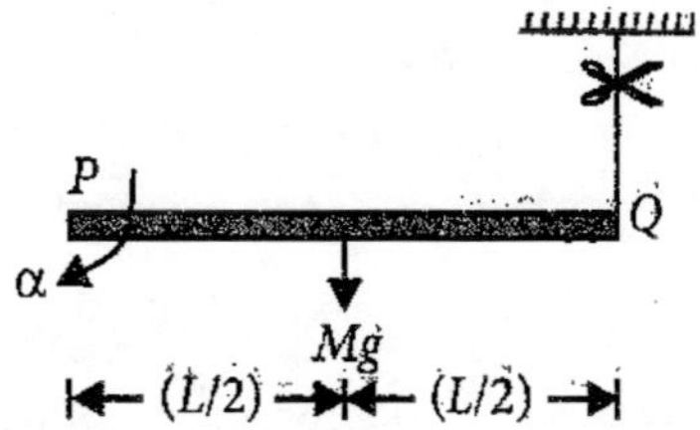

When the string is cut, the rod will rotate about P. Let α be initial angular acceleration of the rod: Then

Torque, $\tau=I\alpha=\frac{ML^2}{3}\alpha$

Also, $\tau=Mg\frac{L}{2}$

Equating (i) and (ii), we get

$$Mg\frac{L}{2}=\frac{ML^2}{3}\alpha\text{ or }\alpha=\frac{3g}{2L}$$

71. **(a) :** Given: $\theta(t)=2t^3-6t^2$

$\therefore \frac{d\theta}{dt} = 6t^2 - 12t \Rightarrow \frac{d^2\theta}{dt^2} = 12t - 12$

Angular acceleration, $\alpha = \frac{d^2\theta}{dt^2} = 12t - 12$

When angular acceleration (α) is zero, then the torque on the wheel becomes zero

$\Rightarrow 12t - 12 = 0$ or $t = 1$ s

$(\because \tau = I\alpha)$

72. **(c) :** Torque about A,

$\tau = mg \times \frac{l}{2} = \frac{mgl}{2}$

Also $\tau = I\alpha$

$\therefore$ Angular acceleration,

$$\alpha = \frac{\tau}{I} = \frac{mgl/2}{ml^2/3} = \frac{3}{2}\frac{g}{l}$$

73. **(c) :** $\omega_f = \omega_i - \alpha t \Rightarrow 0 = \omega_i - \alpha_t$

$\therefore \alpha = \omega_i/t$, where α is retardation.

The torque on the wheel is given by

$$\tau = I\alpha = \frac{I\omega}{t} = \frac{I \cdot 2\pi v}{t} = \frac{2 \times 2 \times \pi \times 60}{60 \times 60}$$

$$= \frac{\pi}{15} \text{ N m}$$

74. **(b) :** $I = 1.2 \text{ kg m}^2, E_r = 1500$ J,

$\alpha = 25 \text{rad/s}^2, \omega_1 = 0, t = ?$

As $E_r = \frac{1}{2}I\omega^2, \omega = \sqrt{\frac{2E_r}{I}} = \sqrt{\frac{2\times1500}{1.2}} = 50 \text{rad/s}$

From $\omega_2 = \omega_1 + \alpha t$

$50 = 0 + 25t$, or $t = 2$ s

75. **(d) :** As there is no external torque acting on a sphere, i.e., $\tau_{ex} = 0$

So, $\frac{dL}{dt} = \tau_{ex} = 0$ i.e., $L =$ constant

So angular momentum remains constant.

76. **(a) :** Initial angular momentum $= I\omega_1 + I\omega_2$ Let ω be angular speed of the combined system.

Final angular momentum = 210

$\therefore$ According to conservation of angular momentum

$$I\omega_1 + I\omega_2 = 2I\omega \text{ or } \omega = \frac{\omega_1 + \omega_2}{2}$$

Initial rotational kinetic energy,

$$E = \frac{1}{2}I(\omega_1^2 + \omega_2^2)$$

Final rotational kinetic energy

$$E_f = \frac{1}{2}(2I)\omega^2 = \frac{1}{2}(2I)\left(\frac{\omega_1 + \omega_2}{2}\right)^2$$

$$= \frac{1}{4}I(\omega_1 + \omega_2)^2$$

$\therefore$ Loss of energy $\Delta E = E_i - E_f$

$$= \frac{I}{2}(\omega_1^2 + \omega_2^2) - \frac{I}{4}(\omega_1^2 + \omega_2^2 + 2\omega_1\omega_2)$$

$$= \frac{I}{4}[\omega_1^2 + \omega_2^2 - 2\omega_1\omega_2] = \frac{I}{4}(\omega_1 - \omega_2)^2$$

77. **(c) :** Here, $m_A = m, m_B = 2m$

Both bodies A and B have equal kinetic energy of rotation

$$K_A - K_B \Rightarrow \frac{1}{2}I_A\omega_A^2 = \frac{1}{2}I_B\omega_B^2$$

$$\Rightarrow \frac{\omega_A^2}{\omega_B^2} = \frac{I_B}{I_A}$$

Ratio of angular momenta,

$$\frac{L_A}{L_B} = \frac{I_A\omega_A}{I_B\omega_B} = \frac{I_A}{I_B} \times \sqrt{\frac{I_B}{I_A}}$$

$$= \sqrt{\frac{I_A}{I_B}} < 1$$

[Using eqn. (i)]

$\therefore L_B > L_A$

78. **(b) :** Moment of inertia of disc D_1 about an axis passing through its centre and normal to its plane is

$$I_1 = \frac{MR^2}{2} = \frac{(2\text{ kg})(0.2\text{ m})^2}{2} = 0.04\text{ kg m}^2$$

Initial angular velocity of disc $D_1, \omega_1 = 50\text{rads}^{-1}$

Moment of inertia of disc D_2 about an axis passing through its centre and normal to its plane is

$$I_2 = \frac{(4\text{ kg})(0.1\text{ m})^2}{2} = 0.02\text{ kg m}^2$$

Initial angular velocity of disc $D_2, \omega_2 = 200\text{rads}^{-1}$

Total initial angular momentum of the two discs is

$$L_i = I_1\omega_1 + I_2\omega_2$$

When two discs are brought in contact face to face (one on the top of the other) and their axes of rotation coincide, the moment of inertia I of the system is equal to the sum of their individual moment of inertia.

$$I = I_1 + I_2$$

Let ω be the final angular speed of the system. The final angular momentum of the system is

$$L_f = I\omega = (I_1 + I_2)\omega$$

According to law of conservation of angular momentum, we get $L_i = L_f$ or,

$I_1\omega_1 + I_2\omega_2 = (I_1 + I_2)\omega$ or, $\omega = \frac{I_1\omega_1 + I_2\omega_2}{I_1 + I_2} = \frac{(0.04\text{ kg m}^2)(50\text{rads}^{-1}) + (0.02\text{ kg m}^2)(200\text{rads}^{-1})}{(0.04+0.02)\text{kgm}^2}$

$$= \frac{(2+4)}{0.06}\text{rads}^{-1} = 100\text{rads}^{-1}$$

79. **(c) :** As the system is initially at rest, therefore, initial angular momentum $L_i = 0$.

According to the principle of conservation of angular momentum, final angular momentum, $L_f = 0$.

$\therefore$ Angular momentum of platform = Angular momentum of man in opposite direction of platform.

i.e., $mvR = I\omega$

or $\omega = \frac{mvR}{I} = \frac{50\times1\times2}{200} = \frac{1}{2}\text{rads}^{-1}$

Angular velocity of man relative to platform is

$$\omega_r = \omega + \frac{v}{R} = \frac{1}{2} + \frac{1}{2} = 1\text{rads}^{-1}$$

Time taken by the man to complete one revolution is

$$T = \frac{2\pi}{\omega_r} = \frac{2\pi}{1} = 2\pi\text{s}$$

80. **(d) :** As no external torque is applied to the system, the angular momentum of the system remains conserved.

$\therefore L_i = L_f$

According to given problem,

$I_t\omega_i = (I_t + I_b)\omega_f$ or $\omega_f = \frac{I_t\omega_i}{(I_t+I_b)}$

Initial energy, $E_i = \frac{1}{2}I_t\omega_i^2$

Final energy, $E_f = \frac{1}{2}(I_t + I_b)\omega_f^2$

Substituting the value of ω_f from equation (i) in equation (iii) we get

Final energy,

$$E_f = \frac{1}{2}(I_t + I_b)\left(\frac{I_t\omega_i}{I_t + I_b}\right)^2 = \frac{1}{2}\frac{I_t^2\omega_i^2}{(I_t + I_b)}$$

Loss of energy, $\Delta E = E_i - E_f$

$$= \frac{1}{2}I_t\omega_i^2 - \frac{1}{2}\frac{I_t^2\omega_i^2}{(I_t + I_b)} \text{ (Using (ii) and (iv))}$$

$$= \frac{\omega_i^2}{2}\left(I_t - \frac{I_t^2}{(I_t + I_b)}\right) = \frac{\omega_i^2}{2}\left(\frac{I_t^2 + I_bI_t - I_t^2}{(I_t + I_b)}\right)$$

$$= \frac{1}{2}\frac{I_bI_t}{(I_t + I_b)}\omega_i^2$$

81. **(d)** : As no external torque is acting about the axis, angular momentum of system remains conserved. $I_1\omega_1 = I_2\omega_2$

$$\Rightarrow \omega_2 = \frac{I_1\omega_1}{I_2} = \frac{Mr^2\omega}{(M + 2m)r^2}$$

$$= \frac{M\omega}{(M + 2m)}$$

82. **(c)** : Applying conservation of angular momentum

$$I_1\omega = (I_1 + I_2)\omega_1 \text{ or } \omega_1 = \frac{I_1}{(I_1 + I_2)}\omega$$

83. **(b)** : According to conservation of angular momentum, $L = I\omega =$ constant

Therefore, $I_2\omega_2 = I_1\omega_1$

or $\omega_2 = \frac{I_1\omega_1}{I_2} = \frac{Mr^2\omega}{(M+4m)r^2} = \frac{M\omega}{M+4m}$

84. **(b)** : When a child sits on a rotating disc, no external torque is introduced. Hence the angular momentum of the system is conserved. But the moment of inertia of the system will increase and as a result, the angular speed of the disc will decrease to maintain constant angular momentum.

85. **(b)** : Required work done $= -(K_f - K_i) = 0 + K_i = K_i$

$$= \frac{1}{2}I\omega^2 + \frac{1}{2}mv^2 = \frac{1}{2}\left(\frac{1}{2}mR^2\right)\frac{v^2}{R^2} + \frac{1}{2}mv^2$$

$$= \frac{3}{4}mv^2 = \frac{3}{4} \times 100 \times (20 \times 10^{-2})^2 = 3 \text{ J}$$

86. **(d)** : Using law of conservation of energy,

$$mgh = \frac{1}{2}mv_{CM}^2 + \frac{1}{4}mr^2\omega^2$$

$$\Rightarrow mgs\sin 30° = \frac{1}{2}mv_{CM}^2 + \frac{1}{4}mv_{CM}^2$$

$$\Rightarrow s = \frac{3}{4}\frac{v_{CM}^2}{g\sin 30°} \Rightarrow s = \frac{3}{4} \times \frac{4^2}{10 \times \frac{1}{2}}$$

$$\Rightarrow s = \frac{3 \times 4 \times 2}{10} = \frac{12}{5} = 2.4 \text{ m}$$

87. **(b)** : Translational kinetic energy, $K_t = \frac{1}{2}mv^2$

Rotational kinetic energy, $K_r = \frac{1}{2}I\omega^2$

$$\therefore K_t + K_r = \frac{1}{2}mv^2 + \frac{1}{2}I\omega^2$$

$$= \frac{1}{2}mv^2 + \frac{1}{2}\left(\frac{2}{5}mr^2\right)\left(\frac{v}{r}\right)^2$$

$\therefore K_t + K_r = \frac{7}{10}mv^2$ $\left[\because I = \frac{2}{5}mr^2\right.$ (for sphere)]

So, $\frac{K_t}{K_t+K_r} = \frac{5}{7}$

88. **(d)** : Time taken by the body to reach the bottom when it rolls down on an inclined plane without slipping is given by

$$t = \sqrt{\frac{2l\left(1 + \frac{k^2}{R^2}\right)}{g\sin\theta}}$$

Since g is constant and l, R and $\sin\theta$ are same for both

$\therefore \frac{t_d}{t_s} = \frac{\sqrt{1+\frac{k_d^2}{R^2}}}{\sqrt{1+\frac{k_s^2}{R^2}}} = \sqrt{\frac{1+\frac{R^2}{2R^2}}{1+\frac{2R^2}{5R^2}}}$

$\left(\because k_d = \frac{R}{\sqrt{2}}, k_s = \sqrt{\frac{2}{5}}R\right)$

$= \sqrt{\frac{3}{2}\times\frac{5}{7}} = \sqrt{\frac{15}{14}} \Rightarrow t_d > t_s$

Hence, the sphere gets to the bottom first.

89. **(a) :** Acceleration of the solid sphere slipping down the incline without rolling is

$a_{\text{slipping}} = g\sin\theta$

Acceleration of the solid sphere rolling down the incline without slipping is

$a_{\text{rolling}} = \frac{g\sin\theta}{1+\frac{k^2}{R^2}} = \frac{g\sin\theta}{1+\frac{2}{5}} = \frac{5}{7}g\sin\theta$

($\because$ For solid sphere, $\frac{k^2}{R^2} = \frac{2}{5}$) Divide eqn. (ii) by eqn. (i), we get

$\frac{a_{\text{rolling}}}{a_{\text{slipping}}} = \frac{5}{7}$

90. **(b) :** The kinetic energy of the rolling object is converted into potential energy at height h and

$h = \frac{3v^2}{4g}$

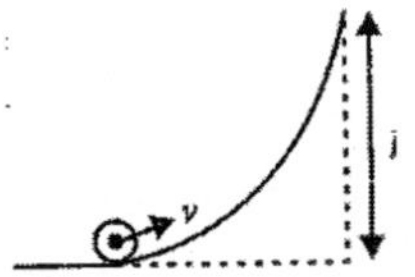

So by the law of conservation of mechanical energy, we have

$\frac{1}{2}Mv^2 + \frac{1}{2}I\omega^2 = Mgh$

$\frac{1}{2}Mv^2 + \frac{1}{2}I\left(\frac{v}{R}\right)^2 = Mg\left(\frac{3v^2}{4g}\right)$

$\frac{1}{2}I\frac{v^2}{R^2} = \frac{3}{4}Mv^2 - \frac{1}{2}Mv^2$

$\frac{1}{2}I\frac{v^2}{R^2} = \frac{1}{4}Mv^2$ or $I = \frac{1}{2}MR^2$

Hence, the object is disc.

91. **(b) :** At maximum compression the solid cylinder will stop.

According to law of conservation of mechanical energy

Loss in kinetic energy of cylinder = Gain in potential of spring

$\frac{1}{2}mv^2 + \frac{1}{2}I\omega^2$

$= \frac{1}{2}kx^2; \frac{1}{2}mv^2 + \frac{1}{2}\left(\frac{mR^2}{2}\right)\left(\frac{v}{R}\right)^2 = \frac{1}{2}kx^2$

($\because v = R\omega$ and for solid cylinder, $I = \frac{1}{2}mR^2$)

$\frac{1}{2}mv^2 + \frac{1}{4}mv^2 = \frac{1}{2}kx^2$ or, $\frac{3}{4}mv^2 = \frac{1}{2}kx^2$

or $x^2 = \frac{3}{2}\frac{mv^2}{k}$

Here, $m = 3\text{ kg}, v = 4\text{ m s}^{-1}, k = 200\text{ N m}^{-1}$

Substituting the given values, we get

$x^2 = \frac{3\times3\times4\times4}{2\times200} \Rightarrow x^2 = \frac{36}{100}$ or $x = 0.6$ m

92. **(d) :** Time taken to reach the bottom of inclined plane.

$t = \sqrt{\frac{2l\left(1+\frac{k^2}{R^2}\right)}{g\sin\theta}}$

Here, l is length of incline plane.

For solid cylinder $k^2 = \frac{R^2}{2}$.

For hollow cylinder $k^2 = R^2$.

Hence, solid cylinder will reach the bottom first.

93. **(d)** : Required frictional force convert some part of translational energy into rotational energy.

94. **(c)** : Total energy

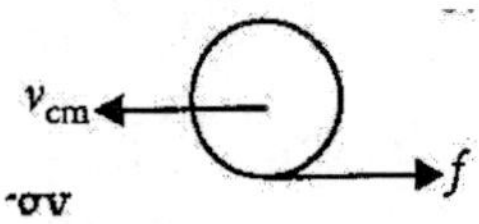

$$= \frac{1}{2} I\omega^2 + \frac{1}{2} mv^2 = \frac{1}{2} mv^2 (1 + K^2/R^2)$$

Required fraction $= \frac{K^2/R^2}{1+K^2/R^2} = \frac{K^2}{R^2+K^2}$.

95. **(c)** : Potential energy of the solid cylinder at height $h = Mgh$

K.E. of centre of mass when it reaches the bottom

$$= \frac{1}{2} Mv^2 + \frac{1}{2} I\omega^2 = \frac{1}{2} Mv^2 + \frac{1}{2} Mk^2 \frac{v^2}{R^2}$$
$$= \frac{1}{2} Mv^2 \left(1 + \frac{k^2}{R^2}\right)$$

For a solid cylinder $\frac{k^2}{R^2} = \frac{1}{2}$ $\therefore$ K.E. $= \frac{3}{4} Mv^2$

$\therefore Mgh = \frac{3}{4} Mv^2,\ v = \sqrt{\frac{4}{3} gh}.$

96. **(b)** :

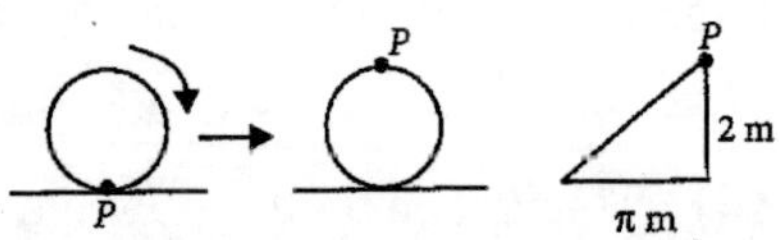

In half rotation point P has moved horizontal distance

$\frac{\pi d}{2} = \pi r = \pi \times 1\text{ m} = \pi\text{m}.$ [$\because$ radius $= 1$ m]

In the same time, it has moved vertical distance which is equal to its diameter = 2 m

$\therefore$ Displacement of point $= \sqrt{\pi^2 + 2^2} = \sqrt{\pi^2 + 4}$ m.

97. **(b)** :

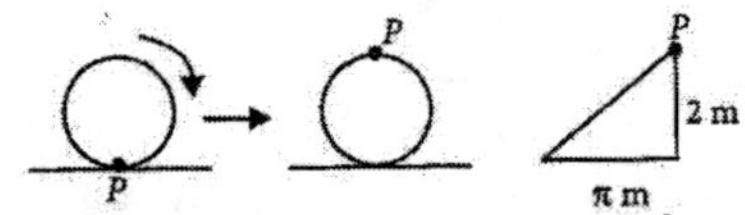

In half rotation point P has moved horizontal distance

$\frac{\pi d}{2} = \pi r = \pi \times 1\text{ m} = \pi\text{m}.$ [$\because$ radius $= 1$ m]

In the same time, it has moved vertical distance which is equal to its diameter = 2 m

$\therefore$ Displacement of point $= \sqrt{\pi^2 + 2^2} = \sqrt{\pi^2 + 4}$ m.

98. **(a)**

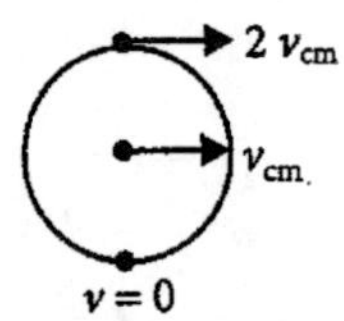

99. **(d)** : Linear K.E. of ball $= \frac{1}{2} mv^2$ and rotational K.E. of ball $= \frac{1}{2} I\omega^2 = \frac{1}{2}\left(\frac{2}{5} mr^2\right)\omega^2 = \frac{1}{5} mv^2$.

Total K.E. $= \frac{1}{2} mv^2 + \frac{1}{5} mv^2 = \frac{7}{10} mv^2$.

Ratio of rotational K.E. and total K.E.

$$= \frac{(1/5)mv^2}{(7/10)mv^2} = \frac{2}{7}$$

100. **(a)** : For solid sphere, $\frac{K^2}{R^2} = \frac{2}{5}$

For disc and solid cylinder, $\frac{K^2}{R^2} = \frac{1}{2}$

As for solid sphere K^2/R^2 is smallest, it takes minimum time to reach the bottom of the incline, disc and cylinder reach together later.

101. **(a)** : P.E. = total K.E.

$$mgh = \frac{7}{10}mv^2, v = \sqrt{\frac{10gh}{7}}$$

102. **(b)** : Angular momentum about the point of contact with the surface includes the angular momentum about the centre. Because of friction, linear momentum will not be conserved.

Chapter: 7 GRAVITATION

Kepler's Laws

1. The kinetic energies of a planet in an elliptical orbit about the Sun, at positions A, B and C are K_A, K_B and K_C, respectively. AC is the major axis and SB is perpendicular to AC at the position of the Sun S as shown in the figure. Then **(2018)**

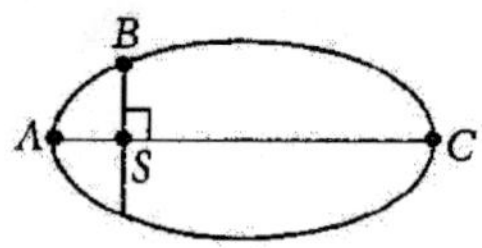

(a) $K_A < K_B < K_C$

(b) $K_A > K_B > K_C$

(c) $K_B < K_A < K_C$

(d) $K_B > K_A > K_C$

2. A planet moving along an elliptical orbit is closest to the sun at a distance r_1 and farthest away at a distance of r_2. If v_1 and v_2 are the linear velocities at these points respectively, then the ratio $\frac{v_1}{v_2}$ is **(2011)**

(a) $(r_1/r_2)^2$ (b) r_2/r_1

(c) $(r_2/r_1)^2$ (d) r_1/r_2

3. The figure shows elliptical orbit of a planet m about the sun S. The shaded area SCD is twice the shaded area SAB. If t_1 is the time for the planet to move from C to D and t_2 is the time to move from A to B then **(2009)**

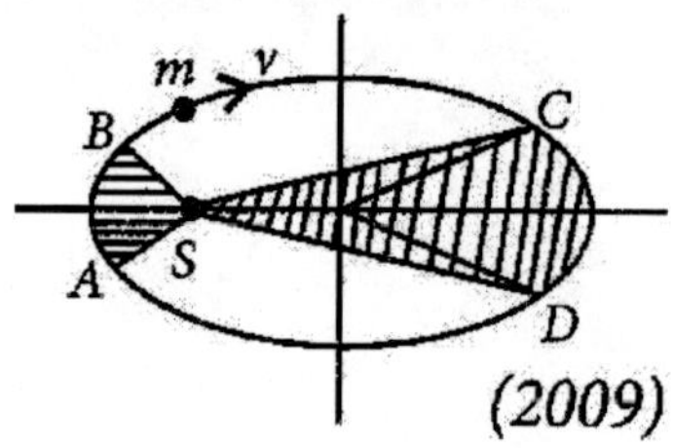

(2009)

(a) $t_1 = 4t_2$ (b) $t_1 = 2t_2$

(c) $t_1 = t_2$ (d) $t_1 > t_2$

4. The period of revolution of planet A around the sun is 8 times that of B. The distance of A from the sun is how many times greater than that of B from the sun? **(1997)**

(a) 4 (b) 5

(c) 2 (d) 3

5. The distance of two planets from the sun are 10^{13} m and 10^{12} m respectively. The ratio of time periods of the planets is **(1994, 1988)**

(a) $\sqrt{10}$ (b) $10\sqrt{10}$

(c) 10 (d) $1/\sqrt{10}$

6. A planet is moving in an elliptical orbit around the sun. If T, V, E and L stand respectively for its kinetic energy, gravitational potential energy, total energy and magnitude of angular momentum about the centre of force, which of the following is correct? **(1990)**

(a) T is conserved.

(b) V is always positive.

(c) E is always negative.

(d) L is conserved but direction of vector L changes continuously.

7. The largest and the shortest distance of the earth from the sun are r_1 and r_2. Its distance from the sun when it is at perpendicular to the major-axis of the orbit drawn from the sun is **(1988)**

(a) $\frac{r_1+r_2}{4}$ (b) $\frac{r_1+r_2}{r_1-r_2}$

(c) $\frac{2r_1r_2}{r_1+r_2}$ (d) $\frac{r_1+r_2}{3}$

Universal Law of Gravitation

8. A body of mass 60 g experiences a gravitational force of 3.0 N, when placed at a particular point. The magnitude of the gravitational field intensity at that point is **(2022)**

(a) 0.05 N/kg

(b) 50 N/kg

(c) 20 N/kg

(d) 180 N/kg

9. Two astronauts are floating in gravitational free space after having lost contact with their spaceship. The two will **(2017)**

(a) move towards each other

(b) move away from each other

(c) will become stationary

(d) keep floating at the same distance between them.

10. Kepler's third law states that square of period of revolution (T) of a planet around the sun, is proportional to third power of average distance r between sun and planet i.e. $T^2 = Kr^3$ here K is constant. If the masses of sun and planet are M and m respectively then as per Newton's law of gravitation force of attraction between them is $F = \frac{GMm}{r^2}$, here G is gravitational constant. The relation between G and K is described as **(2015 Cancelled)**

(a) $K = G$ (b) $K = \frac{1}{G}$

(c) $GK = 4\pi^2$ (d) $GMK = 4\pi^2$

11. Dependence of intensity of gravitational field (E) of earth with distance (r) from centre of earth is correctly represented by **(2014)**

(a) 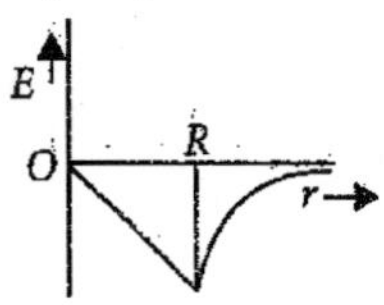

(b) 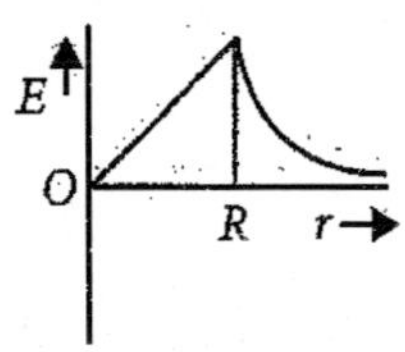

(c) 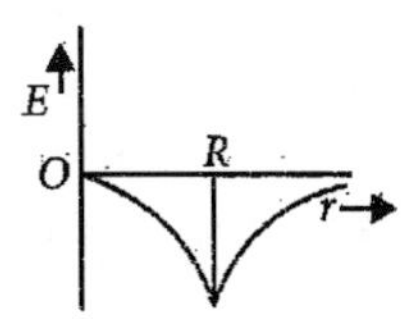

(d) 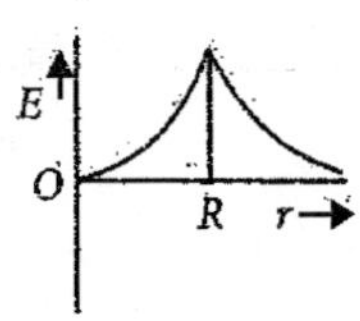

12. Which one of the following plots represents the variation of gravitational field on a particle with distance r due to a thin spherical shell of radius ? (r is measured from the centre of the spherical shell) **(Mains 2012)**

(a) 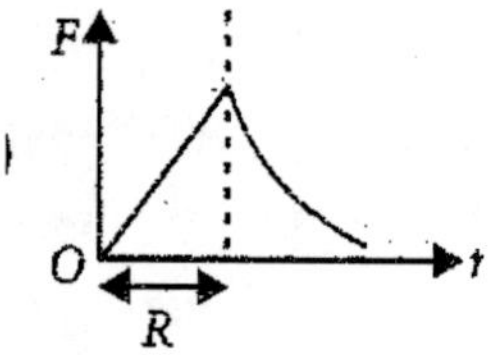

(b) 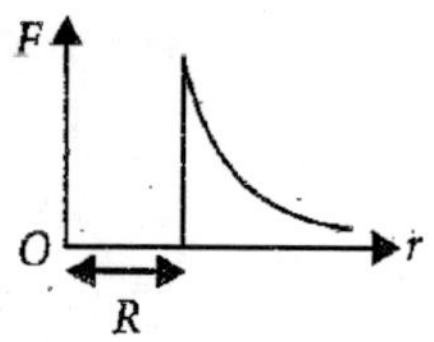

(c) 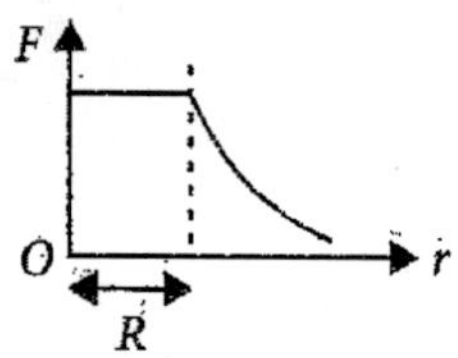

(d) 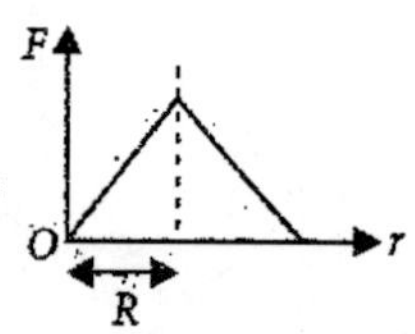

13. Two spheres of masses m and M are situated in air and the gravitational force between them is F. The space around the masses is now filled with a liquid of specific gravity 3 . The gravitational force will now be **(2003)**

(a) $3F$ (b) F

(c) $F/3$ (d) $F/9$

14. Gravitational force is required for **(2000)**

(a) stirring of liquid

(b) convection

(c) conduction

(d) radiation

15. A body of weight 72 N moves from the surface of earth at a height half of the radius of earth, then gravitational force exerted on it will be **(2000)**

(a) 36 N (b) 32 N

(c) 144 N (d) 50 N

16. Two particles of equal mass m go around a circle of radius R under the action of their mutual gravitational attraction. The speed v of each particle is **(1995)**

(a) $\frac{1}{2}\sqrt{\frac{Gm}{R}}$ (b) $\sqrt{\frac{4Gm}{R}}$

(c) $\frac{1}{2R}\sqrt{\frac{1}{Gm}}$ (d) $\sqrt{\frac{Gm}{R}}$

17. The earth (mass $= 6 \times 10^{24}$ kg) revolves around the sun with an angular velocity of 2×10^{-7} rad/s in a circular orbit of radius 1.5×10^{8} km. The force exerted by the sun on the earth, in newton, is **(1995)**

(a) 36×10^{21} (b) 27×10^{39}

(c) zero (d) 18×10^{25}

18. If the gravitational force between two objects were proportional to $1/R$ (and not as $1/R^2$), where R is the distance between them, then a particle in a circular path (under such a force) would have its orbital speed v, proportional to **(1994, 1989)**

(a) R

(b) R^0 (independent of R)

(c) $1/R^2$ (d) $1/R$

Acceleration due to Gravity of the Earth

19. If the mass of the Sun were ten times smaller and the universal gravitational constant were ten times larger in magnitude, which of the following is not correct? **(2018)**

(a) Raindrops will fall faster.

(b) Walking on the ground would become more difficult.

(c) Time period of a simple pendulum on the Earth would decrease.

(d) g on the Earth will not change.

20. A spherical planet has a mass M_p and diameter D_p. A particle of mass m falling freely near the surface of this planet will experience an acceleration due to gravity; equal to **(2012)**

(a) $\frac{4GM_p}{D_p^2}$ (b) $\frac{GM_pm}{D_p^2}$

(c) $\frac{GM_p}{D_p^2}$ (d) $\frac{4GM_pm}{D_p^2}$

21. Imagine a new planet having the same density as that of earth but it is 3 times bigger than the earth in size. If the acceleration due to gravity on the surface of earth is g and that on the surface of the new planet is g', then **(2005)**

(a) $g' = g/9$ (b) $g' = 27g$

(c) $g' = 9g$ (d) $g' = 3g$

22. The density of a newly discovered planet is twice that of earth. The acceleration due to gravity at the surface of the planet is equal to that at the surface of the earth. If the radius of the earth is R, the radius of the planet would be **(2004)**

(a) $2R$ (b) $4R$

(c) $\frac{1}{4}R$ (d) $\frac{1}{2}R$

23. The acceleration due to gravity on the planet A is 9 times the acceleration due to gravity on planet B. A man jumps to a height of 2 m on the surface of A. What is the height of jump by the same person on the planet ? **(2003)**

(a) $(2/9)$m (b) 18 m

(c) 6 m (d) $(2/3)$m

24. What will be the formula of mass of the earth in terms of g, R and ? **(1996)**

(a) $G\frac{R}{g}$ (b) $g\frac{R^2}{G}$

(c) $g^2\frac{R}{G}$ (d) $G\frac{g}{R}$.

25. The acceleration due to gravity g and mean density of the earth ρ are related by which of the following relations? (where G is the gravitational constant and R is the radius of the earth.) **(1995)**

(a) $\rho = \frac{3g}{4\pi GR}$ (b) $\rho = \frac{3g}{4\pi GR^3}$

(c) $\rho = \frac{4\pi gR^2}{3G}$ (d) $\rho = \frac{4\pi gR^3}{3G}$

26. The radius of earth is about 6400 km and that of mars is 3200 km. The mass of the earth is about 10 times mass of mars. An object weighs 200 N on the surface of earth. Its weight on the surface of mars will be **(1994)**

(a) 20 N (b) 8 N

(c) 80 N (d) 40 N

Acceleration due to Gravity Below and Above the Surface of Earth

27. A body weighs 72 N on the surface of the earth. What is the gravitational force on it, at a height equal to half the radius of the earth? **(2020)**

(a) 48 N (b) 32 N

(c) 30 N (d) 24 N

28. A body weighs 200 N on the surface of the earth. How much will it weigh half way down to the centre of the earth? **(2019)**

(a) 100 N (b) 150 N

(c) 200 N (d) 250 N

29. The acceleration due to gravity at a height 1 km above the earth is the same as at a depth d below the surface of earth. Then **(2017)**

(a) $d = 1$ km (b) $d = \frac{3}{2}$ km

(c) $d = 2$ km (d) $d = \frac{1}{2}$ km

30. Starting from the centre of the earth having radius R, the variation of g (acceleration due to gravity) is shown by **(NEET-II 2016)**

(a) 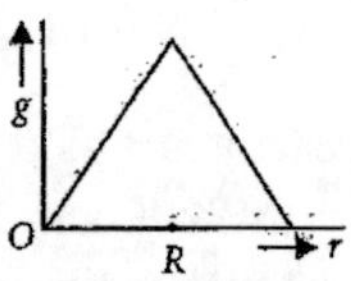

(b) 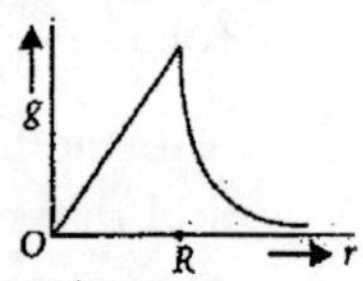

(c) 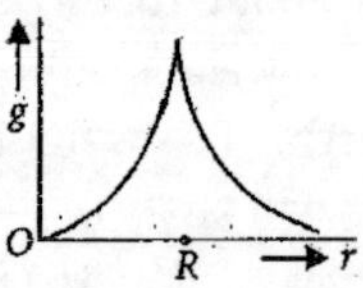

(d) 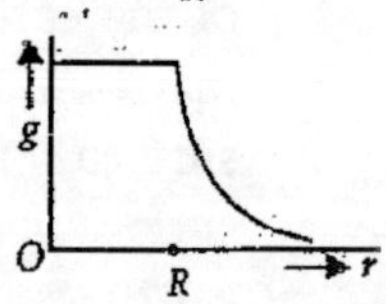

31. The height at which the weight of a body becomes $\left(\frac{1}{16}\right)^{th}$, its weight on the surface of earth (radius R), is **(2012)**

(a) $5R$ (b) $15R$

(c) $3R$ (d) $4R$

32. The dependence of acceleration due to gravity g on the distance r from the centre of the earth, assumed to be a sphere of radius R and of uniform density is as shown in figures. **(Mains 2010)**

(1) 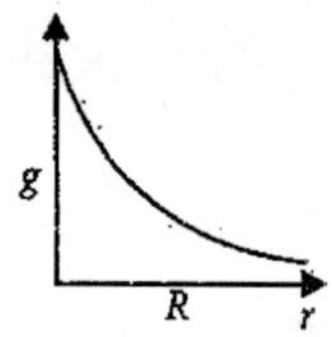

(2) 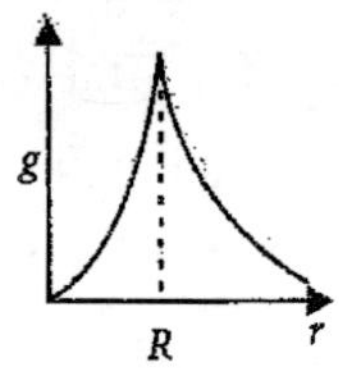

(3) 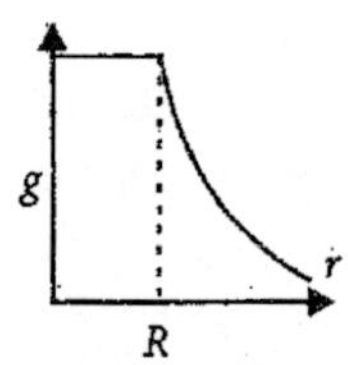

(4) 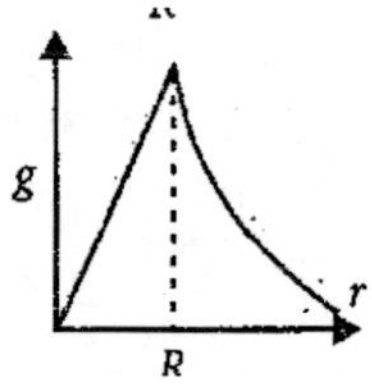

The correct figure is

(a) (4) (b) (1)

(c) (2) (d) (3)

Gravitational Potential Energy

33. Two bodies of mass m and 9m are placed at a distance R. The gravitational potential on the line joining the bodies where the gravitational field equals zero, will be (G = gravitational constant) **(2023)**

(a) $-\frac{12Gm}{R}$ (b) $-\frac{16Gm}{R}$

(c) $-\frac{20Gm}{R}$ (d) $-\frac{8Gm}{R}$

34. Match List-I and List-II :

List-I	List-II
a) Gravitational constant (G)	(i) $[L^2 T^{-2}]$
b) Gravitational potential energy	(ii) $[M^{-1} L^3 T^{-2}]$
c) Gravitational potential	(iii) $[LT^{-2}]$
d) Gravitational intensity	(iv) $[ML^2 T^{-2}]$

Choose the correct answer from the options given below: **(2022)**

(a) (A)-(ii), (B)-(i), (C)-(iv), (D)-(iii)

(b) (A)-(ii), (B)-(iv), (C)-(i), (D)-(iii)

(c) (A)-(ii), (B)-(iv), (C)-(iii), (D)-(i)

(d) (A)-(iv), (B)-(ii), (C)-(i), (D)-(iii)

35. The work done to raise a mass m from the surface of the earth to a height h, which is equal to the radius of the earth, is **(2019)**

(a) $\frac{3}{2}mgR$ (b) mgR

(c) $2mgR$ (d) $\frac{1}{2}mgR$

36. At what height from the surface of earth the gravitation potential and the value of g are -5.4×10^7 J kg^{-1} and 6.0 m s^{-2} respectively? Take the radius of earth as 6400 km : **(NEET-I 2016)**

(a) 1400 km (b) 2000 km

(c) 2600 km (d) 1600 km

37. Infinite number of bodies, each of mass 2 kg are situated on x-axis at distances 1 m, 2 m, 4 m, 8 m, ..., respectively, from the origin. The resulting gravitational potential due to this system at the origin will be **(2013)**

(a) $-\frac{4}{3}G$ (b) $-4G$

(c) $-G$ (d) $-\frac{8}{3}G$

38. A body of mass ' m ' is taken from the earth's surface to the height equal to twice the radius (R) of the earth. The change in potential energy of body will be **(2013)**

(a) $3mgR$ (b) $\frac{1}{3}mgR$

(c) $mg2R$ (d) $\frac{2}{3}mgR$

39. A particle of mass M is situated at the centre of a spherical shell of same mass and radius a. The magnitude of the gravitational potential at a point situated at $a/2$ distance from the centre, will be **(Mains 2011, 2010)**

(a) $\frac{GM}{a}$ (b) $\frac{2GM}{a}$

(c) $\frac{3GM}{a}$ (d) $\frac{4GM}{a}$

40. A body of mass m is placed on earth's surface which is taken from earth surface to a height of $h = 3R$, then change in gravitational potential energy is **(2003)**

(a) $\frac{mgR}{4}$ (b) $\frac{2}{3}mgR$

(c) $\frac{3}{4}mgR$ (d) $\frac{mgR}{2}$

Escape Speed

41. The escape velocity from the Earth's surface is v. The escape velocity from the surface of another planet having a radius, four times that of Earth and same mass density is **(2021)**

(a) $4v$ (b) v (c) $2v$ (d) $3v$

42. A particle of mass ' m ' is projected with a velocity $v = kV_e (k < 1)$ from the surface of the earth. (V_e = escape velocity)
The maximum height above the surface reached by the particle is **(2021)**

(a) $\frac{Rk^2}{1-k^2}$ (b) $R\left(\frac{k}{1-k}\right)^2$

(c) $R\left(\frac{k}{1+k}\right)^2$ (d) $\frac{R^2k}{1+k}$

43. The ratio of escape velocity at earth (v_e) to the escape velocity at a planet (v_p) whose radius and mean density are twice as that of earth is

(NEET-I 2016)

(a) $1:4$ (b) $1:\sqrt{2}$

(c) $1:2$ (d) $1:2\sqrt{2}$

44. A black hole is an object whose gravitational field is so strong that even light cannot escape from it. To what approximate radius would earth (mass $= 5.98 \times 10^{24}$ kg) have to be compressed to be a black hole?

(2014)

(a) 10^{-9} m (b) 10^{-6} m

(c) 10^{-2} m (d) 100 m

45. The radius of a planet is twice the radius of earth. Both have almost equal average mass-densities. V_P and V_E are escape velocities of the planet and the earth, respectively, then

(Karnataka NEET 2013)

(a) $V_P = 1.5V_E$ (b) $V_p = 2V_E$

(c) $V_E = 3V_P$ (d) $V_E = 1.5V_p$

46. A particle of mass ' m ' is kept at rest at a height ' $3R$ ' from the surface of earth, where ' R ' is radius of earth and ' M ' is mass of earth. The minimum speed with which it should be projected, so that it does not return back, is (g is acceleration due to gravity on the surface of earth)

(Karnataka NEET 2013)

(a) $\left(\frac{GM}{2R}\right)^{1/2}$ (b) $\left(\frac{gR}{4}\right)^{1/2}$

(c) $\left(\frac{2g}{R}\right)^{1/2}$ (d) $\left(\frac{GM}{R}\right)^{1/2}$

47. A particle of mass m is thrown upwards from the surface of the earth, with a velocity u. The mass and the radius of the earth are, respectively, M and R. G is gravitational constant and g is acceleration due to gravity on the surface of the earth. The minimum value of u so that the particle does not return back to earth, is

(Mains 2011)

(a) $\sqrt{\frac{2GM}{R^2}}$ (b) $\sqrt{\frac{2GM}{R}}$

(c) $\sqrt{\frac{2gM}{R^2}}$ (d) $\sqrt{2gR^2}$

48. The earth is assumed to be a sphere of radius R. A platform is arranged at a height R from the surface of the earth. The escape velocity of a body from this platform is fv, where v is its escape velocity from the surface of the Earth. The value of f is **(2006)**

(a) ½ (b) $\sqrt{2}$

(c) $1/\sqrt{2}$ (d) $1/3$

49. With what velocity should a particle be projected so that its height becomes equal to radius of earth? **(2001)**

(a) $\left(\frac{GM}{R}\right)^{1/2}$ (b) $\left(\frac{8GM}{R}\right)^{1/2}$

(c) $\left(\frac{2GM}{R}\right)^{1/2}$ (d) $\left(\frac{4GM}{R}\right)^{1/2}$

50. For a planet having mass equal to mass of the earth but radius is one fourth of radius of the earth. The escape velocity for this planet will be **(2000)**

(a) 11.2 km/s (b) 22.4 km/s

(c) 5.6 km/s (d) 44.8 km/s

51. The escape velocity of a sphere of mass m is given by (= Universal gravitational constant; M_e = Mass of the earth and R_e = Radius of the earth) **(1999)**

(a) $\sqrt{\frac{2GM_em}{R_e}}$ (b) $\sqrt{\frac{2GM_e}{R_e}}$

(c) $\sqrt{\frac{GM_e}{R_e}}$ (d) $\sqrt{\frac{2GM_e+R_e}{R_e}}$

52. The escape velocity of a body on the surface of the earth is 11.2 km/s. If the earth's mass increases to twice its present value and radius of the earth becomes half, the escape velocity becomes **(1997)**

(a) 22.4 km/s (b) 44.8 km/s

(c) 5.6 km/s (d) 11.2 km/s

53. The escape velocity from earth is 11.2 km/s. If a body is to be projected in a direction making an angle 45° to the vertical, then the escape velocity is **(1993)**

(a) 11.2×2 km/s

(b) 11.2 km/s

(c) $11.2/\sqrt{2}$ km/s

(d) $11.2\sqrt{2}$ km/s

54. For a satellite escape velocity is 11 km/s. If the satellite is launched at an angle of 60° with the vertical, then escape velocity will be **(1989)**

(a) 11 km/s (b) $1\sqrt{3}$ km/s

(c) $\frac{11}{\sqrt{3}}$ km/s (d) 33 km/s

ANSWER KEY

1.	(b)	2.	(b)	3.	(b)	4.	(a)	5.	(b)	6.	(c)
7.	(c)	8.	(b)	9.	(a)	10.	(d)	11.	(a)	12.	(b)
13.	(b)	14.	(b)	15.	(b)	16.	(a)	17.	(a)	18.	(b)
19.	(d)	20.	(a)	21.	(d)	22.	(d)	23.	(b)	24.	(b)
25.	(a)	26.	(c)	27.	(b)	28.	(a)	29.	(c)	30.	(b)
31.	(c)	32.	(a)	33.	(b)	34.	(b)	35.	(d)	36.	(c)
37.	(b)	38.	(d)	39.	(c)	40.	(c)	41.	(a)	42.	(a)
43.	(d)	44.	(c)	45.	(b)	46.	(a)	47.	(b)	48.	(c)
49.	(a)	50.	(b)	51.	(b)	52.	(a)	53.	(b)	54.	(a)

Hints & Explanations

1. **(b) :**

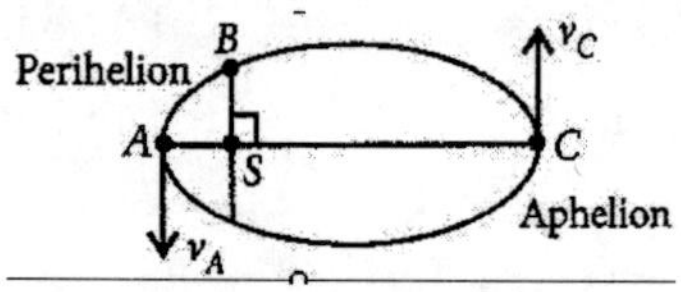

Point A is perihelion and C is aphelion.

So, $v_A > v_B > v_C$

As kinetic energy $K = (1/2)mv^2$ or $K \propto v^2$

So, $K_A > K_B > K_C$.

2. **(b)** : According to the law of conservation of angular momentum $L_1 = L_2$

$mv_1r_1 = mv_2r_2 \Rightarrow v_1r_1 = v_2r_2$ or $\frac{v_1}{v_2} = \frac{r_2}{r_1}$

3. **(b) :** Equal areas are swept in equal time.

As it is given that area $SCD = 2 \times$ area of SAB

The time taken to go from C to $D, t_1 = 2t_2$where t_2 is the time taken to go from A to B.

4. **(a) :** Period of revolution of planet $A, (T_A) = 8T_B$. According to Kcplcr's III law of planetary motion $T^2 \propto R^3$.

Therefore $= \left(\frac{r_A}{r_B}\right)^3 = \left(\frac{T_A}{T_B}\right)^2 = \left(\frac{8T_B}{T_B}\right)^2 = 64$

or $\frac{r_A}{r_B} = 4$ or $r_A = 4r_B$

5. **(b) :** Distance of two planets from sun, $r_1 = 10^{13}$ m and $r_2 = 10^{12}$ m

Relation between time period (T) and distance of the planet from the sun is $T^2 \propto r^3$ or $T \propto r^{3/2}$.

Therefore, $\frac{T_1}{T_2} = \left(\frac{r_1}{r_2}\right)^{\frac{3}{2}} = \left(\frac{10^{13}}{10^{12}}\right)^{\frac{3}{2}}$

$= 10^{3/2} = 10\sqrt{10}$

6. **(c) :** In a circular or elliptical orbital motion a planet, angular momentum is conserved. In attractive field, potential energy and the total energy is negative. Kinetic energy increases with increase in velocity. If the motion is in a plane, the direction of L does not change.

7. **(c) :**

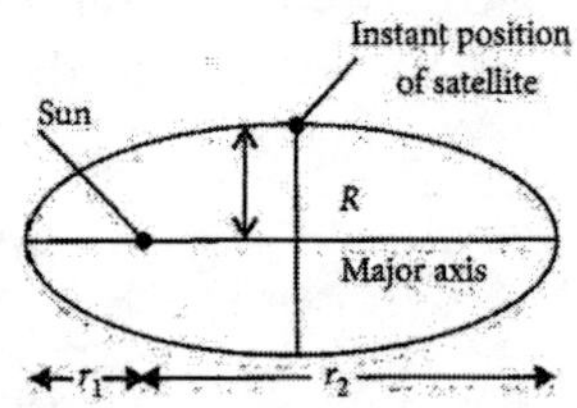

Applying the properties of ellipse, we have

$$\frac{2}{R} = \frac{1}{r_1} + \frac{1}{r_2} = \frac{r_1 + r_2}{r_1r_2}; R = \frac{2r_1r_2}{r_1 + r_2}$$

8. **(b)** : According to universal law of gravitation, gravitational force is

$$F = \frac{GMm}{r^2}$$

$$\text{or } \frac{F}{m} = \frac{GM}{r^2}$$

Given that, $F = 3.0$ N and

$m = 60 \text{ g} = 60 \times 10^{-3}$ kg

We know that, gravitational field intensity at point,

$I_G = \frac{GM}{r^2}$

$\therefore$ From eq. (i), we have

$$I_G = \frac{F}{m} = \frac{3.0}{60 \times 10^{-3}} = 50 \text{ N/kg}$$

9. **(a)** : Since two astronauts are floating in gravitational free space. The only force acting on the two astronauts is the gravitational pull of their masses, $F = \frac{Gm_1m_2}{r^2}$, which is attractive in nature.
Hence they move towards each other.

10. **(d)** : Gravitational force of attraction between sun and planet provides centripetal force for the orbit of planet.

$$\therefore \frac{GMm}{r^2} = \frac{mv^2}{r}; v^2 = \frac{GM}{r}$$

Time period of the planet is given by

$$T = \frac{2\pi r}{v}, T^2 = \frac{4\pi^2r^2}{v^2} = \frac{4\pi^2r^2}{\left(\frac{GM}{r}\right)}$$

$$T^2 = \frac{4\pi^2r^3}{GM}$$

According to question, $T^2 = Kr^3$

Comparing equations (ii) and (iii), we get

$$K = \frac{4\pi^2}{GM}, \therefore GMK = 4\pi^2$$

11. **(a)** : For a point inside the earth i.e. $r < R$

$$E = -\frac{GM}{R^3}r$$

where M and R be mass and radius of the earth respectively. At the centre, $r = 0$

$\therefore E = 0$

For a point outside the earth i.e. $r > R$,

$$E = -\frac{GM}{r^2}$$

On the surface of the earth i.e. $r = R$,

$$E = -\frac{GM}{R^2}$$

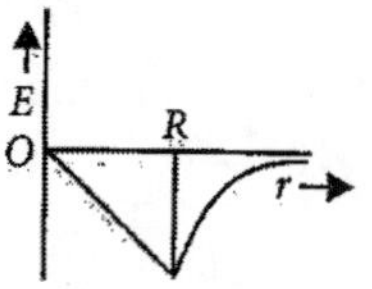

The variation of E with distance r from the centre is as shown in the figure.

12. **(b)** : Gravitational field due to the thin spherical shell Inside the shell,

(for r<R) F = 0

On the surface of the shell, (for r = R)

$$F = \frac{GM}{R^2}$$

Outside the shell, (for r>R)

$$F = \frac{GM}{r^2}$$

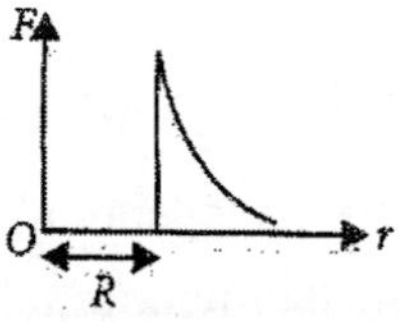

The variation of F with distance r from the centre is as shown in the figure.

13. **(b)** : The gravitational force does not depend upon the medium in which objects are placed.

14. **(b)**

15. **(b)** : $F_{\text{surface}} = G\frac{Mm}{R_e^2}$

$$F_{\frac{R_e}{2}} = G\frac{Mm}{\left(R_e + \frac{R_e}{2}\right)^2}$$

$$= \frac{4}{9} \times F_{\text{surface}} = \frac{4}{9} \times 72 = 32 \text{ N}$$

16. (a) : Force between the two masses, $F = -G\frac{mm}{4R^2}$

This force will provide the necessary centripetal force for the masses to go around a circle, then

$$\frac{Gmm}{4R^2} = \frac{mv^2}{R} \Rightarrow v^2 = \frac{Gm}{4R} \Rightarrow v = \frac{1}{2}\sqrt{\frac{Gm}{R}}$$

17. (a) : Given: mass $(m) = 6 \times 10^{24}$ kg; angular velocity $(\omega) = 2 \times 10^{-7}$ rad/s and radius $(r) = 1.5 \times 10^8$ km $= 1.5 \times 10^{11}$ m Force exerted on the earth $= mR\omega^2$

$= (6 \times 10^{24}) \times (1.5 \times 10^{11}) \times (2 \times 10^{-7})^2$

$= 36 \times 10^{21}$ N

18. (b) : Centripetal force $(F) = \frac{mv^2}{R}$ and the gravitational force $(F) = \frac{GMm}{R^2} = \frac{GMm}{R}$

(where $R^2 \to R$).

Since $\frac{mv^2}{R} = \frac{GMm}{R}$ therefore $v = \sqrt{GM}$.

Thus velocity v is independent of R.

19. (d) : If universal gravitational constant becomes ten times, then $G' = 10G$.

So, acceleration due to gravity increases. i.e, (d) is the wrong option.

20.(a) : Gravitational force acting on particle of mass m is

$$F = \frac{GM_pm}{(D_p/2)^2}$$

Acceleration due to gravity experienced by the particle is

$$g = \frac{F}{m} = \frac{GM_p}{(D_p/2)^2} = \frac{4GM_p^1}{D_p^2}$$

21. (d) : $g = \frac{GM}{r^2} = \frac{G}{r^2}\left(\frac{4}{3} \times \pi r^3 \rho\right) = \frac{4}{3} \times \pi\rho G r$

$$\frac{g'}{g} = \frac{3R}{R} \Rightarrow g' = 3g$$

22. (d) : From equation of acceleration due to gravity.

$$g_e = \frac{GM_e}{R_e^2} = \frac{G(4/3)\pi R_e^3}{R_e^2}\rho_e$$

$$g_e \propto R_e\rho_e$$

Acceleration due to gravity of planet $g_p \propto R_p\rho_p$

$$R_e\rho_e = R_p\rho_p \Rightarrow R_e\rho_e = R_p 2\rho_e$$

$$\Rightarrow R_p = \frac{1}{2}R \; (\because R_e = R)$$

23. (b) : Initial velocity of the mass on both the planets is same.

i.e., $\sqrt{2g'h'} = \sqrt{2gh}$

$\sqrt{2 \times g' \times h'} = \sqrt{2 \times 9g' \times 2} \Rightarrow 2h' = 36$

$\Rightarrow h' = 18$ m

24. (b): $\frac{GM}{R^2} = g$ [acceleration due to gravity near earth surface]

$$M = \frac{gR^2}{G}$$

25. (a) : Acceleration due to gravity

$$g = G \times \frac{M}{R^2} = G\frac{(4/3)\pi R^3 \times \rho}{R^2}$$

$$= G \times \frac{4}{3}\pi R \times \rho$$

or $\rho = \frac{3g}{4\pi GR}$

26. (c) : Given : radius of earth $(R_e) =$ 6400 km; radius of mars $(R_m) =$ 3200 km; mass of earth $(M_e) = 10M_m$ and weight of the object on earth $(W_e) = 200$ N.

$$\frac{W_m}{W_e} = \frac{mg_m}{mg_e} = \frac{M_m}{M_e} \times \left(\frac{R_e}{R_m}\right)^2 = \frac{1}{10} \times (2)^2$$
$$= \frac{2}{5}$$

or $W_m = W_e \times \frac{2}{5} = 200 \times 0.4 = 80$ N

27. (b) : Gravitational force at a height h,

$$mg_h = \frac{mg_0}{\left(1+\frac{h}{r}\right)^2} = \frac{72}{\left(1+\frac{R/2}{R}\right)^2} \text{ or } mg_h = 32 \text{ N}$$

or $F_g = 32$ N

28. (a) : Acceleration due to gravity at a depth $d, g_d = g\left(1-\frac{d}{R}\right)$

For $d = R/2 \Rightarrow g_d = g\left(1-\frac{R/2}{R}\right) = \frac{g}{2}$

Required weight $W' = mg_d = \frac{mg}{2} = \frac{W}{2} = \frac{200}{2} = 100$ N

29. (c) : The acceleration due to gravity at a height h is given as

$$g_h = g\left(1-\frac{2h}{R_e}\right)$$

where R_e is radius of earth.

The acceleration due to gravity at a depth d is given as

$$g_d = g\left(1-\frac{d}{R_e}\right)$$

Given, $g_h = g_d$ $\therefore g\left(1-\frac{2h}{R_e}\right) = g\left(1-\frac{d}{R_e}\right)$ or, $d = 2h = 2 \times 1 = 2$ km ($\because h = 1$ km)

30.(b) : Acceleration due to gravity is given by

$$g = \begin{cases} \frac{4}{3}\pi\rho G r & ; r \le R \\ \frac{4}{3}\frac{\pi\rho R^3 G}{r^2} & ; r > R \end{cases}$$

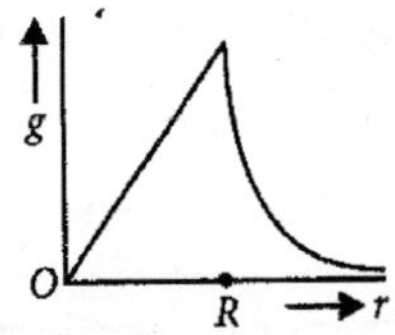

31. (c) : Acceleration due to gravity at a height h from the surface of earth is

$$g' = \frac{g}{\left(1+\frac{h}{R}\right)^2}$$

where g is the acceleration due to gravity at the surface of earth and R is the radius of earth.

Multiplying m (mass of the body) on both sides in (i), we get

$$mg' = \frac{mg}{\left(1+\frac{h}{R}\right)^2}$$

$\therefore$ Weight of body at height $h, W' = mg'$

Weight of body at surface of earth, $W = mg$

$$\because W' = \frac{1}{16}W \therefore \frac{1}{16} = \frac{1}{\left(1+\frac{h}{R}\right)^2}$$

$$\left(1+\frac{h}{R}\right)^2 = 16 \text{ or } 1+\frac{h}{R} = 4$$

or $\frac{h}{R} = 3$ or $h = 3R$

32. (a) : for r < R

$g = \frac{GM_e r}{R^3}$ [which is straight line (linear) equation]

for r ≥ R

$g = \frac{GM_e}{R^2}$

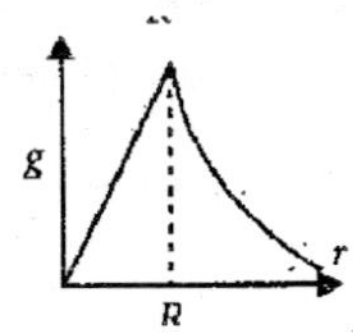

Hence 4th figure is correct

33. (b):

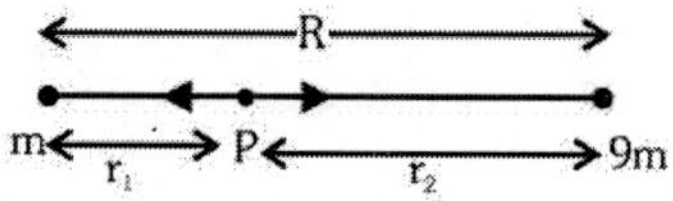

Position of Neutral point (Zero Gravitational Field)

$$r_1 = \frac{\sqrt{m_1}R}{\sqrt{m_1}+\sqrt{m_2}} = \frac{\sqrt{m}R}{\sqrt{m}+\sqrt{9m}} = \frac{R}{4}$$

$$r_2 = R - R/4 = 3R/4$$

Now Gravitational potential at point P

$$V_P = -\frac{GM}{R/4} - \frac{9(GM)}{3R/4}$$

$$= \frac{-16GM}{R}$$

34. (b) : Here, $F = G\frac{M_1M_2}{r^2}$

Gravitational constant,

$$G = \frac{F \times r^2}{M_1 \times M_2} = [\mathrm{M^{-1}\,L^3\,T^{-2}}]$$

Gravitational potential energy,

$U = \frac{-GM_1M_2}{r} = [\mathrm{M^1\,L^2\,T^{-2}}]$

Gravitational potential,

$V = -\frac{GM}{r} = [\mathrm{M^0\,L^2\,T^{-2}}]$

Gravitational intensity, $I = \frac{GM}{r^2} =$ $[\mathrm{M^0\,L^1\,T^{-2}}]$

So, (A)-(ii), (B)-(iv), (C)-(i), (D) - (iii)

35. (d) : Work done = Change in potential energy

$$= u_f - u_i = \frac{-GMm}{(R+h)} - \left(\frac{-GMm}{R}\right)$$

where M is the mass of earth and R is the radius of earth.

$$\therefore W = GMm\left[\frac{1}{R} - \frac{1}{(R+h)}\right]$$

Now, $h = R$

$$\therefore W = GMm\left[\frac{1}{R} - \frac{1}{2R}\right] = \frac{GMm}{2R}$$

$$\Rightarrow W = \frac{mgR}{2}\left[\because g = \frac{GM}{R^2}\right]$$

36. (c) : Gravitation potential at a height h from the surface of earth, $V_h = -5.4 \times 10^7\ \mathrm{J\,kg^{-1}}$

At the same point acceleration due to gravity, $g_h = 6\ \mathrm{m\,s^{-2}}$ $R = 6400\ \mathrm{km} = 6.4 \times 10^6\ \mathrm{m}$

We know, $V_h = -\frac{GM}{(R+h)}$,

$$g_h = \frac{GM}{(R+h)^2} = -\frac{V_h}{R+h} \Rightarrow R + h = -\frac{V_h}{g_h}$$

$$\therefore \quad h = -\frac{V_h}{g_h} - R = -\frac{(-5.4 \times 10^7)}{6} - 6.4 \times 10^6$$

$$= 9 \times 10^6 - 6.4 \times 10^6 = 2600\ \mathrm{km}$$

37. (b) : The resulting gravitational potential at the origin O due to each of mass 2 kg located at positions as shown in figure is

$x = 0\ 2$ kg

$$V = -\frac{G\times 2}{1} - \frac{G\times 2}{2} - \frac{G\times 2}{4} - \frac{G\times 2}{8} - \cdots$$

$$= -2G\left[1 + \frac{1}{2} + \frac{1}{4} + \frac{1}{8} + \cdots..\right] = -2G\left[\frac{1}{1-\frac{1}{2}}\right]$$

$$= -2G\left[\frac{2}{1}\right] = -4G$$

38. (d) : Gravitational potential energy at any point at a distance r from the centre of the earth is

$\Rightarrow\ U = -\frac{GMm}{r}$

where M and m be masses of the earth and the body respectively. At the surface of the earth, $r = R; U_i = -\frac{GMm}{R}$

At a height h from the surface,

$$r = R + h = R + 2R = 3R$$

$$(h = 2R(\text{ Given }))$$

$$\therefore U_f = -\frac{GMm}{3R}$$

Change in potential energy, $\Delta U = U_f - U_i$

$$= -\frac{GMm}{3R} - \left(-\frac{GMm}{R}\right) = \frac{GMm}{R}\left(1 - \frac{1}{3}\right)$$

$$= \frac{2}{3}\frac{GMm}{R} = \frac{2}{3}mgR\left(\because g = \frac{GM}{R^2}\right)$$

39. (c) : Here, Mass of a particle $= M$

Mass of a spherical shell $= M$

Radius of a spherical shell $= a$

Let O be centre of a spherical shell.

Gravitational potential at point P due to particle at O is

$$V_1 = -\frac{GM}{a/2}$$

Gravitational potential at point P due to spherical shell is

$$V_2 = -\frac{GM}{a}$$

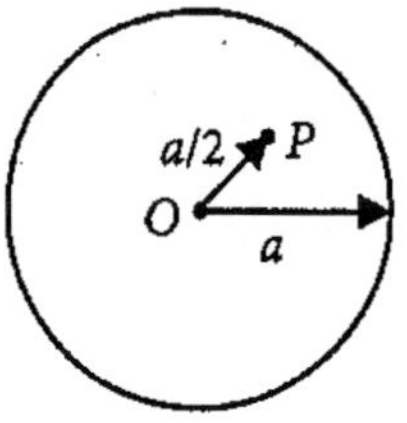

Hence, total gravitational potential at point P is $V = V_1 + V_2$

$$= \frac{-GM}{a/2} + \left(\frac{-GM}{a}\right) = \frac{-2GM}{a} - \frac{GM}{a}$$

$$= \frac{-3GM}{a}$$

$$|V| = \frac{3GM}{a}$$

40. (c) : Gravitational potential energy on earth's surface $= -\frac{GMm}{R}$, where M and R are the mass and radius of the earth respectively, m is the mass of the body and G is the universal gravitational constant.

Gravitational potential energy at a height $h = 3R$

$$= -\frac{GMm}{R+h} = -\frac{GMm}{R+3R} = -\frac{GMm}{4R}$$

$\therefore$ Change in potential energy

$$= -\frac{GMm}{4R} - \left(-\frac{GMm}{R}\right)$$

$$= -\frac{GMm}{4R} + \frac{GMm}{R} = \frac{3}{4}\frac{GMm}{R} = \frac{3}{4}mgR$$

41. (a) : The formula of escape velocity is

$$v = \sqrt{\frac{2GM}{R}}$$

where, $G =$ gravitational constant, $M =$ mass and $R =$ radius.

Mass, $M = \frac{4}{3}\pi R^3 \rho$ where, ρ is density of planet

$$v = \sqrt{\frac{2 \times G}{R} \times \frac{4}{3}\pi R^3 \rho}$$

$$v = \sqrt{\frac{8G\pi}{3} R^2 \rho}$$

Let the escape velocity on planet is v'. For planet, $R' = 4R, \rho' = \rho$

$$v' = \sqrt{\frac{8G\pi}{3} R'^2 \rho'}$$

Divide eqn. (i) by (ii), we get

So, $\frac{v'}{v} = \sqrt{\frac{R'^2}{R^2} \times \frac{\rho'}{\rho}}$

$$\frac{v'}{v} = \sqrt{\frac{16R^2}{R^2} \times \frac{\rho}{\rho}} = 4$$

$$v' = 4v$$

42. (a) : The particle is fired vertically upwards from the Earth's surface with a velocity v and reaches a height h. Energy of the particle at the surface of the Earth is

$$E_i = \frac{1}{2}mv^2 - \frac{GM_E m}{R_E}$$

Energy of the particle at a height h

$$E_f = -\frac{GM_E m}{R_E + h}$$

($\because$ At height h velocity of the particle is zero.)

According to law of conservation of energy,

$E_i = E_f$

$$\frac{1}{2}mv^2 - \frac{GM_E m}{R_E} = -\frac{GM_E m}{R_E + h}$$

$$\frac{1}{2}mv^2 = GM_E m\left[\frac{1}{R_E} - \frac{1}{R_E + h}\right] = \frac{GM_E mh}{(R_E)(R_E + h)}$$

$$\frac{1}{2}mv^2 = \frac{mghR_E}{R_E + h} \text{ ... (i) } \left(\because g = \frac{GM_E}{R_E^2}\right)$$

As per question,

$$v = kv_e = k\sqrt{2gR_E}$$

$$\left(\because v_e = V_e = \sqrt{2gR_E}\right)$$

Using (i) and (ii), we get

$$h = \frac{R_E k^2}{1 - k^2}$$

If $R_E = R$, then $h = \frac{Rk^2}{1-k^2}$

43. (d) : As escape velocity, $v = \sqrt{\frac{2GM}{R}}$

$$= \sqrt{\frac{2G}{R} \cdot \frac{4\pi R^3}{3} \rho} = R\sqrt{\frac{8\pi G}{3}\rho}$$

$$\therefore \frac{v_e}{v_p} = \frac{R_e}{R_p} \times \sqrt{\frac{\rho_e}{\rho_p}} = \frac{1}{2} \times \sqrt{\frac{1}{2}} = \frac{1}{2\sqrt{2}}$$

$$(\therefore R_p = 2R_e \text{ and } \rho_p = 2\rho_e)$$

44. (c) : Light cannot escape from a black hole,

$$v_e = c \Rightarrow \sqrt{\frac{2GM}{R}} = c \text{ or } R = \frac{2GM}{c^2}$$

$$R = \frac{2 \times 6.67 \times 10^{-11} \text{ N m}^2 \text{ kg}^{-2} \times 5.98 \times 10^{24} \text{ kg}}{(3 \times 10^8 \text{ m s}^{-1})^2}$$

$$= 8.86 \times 10^{-3} \text{ m} \propto 10^{-2} \text{ m}$$

45. (b) : Here, $R_P = 2R_E, \rho_E = \rho_P$

Escape velocity of the earth,

$$V_E = \sqrt{\frac{2GM_E}{R_E}} = \sqrt{\frac{2G}{R_E}\left(\frac{4}{3}\pi R_E^3 \rho_E\right)}$$

$$= R_E\sqrt{\frac{8}{3}\pi G\rho_E}$$

Escape velocity of the planet,

$$V_P = \sqrt{\frac{2GM_P}{R_P}} = \sqrt{\frac{2G}{R_P}\left(\frac{4}{3}\pi R_P^3 \rho_P\right)}$$

$$= R_P\sqrt{\frac{8}{3}\pi G\rho_P}$$

Divide (i) by (ii), we get

$\frac{V_E}{V_P} = \frac{R_E}{R_P}\sqrt{\frac{\rho_E}{\rho_P}} = \frac{R_E}{2R_E}\sqrt{\frac{\rho_E}{\rho_E}} = \frac{1}{2}$ or $V_P = 2V_E$

46. (a) : The minimum speed with which the particle should be projected from the surface of the earth so that it does not return back is known as escape speed and it is given by

$$v_e = \sqrt{\frac{2GM}{(R+h)}}$$

Here, $h = 3R$

$$\therefore\ v_e = \sqrt{\frac{2GM}{(R+3R)}} = \sqrt{\frac{2GM}{4R}} = \sqrt{\frac{GM}{2R}}$$

47. (b) : According to law of conservation of mechanical energy,

$$\frac{1}{2}mu^2 - \frac{GMm}{R} = 0 \text{ or } u^2 = \frac{2GM}{R}$$

$$u = \sqrt{\frac{2GM}{R}} = \sqrt{2gR}\ \left(\because g = \frac{GM}{R^2}\right)$$

48. (c) : Escape velocity of the body from the surface of earth is $v = \sqrt{2gR}$

For escape velocity of the body from the platform, potential energy + kinetic energy = 0

$$-\frac{GMm}{2R} + \frac{1}{2}mv_e^2 = 0$$

$$\Rightarrow v_e = \sqrt{\frac{GM}{R^2}\cdot R} = \sqrt{gR} \Rightarrow fv = \sqrt{gR}$$

From equation (i) and (ii), we get $f = \frac{1}{\sqrt{2}}$

49. (a) : Use $v^2 = \frac{2gh}{1+\frac{h}{R}}$ given $h = R$.

$$\therefore\ v = \sqrt{gR} = \sqrt{\frac{GM}{R}}$$

50. (b) : $v_e = \sqrt{2gR_e} = \sqrt{\frac{2GM}{R_e}}$

$\because\ R_P = \frac{1}{4}R_e\ v_P = 2v_e = 2 \times 11.2 = 22.4$ km/s.

51. (b) $B.E. = \frac{GM_e m}{R_e}$

$$\frac{1}{2}mv_e^2 = \frac{GM_e m}{R_e}$$

$$V_e^2 = \frac{2GM_e}{R_e}$$

$$\therefore\quad V_e = \sqrt{\frac{2GM_e}{R_e}}$$

52. (a) : Escape velocity of a body (v_e) = 11.2 km/s; New mass of the earth $M_e' = 2M_e$ and new radius of the earth $R_e' = 0.5R_e$. Escape velocity $(v_e) = \sqrt{\frac{2GM_e}{R_e}} \propto \sqrt{\frac{M_e}{R_e}}$

Therefore $\frac{v_e}{v_e'} = \sqrt{\frac{M_e}{R_e} \times \frac{0.5R_e}{2M_e}} = \sqrt{\frac{1}{4}} = \frac{1}{2}$

or, $v_e' = 2v_e = 22.4$ km/s

53. (b) : Escape velocity does not depend on the angle of projection.

54. (a)

Chapter: 8 MECHANICAL PROPERTIES OF SOLIDS

Stress-Strain Curve

1. The stress-strain curves are drawn for two different materials X and Y. It is observed that the ultimate strength point and the fracture point are close to each other for material X but are far apart for material Y. We can say that materials X and Y are likely to be (respectively)

(Odisha NEET 2019)

(a) ductile and brittle

(b) brittle and ductile

(c) brittle and plastic

(d) plastic and ductile

Elastic Moduli

2. Given below are two statements: One is labelled as Assertion (A) and the other is labelled as Reason (R). Assertion (A): The stretching of a spring is determined by the shear modulus of the material of the spring.

Reason (R): A coil spring of copper has more tensile strength than a steel spring of same dimensions. In the light of the above statements, choose the most appropriate answer from the options given below:

(2022)

(a) Both (A) and (R) are true and (R) is the correct explanation of (A)

(b) Both (A) and (R) are true and (R) is not the correct explanation of (A)

(c) (A) is true but (R) is false

(d) (A) is false but (R) is true

3. A wire of length L, area of cross section A is hanging from a fixed support. The length of the wire changes to L_1 when mass M is suspended from its free end. The expression for Young's modulus is

(2020)

(a) $\frac{MgL_1}{AL}$ (b) $\frac{Mg(L_1-L)}{AL}$

(c) $\frac{MgL}{AL_1}$ (d) $\frac{MgL}{A(L_1-L)}$

4. When a block of mass M is suspended by a long wire of length L, the length of the wire becomes $(L+l)$. The elastic potential energy stored in the extended wire is

(a) $\frac{1}{2}MgL$ (b) Mgl

(c) MgL (d) $\frac{1}{2}Mgl$

5. Two wires are made of the same material and have the same volume. The first wire has cross-sectional area A and the second wire has cross-sectional area $3A$. If the length of the first wire is increased by Δl on applying a force F, how much force is needed to stretch the second wire by the same amount? **(2018)**

(a) $9F$ (b) $6F$ (c) 4 F (d) F

6. The bulk modulus of a spherical object is 'B'. If it is subjected to uniform pressure 'p', the fractional decrease in radius is **(2017)**

(a) $\frac{B}{3p}$ (b) $\frac{3p}{B}$ (c) $\frac{p}{3B}$ (d) $\frac{p}{B}$

7. The Young's modulus of steel is twice that of brass. Two wires of same length and of same area of cross section, one of steel and another of brass are suspended from the same roof. If we want the lower ends of the wires to be at the same level, then the weights added to the steel and brass wires must be in the ratio of **(2015)**

(a) 4: 1 (b) 1: 1

(c) 1: 2 (d) 2: 1

8. The approximate depth of an ocean is 2700 m. The compressibility of water is 45.4×10^{-11} Pa^{-1} and density of water is 10^3 kg/m^3. What fractional compression of water will be obtained at the bottom of the ocean? **(2015 Cancelled)**

(a) 1.2×10^{-2}

(b) 1.4×10^{-2}

(c) 0.8×10^{-2}

(d) 1.0×10^{-2}

9. Copper of fixed volume V is drawn into wire of length l. When this wire is subjected to a constant force F, the extension produced in the wire is Δl. Which of the following graphs is a straight line? **(2014)**

(a) Δl versus $1/l$ (b) Δl versus l^2

(c) Δl versus $1/l^2$ (d) Δl versus l

10. The following four wires are made of the same material. Which of these will have the largest extension when the same tension is applied? **(2013)**

(a) length = 200 cm, diameter = 2 mm

(b) length = 300 cm, diameter = 3 mm

(c) length = 50 cm, diameter = 0.5 mm

(d) length = 100 cm, diameter = 1 mm

11. If the ratio of diameters, lengths and Young's modulus of steel and copper wires shown in the figure are p, q and s respectively, then the corresponding ratio of increase in their lengths would be

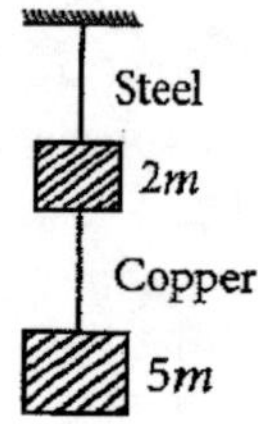

(a) $\frac{5q}{(7sp^2)}$ (b) $\frac{7q}{(5sp^2)}$

(c) $\frac{2q}{(5sp)}$ (d) $\frac{7q}{(5sp)}$

ANSWER KEY

1.	(b)	2.	(c)	3.	(d)	4.	(d)	5.	(a)	6.	(c)
7.	(d)	8.	(a)	9.	(b)	10.	(c)	11.	(b)		

Hints & Explanations

1. **(b) :** Ultimate strength point in that point of solids after which if applied force get increased then-after solid be have as plastic body fracture point as name suggest it's a point at which body will break if applied force-increased ultimate strength point is close to fracture point are in nearer position for 'x' which means it's Brittle in nature.

Ultimate strength point is for way from fracture point for 'y' which means it's ductile in Nature.

2. **(c)** The stretching of a coiled spring is determined by its shear modulus because neither its length nor its volume changes but only the shape of the spring is changed. Elasticity of steel is more than copper.

3. **(d)** Given : initial length $= L$, area of cross section $= A$

New length after mass M is suspended on the wire $= L_1$

$\therefore$ Change in length, $\Delta L = L_1 - L$.

Now Young's modulus, $Y = \frac{\text{Stress}}{\text{Strain}} = \frac{F}{A} \times \frac{L}{\Delta L}$

$$= \frac{mg}{A}\frac{L}{\Delta L} \text{ or } \frac{MgL}{A(L_1 - L)}$$

4. **(d) :** Stress $= \frac{F}{A} = \frac{Mg}{A}$,

Strain $= \frac{\Delta L}{L} = \frac{L+l-L}{L} = \frac{l}{L}$

Energy stored in the wire is,

$U = \frac{1}{2} \times \text{Stress} \times \text{Strain} \times \text{Volume}$

$$= \frac{1}{2} \times \frac{Mg}{A} \times \frac{l}{L} \times A \times L = \frac{1}{2} Mgl$$

5. **(a) :** Young's modulus, $Y = \frac{Fl}{A\Delta l}$

Since initial volume of wires are same and their areas of cross- sections are A and $3A$ so lengths are $3l$ and l respectively. For wire 1,

$$\Delta l = \left(\frac{F}{AY}\right) 3l$$

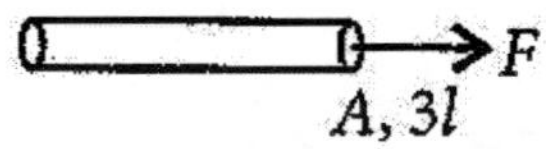

For wire 2, let F' force is applied

$$\frac{F'}{3A} = Y\frac{\Delta l}{l}$$

$$\Rightarrow \Delta l = \left(\frac{F'}{3AY}\right) l$$

From eqns (i) and (ii)

$$\left(\frac{F}{AY}\right) 3l = \left(\frac{F'}{3AY}\right) l \Rightarrow F' = 9F$$

6. **(c) :** Bulk modulus B is given as

$$B = \frac{-pV}{\Delta V}$$

The volume of a spherical object of radius r is given as $V = \frac{4}{3}\pi r^3, \Delta V = \frac{4}{3}\pi(3r^2)\Delta r$

$$\therefore -\frac{V}{\Delta V} = \frac{\frac{4}{3}\pi r^3}{\frac{4}{3}\pi 3r^2 \Delta r} \text{ or } -\frac{V}{\Delta V} = -\frac{r}{3\Delta r}$$

Put this value in eqn. (i), we get $B = -\frac{pr}{3\Delta r}$

Fractional decrease in radius is $-\frac{\Delta r}{r} = \frac{p}{3B}$

7. **(d)** : Let L and A be length and area of cross section of each wire. In order to have the lower ends of the wires to be at the same level (i.e. same elongation is produced in both wires), let

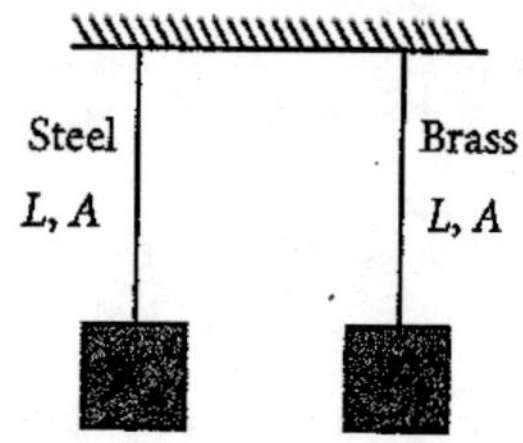

weights W_s and W_b are added to steel and brass wires respectively. Then, by definition of Young's modulus, the elongation produced in the steel wire is

$$\Delta L_s = \frac{W_s L}{Y_s A}$$

$$\left(\text{as } Y = \frac{W/A}{\Delta L/L}\right)$$

and that in the brass wire is $\Delta L_b = \frac{W_b L}{Y_b A}$

But $\Delta L_s = \Delta L_b$

(given)

$\therefore \frac{W_s L}{Y_s A} = \frac{W_b L}{Y_b A}$ or $\frac{W_s}{W_b} = \frac{Y_s}{Y_b}$

As $\frac{Y_s}{Y_b} = 2; \therefore \frac{W_s}{W_b} = \frac{2}{1}$

8. **(a)** : Depth of ocean, $d = 2700$ m

Density of water, $\rho = 10^3$ kg m^{-3}

Compressibility of water, $K = 45.4 \times 10^{-11}$ Pa^{-1}

$\frac{\Delta V}{V} = ?$

Excess pressure at the bottom, $\Delta P = \rho g d$

$$= 10^3 \times 10 \times 2700 = 27 \times 10^6 \text{ Pa}$$

We know, $B = \frac{\Delta P}{(\Delta V/V)}$

$$\left(\frac{\Delta V}{V}\right) = \frac{\Delta P}{B} = K.\Delta P \left(\because K = \frac{1}{B}\right)$$

$$= 45.4 \times 10^{-11} \times 27 \times 10^6 = 1.2 \times 10^{-2}$$

9. (b) : As $V = Al$

where A is the area of cross-section of the wire.

Young's modulus, $Y = \frac{(F/A)}{(\Delta l/l)} = \frac{Fl}{A\Delta l}$

$$\Delta l = \frac{Fl}{YA} = \frac{Fl^2}{YV}$$

$$\Delta l \propto l^2$$

Hence, the graph between Δl and l is a straight line.

10. **(c)** : Young's modulus,

$$Y = \frac{FL}{A\Delta L} = \frac{4FL}{\pi D^2 \Delta L} \text{ or } \Delta L = \frac{4FL}{\pi D^2 Y}$$

where F is the force applied, L is the length, D is the diameter and ΔL is the extension of the wire respectively.

As each wire is made up of same material therefore their Young's modulus is same for each wire.

For all the four wires, $Y, F (=\text{tension})$ are the same.

$$\therefore \Delta L \propto \frac{L}{D^2}$$

In (a) $\frac{L}{D^2} = \frac{200\text{ cm}}{(0.2\text{ cm})^2} = 5 \times 10^3\text{ cm}^{-1}$

In (b) $\frac{L}{D^2} = \frac{300\text{ cm}}{(0.3\text{ cm})^2} = 3.3 \times 10^3\text{ cm}^{-1}$

In (c) $\frac{L}{D^2} = \frac{50\text{ cm}}{(0.05\text{ cm})^2} = 20 \times 10^3\text{ cm}^{-1}$

In (d) $\frac{L}{D^2} = \frac{100\text{ cm}}{(0.1\text{ cm})^2} = 10 \times 10^3\text{ cm}^{-1}$

Hence, ΔL is maximum in (c).

11. **(b) :** As $Y = \frac{FL}{A\Delta L} = \frac{4FL}{\pi D^2 \Delta L}$

$$\Delta L = \frac{4FL}{\pi D^2 Y}$$

$$\therefore \frac{\Delta L_S}{\Delta L_C} = \frac{F_S}{F_C}\frac{L_S}{L_C}\frac{D_C^2}{D_S^2}\frac{Y_C}{Y_S}$$

where subscripts S and C refer to copper and steel respectively.

Here, $F_S = (5m + 2m)g = 7mg$

$F_C = 5mg$

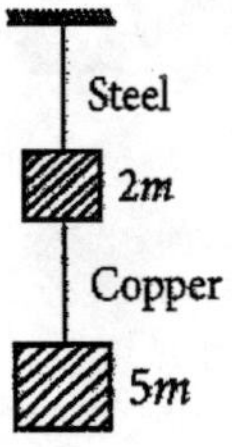

$$\frac{L_S}{L_C} = q, \frac{D_S}{D_C} = p, \frac{Y_S}{Y_C} = s$$

$$\therefore \frac{\Delta L_S}{\Delta L_C} = \left(\frac{7mg}{5mg}\right)(q)\left(\frac{1}{p}\right)^2\left(\frac{1}{s}\right) = \frac{7q}{5p^2 s}$$

Pressure

1. A U tube with both ends open to the atmosphere, is partially filled with water. Oil, which is immiscible with water, is poured into one side until it stands at a distance of 10 mm above the water level on the other side. Meanwhile the water rises by 65 mm from its original level (see diagram). The density of the oil is

(2017)

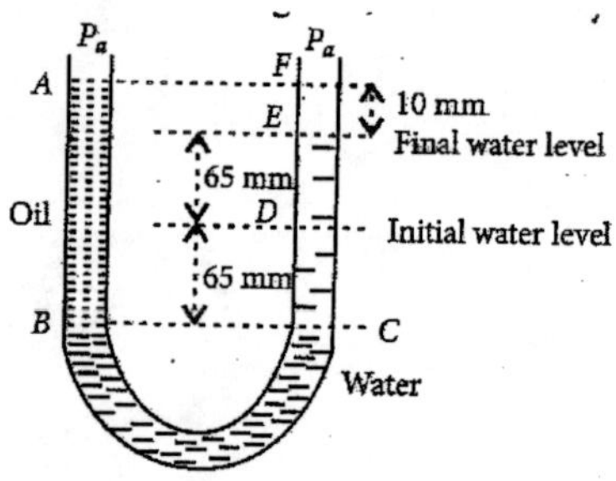

(a) 425 kg m^{-3} (b) 800 kg m^{-3}

(c) 928 kg m^{-3} (d) 650 kg m^{-3}

2. Two non-mixing liquids of densities ρ and $n\rho$ $(n > 1)$ are put in a container. The height of each liquid is h. A solid cylinder of length L and density d is put in this container. The cylinder floats with its axis vertical and length $pL(p < 1)$ in the denser liquid. The density d is equal to

(NEET-I 2016)

(a) $\{2 + (n - 1)p\}\rho$

(b) $\{1 + (n - 1)p\}\rho$

(c) $\{1 + (n + 1)p\}\rho$

(d) $\{2 + (n + 1)p\}\rho$

Streamline Flow

3. The cylindrical tube of a spray pump has radius R, one end of which has n fine holes, each of radius r. If the speed of the liquid in the tube is V, the speed of the ejection of the liquid through the holes is

(2015)

(a) $\frac{VR^2}{n^3r^2}$ (b) $\frac{V^2R}{nr}$

(c) $\frac{VR^2}{n^2r^2}$ (d) $\frac{VR^2}{nr^2}$

Bernoulli's Principle

4. The venturi-meter works on **(2023)**

(a) Bernoulli's principle

(b) The principle of parallel axes

(c) The principle of perpendicular axes

(d) Huygen's principle

5. A small hole of area of cross-section 2 mm^2 is present near the bottom of a fully filled open tank of height 2 m. Taking $g = 10 \text{ m/s}^2$, the rate of flow of water through the open hole would be nearly **(2019)**

(a) $6.4 \times \frac{10^{-6} \text{ m}^3}{\text{s}}$ (b) $12.6 \times 10^{-6} \text{ m}^3/\text{s}$

(c) $8.9 \times 10^{-6} \text{ m}^3/\text{s}$ (d) $2.23 \times 10^{-6} \text{ m}^3/\text{s}$

6. A wind with speed 40 m/s blows parallel to the roof of a house. The area of the roof is 250 m^2. Assuming that the pressure inside the house is atmospheric pressure, the force exerted by the wind on the roof and the direction of the force will be ($\rho_{air} = 1.2 \text{ kg/m}^3$) **(2015 celled)**

(a) 2.4×10^5 N, upwards

(b) 2.4×10^5 N, downwards

(c) 4.8×10^5 N, downwards

(d) 4.8×10^5 N, upwards

7. A fluid is in streamline flow across a horizontal pipe of variable area of cross section. For this which of the following statements is correct?

(Karnataka NEET 2013)

(a) The velocity is maximum at the narrowest part of the pipe and pressure is maximum at the widest part of the pipe.

(b) Velocity and pressure both are maximum at the narrowest part of the pipe.

(c) Velocity and pressure both are maximum at the widest part of the pipe.

(d) The velocity is minimum at the narrowest part of the pipe and the pressure is minimum at the widest part of the pipe.

Viscosity

8. A spherical ball is dropped in a long column of a highly viscous liquid. The curve in the graph shown, which represents the speed of the ball (v) as a function of time (t) is **(2022)**

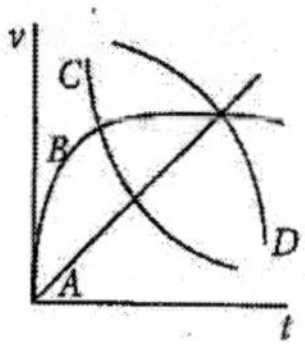

(a) A (b) B (c) C (d) D

9. The velocity of a small ball of mass M and density d, when dropped in a container filled with glycerine becomes constant after some time. If the density of glycerine is $\frac{d}{2}$, then the viscous force acting on the ball will be **(2021)**

(a) 2Mg (b) $\frac{Mg}{2}$

(c) Mg (d) $\frac{3}{2}Mg$

10. Two small spherical metal balls, having equal masses, are made from materials of densities ρ_1 and $\rho_2 (\rho_1 = 8\rho_2)$ and have radii of 1 mm and 2 mm, respectively. They are made to fall vertically (from rest) in a viscous medium whose coefficient of viscosity equals η and whose density is $0.1\rho_2$. The ratio of their terminal velocities would be **(Odisha NEET 2019)**

(a) $\frac{79}{72}$ (b) $\frac{19}{36}$

(c) $\frac{39}{72}$ (d) $\frac{79}{36}$

11. A small sphere of radius 'r' falls from rest in a viscous liquid. As a result, heat is produced due to viscous force. The rate of production of heat when the sphere attains its terminal velocity, is proportional to

(2018)

(a) r^3 (b) r^2 (c) r^5 (d) r^4

Surface Tension

12. The amount of energy required to form a soap bubble of radius 2 cm from a soap solution is nearly (surface tension of soap solution = 0.03 N m^{-1}) **(2023)**

(a) 5.06×10^{-4} J

(b) 3.01×10^{-4} J

(c) 50.1×10^{-4} J

(d) 30.16×10^{-4} J

13. If a soap bubble expands, the pressure inside the bubble **(2022)**

(a) decreases

(b) increases

(c) remains the same

(d) is equal to the atmospheric pressure

14. A capillary tube of radius r is immersed in water and water rises in it to a height h. The mass of the water in the capillary is 5 g. Another capillary tube of radius $2r$ is immersed in water. The mass of water that will rise in this tube is **(2020)**

(a) 2.5 g (b) 5.0 g

(c) 10.0 g (d) 20.0 g

15. A soap bubble, having radius of 1 mm, is blown from a detergent solution having a surface tension of 2.5×10^{-2} N/m. The pressure inside the bubble equals at a point Z_0 below the free surface of water in a container. Taking $g = 10\ \text{m/s}^2$, density of water $= 10^3\ \text{kg/m}^3$, the value of Z_0 is **(2019)**

(a) 0.5 cm (b) 100 cm

(c) 10 cm (d) 1 cm

16. A rectangular film of liquid is extended from (4 cm × 2 cm) to (5 cm × 4 cm). If the work done is 3×10^{-4} J, the value of the surface tension of the liquid is **(NEET-II 2016)**

(a) 0.250 N m^{-1} (b) 0.125 N m^{-1}

(c) 0.2 N m^{-1} (d) 8.0 N m^{-1}

17. Three liquids of densities ρ_1, ρ_2 and ρ_3 (with $\rho_1 > \rho_2 > \rho_3$), having the same value of surface tension T, rise to the same height in three identical capillaries. The angles of contact θ_1, θ_2 and θ_3 obey **(NEET-II 2016)**

(a) $\pi/2 > \theta_1 > \theta_2 > \theta_3 \geq 0$

(b) $0 \leq \theta_1 < \theta_2 < \theta_3 < \pi/2$

(c) $\pi/2 < \theta_1 < \theta_2 < \theta_3 < \pi$

(d) $\pi > \theta_1 > \theta_2 > \theta_3 > \pi/2$

18. Water rises to a height h in capillary tube. If the length of capillary tube above the surface of water is made less than h, then **(2015)**

(a) water rises upto a point a little below the top and stays there

(b) water does not rise at all

(c) water rises upto the tip of capillary tube and then starts overflowing like a fountain

(d) water rises upto the top of capillary tube and stays there without overflowing.

19. A certain number of spherical drops of a liquid of radius r coalesce to form a single drop of radius R and volume V. If T is the surface tension of the liquid, then

(2014)

(a) energy $= 4VT\left(\frac{1}{r}-\frac{1}{R}\right)$ is released

(b) energy $= 3VT\left(\frac{1}{r}+\frac{1}{R}\right)$ is absorbed

(c) energy $= 3VT\left(\frac{1}{r}-\frac{1}{R}\right)$ is released

(d) energy is neither released nor absorbed.

20. The wettability of a surface by a liquid depends primarily on **(2013)**

(a) density

(b) angle of contact between the surface and the liquid

(c) viscosity

(d) surface tension.

ANSWER KEY

1.	(c)	2.	(b)	3.	(d)	4.	(a)	5.	(b)	6.	(a)
7.	(a)	8.	(b)	9.	(b)	10.	(d)	11.	(c)	12.	(b)
13.	(a)	14.	(c)	15.	(d)	16.	(b)	17.	(b)	18.	(d)
19.	(c)	20.	(b)								

Hints & Explanations

1. (c) : Pressure at point C,

$$P_C = P_a + \rho_{\text{water}}\, g h_{\text{water}}\cdot$$

where $h_{\text{water}} = CE = (65+65)\text{mm} = 130\text{ mm}$

Pressure at point B, $P_B = P_a + \rho_{\text{oil}}\, g h_{\text{oil}}$

where $h_{\text{oil}} = AB = (65+65+10)\text{mm} = 140\text{ mm}$

In liquid, pressure is same at same liquid level,

$$P_B = P_C \Rightarrow \rho_{\text{oil}}\, g h_{\text{oil}} = \rho_{\text{water}}\, g h_{\text{water}}$$

$$\rho_{\text{oil}} = \frac{130\times10^3}{140} = \frac{13}{14}\times10^3$$

$$= 928.57\text{ kg m}^{-3}$$

2. (b):

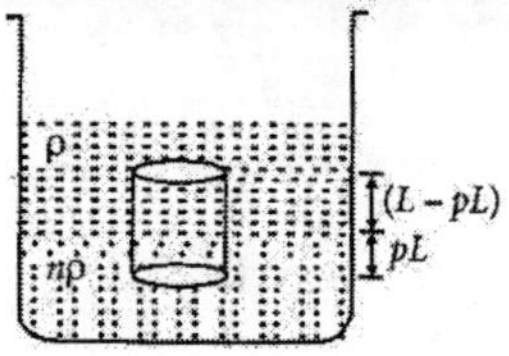

d = density of cylinder

A = area of cross-section of cylinder

Using law of floatation,

weight of cylinder = upthrust by two liquids

$$L\times A\times d\times g$$

$$= n\rho\times(pL\times A)g + \rho(L-pL)Ag$$

$$d = np\rho + \rho(1-p)$$

$$= (np+1-p)\rho$$

$$d = \{1+(n-1)p\}\rho$$

3. **(d) :** Let the speed of the ejection of the liquid through the holes be v. Then according to the equation of continuity,

$\pi R^2 V = n\pi r^2 v$ or $v = \frac{\pi R^2 V}{n\pi r^2} = \frac{VR^2}{nr^2}$

4. **(a) :** Venturimeter works an Bernoulli's principle

5. **(b) :** According to Torricelli's theorem,

Velocity, $= \sqrt{2gh} = \sqrt{2 \times 10 \times 2} =$ 6.32 m/s.

From equation of continuity,

Volume of liquid flowing per second, $Q = Av$

$= 2 \times 10^{-6} \times 6.32 = 12.6 \times 10^{-6}\ \mathrm{m^3/s}$

6. **(a) :** Applying Bernoulli's theorem at two points just inside house and out side house

$$p + \frac{1}{2}\rho v^2 = \text{constant}$$

inside pressure = P_{atm}, V = 0 (inside)

outside pressure = P, V = 40 m / s

$$P - P_{atm} = \frac{1}{2}\rho V^2 = \frac{1}{2} \times 1.2 \times 40 \times 40 = 960$$

Force is = $(P - P_{atm}) \times$ Area

$= 960 \times 250 = 2.4 \times 10^5$ (upward)

Force is in upward direction as pressure goes from higher to lower pressure area.

7. **(a) :** According to equation of continuity,

$Av =$ constant

Therefore, velocity is maximum at the narrowest part and minimum at the widest part of the pipe.

According to Bernoulli's theorem for a horizontal pipe,

$$P + \frac{1}{2}\rho v^2 = \text{constant}$$

Hence, when a fluid flow across a horizontal pipe of variable area of cross-section its velocity is maximum and pressure is minimum at the narrowest part and vice versa.

Viscosity

8. **(b) :** Initially, when the ball starts falling down, due to the force of gravity, the speed of ball increases and the viscous drag force increases also (it depends on speed $F = 6\pi\eta r v$). As the viscous force balances the force of gravity, the net acceleration of the ball is zero, and it starts moving with constant veleocty called terminal velocity. So, option (b) is correct.

9. **(b) :** Given, Mass of ball = M

Density of ball = d

Density of given wire = $\frac{d}{2}$

Viscous force = weight - buoyant force

$= vdg - v\left(\frac{d}{2}\right)g$

$= vdg\left(1 - \frac{1}{2}\right) = \frac{vdg}{2}$

Also mass, $M = vd$

So, from equation (i),

Viscous force = $\frac{Mg}{2}$

10. (d) : Terminal velocity, $v = \frac{2r^2(\rho-\sigma)g}{9\eta}$

Ratio of terminal velocity of spherical metal balls,

$$\frac{v_1}{v_2} = \frac{\frac{2}{9}(1)^2(8\rho_2 - 0.1\rho_2)}{\frac{2}{9}(2)^2(\rho_2 - 0.1\rho_2)} \Rightarrow \frac{v_1}{v_2} = \frac{7.9\rho_2}{4(0.9\rho_2)}$$

$$= \frac{79}{36}$$

11. (c) : The viscous drag force, $F = 6\pi\eta r v$;

where v = terminal velocity

$\therefore$ The rate of production of heat = power = force × terminal velocity

$\Rightarrow$ Power $= 6\pi\eta r v \cdot v = 6\pi\eta r v^2$

$\because$ Terminal velocity $v = \frac{2r^2(\rho-\sigma)g}{9\eta}$;

Now, power $= 6\pi\eta r\left[\frac{4r^4(\rho-\sigma)^2}{81\eta^2}g^2\right]$

or Power $\propto r^5$

12. (b) :

$$E = 2T\left(4\pi R^2\right)$$

$$= 2(0.03)(4)(3.14)\left(2\times10^{-2}\right)^2$$

$$= 3.01\times10^{-4} J$$

13. (a) : The excess pressure inside a soap bubble is

$$P_i = \frac{4T}{R} + P_0$$

where, $P_i \rightarrow$ inside pressure, $P_0 \rightarrow$ outside pressure

T = surface tension and R is radius.

Here, P_0, T is constant, so when R increases, P_i decreases.

So, the pressure inside the bubble decreases.

14. (c) : Force of surface tension balances the weight of water in capillary tube,

$$F_s = T\cos\theta(2\pi r) = mg$$

$m \propto r$

Hence, $\frac{m'}{m} = \frac{r'}{r} \Rightarrow \frac{m'}{5\text{ g}} = \frac{2r}{r} \Rightarrow m' = 10\text{ g}$

15. (d) : The pressure at a point Z_0 below the surface of water, $P_{Z_0} = P_0 + \rho g Z_0$

Also, pressure inside a soap bubble,

$P = P_0 + \frac{4T}{R}$ As per question, $P_{Z_0} = P$

$$\therefore P_0 + \frac{4T}{R} = P_0 + \rho g Z_0$$

$$Z_0 = \frac{4T}{R\rho g} = \frac{4\times2.5\times10^{-2}}{1\times10^{-3}\times10^3\times10}$$

$$= 1\times10^{-2}\text{ m} = 1\text{ cm}$$

16. (b) : Work done = Surface tension of film × Change in area of the film

or, $W = T \times \Delta A$

Here, $A_1 = 4\text{ cm}\times2\text{ cm} = 8\text{ cm}^2, A_2 = 5\text{ cm}\times4\text{ cm} = 20\text{ cm}^2$

$\Delta A = 2(A_2 - A_1) = 24\text{ cm}^2$

$= 24\times10^{-4}\text{ m}^2$

$W = 3\times10^{-4}\text{ J}, T = ?$

$$\therefore T = \frac{W}{\Delta A} = \frac{3\times10^{-4}}{24\times10^{-4}} = \frac{1}{8} = 0.125\text{ N m}^{-1}$$

17. (b) : Capillary rise, $h = \frac{2T\cos\theta}{r\rho g}$

For given value of T and r, $h \propto \frac{\cos\theta}{\rho}$

Also, $h_1 = h_2 = h_3$ or $\frac{\cos\theta_1}{\rho_1} = \frac{\cos\theta_2}{\rho_2} = \frac{\cos\theta_3}{\rho_3}$

Since, $\rho_1 > \rho_2 > \rho_3$, so $\cos\theta_1 > \cos\theta_2 > \cos\theta_3$

For $0 \leq \theta < \pi/2, \theta_1 < \theta_2 < \theta_3$

Hence, $0 \leq \theta_1 < \theta_2 < \theta_3 < \pi/2$

18. (d) : Water will not overflow but will change its radius of curvature.

19. (c) : Let n droplets each of radius r coalesce to form a big drop of radius R.

$\therefore$ Volume of n droplets = Volume of big drop

$$n \times \frac{4}{3}\pi r^3 = \frac{4}{3}\pi R^3 \Rightarrow n = \frac{R^3}{r^3}$$

Volume of big drop, $V = \frac{4}{3}\pi R^3$

Initial surface area of n droplets,

$$A_i = n \times 4\pi r^2 = \frac{R^3}{r^3} \times 4\pi r^2$$

$$= 4\pi \frac{R^3}{r} = \left(\frac{4}{3}\pi R^3\right)\frac{3}{r} = \frac{3V}{r}$$

Final surface area of big drop

$$A_f = 4\pi R^2 = \left(\frac{4}{3}\pi R^3\right)\frac{3}{R} = \frac{3V}{R}$$

Decrease in surface area

$$\Delta A = A_i - A_f = \frac{3V}{r} - \frac{3V}{R} = 3V\left(\frac{1}{r} - \frac{1}{R}\right)$$

$\therefore$ Energy released = Surface tension

$$= T \times \Delta A = 3VT\left(\frac{1}{r} - \frac{1}{R}\right)$$

$\times$ Decrease in surface area

20. (b) : The wettability of a surface by a liquid depends primarily on angle of contact between the surface and the liquid.

Chapter: 10 THERMAL PROPERTIES OF MATTER

Measurement of Temperature

1. On a new scale of temperature (which is linear) and called the W scale, the freezing and boiling points of water are 39°W and 239°W respectively. What will be the temperature on the new scale, corresponding to a temperature of 39°C on the Celsius scale? **(2008)**

(a) 200°W (b) 139°W

(c) 78°W (d) 117°W

2. Mercury thermometer can be used to measure temperature upto **(1992)**

(a) 260°C (b) 100°C

(c) 360°C (d) 500°C

3. A Centigrade and a Fahrenheit thermometer are dipped in boiling water. The water temperature is lowered until the Fahrenheit thermometer registers 140°F. What is the fall in temperature as registered by the centigrade thermometer? **(1990)**

(a) 80°C (b) 60°C

(c) 40°C (d) 30°C

Thermal Expansion

4. A copper rod of 88 cm and an aluminium rod of unknown length have their increase in length independent of increase in temperature. The length of aluminium rod is ($\alpha_{Cu} = 1.7 \times 10^{-5}\ K^{-1}, \alpha_{Al} = 2.2 \times 10^{-5}\ K^{-1}$) **(2019)**

(a) 68 cm (b) 6.8 cm

(c) 113.9 cm (d) 88 cm

5. Coefficient of linear expansion of brass and steel rods are α_1 and α_2. Lengths of brass and steel rods are l_1 and l_2 respectively. If $(l_2 - l_1)$ is maintained same at all temperatures, which one of the following relations holds good? **(NEET-I 2016, 1999)**

(a) $\alpha_1^2 l_2 = \alpha_2^2 l_1$

(b) $\alpha_1 l_1 = \alpha_2 l_2$

(c) $\alpha_1 l_2 = \alpha_2 l_1$

(d) $\alpha_1 l_2^2 = \alpha_2 l_1^2$

6. The value of coefficient of volume expansion of glycerin is $5 \times 10^{-4}\ K^{-1}$. The fractional change in the density of glycerin for a rise of 40°C in its temperature, is **(2015)**

(a) 0.025 (b) 0.010

(c) 0.015 (d) 0.020

7. The density of water at 20°C is 998 kg/m^3 and at 40°C is 992 kg/m^3. The coefficient of volume expansion of water is **(Karnataka NEET 2013)**

(a) $3 \times 10^{-4}/°C$

(b) $2 \times 10^{-4}/°C$

(c) $6 \times 10^{-4}/°C$

(d) $10^{-4}/°C$

Specific Heat Capacity

8. The quantities of heat required to raise the temperature of two solid copper spheres of radii r_1 and $r_2 (r_1 = 1.5r_2)$ through 1 K are in the ratio **(2020)**

(a) $\frac{27}{8}$ (b) $\frac{9}{4}$

(c) $\frac{3}{2}$ (d) $\frac{5}{3}$

9. Thermal capacity of 40 g of aluminium ($s = 0.2 \text{cal/gK}$) is **(1990)**

(a) 168 J/K (b) 672 J/K

(c) 840 J/K (d) 33.6 J/K

Calorimetry

10. Two identical bodies are made of a material for which the heat capacity increases with temperature. One of these is at 100°C, while the other one is at 0°C. If the two bodies are brought into contact, then, assuming no heat loss, the final common temperature is

(NEET-II 2016)

(a) 50°C
(b) more than 50°C
(c) less than 50°C but greater than 0°C
(d) 0 °C

Change of State

11. A piece of ice falls from a height h so that it melts completely. Only one-quarter of the heat produced is absorbed by the ice and all energy of ice gets converted into heat during its fall. The value of h is [Latent heat of ice is 3.4×10^5 J/kg and $g = 10$ N/kg] **(NEET-I 2016)**

(a) 136 km (b) 68 km

(c) 34 km (d) 544 km

12. Steam at 100°C is passed into 20 g of water at 10°C. When water acquires a temperature of 80°C, the mass of water present will be [Take specific heat of water $= 1 \text{calg}^{-1}\,°\text{C}^{-1}$ and latent heat of steam $= 540 \text{calg}^{-1}$] **(2014)**

(a) 24 g (b) 1.5 g

(c) 42.5 g (d) 22.5 g

13. Liquid oxygen at 50 K is heated to 300 K at constant pressure of 1 atm. The rate of heating is constant. Which one of the following graphs represents the variation of temperature with time? **(2012)**

(a) 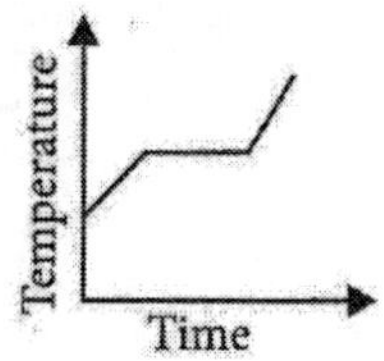

(b) 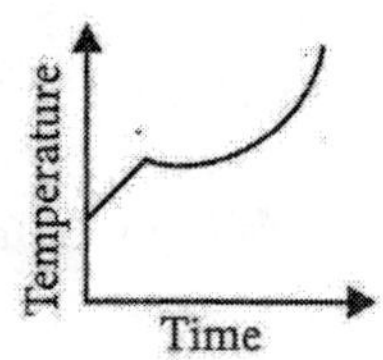

(c) 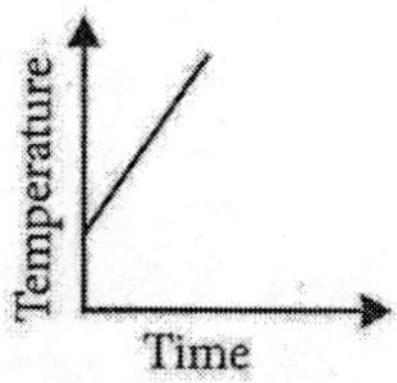

(d) 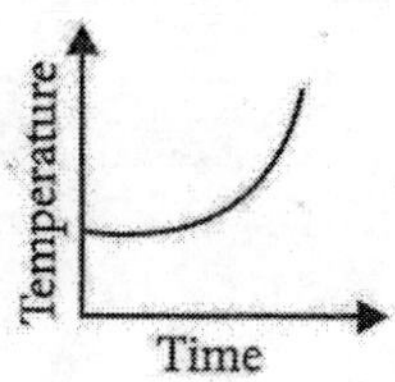

14. If 1 g of steam is mixed with 1 g of ice, then resultant temperature of the mixture is **(1999)**

(a) $100^{\circ}C$ (b) $230^{\circ}C$

(c) $270^{\circ}C$ (d) $50^{\circ}C$

15. 10gm of ice cubes at $0^{\circ}C$ are released in a tumbler (water equivalent $55\ g$) at $40^{\circ}C$. Assuming that negligible heat is taken from the surroundings, the temperature of water in the tumbler becomes nearely ($L = 80 cal/g$) **(1988)**

(a) $31^{\circ}C$ (b) $22^{\circ}C$

(c) $19^{\circ}C$ (d) $15^{\circ}C$

Heat Transfer

16. The energy that will be ideally radiated by a 100 kW transmitter in 1 hour is **(2022)**

(a) 36×10^{7} J (b) 36×10^{4} J

(c) 36×10^{5} J (d) 1×10^{5} J

17. Two rods A and B of different materials are welded together as shown in figure. Their thermal conductivities are K_1 and K_2. The thermal conductivity of the composite rod w'ill be **(2017)**

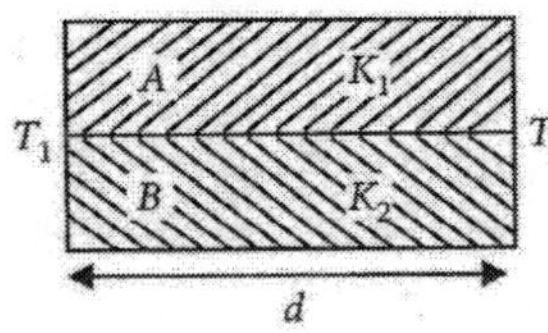

(a) $\frac{3(K_1+K_2)}{2}$ (b) $K_1 + K_2$

(c) $2(K_1 + K_2)$ (d) $\frac{K_1+K_2}{2}$

18. The two ends of a metal rod are maintained at temperatures $100^{\circ}C$ and $110^{\circ}C$. The rate of heat flow in the rod is found to be $4.0\ J/s$. If the ends are maintained at temperatures $200^{\circ}C$ and $210^{\circ}C$, the rate of heat flow will be

(2015 Cancelled)

(a) $8.0\ J/s$ (b) $4.0\ J/s$

(c) $44.0\ J/s$ (d) $16.8\ J/s]$

19. Two metal rods 1 and 2 of same lengths have same temperature difference between their ends. Their thermal conductivities are K_1 and K_2 and cross sectional areas A_1 and A_2, respectively. If the rate of heat conduction in 1 is four times that in 2 , then

(Karnataka NEET 2013)

(a) $K_1A_1 = 4K_2A_2$

(b) $K_1A_1 = 2K_2A_2$

(c) $4K_1A_1 = K_2A_2$

(d) $K_1A_1 = K_2A_2$

20. A slab of stone of area $0.36\ m^2$ and thickness $0.1\ m$ is exposed on the lower surface to steam at $100^{\circ}C$. A block of ice at $0^{\circ}C$ rests on the upper surface of the slab. In one hour 4.8 kg of ice is melted. The thermal conductivity of slab is

(Given latent heat of fusion of ice $= 3.36 \times 10^{5}\ J\ kg^{-1}$)

(Mains 2012)

(a) $1.24\ J/m/s/{}^{\circ}C$

(b) $1.29\ J/m/s/{}^{\circ}C$

(c) $2.05\ J/m/s/{}^{\circ}C$

(d) $1.02\ J/m/s/{}^{\circ}C$

21. A cylindrical metallic rod in thermal contact with two reservoirs of heat at its two ends conducts an amount of heat Q in time t. The metallic rod is melted and the material is formed into a rod of half the radius of the original rod. What is the amount of heat conducted by the new rod, when placed in thermal contact with the two reservoirs in time ? **(2010)**

(a) $\frac{Q}{4}$ (b) $\frac{Q}{16}$

(c) $2Q$ (d) $\frac{Q}{2}$

22. The two ends of a rod of length L and a uniform cross-sectional area A are kept at two temperatures T_1 and $T_2 (T_1 > T_2)$. The rate of heat transfer, $\frac{dQ}{dt}$, through the rod in a steady state is given by **(2009)**

(a) $\frac{dQ}{dt} = \frac{k(T_1-T_2)}{LA}$

(b) $\frac{dQ}{dt} = kLA(T_1 - T_2)$

(c) $\frac{dQ}{dt} = \frac{kA(T_1-T_2)}{L}$

(d) $\frac{dQ}{dt} = \frac{kL(T_1-T_2)}{A}$

23. Which of the following rods, (given radius r and length l) each made of the same material and whose ends are maintained at the same temperature will conduct most heat? **(2005)**

(a) $r = r_0, l = l_0$

(b) $r = 2r_0, l = l_0$

(c) $r = r_0, l = 2l_0$

(d) $r = 2r_0, l = 2l_0$.

24. Consider a compound slab consisting of two different materials having equal thicknesses and thermal conductivities K and $2K$, respectively. The equivalent thermal conductivity of the slab is **(2003)**

(a) $\frac{2}{3}K$ (b) $\sqrt{2}K$ (c) $3K$ (d) $\frac{4}{3}K$

25. Consider two rods of same length and different specific heats (S_1, S_2), conductivities (K_1, K_2) and area of cross-sections (A_1, A_2) and both having temperatures T_1 and T_2 at their ends. If rate of loss of heat due to conduction is equal, then **(2002)**

(a) $K_1A_1 = K_2A_2$

(b) $\frac{K_1A_1}{S_1} = \frac{K_2A_2}{S_2}$

(c) $K_2A_1 = K_1A_2$

(d) $\frac{K_2A_1}{S_2} = \frac{K_1A_2}{S_1}$

26. A cylindrical rod having temperature T_1 and T_2 at its end. The rate of flow of heat Q_1 cal/sec. If all the linear dimension are doubled keeping temperature constant, then rate of flow of heat Q_2 will be **(2001)**

(a) $4Q_1$ (b) $2Q_1$

(c) $Q_1/4$ (d) $Q_1/2$

27. Heat is flowing through two cylindrical rods of the same material. The diameters of the rods are in the ratio $1:2$ and the lengths in the ratio $2:1$. If the temperature difference between the ends is same, then ratio of the rate of flow of heat through them will be **(1995)**

(a) $2:1$ (b) $8:1$

(c) $1:1$ (d) $1:8$

28. If the temperature of the sun is doubled, the rate of energy recieved on earth will be increased by a factor of **(1993)**

(a) 2 (b) 4

(c) 8 (d) 16

ANSWER KEY

1.	(d)	2.	(c)	3.	(c)	4.	(a)	5.	(b)	6.	(d)
7.	(a)	8.	(a)	9.	(d)	10.	(b)	11.	(a)	12.	(d)
13.	(a)	14.	(a)	15.	(b)	16.	(a)	17.	(d)	18.	(c)
19.	(a)	20.	(a)	21.	(b)	22.	(c)	23.	(b)	24.	(a)
25.	(a)	26.	(b)	27.	(d)	28.	(d)				

Hints & Explanations

1. (d) :

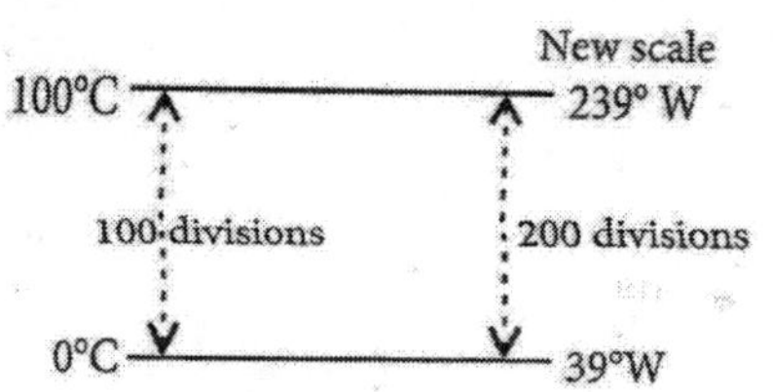

$\therefore$ $39°C = 39 \times 2 + 39 = (78 + 39)°W$

$= 117°W$

2. (c) : Mercury thermometer is based on the principle of change of volume with rise of temperature and can measure temperatures ranging from $-30°C$ to $357°C$

3. (c) : Here, $F = 140°$

Using $\frac{F-32}{180} = \frac{C}{100}$, or, $\therefore \frac{140-32}{180} = \frac{C}{100} \Rightarrow C = 60°C$

we get, fall in temperature $= 40°C$

4. (a) : As per question, $\Delta l_{Cu} = \Delta l_{Al}$

or, $l_{Cu}\alpha_{Cu}\Delta T = l_{Al}\alpha_{Al}\Delta T$

$$l_{Al} = \frac{l_{Cu}\alpha_{Cu}}{\alpha_{Al}} = \frac{88 \times 1.7 \times 10^{-5}}{2.2 \times 10^{-5}} = 68 \text{ cm}$$

5. (b) : Linear expansion of brass $= \alpha_1$

Linear expansion of steel $= \alpha_2$

Length of brass rod $= l_1$, Length of steel rod $= l_2$

On increasing the temperature of the rods by ΔT, new lengths would be

$$l_1' = l_1(1 + \alpha_1\Delta T)$$
$$l_2' = l_2(1 + \alpha_2\Delta T)$$

Subtracting eqn. (i) from eqn. (ii), we get

$$l_2' - l_1' = (l_2 - l_1) + (l_2\alpha_2 - l_1\alpha_1)\Delta T$$

According to question,

$$l_2' - l_1' = l_2 - l_1 \text{ (for all temperatures)}$$

$\therefore$ $l_2\alpha_2 - l_1\alpha_1 = 0$ or $l_1\alpha_1 = l_2\alpha_2$

6. (d) : Let ρ_0 and ρ_T be densities of glycerin at $0°C$ and $T°C$ respectively. Then,

$$\rho_T = \rho_0(1 - \gamma\Delta T)$$

where γ is the coefficient of volume expansion of glycerine and ΔT is rise in temperature.

$\frac{\rho_T}{\rho_0} = 1 - \gamma\Delta T$ or $\gamma\Delta T = 1 - \frac{\rho_T}{\rho_0}$

Thus, $\frac{\rho_0 - \rho_T}{\rho_0} = \gamma\Delta T$

Here, $\gamma = 5 \times 10^{-4}\ \text{K}^{-1}$ and $\Delta T = 40°\text{C} = 40\ \text{K}$

$\therefore$ The fractional change in the density of glycerin

$$= \frac{\rho_0 - \rho_T}{\rho_0} = \gamma\Delta T = (5 \times 10^{-4}\ \text{K}^{-1})(40\ \text{K})$$

$$= 0.020$$

7. (a) : As $\rho_{T_2} = \frac{\rho_{T_1}}{(1+\gamma\Delta T)} = \frac{\rho_{T_1}}{1+\gamma(T_2 - T_1)}$

Here, $T_1 = 20°\text{C}, T_2 = 40°\text{C}$

$\rho_{20} = 998\ \text{kg/m}^3, \rho_{40} = 992\ \text{kg/m}^3$

$$\therefore 992 = \frac{998}{1 + \gamma(40 - 20)} \text{ or, } 992 = \frac{998}{1 + 20\gamma}$$

$$1 + 20\gamma = \frac{998}{992} \text{ or } 20\gamma = \frac{998}{992} - 1 = \frac{6}{992}$$

$$\gamma = \frac{6}{992} \times \frac{1}{20} = 3 \times 10^{-4}/°\text{C}$$

8. (a) : Heat required, $\Delta Q = ms\Delta T$

$\Delta Q = (V \times \rho \times s \times \Delta T)$

$= \frac{4}{3}\pi r^3 \rho \cdot s\Delta T$

$$\frac{\Delta Q_1}{\Delta Q_2} = \frac{r_1^3}{r_2^3} = \left(\frac{r_1}{r_2}\right)^3 = (1.5)^3 = \frac{27}{8}$$

9. (d) : Thermal capacity $= ms = 40 \times 0.2$

$= 8\text{cal/K} = 33.6\ \text{J/K}$.

10. (b) : Since, heat capacity of material increases with increase in temperature so, body at 100°C has more heat capacity than body at 0°C. Hence, final common temperature of the system will be closer to 100°C.

$\therefore T_c > 50°\text{C}$

11. (a) : Gravitational potential energy of a piece of ice at a height $(h) = mgh$

Heat absorbed by the ice to melt completely

$$\Delta Q = \frac{1}{4}mgh$$

Also, $\Delta Q = mL$

From eqns. (i) and (ii), $mL = \frac{1}{4}mgh$ or,

$h = \frac{4L}{g}$

Here $L = 3.4 \times 10^5\ \text{J kg}^{-1}, g = 10\ \text{N kg}^{-1}$

$$\therefore h = \frac{4 \times 3.4 \times 10^5}{10} = 4 \times 34 \times 10^3$$

$$= 136\ \text{km}$$

12. (d) : Specific heat of water, $s_w = 1\text{calg}^{-1}\,°\text{C}^{-1}$

Latent heat of steam, $L_s = 540\text{calg}^{-1}$

Heat lost by m g of steam at 100°C to change into water at 80°C is

$Q_1 = mL_s + ms_w\Delta T_w$

$= m \times 540 + m \times 1 \times (100 - 80)$

$= 540\ \text{m} + 20\ \text{m} = 560\ \text{m}$

Heat gained by 20 g of water to change its temperature from 10°C to 80°C is

$Q_2 = m_w s_w \Delta T_w = 20 \times 1 \times (80 - 10)$

$$= 1400$$

According to principle of calorimetry,

$Q_1 = Q_2$

$\therefore 560m = 1400$ or $m = 2.5$ g

Total mass of water present

$= (20 + m)\text{g} = (20 + 2.5)\text{g} = 22.5 \text{ g}$

13. (a) : Temperature of liquid oxygen will first increase in the same phase. Then, the liquid oxygen will change to gaseous phase during which temperature will remain constant. After that temperature of oxygen in gaseous state will increase. Hence option (a) represents corresponding temperature-time graph.

14. (a) : Heat Required to melt 1gm of ice at 0°C is 80 calorie

Heat required to convert 1gm of steam at 0°C into 1gm of water at 100°C = 1 × 1× 100 = 100 calorie

Heat Required for condensing 1 gm of steam

= 1 × 540 = 540 calorie.

Clearly whole of steam is not condensed so, temperature after mixture is 100°C.

15. (b) : Let the final temperature be T

Heat required by ice $= mL + m \times s \times (T - 0)$

$= 10 \times 80 + 10 \times 1 \times T$

Heat lost by tumbler $= 55 \times (40 - T)$

By using law of calorimetry,

heat gained = heat lost

$800 + 10\text{ T} = 55 \times (40 - T)$

$\Rightarrow T = 21.54°\text{C} = 22°\text{C}$

16. (a) : Power, $P = 100\text{KW} = 1{,}00 \times 10^3 \text{ W}$

time, $t = 1\text{hr} = 3600 \text{ s}$

Energy, E = power × time

$E = 100 \times 10^3 \times 3600$

$E = 36 \times 10^7 \text{ J}$

17. (d) : Equivalent thermal conductivity of the composite rod in parallel combination will be,

$$K = \frac{K_1A_1 + K_2A_2}{A_1 + A_2} = \frac{K_1 + K_2}{2}$$

18. (c) : $Q \propto \Delta T$

$\square T_1 = 110 - 100 = 10^oC$

$\square T_2 = 210 - 200 = 10^oC$

$$\frac{Q_1}{Q_2} = \frac{\Delta T_1}{\Delta T_2} \Rightarrow \frac{4}{Q_2} = \frac{10}{10}$$

$$Q_2 = 4J/S$$

19. (a) : Let L be length of each rod.

Rate of heat flow in rod 1 for the temperature difference ΔT is

$$H_1 = \frac{K_1A_1\Delta T}{L}$$

Rate of heat flow in rod 2 for the same difference ΔT is

$$H_2 = \frac{K_2A_2\Delta T}{L}$$

As per question, $H_1 = 4H_2$

$$\frac{K_1A_1\Delta T}{L} = 4\frac{K_2A_2\Delta T}{L}; K_1A_1 = 4K_2A_2$$

20. (a) : 0.1 m

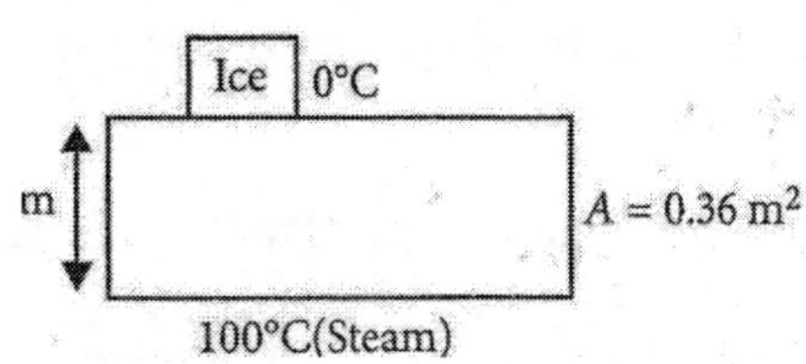

Heat flows through the slab in t s is

$$Q = \frac{KA(T_1 - T_2)t}{L} = \frac{K \times 0.36 \times (100 - 0) \times 3600}{0.1}$$
$$= \frac{K \times 0.36 \times 100 \times 3600}{0.1}$$

So ice melted by this heat is $m_{ice} = \frac{Q}{L_f}$

or $Q = m_{ice} L_f = 4.8 \times 3.36 \times 10^5$ J

From (i) and (ii), we get

$$\frac{K \times 0.36 \times 100 \times 3600}{0.1} = 4.8 \times 3.36 \times 10^5$$
$$K = \frac{4.8 \times 3.36 \times 10^5 \times 0.1}{0.36 \times 100 \times 3600}$$
$$= 1.24 \text{ J/m/s/ °C}$$

21. (b) : The amount of heat flows in time t through a cylindrical metallic rod of length L and uniform area of crosssection $A(= \pi R^2)$ with its ends maintained at temperatures T_1 and $T_2 (T_1 > T_2)$ is given by

$$Q = \frac{KA(T_1 - T_2)t}{L}$$

where K is the thermal conductivity of the material of the rod. Area of cross-section of new rod

$$A' = \pi \left(\frac{R}{2}\right)^2 = \frac{\pi R^2}{4} = \frac{A}{4}$$

As the volume of the rod remains unchanged $\therefore AL = A'L'$

where L' is the length of the new rod

or $L' = L\frac{A}{A'} = 4L$

Now, the amount of heat flows in same time t in the new rod with its ends maintained at the same temperatures T_1 and T_2 is given by

$$Q' = \frac{KA'(T_1 - T_2)t}{L'}$$

Substituting the values of A' and L'

$$Q' = \frac{K(A/4)(T_1 - T_2)t}{4L} = \frac{1}{16}\frac{KA(T_1 - T_2)t}{L}$$
$$= \frac{1}{16}Q$$

(Using (i))

22. (c) : Similar to $I = V/R$

$$\frac{dQ}{dt} = \frac{kA}{L}(T_1 - T_2)$$

k = conductivity of the rod.

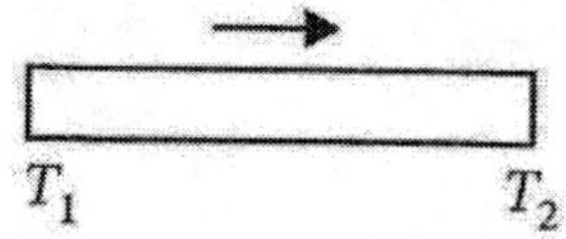

23. (b) : Heat conducted

$$= \frac{KA(T_1 - T_2)t}{l} = \frac{K\pi r^2(T_1 - T_2)t}{l}$$

The rod with the maximum ratio of r^2/l will conduct most. Here the rod with $r = 2r_0$ and $l = l_0$ will conduct most.

24. (a) : The slabs are in series.

Total resistance $R = R_1 + R_2$

$$\Rightarrow \frac{l}{AK_{effective}} = \frac{l}{A \cdot K} + \frac{l}{A2K}$$

$$\Rightarrow \frac{1}{K_{effective}} = \frac{1}{K} + \frac{1}{2K} = \frac{3}{2K} \therefore K_{effective} = \frac{2K}{3}$$

25. (a) :

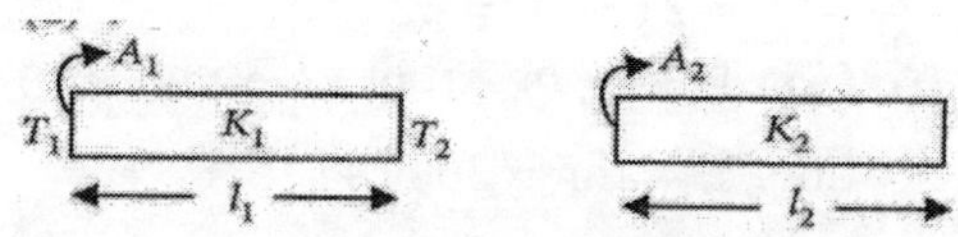

Rate of heat loss in rod $1 = Q_1 = \frac{K_1A_1(T_1-T_2)}{l_1}$

Rate of heat loss in rod $2 = Q_2 = \frac{K_2A_2(T_1-T_2)}{l_2}$

By problem, $Q_1 = Q_2$.

$$\therefore \frac{K_1A_1(T_1-T_2)}{l_1} = \frac{K_2A_2(T_1-T_2)}{l_2}$$

$\therefore K_1A_1 = K_2A_2$

$[\because l_1 = l_2]$

26. (b) : Heat flow rate $\frac{dQ}{dt} = \frac{KA(T_1-T_2)}{L} = Q_1$

When linear dimensions are double.

$A_1 \propto r_1^2, L_1 = L$

$A_2 \propto 4r_1^2, L_2 = 2L$ so $Q_2 = 2Q_1$

27. (d) : Ratio of diameters of rod = 1: 2 and ratio of their lengths 2: 1.

The rate of flow of heat, $(Q) = \frac{KA\Delta T}{l} \propto \frac{A}{l}$.

Therefore, $\frac{Q_1}{Q_2} = \frac{A_1}{A_2} \times \frac{l_2}{l_1} = \left(\frac{1}{2}\right)^2 \times \frac{1}{2} = \frac{1}{8}$

or $Q_1 : Q_2 = 1:8$

28. (d) : Amount of energy radiated $\propto T^4$.

Chapter: 11

THERMODYNAMICS

First Law of Thermodynamics

1. A sample of 0.1 g of water at 100°C and normal pressure $(1.013 \times 10^5 \text{ N m}^{-2})$ requires 54cal of heat energy to convert to steam at 100°C. If the volume of the steam produced is 167.1cc, the change in internal energy of the sample, is **(2018)**
(a) 104.3 J (b) 208.7 J
(c) 42.2 J (d) 84.5 J

2. A system is taken from state a to state c by two paths adc and abc as shown in the figure. The internal energy at a is $U_a = 10$ J. Along the path adc the amount of heat absorbed $dQ_1 = 50$ J and the work

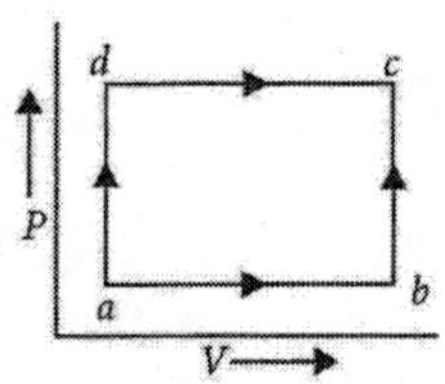

obtained $dW_1 = 20$ J whereas along the path abc the heat absorbed $dQ_2 = 36$ J. The amount of work along the path abc is **(Karnataka NEET 2013)**
(a) 10 J (b) 12 J
(c) 36 J (d) 6 J

3. The internal energy change in a system that has absorbed 2kcal of heat and done 500 J of work is **(2009)**
(a) 6400 J (b) 5400 J
(c) 7900 J (d) 8900 J

4. 110 joule of heat is added to a gaseous system whose internal energy is 40 J, then the amount of external work done is
(a) 150 J (b) 70 J
(c) 110 J (d) 40 J

5. First law of thermodynamics is consequence of conservation of **(1988)**
(a) work (b) energy
(c) heat (d) all of these

Specific Heat Capacity

6. One mole of an ideal diatomic gas undergoes a transition from A to B along a path AB as shown in the figure. The change in internal energy of the gas during the transition is **(2015 Canceled)**

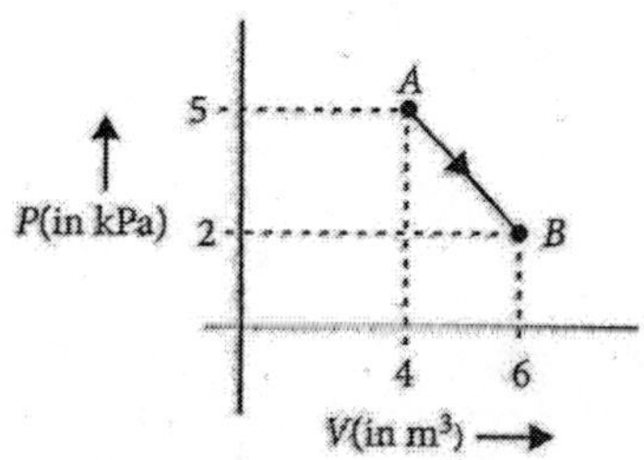

(a) 20 J (b) −12 kJ
(c) 20 kJ (d) −20 kJ

7. If c_p and c_v denote the specific heats per unit mass of an ideal gas of molecular weight M, then **(Mains 2010)**
(a) $c_p - c_v = R/M^2$
(b) $c_p - c_v = R$
(c) $c_p - c_v = R/M$

(d) $c_p - c_v = MR$
where R is the molar gas constant.

8. If the ratio of specific heat of a gas at constant pressure to that at constant volume is γ, the change in internal energy of a mass of gas, when the volume changes from V to $2V$ at constant pressure P, is **(1998)**

(a) $\frac{PV}{(\gamma-1)}$ (b) PV
(c) $\frac{R}{(\gamma-1)}$ (d) $\frac{\gamma PV}{(\gamma-1)}$

9. One mole of an ideal gas requires 207 J heat to rise the temperature by 10 K when heated at constant pressure. If the same gas is heated at constant volume to raise the temperature by the same 10 K, the heat required is **(1990)**

(Given the gas constant $R = 8.3$ J/moleK)
(a) 198.7 J (b) 29 J
(c) 215.3 J (d) 124 J

Thermodynamic State Variables and Equation of State

10. A cylinder contains hydrogen gas at pressure of 249kPa and temperature 27°C. Its density is ($R = 8.3\ \text{J mol}^{-1}\ \text{K}^{-1}$) **(2020)**

(a) $0.5\ \text{kg/m}^3$
(b) $0.2\ \text{kg/m}^3$
(c) $0.1\ \text{kg/m}^3$
(d) $0.02\ \text{kg/m}^3$

11. Which of the following is not thermodynamical function? **(1993)**
(a) Enthalpy (b) Work done
(c) Gibb's energy
(d) Internal energy

Thermodynamic Processes

12. An ideal gas undergoes four different processes from the same initial state as shown in the figure below. Those processes are adiabatic, isothermal, isobaric and isochoric. The curve which represents the adiabatic process among 1,2,3 and 4 is **(2022)**

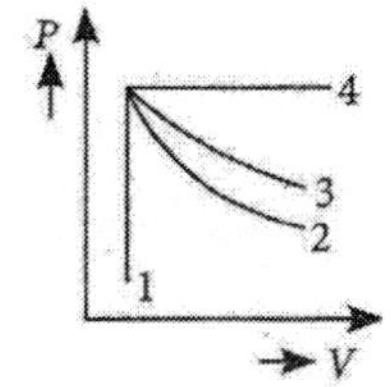

(a) 1 (b) 2
(c) 3 (d) 4

13. Two cylinders A and B of equal capacity are connected to each other via a stopcock. A contains an ideal gas at standard temperature and pressure. B is completely evacuated. The entire system is thermally insulated. The stopcock is suddenly opened. The process is **(2020)**

(a) isothermal (b) adiabatic
(c) isochoric (d) isobaric

14. In which of the following processes, heat is neither absorbed nor released by a system? **(2019)**

(a) isochoric (b) isothermal
(c) adiabatic (d) isobaric

15. The volume (V) of amonatomic gas varies with its temperature (T), as shown in the graph. The ratio of work done by the gas, to the heat absorbed by it, when it undergoes a change from state A to state B, is **(2018)**

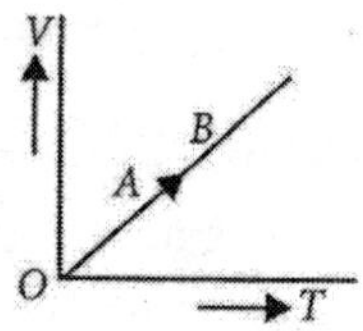

(a) 2/5 (b) 2/3

(c) 1/3 (d) 2/7

16. Thermodynamic processes are indicated in the following diagram.

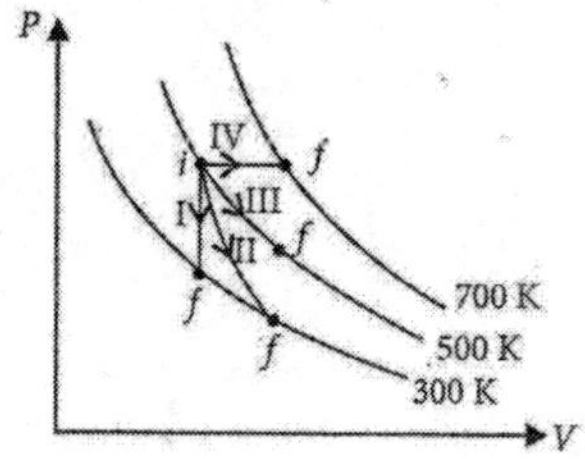

Match the following. **(2017)**

Coloumn-1	**Coloumn-1**
P. Process I	A. Adiabatic
Q. Process II	B. Isobaric
R. Process III	C. Isochoric
S. Process IV	D. Isothermal

(a) $P \to C, Q \to A, R \to D, S \to B$

(b) $P \to C, Q \to D, R \to B, S \to A$

(c) $P \to D, Q \to B, R \to A, S \to C$

(d) $P \to A, Q \to C, R \to D, S \to B$

17. One mole of an ideal monatomic gas undergoes a process described by the equation $PV^3 =$ constant. The heat capacity of the gas during this process is

(NEET-II 2016)

(a) $\frac{3}{2}R$ (b) $\frac{5}{2}R$

(c) $2R$ (d) R

18. A gas is compressed isothermally to half its initial volume. The same gas is compressed separately through an adiabatic process until its volume is again reduced to half. Then **(NEET-I 2016)**

(a) Compressing the gas isothermally or adiabatically will require the same amount of work.

(b) Which of the case (whether compression through isothermal or through adiabatic process) requires more work will depend upon the atomicity of the gas.

(c) Compressing the gas isothermally will require more work to be done.

(d) Compressing the gas through adiabatic process will require more work to be done.

19. An ideal gas is compressed to half its initial volume by means of several processes. Which of the process results in the maximum work done on the gas? **(2015)**

(a) Isochoric (b) Isothermal

(c) Adiabatic (d) Isobaric

20. Figure below shows two paths that may be taken by a gas to go from a state A to a state C. In process AB, 400 J of heat is added to the system and in process

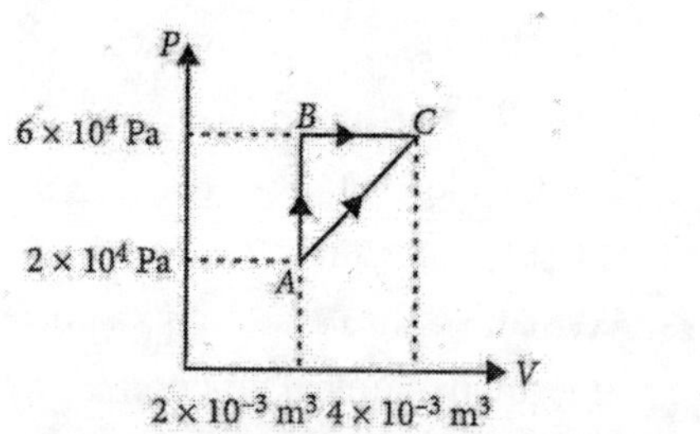

BC, 100 J of heat is added to the system. The heat absorbed by the system in the process AC will be **(2015 Cancelled)**

(a) 460 J (b) 300 J
(c) 380 J (d) 500 J

21. A monatomic gas at a pressure P, having a volume V expands isothermally to a volume $2V$ and then adiabatically to a volume 16 V. The final pressure of the gas is (Take = 5/3) **(2014)**

(a) $64P$ (b) $32P$
(c) $P/64$ (d) $16P$

22. A thermodynamic system undergoes cyclic process $ABCDA$ as shown in figure. The work done by the system in the cycle is **(2014)**

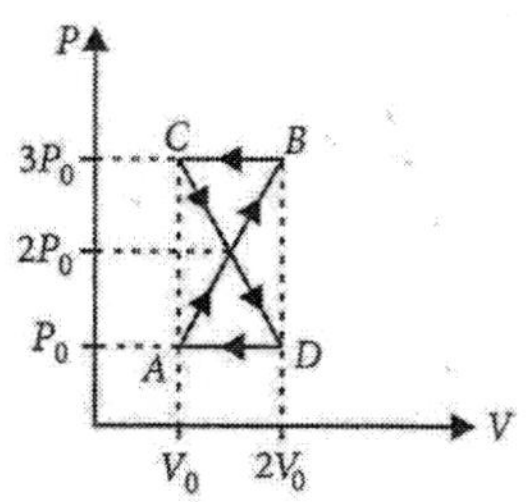

(a) P_0V_0 (b) $2P_0V_0$
(c) $\frac{P_0V_0}{2}$ (d) zero

23. A gas is taken through the cycle $A \to B \to C \to A$, as shown. What is the net work done by the gas? **(2013)**

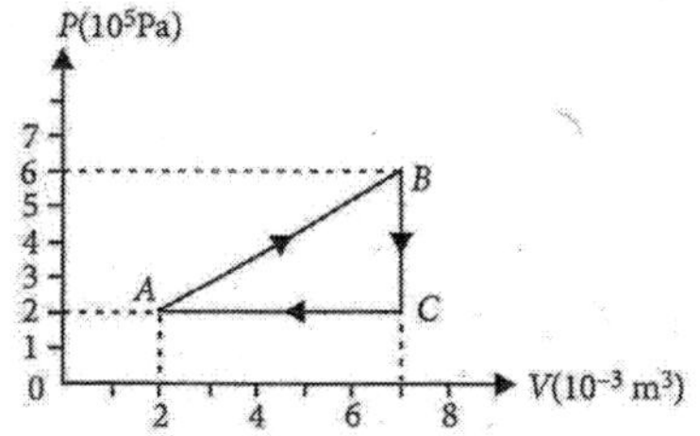

(a) Zero (b) −2000 J
(c) 2000 J (d) 1000 J

24. During an adiabatic process, the pressure of a gas is found to be proportional to the cube of its temperature. The ratio of $\frac{C_p}{C_v}$ for the gas is **(2013)**

(a) 5/3 (b) 3/2
(c) 4/3 (d) 2

25. Which of the following relations does not give the equation of an adiabatic process, where terms have their usual meaning? **(Karnataka NEET 2013)**

(a) $P^{1-\gamma}T^{\gamma}$ = constant
(b) PV^{γ} = constant
(c) $TV^{\gamma-1}$ = constant
(d) $P^{\gamma}T^{1-\gamma}$ = constant

26. A thermodynamic system is taken through the cycle $ABCD$ as shown in figure. Heat rejected by the gas during the cycle is **(2012)**

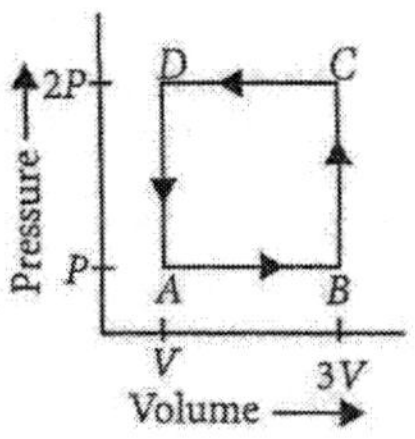

(a) $2PV$ (b) $4PV$
(c) $\frac{1}{2}PV$ (d) PV

27. An ideal gas goes from state A to state B via three different processes as indicated in the $P-V$ diagram. If Q_1, Q_2, Q_3 indicate the heat absorbed by the gas along the three

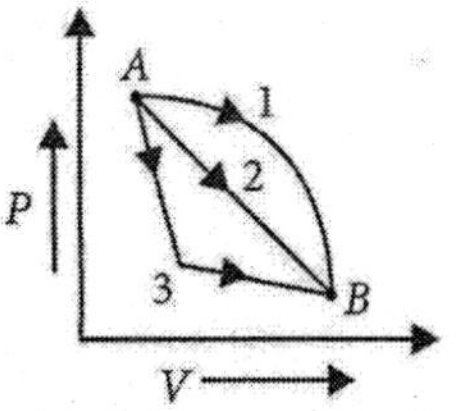

processes and $\Delta U_1, \Delta U_2, \Delta U_3$ indicate the change in internal energy along the three processes respectively, then

(Mains 2012)

(a) $Q_1 > Q_2 > Q_3$ and $\Delta U_1 = \Delta U_2 = \Delta U_3$
(b) $Q_3 > Q_2 > Q_1$ and $\Delta U_1 = \Delta U_2 = \Delta U_3$
(c) $Q_1 = Q_2 = Q_3$ and $\Delta U_1 > \Delta U_2 > \Delta U_3$
(d) $Q_3 > Q_2 > Q_1$ and $\Delta U_1 > \Delta U_2 > \Delta U_3$

28. One mole of an ideal gas goes from an initial state A to final state B via two processes : It first undergoes isothermal expansion from volume V to $3V$ and then its volume is reduced from $3V$ to V at constant pressure. The correct $P - V$ diagram representing the two processes is

(2012)

(a)
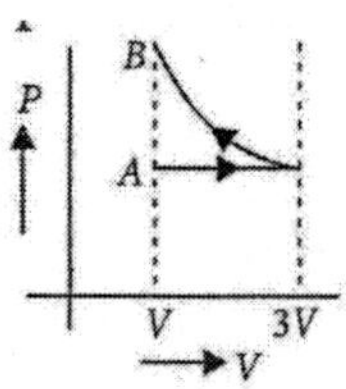

(b)
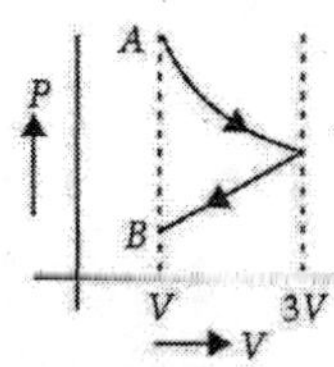

(c)
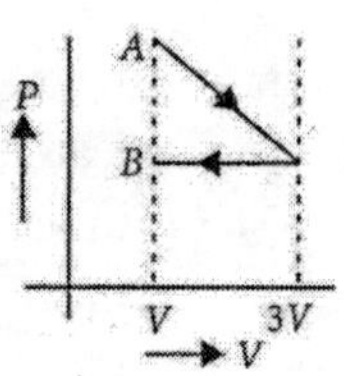

(d)
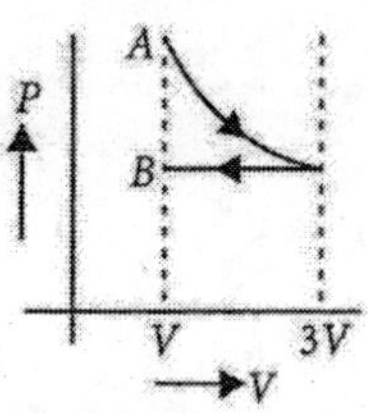

29. During an isothermal expansion, a confined ideal gas does $-150\,\text{J}$ of work against its surroundings. This implies that

(2011)

(a) 150 J of heat has been removed from the gas

(b) 300 J of heat has been added to the gas

(c) no heat is transferred because the process is isothermal

(d) 150 J of heat has been added to the gas.

30. A mass of diatomic gas ($\gamma = 1.4$) at a pressure of 2 atmospheres is compressed adiabatically so that its temperature rises from 27°C to 927°C. The pressure of the gas in the final state is **(Mains 2011)**

(a) 8 atm (b) 28 atm
(c) 68.7 atm (d) 256 atm

31. If ΔU and ΔW represent the increase in internal energy and work done by the system respectively in a thermodynamical process, which of the following is true?

(2010)

(a) $\Delta U = -\Delta W$, in an adiabatic process
(b) $\Delta U = \Delta W$, in an isothermal process
(c) $\Delta U = \Delta W$, in an adiabatic process
(d) $\Delta U = -\Delta W$, in an isothermal process

32. A monatomic gas at pressure P_1 and volume V_1 is compressed adiabatically to $\frac{1}{8}^{\text{th}}$ of its original volume. What is the final pressure of the gas?

(Mains 2010)

(a) $64P_1$ (b) P_1
(c) $16P_1$ (d) $32P_1$

33. In thermodynamic processes which of the following statements is not true? **(2009)**

(a) In an isochoric process pressure remains constant.

(b) In an isothermal process the temperature remains constant.

(c) In an adiabatic process $PV^{\gamma} =$ constant.

(d) In an adiabatic process the system is insulated from the surroundings.

34. If Q, E and W denote respectively the heat added, change in internal energy and the work done in a closed cyclic process, then **(2008)**

(a) $E = 0$ (b) $Q = 0$
(c) $W = 0$ (d) $Q = W = 0$

35. One mole of an ideal gas at an initial temperature of T K does $6R$ joule of work adiabatically. If the ratio of specific heats of this gas at constant pressure and at constant volume is $5/3$, the final temperature of gas will be **(2004)**

(a) $(T + 2.4)$K

(b) $(T - 2.4)$K

(c) $(T + 4)$K

(d) $(T - 4)$K

36. An ideal gas at $27°C$ is compressed adiabatically to $8/27$ of its original volume. The rise in temperature is (Take = $5/3$) **(1999)**

(a) 275 K (b) 375 K
(c) 475 K (d) 175 K

37. We consider a thermodynamic system. If ΔU represents the increase in its internal energy and W the work done by the system, which of the following statements is true? **(1998)**

(a) $\Delta U = -W$ in an isothermal process

(b) $\Delta U = W$ in an isothermal process

(c) $\Delta U = -W$ in an adiabatic process

(d) $\Delta U = W$ in an adiabatic process

38. A sample of gas expands from volume V_1 to V_2. The amount of work done by the gas is greatest, when the expansion is **(1997)**

(a) adiabatic

(b) equal in all cases

(c) isothermal

(d) isobaric.

39. An ideal gas, undergoing adiabatic change, has which of the following pressure temperature relationship? **(1996)**

(a) $P^{\gamma}T^{1-\gamma}$ = constant

(b) $P^{1-\gamma}T^{\gamma}$ = constant

(c) $P^{\gamma-1}T^{\gamma}$ = constant

(d) $P^{\gamma}T^{\gamma-1}$ = constant.

40. A diatomic gas initially at $18°C$ is compressed adiabatically to one eighth of its original volume. The temperature after compression will be **(1996)**

(a) $395.4°C$ (b) $144°C$
(c) $18°C$ (d) $887.4°C$

41. In an adiabatic change, the pressure and temperature of a monatomic gas are related as $P \propto T^{C}$, where C equals **(1994)**

(a) $3/5$ (b) $5/3$
(c) $2/5$ (d) $5/2$

42. An ideal gas A and a real gas B have their volumes increased from V to $2V$ under isothermal conditions. The increase in internal energy **(1993)**

(a) will be same in both A and B

(b) will be zero in both the gases

(c) of B will be more than that of A

(d) of A will be more than that of B.

43. A thermodynamic system is taken from state A to B along ACB and is brought back to A along BDA as shown in the PV diagram. The net work done during the complete cycle is given by the area **(1992)**

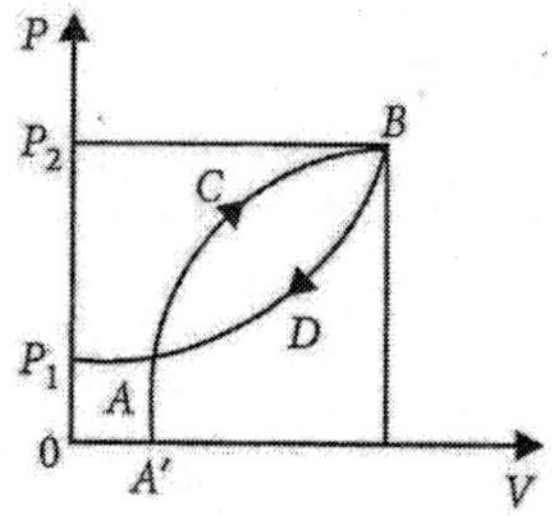

(a) $P_1ACBP_2P_1$ (b) $ACBB'A'A$

(c) $ACBDA$ (d) $ADBB'A'A$

44. A thermodynamic process is shown in the figure. The pressure and volumes corresponding to some points in the figure are

$P_A = 3 \times 10^4$ Pa; $V_A = 2 \times 10^{-3}$ m^3;

$P_B = 8 \times 10^4$ Pa; $V_D = 5 \times 10^{-3}$ m^3.

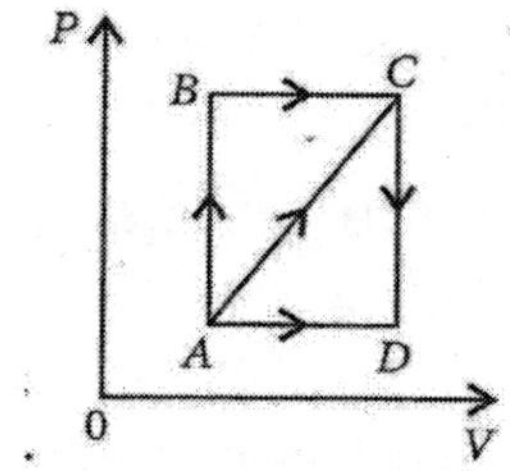

In the process AB, 600 J of heat is added to the system and in process BC, 200 J of heat is added to the system. The change in internal energy of the system is process AC would be **(1991)**

(a) 560 J (b) 800 J

(c) 600 J (d) 640 J

45. The efficiency of an ideal heat engine working between the freezing point and boiling point of water, is **(2018)**

(a) 26.8% (b) 20%

(c) 6.25% (d) 12.5%

Reversible and Irreversible Processes

46. Which of the following processes is reversible? **(2005)**

(a) Transfer of heat by conduction

(b) Transfer of heat by radiation

(c) Isothermal compression

(d) Electrical heating of a nichrome wire

ANSWER KEY

1. (b)	2. (d)	3. (c)	4. (b)	5. (b)	6. (d)	7. (c)
8. (a)	9. (d)	10. (b)	11. (b)	12. (b)	13. (b)	14. (c)
15. (a)	16. (a)	17. (d)	18. (d)	19. (c)	20. (a)	21. (c)
22. (d)	23. (d)	24. (b)	25. (d)	26. (a)	27. (a)	28. (d)
29. (d)	30. (d)	31. (a)	32. (d)	33. (a)	34. (a)	35. (d)
36. (b)	37. (c)	38. (d)	39. (b)	40. (a)	41. (d)	42. (b)
43. (c)	44. (a)	45. (a)	46. (c)			

Hints & Explanations

1. **(b) :** Using first law of thermodynamics, $\Delta Q = \Delta U + \Delta W$

$\Rightarrow 54 \times 4.18$

$= \Delta U + 1.013 \times 10^5 (167.1 \times 10^{-6} - 0)$

$\Rightarrow \Delta U = 208.7 \text{ J}$

2. (d) : According to first law of thermodynamics, $\delta Q = \delta U + \delta W$

Along the path adc, change in internal energy, $\delta U_1 = \delta Q_1 - \delta W_1$
$= 50J - 20J = 30J$

Along the path abc,

Change in internal energy,

$$\delta U_2 = \delta Q_2 - \delta W_2$$
$$\delta U_2 = 36 \text{ J} - \delta W_2$$

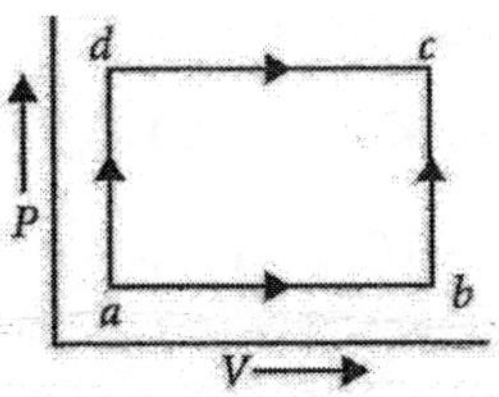

As change in internal energy is path independent.

$\therefore \delta U_1 = \delta U_2 \Rightarrow 30 \text{ J} = 36 \text{ J} - \delta W_2$

$\delta W_2 = 36 \text{ J} - 30 \text{ J} = 6 \text{ J}$

3. **(c) :** Heat energy given $dQ = dU + dW$ where dU is the change in internal energy and dW is the work done.

Given $dQ = 2\text{kcal} = 2000 \times 4.2 \text{ J}$ and $dW = 500 \text{ J}$

$\therefore 2000 \times 4.2 = dU + 500 \Rightarrow dU = 7900 \text{ J}$

4. **(b) :** $\Delta Q = \Delta U + \Delta W$

$\Rightarrow \Delta W = \Delta Q - \Delta U = 110 - 40 = 70 \text{ J}$

5. **(b) :** The first law of thermodynamics is just a conservation of energy.

6. **(d) :**

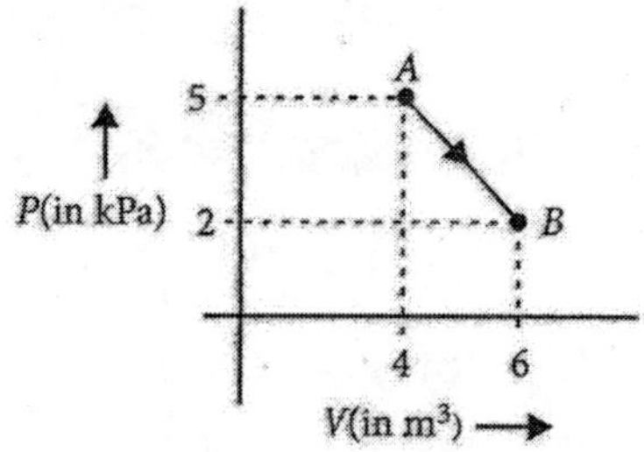

We know, $\Delta U = nC_V\Delta T$

$= n\left(\frac{5R}{2}\right)(T_B - T_A)$ [for diatomic gas, $C_v = \frac{5R}{2}$]

$= \frac{5nR}{2}\left(\frac{P_BV_B}{nR} - \frac{P_AV_A}{nR}\right)$ [$\because PV = nRT$]

$= \frac{5}{2}(P_BV_B - P_AV_A) = \frac{5}{2}(2 \times 10^3 \times 6 - 5 \times 10^3 \times 4)$

$= \frac{5}{2}(-8 \times 10^3) = -20$ kJ

7. **(c)** : Let C_V and C_P be molar specific heats of the ideal gas at constant volume and constant pressure, respectively, then

$C_P = Mc_P$ and $C_V = Mc_V$; $C_P - C_V = R$

$\therefore Mc_p - Mc_V = R \Rightarrow c_P - c_V = R/M$

8. **(a) :** Change in internal energy,

$\Delta U = nC_V\Delta T$

$$= \frac{nR\Delta T}{(\gamma - 1)} = \frac{nP\Delta V}{(\gamma - 1)} = \frac{nP(2V - V)}{\gamma - 1}$$

For one mole, $n = 1$ $\therefore \Delta U = PV/(\gamma - 1)$

9. **(d) :** Using $C_P - C_V = R$,

C_P is heat needed for raising by 10 K.

$\therefore C_P = 20.7$ J/moleK

Given $R = 8.3$ J/moleK

$\therefore C_V = 20.7 - 8.3 = 12.4$ J/moleK

$\therefore$ For raising by 10 K = 124 J.

10. **(b) :** Here, $P = 249\text{kPa} = 249 \times 10^3$ Pa

$T = 27°\text{C} = 27 + 273 = 300$ K, $M = 2 \times 10^{-3}$ kg

Equation of state, $PV = nRT$

or $PM = \rho RT$

or $\rho = \frac{PM}{RT}$

$\left[\because n = \frac{m}{M}\right]$

Substituting the values,

$$\rho = \frac{(249 \times 10^3)(2 \times 10^{-3})}{8.3 \times 300} = 0.2 \text{ kg/m}^3$$

11. **(b)** : Work done is not a thermodynamical function.

12. **(b)** : When a thermodynamic system undergoes a change in such a way that there is no exchange of heat P with the surrounding, then the process is known as adiabatic process and the slope of adiabatic is more than isothermal.

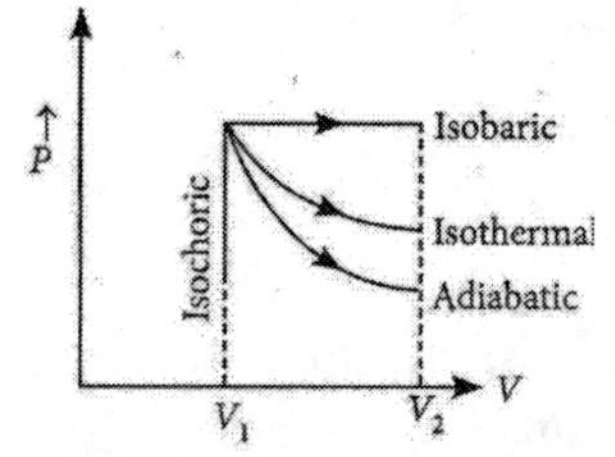

13. **(b) :** Since, the entire system is thermally insulated, no heat flows into the system. When the stopcock is removed, the gas expands adiabatically.

14. **(c) :** Adiabatic process is the process in which no exchange of heat energy takes place between the gas and the surroundings,

i.e., $\Delta Q = 0$.

15. **(a) :** Given process is isobaric.

$\therefore dQ = nC_PdT$; where C_P is specific heat at constant pressure.

or $dQ = n\left(\frac{5}{2}R\right)dT$

Also, $dW = PdV = nRdT$ ($\because PV = nRT$)

Required ratio $= \frac{dW}{dQ} = \frac{nRdT}{n\left(\frac{5}{2}R\right)dT} = \frac{2}{5}$

16. **(a) :** In process I, volume is constant.

$\therefore$ Process I $\rightarrow$ Isochoric; P $\rightarrow$ C

As slope of curve II is more than the slope of curve III.

Process II $\rightarrow$ Adiabatic and Process III $\rightarrow$ Isothermal

$\therefore$ Q $\rightarrow$ A, R $\rightarrow$ D

In process IV, pressure is constant. Process IV $\rightarrow$ Isobaric; $S \rightarrow B$

17. (d) : Process described by the equation,

$PV^3 =$ constant

For a polytropic process, $PV^{\alpha} =$ constant

$$C = C_V + \frac{R}{1-\alpha} = \frac{3}{2}R + \frac{R}{1-3} = R$$

18. **(d):** $V_1 = V, V_2 = V/2$

On $P - V$ diagram, Area under adiabatic curve > Area under isothermal curve. So, compressing the gas through adiabatic process will require more work to be done.

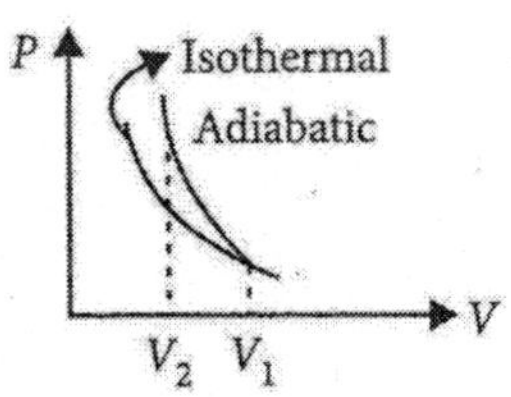

19. **(c)**

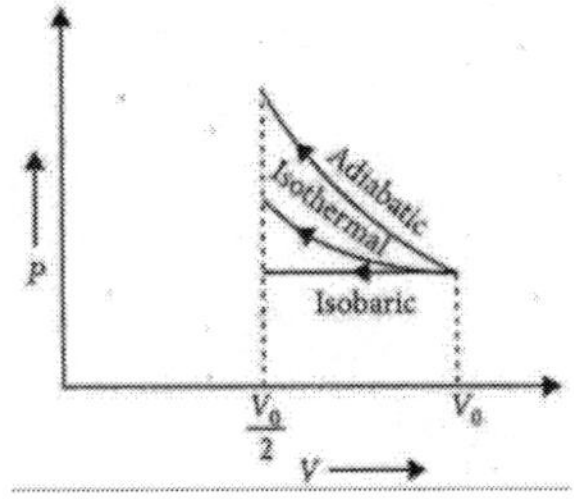

The $P - V$ diagram of an ideal gas compressed from its initial volume V_0 to $\frac{V_0}{2}$ by several processes is shown in the figure. Work done on the gas = Area under $P - V$ curve.

As area under the $P - V$ curve is maximum for adiabatic process, so work done on the gas is maximum for adiabatic process.

20. **(a)** : As initial and final points for two paths are same so $\Delta U_{ABC} = \Delta U_{AC}$

AB is isochoric process.

$\Delta W_{AB} = 0$

$\Delta Q_{AB} = \Delta U_{AB} = 400$ J

BC is isobaric process.

$\Delta Q_{BC} = \Delta U_{BC} + \Delta W_{BC}$

$$100 = \Delta U_{BC} + 6 \times 10^4 (4 \times 10^{-3} - 2 \times 10^{-3})$$

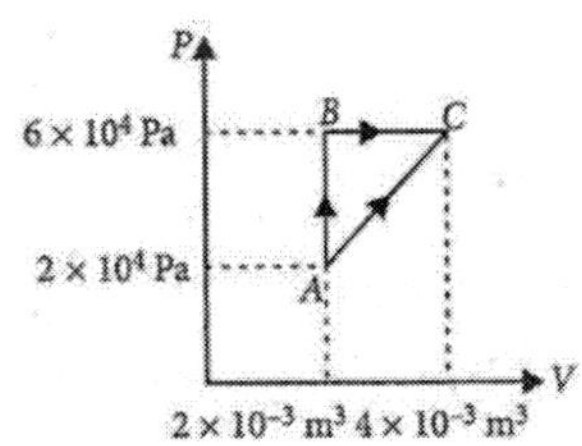

$100 = \Delta U_{BC} + 12 \times 10$

$\Delta U_{BC} = 100 - 120 = -20$ J

As, $\Delta U_{ABC} = \Delta U_{AC}, \Delta U_{AB} + \Delta U_{BC} = \Delta Q_{AC} - \Delta W_{AC}$

$$400 - 20 = \Delta Q_{AC}$$
$$-\left(2 \times 10^4 \times 2 \times 10^{-3} + \frac{1}{2} \times 2 \times 10^{-3} \times 4 \times 10^4\right)$$

$$\Delta Q_{AC} = 460 \text{ J}$$

21. (c) : First, isothermal expansion

$$PV = P'(2V); P' = \frac{P}{2}$$

Then, adiabatic expansion, $P'(2V)^\gamma = P_f(16V)^\gamma$

(For adiabatic process, PV^N = constant)

$$\frac{P}{2}(2V)^{5/3} = P_f(16V)^{5/3}$$

$$P_f = \frac{P}{2}\left(\frac{2V}{16V}\right)^{5/3} = \frac{P}{2}\left(\frac{1}{8}\right)^{5/3} = \frac{P}{2}\left(\frac{1}{2^3}\right)^{5/3} = \frac{P}{64}$$

22. (d) : In a cyclic process work done is equal to the area under the cycle and is positive if the cycle is clockwise and negative if cycle is anticlockwise.

As is clear from figure,

W_{AEDA} = + area of $\triangle AED = +\frac{1}{2}P_0V_0$

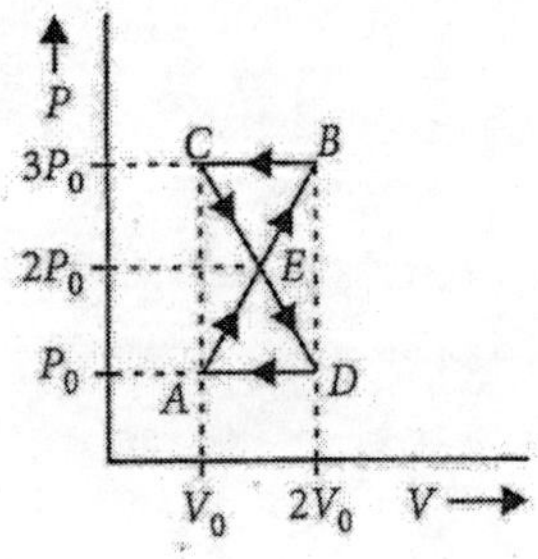

W_{BCEB} = − Area of $\triangle BCE = -\frac{1}{2}P_0V_0$

The net work done by the system is

$$W_{\text{net}} = W_{AEDA} + W_{BCEB}$$
$$= +\frac{1}{2}P_0V_0 - \frac{1}{2}P_0V_0$$
$$= \text{zero}$$

23. (d):

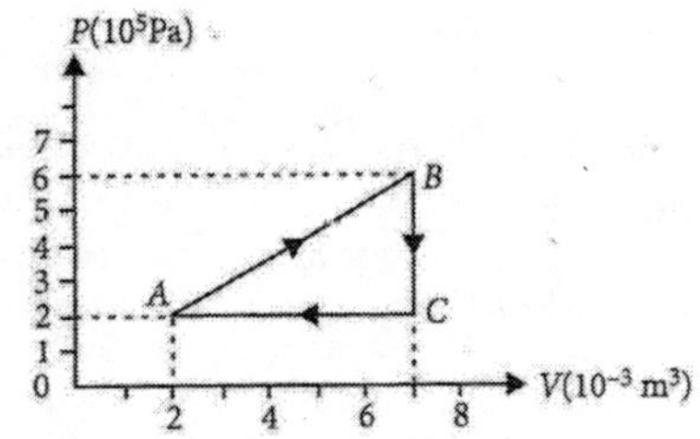

In a cyclic process, work done is equal to the area under the cycle and is positive if the cycle is clockwise and negative if the cycle is anticlockwise.

∴ The net work done by the gas is

W = Area of the cycle $ABCA$

$$= \frac{1}{2} \times (7-2) \times 10^{-3} \times (6-2) \times 10^5$$
$$= \frac{1}{2} \times 5 \times 10^{-3} \times 4 \times 10^5 = 10 \times 10^2 \text{ J} = 1000 \text{ J}$$

24. (b) : $P \propto T^3; PT^{-3}$ = constant

For an adiabatic process; $PT^{\gamma/1-\gamma}$ = constant

Comparing (i) and (ii), we get

$$\frac{\gamma}{1-\gamma} = -3; \gamma = -3 + 3\gamma \text{ or } \gamma = \frac{3}{2}$$

$$\text{As } \gamma = \frac{C_P}{C_V} \quad \therefore \quad \frac{C_P}{C_V} = \frac{3}{2}$$

25. (d) : For an adiabatic process, PV' = constant

According to ideal gas equation

$PV = nRT \Rightarrow P = \frac{nRT}{V}$

Putting value of P in (i), we get

$\frac{nRT}{V} V^{\gamma} = \text{constant}\,;\ \therefore TV^{\gamma-1}$

$= \text{constant}$

Again from the ideal gas equation, $V = \frac{nRT}{P}$

Putting value of V in (i), we get

$P\left(\frac{nRT}{P}\right)^{\gamma} = \text{constant}\,; P^{1-\gamma}T^{\gamma}$

$= \text{constant}$

26. **(a):** In a cyclic process, $\Delta U = 0$. In a cyclic process work done is equal to the area under the cycle and is positive if the cycle is clockwise and negative if anticlockwise.

$\therefore\ \triangle W = -$ Area of rectangle

$ABCD = -P(2V) = -2PV$

According to first law of thermodynamics

$\Delta Q = \Delta U + \Delta W$ or $\Delta Q = \Delta W$

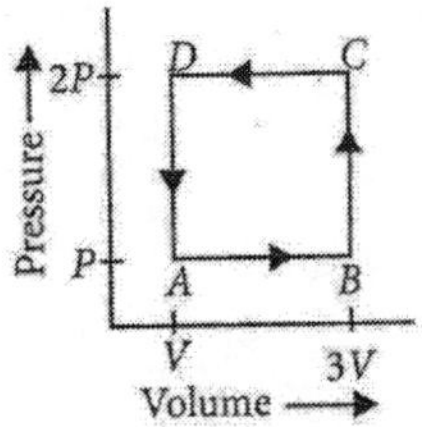

So, $\Delta Q = \Delta W = -2PV$

(As $\Delta U = 0$)

$\therefore$ Heat rejected by the gas $= 2PV$

27. **(a) :** Change in internal energy is path independent and depends only on the initial and final states.

As the initial and final states in the three processes are same. Therefore,

$$\Delta U_1 = \Delta U_2 = \Delta U_3$$

Workdone, $W =$ Area under $P - V$ graph

As area under curve 1 > area under curve 2 > area under curve 3 $\therefore\ W_1 > W_2 > W_3$

According to first law of thermodynamics, $Q = W + \Delta U$

As $W_1 > W_2 > W_3$ and $\Delta U_1 = \Delta U_2 = \Delta U_3$

$\therefore\ Q_1 > Q_2 > Q_3$

28. **(d)**

29. **(d) :** In isothermal expansion work done against surroundings is negative but work done by gas is positive.

$\Delta W = +150J$

$dU = 0$

From F.L.O.T.

$\Delta Q = \Delta W + dU \Rightarrow \qquad \Delta Q = +150J$

heat is +ve it means heat absorb by gas

30. **(d) :** For an adiabatic process, $\frac{T^{\gamma}}{P^{\gamma-1}} =$ constant

$\therefore \left(\frac{T_i}{T_f}\right)^{\gamma} = \left(\frac{P_i}{P_f}\right)^{\gamma-1}\,;\ P_f = P_i\left(\frac{T_f}{T_i}\right)^{\frac{\gamma}{\gamma-1}}$

Here, $\quad T_i = 27°\text{C} = 300\text{ K}, T_f = 927°\text{C} = 1200\text{ K}$

$$P_i = 2\text{ atm}, \gamma = 1.4$$

Substituting these values in eqn. (i), we get

$$P_f = (2)\left(\frac{1200}{300}\right)^{\frac{1.4}{1.4-1}} = (2)(4)^{1.4/0.4}$$
$$= 2(2^2)^{7/2} = (2)(2)^7 = 2^8 = 256 \text{ atm}$$

31. (a) : According to first law of thermodynamics $\Delta Q = \Delta U + \Delta W$

where, ΔQ = Heat supplied to the system

ΔU = Increase in internal energy of the system

ΔW = Work done by the system

For an adiabatic process

$\Delta Q = 0 \therefore \Delta U = -\Delta W$

For an isothermal process, $\Delta U = 0 \therefore \Delta Q = \Delta W$

32. (d) : Ideal gas equation, for an adiabatic process is

$PV^\gamma =$ constant or $P_1V_1^\gamma = P_2V_2^\gamma$

For monoatomic gas, $\gamma = \frac{5}{3}$

$$\therefore P_1V_1^{5/3} = P_2\left(\frac{V_1}{8}\right)^{5/3}$$

$\Rightarrow P_2 = P_1 \times (2)^5 = 32P_1$.

33. (a) : In isochoric process, it is volume that is kept constant. If pressure is kept constant, it is an isobaric process.

34. (a) : Internal energy depends only on the initial and final states of temperature and not on the path. In a cyclic process, as initial and final states are the same, change in internal energy is zero. Hence E is zero.

35. (d) : Work done in adiabatic process is given as

$$W = \frac{-1}{\gamma - 1}(P_fV_f - P_iV_i)$$

$$6R = \frac{-1}{5/3 - 1}R(T_f - T_i)$$

[using = RT]

$\Rightarrow T_f - T_i = -4 \therefore T_f = (T - 4)$K

36. (b) : $TV^{\gamma-1}$ = constant (adiabatic)

$\therefore (300)(V_0)^{2/3} = (V_f)^{2/3}T$

$$T = 300\left(\frac{27}{8}\right)^{2/3} = 300 \times \left(\frac{3}{2}\right)^{3\times\frac{2}{3}}$$
$$= \frac{300 \times 9}{4} = 675 \text{ K}$$

Temperature rise = $675 - 300 = 375$ K

37. (c) : $\Delta U = -W$ in an adiabatic process

According to the first law of thermodynamics,

$Q = \Delta U + W$

In adiabatic process,

$Q = 0$

Hence,

$\Delta U = -W$

Therefore option (c) is correct

For isothermal process,

$\Delta U = 0$

Hence option (b) and (c) are wrong

38. (d) : During expansion, work is performed by the gas. The isobaric expansion is represented by the horizontal straight line AB_1, since the adiabatic curve is steeper than the isothermal curve, the adiabatic expansion curve (AB_3) must lie below

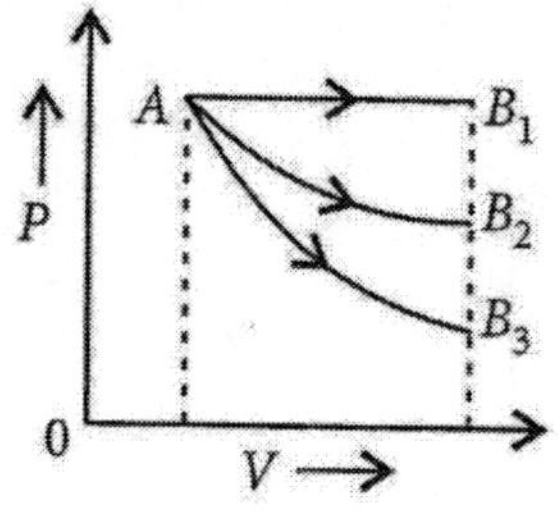

the isothermal curve (AB_2) as shown in the given figure

Since area under AB_1, is maximum, the work done is maximum in case of isobaric expansion.

39. **(b)** : For the adiabatic change, PV^{γ} = constant.

And for ideal gas, $V = \frac{RT}{P} \propto \frac{T}{P}$.

Therefore $P^{1-\gamma}T^{\gamma}$ = constant.

40. **(a)** : Initial temperature $(T_1) = 18°C = 291$ K and $V_2 = (1/8)V_1$

For adiabatic compression, $TV^{\gamma-1}$ = constant

or $T_1V_1^{\gamma-1} = T_2V_2^{\gamma-1}$.

Therefore $T_2 = T_1\left(\frac{V_1}{V_2}\right)^{\gamma-1}$

$$= 291 \times (8)^{1.4-1} = 291 \times (8)^{0.4}$$
$$= 291 \times 2.297 = 668.4 \text{ K} = 395.4°C$$

41. **(d)** : For adiabatic change, PV^{γ} = constant

$\Rightarrow P\left(\frac{RT}{P}\right)^{\gamma}$ = constant

$\Rightarrow P^{1-\gamma}T^{\gamma}$ = constant $\Rightarrow$ $P \propto T^{\frac{-\gamma}{1-\gamma}}$

Therefore, the value of constant, $C = \frac{\gamma}{(\gamma-1)}$.

For monoatomic gas, $\gamma = 5/3$.

Therefore $C = \frac{5/3}{(5/3)-1} = \frac{5/3}{2/3} = \frac{5}{2}$.

42. **(b)** : Under isothermal conditions, there is no change in internal energy.

43. **(c)** : Work done = Area under curve $ACBDA$

44. **(a)** : Since AB is a isochoric process. So no work is done.

BC is isobaric process,

$W = P_B \times (V_D - V_A) = 240$ J

Therefore $\Delta Q = 600 + 200 = 800$ J

Using $\Delta Q = \Delta U + \Delta W$

$\Rightarrow \Delta U = \Delta Q - \Delta W = 800 - 240 = 560$ J

45. **(a)** : Efficiency of an ideal heat engine,

$$\eta = \left(1 - \frac{T_2}{T_1}\right)$$

Freezing point of water = 0°C = 273 K

Boiling point of water = 100°C = (100 + 273)K = 373 K

T_2: Sink temperature = 273 K

T_1: Source temperature = 373 K

$$\%\eta = \left(1 - \frac{T_2}{T_1}\right) \times 100 = \left(1 - \frac{273}{373}\right) \times 100$$
$$= \left(\frac{100}{373}\right) \times 100 = 26.8\%$$

46. **(c)** : Isothermal compression is reversible, for example, Carnot cycle, heat engine.

Chapter: 12

KINETIC THEORY

Behaviour of Gases

1. The volume occupied by the molecules contained in 4.5 kg water at STP, if the intermolecular forces vanish away is **(2022)**

(a) 5.6×10^6 m^3 (b) 5.6×10^3 m^3

(c) 5.6×10^{-3} m^3 (d) 5.6 m^3

2. A given sample of an ideal gas occupies a volume V at a pressure P and absolute temperature T. The mass of each molecule of the gas is m. Which of the following gives the density of the gas? **(NEET-II 2016)**

(a) $P/(kT)$ (b) $Pm/(kT)$

(c) $P/(kTV)$ (d) mkT

3. Two vessels separately contain two ideal gases A and B at the same temperature, the pressure of A being twice that of B. Under such conditions, the density of A is found to be 1.5 times the density of B. The ratio of molecular weight of A and B is **(2015)**

(a) 2 (b) 1/2

(c) 2/3 (d) ¾

4. In the given $(V - T)$ diagram, what is the relation between pressures P_1 and P_2? **(2013)**

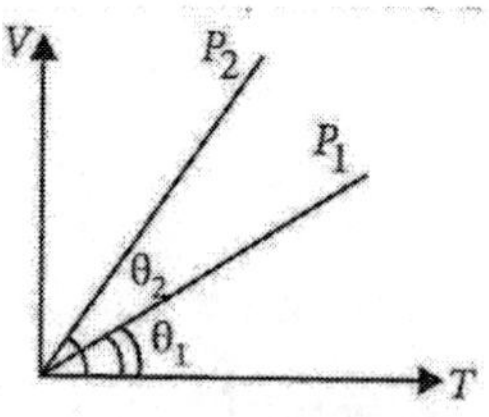

(a) $P_2 < P_1$

(b) Cannot be predicted

(c) $P_2 = P_1$ (d) $P_2 > P_1$

5. At 10°C the value of the density of a fixed mass of an ideal gas divided by its pressure is x. At 110°C this ratio is **(2008)**

(a) $\frac{10}{110}x$ (b) $\frac{283}{383}x$

(c) x (d) $\frac{383}{283}x$

6. The equation of state for 5 g of oxygen at a pressure P and temperature T, when occupying a volume V, will be **(2004)**

(a) $PV = (5/32)RT$

(b) $PV - 5RT$

(c) $PV = (5/2)RT$

(d) $PV = (5/16)RT$

(where R is the gas constant)

7. The value of critical temperature in terms of van der Waals' constant a and b is given by **(1996)**

(a) $T_C = \frac{8a}{27Rb}$ (b) $T_C = \frac{27a}{8Rb}$

(c) $T_C = \frac{a}{2Rb}$ (d) $T_C = \frac{a}{27Rb}$

8. Three containers of the same volume contain three different gases. The masses of the molecules are m_1, m_2 and m_3 and the number of molecules in their respective containers are N_1, N_2 and N_3. The gas pressure in the containers are P_1, P_2 and P_3 respectively. All the gases are now mixed and put in one of these containers. The pressure P of the mixture will be **(1991)**

(a) $P < (P_1 + P_2 + P_3)$

(b) $P = \frac{P_1+P_2+P_3}{3}$

(c) $P = P_1 + P_2 + P_3$

(d) $P > (P_1 + P_2 + P_3)$

9. Two containers A and B are partly filled with water and closed. The volume of A is twice that of B and it contains half the amount of water in B. If both are at the same temperature, the water vapour in the containers will have pressure in the ratio of **(1988)**

(a) $1:2$ (b) $1:1$

(c) $2:1$ (d) $4:1$

Kinetic Theory of an Ideal Gas

10. The temperature of a gas is –50°C. To what temperature the gas should be heated so that the rms speed is increased by 3 times? **(2023)**

(a) 3295°C (b) 3097 K

(c) 223 K (d) 669°C

11. Increase in temperature of a gas filled in a container would lead to **(2019)**

(a) decrease in intermolecular distance

(b) increase in its mass

(c) increase in its kinetic energy

(d) decrease in its pressure

12. At what temperature will the rms speed of oxygen molecules become just sufficient for escaping from the Earth's atmosphere?

(Given: Mass of oxygen molecule $(m) = 2.76 \times 10^{-26}$ kg, Boltzmann's constant $k_B = 1.38 \times 10^{-23}\ \text{J K}^{-1}$) **(2018)**

(a) 2.508×10^4 K

(b) 8.360×10^4 K

(c) 5.016×10^4 K

(d) 1.254×10^4 K

13. The molecules of a given mass of a gas have r.m.s. velocity of $200\ \text{m s}^{-1}$ at 27°C and $1.0 \times 10^5\ \text{N m}^{-2}$ pressure. When the temperature and pressure of the gas are respectively, 127°C and $0.05 \times 10^5\ \text{N m}^{-2}$, the r.m.s. velocity of its molecules in ms^{-1} is **(NEET-I 2016)**

(a) $\frac{100\sqrt{2}}{3}$ (b) $\frac{100}{3}$

(c) $100\sqrt{2}$ (d) $\frac{400}{\sqrt{3}}$

14. In a vessel, the gas is at pressure P. If the mass of all the molecules is halved and their speed is doubled, then the resultant pressure will be

(Karnataka NEET 2013)

(a) $2P$ (b) P

(c) $P/2$ (d) $4P$

15. At 0 K which of the following properties of a gas will be zero? **(1996)**

(a) vibrational energy

(b) density

(c) kinetic energy

(d) potential energy

16. Relation between pressure (P) and kinetic energy per unit volume (E) of a gas is **(1991)**

(a) $P = \frac{2}{3}E$ (b) $P = \frac{1}{3}E$

(c) $P = E$ (d) $P = 3E$

17. According to kinetic theory of gases, at absolute zero of temperature **(1990)**

(a) water freezes

(b) liquid helium freezes

(c) molecular motion stops

(d) liquid hydrogen freezes.

18. At constant volume temperature is increased then **(1989)**

(a) collission on walls will be less

(b) number of collisions per unit time will increase

(c) collisions will be in straight lines

(d) collisions will not change.

Law of Equipartition of Energy

19. Match Column-I and Column-II and choose the correct match from the given choices. **(2021)**

Column-I	Column-II
(A) Root mean square speed of gas molecules	(P) $\frac{1}{3}nm\bar{v}^2$
(B) Pressure exerted by ideal gas	(Q) $\sqrt{\frac{3RT}{M}}$
(C) Average kinetic energy of a molecule	(R) $\frac{5}{2}RT$
(D) Total internal energy of 1 mole of a diatomic gas	(S) $\frac{3}{2}k_BT$

(a) (A)-(R), (B)-(Q), (C)-(P), (D) -(S)

(b) (A)-(R), (B)-(P), (C)-(S), (D)-(Q)

(c) (A)-(Q), (B)-(R), (C)-(S), (D) - (P)

(d) (A)-(Q), (B)-(P), (C)-(S), (D) - (R)

20. The average thermal energy for a mono-atomic gas is (k_B is Boltzmann constant and T, absolute temperature) **(2020)**

(a) $\frac{1}{2}k_BT$ (b) $\frac{3}{2}k_BT$

(c) $\frac{5}{2}k_BT$ (d) $\frac{7}{2}k_BT$

21. The degrees of freedom of a triatomic gas is **(1999)**

(a) 6 (b) 4

(c) 2 (d) 8

22. The number of translational degrees of freedom for a diatomic gas is **(1993)**

(a) 2 (b) 3

(c) 5 (d) 6

23. A polyatomic gas with n degrees of freedom has a mean energy per molecule given **(1989)**

(a) $\frac{nkT}{N}$ (b) $\frac{nkT}{2N}$

(c) $\frac{nkT}{2}$ (d) $\frac{3kT}{2}$

Specific Heat Capacity

24. The value of $\gamma\left(=\frac{C_p}{C_v}\right)$, for hydrogen, helium and another ideal diatomic gas X (whose molecules are not rigid but have an additional vibrational mode), are respectively equal to **(Odisha NEET 2019)**

(a) $\frac{7}{5},\frac{5}{3},\frac{9}{7}$ (b) $\frac{5}{3},\frac{7}{5},\frac{9}{7}$
(c) $\frac{5}{3},\frac{7}{5},\frac{7}{5}$ (d) $\frac{7}{5},\frac{5}{3},\frac{7}{5}$

25. A gas mixture consists of 2 moles of O_2 and 4 moles of Ar at temperature T. Neglecting all vibrational modes, the total internal energy of the system is **(2017)**

(a) 15RT (b) $9RT$
(c) $11RT$ (d) $4RT$

26. The amount of heat energy required to raise the temperature of 1 g of Helium at NTP, from T_1 K to T_2 K is **(2013)**

(a) $\frac{3}{4}N_a k_B(T_2 - T_1)$

(b) $\frac{3}{4}N_a k_B\left(\frac{T_2}{T_1}\right)$

(c) $\frac{3}{8}N_a k_B(T_2 - T_1)$

(d) $\frac{3}{2}N_a k_B(T_2 - T_1)$

27. The molar specific heat at constant pressure of an ideal gas is $(7/2)R$. The ratio of specific heat at constant pressure to that at constant volume is **(2006)**

(a) $9/7$ (b) $7/5$
(c) $8/7$ (d) $5/7$

28. To find out degree of freedom, the expression is **(2000)**

(a) $f = \frac{2}{\gamma-1}$ (b) $f = \frac{\gamma+1}{2}$
(c) $f = \frac{2}{\gamma+1}$ (d) $f = \frac{1}{\gamma+1}$

29. If for a gas, $\frac{R}{C_V} = 0.67$, this gas is made up of molecules which are **(1992)**

(a) diatomic

(b) mixture of diatomic and polyatomic molecules

(c) monoatomic (d) polyatomic.

30. For hydrogen gas $C_P - C_V = a$ and for oxygen gas $C_P - C_V = b$, so the relation between a and b is given by **(1991)**

(a) $a = 16b$ (b) $16b = a$
(c) $a = 4b$ (d) $a = b$

31. For a certain gas the ratio of specific heats is given to be $\gamma = 1.5$. For this gas **(1990)**

(a) $C_V = 3R/J$ (b) $C_P = 3R/J$
(c) $C_P = 5R/J$ (d) $C_V = 5R/J$

Mean Free Path

32. The mean free path for a gas, with molecular diameter d and number density n can be expressed as **(2020)**

(a) $\frac{1}{\sqrt{2}n\pi d}$ (b) $\frac{1}{\sqrt{2}n\pi d^2}$

(c) $\frac{1}{\sqrt{2}n^2\pi d^2}$ (d) $\frac{1}{\sqrt{2}n^2\pi^2 d^2}$

33. The mean free path of molecules of a gas, (radius) is inversely proportional to **(2014)**

(a) r^3 (b) r^2

(c) r (d) $\sqrt{r}$

ANSWER KEY

1.	(d)	2.	(b)	3.	(d)	4.	(a)	5.	(b)	6.	(a)	7.	(a)
8.	(c)	9.	(b)	10.	(b)	11.	(c)	12.	(b)	13.	(d)	14.	(a)
15.	(c)	16.	(a)	17.	(c)	18.	(b)	19.	(d)	20.	(b)	21.	(a)
22.	(b)	23.	(c)	24.	(a)	25.	(c)	26.	(c)	27.	(b)	28.	(a)
29.	(c)	30.	(d)	31.	(b)	32.	(b)	33.	(b)				

Hints & Explanations

1. **(d)** : $\mu = \frac{\text{Mass of water}}{\text{Molecular weight of water}} = \frac{4.5\text{ kg}}{18\times10^{-3}\text{ kg}} = 250$

At STP, $T = 273$ K and $P = 10^5\ \text{N/m}^2$

From, $PV = \mu RT \Rightarrow V = \frac{\mu RT}{P}$

$$V = \frac{250\times 8.3\times 273}{10^5}$$

$V = 5.66\ \text{m}^3$

2. **(b)** : As $PV = nRT$

or $n = \frac{PV}{RT} = \frac{\text{mass}}{\text{molar mass}}$

Density, $\rho = \frac{\text{mass}}{\text{volume}} = \frac{(\text{molar mass})P}{RT} = \frac{(mN_A)P}{RT}$

$\therefore \rho = \frac{mP}{kT}$ $\quad (\because R = N_A k)$

3. **(d)** : According to an ideal gas equation, the molecular weight of an ideal gas is

$$M = \frac{\rho RT}{P}\left(\text{as } P = \frac{\rho RT}{M}\right)$$

where P, T and ρ are the pressure, temperature and density of the gas respectively and R is the universal gas constant.

$\therefore$ The molecular weight of A is

$M_A = \frac{\rho_A RT_A}{P_A}$ and that of B is M_B

$$= \frac{\rho_B RT_B}{P_B}$$

Hence, their corresponding ratio is

$$\frac{M_A}{M_B} = \left(\frac{\rho_A}{\rho_B}\right)\left(\frac{T_A}{T_B}\right)\left(\frac{P_B}{P_A}\right)$$

Here, $\frac{\rho_A}{\rho_B} = 1.5 = \frac{3}{2}, \frac{T_A}{T_B} = 1$ and $\frac{P_A}{P_B} = 2$

$$\therefore \frac{M_A}{M_B} = \left(\frac{3}{2}\right)(1)\left(\frac{1}{2}\right) = \frac{3}{4}$$

4. **(a)** : According to ideal gas equation

$PV = nRT$

or $V = \frac{nRT}{P}$

For an isobaric process,

$P =$ constant and $V \propto T$

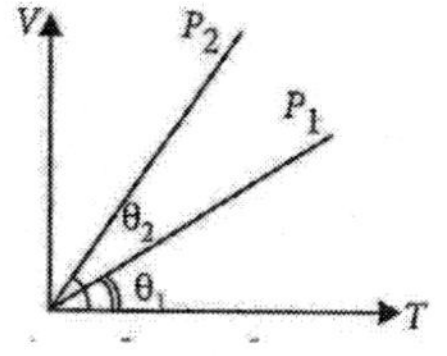

Therefore, $V - T$ graph is a straight line passing through origin. Slope of this line is inversely proportional to P. In the given figure,

$(\text{Slope})_2 > (\text{Slope})_1 \therefore P_2 < P_1$

5. **(b) :** Mass of the gas $= m$.

At a fixed temperature and pressure, volume is fixed.

Density of the gas $\rho = \frac{m}{V} \Rightarrow \frac{\rho}{P} = \frac{m}{V \cdot P} \Rightarrow \frac{m}{nRT} =$

$\therefore xT =$ constant.

At $10°C$ i.e., $283 \text{ K}, xT = x \cdot 283 \text{ K}$

At $110°C, xT = x' \cdot 383 \text{ K}$

From eq. (i) and (ii) we get $x' = \frac{283}{383}x$

6. **(a) :** As $PV = nRT$

$n = \frac{m}{\text{molecular mass}} = \frac{5}{32} \Rightarrow PV$

$= \left(\frac{5}{32}\right) RT$

7. **(a):** Vander weal's equation is given by

$\left(p + \frac{q}{V^2}\right)(v - b) = RT$

a and b are constants

solving above questions $\left(p + \frac{RT}{V-b} - \frac{a}{V^2}\right)$

taking derivation of p w.r.t. volume

$\frac{\partial P}{\partial V} = 0$

$\frac{\partial^2 P}{\partial V^2} = 0$

so, P becomes $\frac{\partial^2 P}{\partial V} = -\frac{RT}{(v-b)^2} + \frac{2a}{v^3} = 0$

$\frac{2a}{V^3} = \frac{RT}{(v-b)^2} \dots (i)$

$\frac{a}{V^4} = \frac{RT}{2v(v-b)^2} \dots (ii)$

$\frac{\partial^2 P}{\partial V^2} = \frac{2RT}{(v-b)^3} - \frac{6a}{v^4} = 0$ or $\frac{RT}{(V-b)^3} = \frac{3a}{(V)^4}$

[putting equation in this equation]

$\Rightarrow \frac{RT}{(V-b)^3} = \frac{3a}{2V(v-g)^2}$

$\Rightarrow 3v - 3b = 2v$

$\Rightarrow V_C = 3b$ (Critical volume)

using V_C in equation (i)

$\frac{RT}{4b^2} = \frac{2a}{27b^3}$

$\Rightarrow T_C = \frac{8a}{27Rb}$ [critical temperature]

8. **(c)** : According to Dalton's law of partial pressure, we have $P = P_1 + P_2 + P_3$

9. **(b)** : Vapour pressure does not depend on the amount of substance. It depends on the temperature alone.

10. **(a)** : $v_{rms} \propto \sqrt{T}$

$$\frac{v_1}{v_2} = \sqrt{\frac{T_1}{T_2}}$$

= let initial speed is V

As speed is increased by 3 times so final speed become 4 v

$$\Rightarrow \frac{v}{4v} = \sqrt{\frac{223}{T}}$$

T =3568 K

So temp. in $^{\circ}C = 3568 - 273 = 3295^{\circ}C$

11. **(c)** : As per kinctic theory of gases, kinetic energy of gas molecules is directly proportional to the temperature of the gas.

12. **(b)** : Escape velocity from the Earth's surface is $v_{\text{escape}} = 11200 \text{ m s}^{-1}$

Say at temperature T, oxygen molecule attains escape velocity.

So, $v_{\text{escape}} = \sqrt{\frac{3k_BT}{m_{O_2}}} \Rightarrow 11200 = \sqrt{\frac{3\times1.38\times10^{-23}\times T}{2.76\times10^{-26}}}$

On solving, $T = 8.360 \times 10^4$ K

13. **(d)**

As, $v_{\text{rms}} = \sqrt{\frac{3k_BT}{m}}$

$$\therefore \frac{v_{27}}{v_{127}} = \sqrt{\frac{27+273}{127+273}} = \sqrt{\frac{300}{400}} = \frac{\sqrt{3}}{2}$$

or

$v_{127} = \frac{2}{\sqrt{3}} \times v_{27} = \frac{2}{\sqrt{3}} \times 200 \text{ m s}^{-1} = \frac{400}{\sqrt{3}} \text{ m s}^{-1}$

14. **(a)** : As $P = \frac{1}{3}\frac{mN}{V} v_{\text{rms}}^2$

where m is the mass of each molecule, N is the total number of molecules, V is the volume of the gas.

When mass of all the molecules is halved and their speed is doubled, then the pressure will be

$$P' = \frac{1}{3}\left(\frac{m}{2}\right) \times \frac{N}{V} \times (2v_{\text{rms}})^2$$

$$= \frac{2}{3}\frac{mN}{V} v_{\text{rms}}^2 = 2P$$

(Using (i))

15. **(c) :** The kinetic energy of gas molecules is directly proportional to absolute temperature.

K. $E \propto T$

i.e. $KE = cT$

at OK, the kinetic energy of the gas molecules would be zero

16. **(a) :** $PV = \frac{1}{3}Nmv^2 = \frac{2}{3}\left(\frac{1}{2}Nm\right)v^2 \Rightarrow$ $P = \frac{2}{3}E$

17. **(c) :** According to classical theory all motion of molecules stop at 0 K.

18. **(b) :** As the temperature increases, the average velocity increases. So, the number collisions per unit time will increase.

19. **(d) :** The rms velocity is, $v_{\text{rms}} = \sqrt{\frac{3RT}{M}}$

where, R is a gas constant, M = molecular mass,

T = absolute temperature. So, $A \rightarrow Q$

Pressure exerted by ideal gas is $\frac{1}{3}mn\bar{v}^2$, where m is mass of each molecule, n = number of molecules, $\bar{v}^2$ = rms speed. So, B → P.

Average kinetic energy of a molecule $\frac{3}{2}k_BT$

where, k_B = Boltzmann's constant, T = absolute temperature. So, C → S.

Total internal energy of 1 mole of a diatomic gas, $U = \frac{5}{2}RT$ So, D → R.

20. **(b) :** For mono-atomic gas, degree of freedom = 3

Energy associated with each degree of freedom $= \frac{1}{2}k_BT$ So, energy is $\frac{3}{2}k_BT$.

21. **(a) :** 3 translational, 3 rotational.

22. **(b):** Number of translational degrees of freedom are same for all types of gases that is 3 .

23. **(c) :** According to law of equipartition of energy, the energy per degree of freedom is $\frac{1}{2}kT$. For a polyatomic gas with n degrees of freedom, the mean energy per molecule $= \frac{1}{2}nkT$

24. **(a) :** $\gamma = 1 + \frac{2}{n}$; For $H_2, \gamma = 1 + \frac{2}{5} = \frac{7}{5}$

For He, $\gamma = 1 + \frac{2}{3} = \frac{5}{3}$; For $X, \gamma = 1 + \frac{2}{7} = \frac{9}{7}$

25. **(c) :** The internal energy of 2 moles of O_2 atom is

$U_{O_2} = \frac{n_1 f_1}{2} RT = 2 \times \frac{5}{2} \times RT = 5RT$

The internal energy of 4 moles of Ar atom is

$U_{Ar} = \frac{n_2 f_2 RT}{2} = 4 \times \frac{3}{2} \times RT = 6RT$

$\therefore$ The total internal energy of the system is

$U = U_{O_2} + U_{Ar} = 5RT + 6RT = 11RT$

26. **(c) :** As here volume of the gas remains constant, therefore the amount of heat energy required to raise the temperature of the gas is

$\Delta Q = nC_V \Delta T$

Here, number of moles, $n = \frac{1}{4}$

$C_V = \frac{3}{2} R$ ($\because$ He is a monatomic.)

$\Delta T = T_2 - T_1$

$\therefore \Delta Q = \frac{1}{4} \times \frac{3}{2} R (T_2 - T_1)$

$= \frac{3}{8} N_a k_B (T_2 - T_1) \qquad \left(\because k_B = \frac{R}{N_a}\right)$

27. **(b) :** Molar specific heat at constant pressure

$C_P = \frac{7}{2} R \therefore C_V = C_P - R = \frac{7}{2} R - R = \frac{5}{2} R.$

$\therefore \frac{C_P}{C_V} = \frac{(7/2)R}{(5/2)R} = \frac{7}{5}$

28. **(a) :** Here, $\gamma = 1 + \frac{2}{f}$ where f is the degree of freedom

$\therefore \frac{2}{f} = \gamma - 1$ or $f = \frac{2}{\gamma - 1}$

29. **(c) :** Since $\frac{R}{C_V} = 0.67 \Rightarrow \frac{C_P - C_V}{C_V} = 0.67$

$\Rightarrow \gamma = 1.67 = \frac{5}{3}$ Hence gas is monoatomic.

30. **(d) :** $C_P - C_V = R$ for all gases.

31. **(b) :** $\gamma = \frac{C_P}{C_V} = \frac{15}{10} = \frac{3}{2} \Rightarrow C_V = \frac{2}{3} C_P$

$C_P - C_V = \frac{R}{J}$ or $C_P - \frac{2}{3} C_P = \frac{R}{J}$

or $\frac{C_P}{3} = \frac{R}{J}$ or $C_P = \frac{3R}{J}$

32. **(b) :** Mean free path for a gas, $\lambda = \frac{1}{\sqrt{2} n \pi d^2}$

33. **(b) :** Mean free path, $\lambda = \frac{1}{\sqrt{2} n \pi d^2}$

where n is the number density and d is the diameter of the molecule.

As $d = 2r$, $\therefore \lambda = \frac{1}{4\sqrt{2} n \pi r^2}$ or $\lambda \propto \frac{1}{r^2}$

Chapter: 13

OSCILLATIONS

Simple Harmonic Motion

1. The displacement of a particle executing simple harmonic motion is given by $y = A_0 + A\sin\omega t + B\cos\omega t$. Then the amplitude of its oscillation is given by **(2019)**

(a) $A + B$

(b) $A_0 + \sqrt{A^2 + B^2}$

(c) $\sqrt{A^2 + B^2}$

(d) $\sqrt{A_0^2 + (A + B)^2}$

2. The distance covered by a particle undergoing SHM in one time period is (amplitude = A) **(Odisha NEET 2019)**

(a) zero (b) A

(c) $2A$ (d) 4 A

3. Out of the following functions representing motion of a particle, which represents SHM ? **(2011)**

(1) $y = \sin\omega t - \cos\omega t$
(2) $y = \sin^3\omega t$
(3) $y = 5\cos\left(\frac{3\pi}{4} - 3\omega t\right)$
(4) $y = 1 + \omega t + \omega^2 t^2$

(a) Only (1)

(b) Only (4) does not represent SHM

(c) Only (1) and (3)

(d) Only (1) and (2)

4. Two particles are oscillating along two close parallel straight lines side by side, with the same frequency and amplitudes. They pass each other, moving in opposite directions when their displacement is half of the amplitude. The mean positions of the two particles lie on a straight line perpendicular to the paths of the two particles. The phase difference is **(Mains 2011)**

(a) $\frac{\pi}{6}$ (b) 0

(c) $\frac{2\pi}{3}$ (d) π

5. The displacement of a particle along the x-axis is given by $x = a\sin^2\omega t$. The motion of the particle corresponds to **(2010)**

(a) simple harmonic motion of frequency ω/π

(b) simple harmonic motion of frequency $3\omega/2\pi$

(c) non simple harmonic motion

(d) simple harmonic motion of frequency $\omega/2\pi$

6. A particle executes simple harmonic oscillation with an amplitude a. The period of oscillation is T. The minimum time taken by the particle to travel half of the amplitude from the equilibrium position is **(2007)**

(a) $T/8$ (b) $T/12$

(c) $T/2$ (d) $T/4$

7. The circular motion of a particle with constant speed is **(2005)**
(a) periodic but not simple harmonic
(b) simple harmonic but not periodic
(c) period and simple harmonic
(d) neither periodic nor simple harmonic.

8. Two SHM's with same amplitude and time period, when acting together in perpendicular directions with a phase difference of $\pi/2$, give rise to **(1997)**
(a) straight motion
(b)elliptical motion
(c) circular motion
(d) none of these.

9. A simple harmonic oscillator has an amplitude A and time period T. The time required by it to travel from $x = A$ to $x = A/2$ is **(1992)**
(a) $T/6$
(b) $T/4$
(c) $T/3$
(d) $T/2$

10. The composition of two simple harmonic motions of equal periods at right angle to each other and with a phase difference of π results in the displacement of the particle along **(1990)**
(a) circle
(b) figure of eight
(d) ellipse
(c) straight line

Simple Harmonic Motion and Uniform Circular Motion

11. The radius of circle, the period of revolution, initial position and sense of revolution are indicated in the figure. y-projection of the radius vector of rotating particle P is

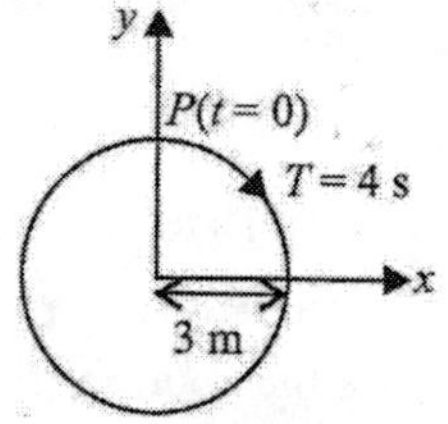

(a) $y(t) = 3\cos\left(\frac{\pi t}{2}\right)$, where y in m
(b) $y(t) = -3\cos 2\pi t$, where y in m
(c) $y(t) = 4\sin\left(\frac{\pi t}{2}\right)$, where y in m
(d) $y(t) = 3\cos\left(\frac{3\pi t}{2}\right)$, where y in m

Velocity and Acceleration in Simple Harmonic Motion

12. The x –t graphy of a particle performing simple harmonic motion is shown in the figure. The acceleration of the particle at t = 2 s is : **(2023)**

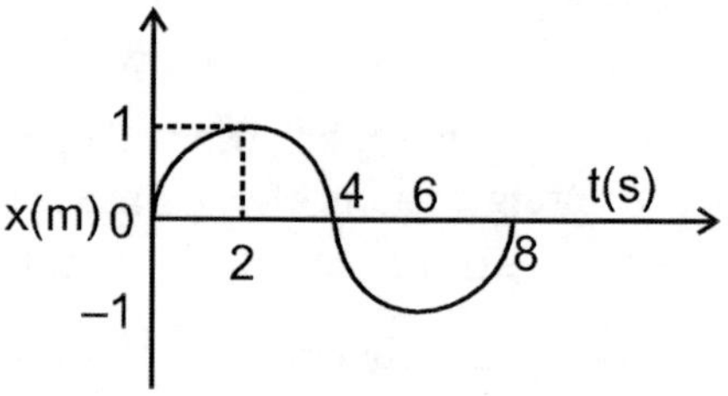

(a) $-\frac{\pi^2}{8}ms^{-2}$
(b) $\frac{\pi^2}{16}ms^{-2}$
(c) $-\frac{\pi^2}{16}ms^{-2}$
(d) $\frac{\pi^2}{8}ms^{-2}$

13. The phase difference between displacement and acceleration of a particle in a simple harmonic motion is **(2020)**

(a) πrad (b) $3\pi/2$rad

(c) $\pi/2$rad (d) zero

14. Average velocity of a particle executing SHM in one complete vibration is **(2019)**

(a) zero (b) $\frac{A\omega}{2}$

(c) $A\omega$ (d) $\frac{A\omega^2}{2}$

15. A particle executes linear simple harmonic motion with an amplitude of 3 cm. When the particle is at 2 cm from the mean position, the magnitude of its velocity is equal to that of its acceleration. Then its time period in seconds is **(2017)**

(a) $\frac{\sqrt{5}}{2\pi}$ (b) $\frac{4\pi}{\sqrt{5}}$

(c) $\frac{2\pi}{\sqrt{3}}$ (d) $\frac{\sqrt{5}}{\pi}$

16. A particle is executing a simple harmonic motion. Its maximum acceleration is α and maximum velocity is β. Then, its time period of vibration will be **(2015)**

(a) $\frac{\beta^2}{\alpha}$ (b) $\frac{2\pi\beta}{\alpha}$

(c) $\frac{\beta^2}{\alpha^2}$ (d) $\frac{\alpha}{\beta}$

17. A particle is executing SHM along a straight line. Its velocities at distances x_1 and x_2 from the mean position are V_1 and V_2, respectively. Its time period is

(2015 Cancelled)

(a) $2\pi\sqrt{\frac{V_1^2+V_2^2}{x_1^2+x_2^2}}$

(b) $2\pi\sqrt{\frac{V_1^2-V_2^2}{x_1^2-x_2^2}}$

(c) $2\pi\sqrt{\frac{x_1^2+x_2^2}{V_1^2+V_2^2}}$

(d) $2\pi\sqrt{\frac{x_2^2-x_1^2}{V_1^2-V_2^2}}$

18. The oscillation of a body on a smooth horizontal surface is represented by the equation, $X = A\cos(\omega t)$ where $X =$ displacement at time t

$\omega =$ frequency of oscillation

Which one of the following graphs shows correctly the variation of a with ?

Here $a =$ acceleration at time $t, T =$ time period **(2014)**

(a) 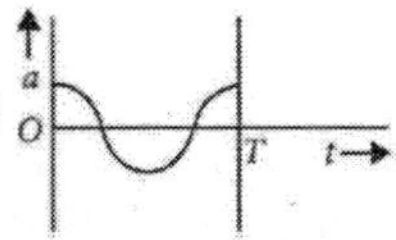

(b) 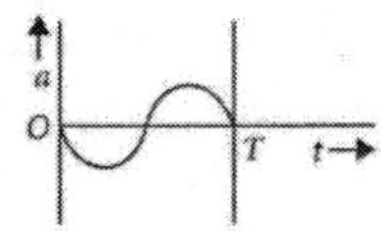

(c) 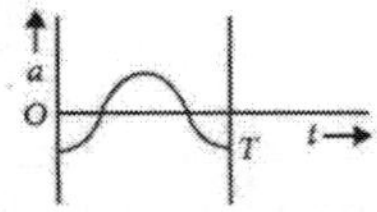

(d) 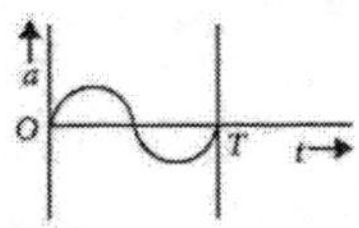

19. A particle of mass m oscillates along x-axis according to equation $x = a\sin\omega t$. The nature of the graph between momentum and displacement of the particle is

(Karnataka NEET 2013)

(a) Circle

(b) Hyperbola

(c) Ellipse

(d) Straight line passing through origin.

20. Two simple harmonic motions of angular frequency 100 and 1000rads^{-1} have the same displacement amplitude. The ratio of their maximum acceleration is **(2008)**

(a) $1:10^3$ (b) $1:10^4$

(c) $1:10$ (d) $1:10^2$

21. A point performs simple harmonic oscillation of period T and the equation of motion is given by $x = a\sin(\omega t + \pi/6)$. After the elapse of what fraction of the time period, the velocity of the point will be equal to half of its maximum velocity?

(2008)

(a) $T/3$ (b) $T/12$

(c) $T/8$ (d) $T/6$

22. The phase difference between the instantaneous velocity and acceleration of a particle executing simple harmonic motion is **(2007)**

(a) π (b) 0.707π

(c) zero (d) 0.5π

23. A particle executing simple harmonic motion of amplitude 5 cm has maximum speed of $31.4\ \text{cm/s}$. The frequency of its oscillation is **(2004)**

(a) 4 Hz (b) 3 Hz

(c) 2 Hz (d) 1 Hz

24. Which one of the following statements is true for the speed v and the acceleration a of a particle executing simple harmonic motion? **(2003)**

(a) When v is maximum, a is maximum.

(b) Value of a is zero, whatever may be the value of v.

(c) When v is zero, a is zero.

(d) When v is maximum, a is zero.

25. A particle starts with S.H.M. from the mean position as shown in the figure. Its amplitude is A and its time period is T. At one time, its speed is half that of the maximum speed.

What is its displacement? **(1996)**

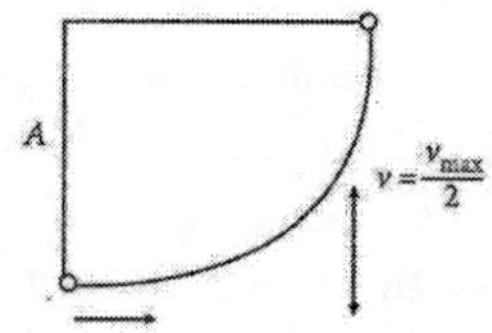

(a) $\frac{2A}{\sqrt{3}}$ (b) $\frac{3A}{\sqrt{2}}$

(c) $\frac{\sqrt{2}A}{3}$ (d) $\frac{\sqrt{3}A}{2}$

26. If a simple harmonic oscillator has got a displacement of $0.02\ \text{m}$ and acceleration equal to $2.0\ \text{m/s}^2$ at any time, the angular frequency of the oscillator is equal to

(1992)

(a) 10rad/s (b) 0.1rad/s

(c) 100rad/s (d) 1rad/s

27. A body is executing simple harmonic motion. When the displacements from the mean position is 4 cm and 5 cm, the corresponding velocities of the body is $10\ \text{cm/sec}$ and $8\ \text{cm/sec}$. Then the time period of the body is **(1991)**

(a) $2\pi\text{sec}$ (b) $\pi/2\text{sec}$

(c) πsec (d) $3\pi/2\text{sec}$

Force Law for Simple Harmonic Motion

28. Which one of the following equations of motion represents simple harmonic motion? **(2009)**

(a) Acceleration $= -k(x+a)$

(b) Acceleration $= k(x+a)$

(c) Acceleration $= -\omega^2 x$

(d) Acceleration $= -k_0 x + k_1 x^2$

where k, k_0, k_1 and a are all positive

29. A particle executes S.H.M. along x-axis. The force acting on it is given by **(1994, 1988)**

(a) $A\cos(kx)$ (b) Ae^{-kx}

(c) Akx (d) $-Akx$.

Energy in Simple Harmonic Motion

30. A body is executing simple harmonic motion with frequency ' n ', the frequency of its potential energy is **(2021)**

(a) $4n$ (b) n

(c) $2n$ (d) $3n$

31. A particle of mass m is released from rest and follows a parabolic path as shown. Assuming that the displacement of the mass from the origin is small, which graph correctly depicts the position of the particle as a function of time? **(2011)**

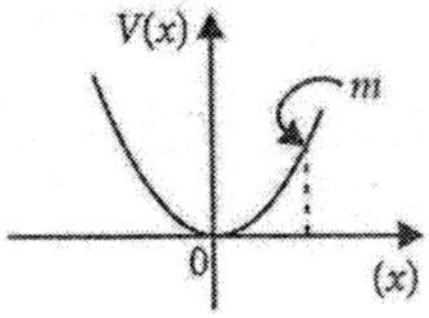

(a) 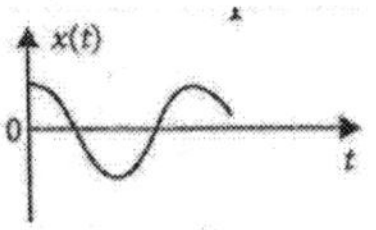

(b) 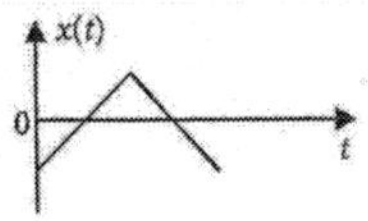

(c) 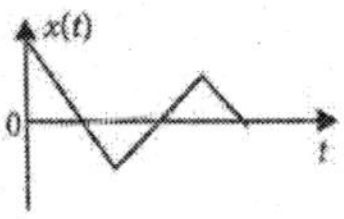

(d) 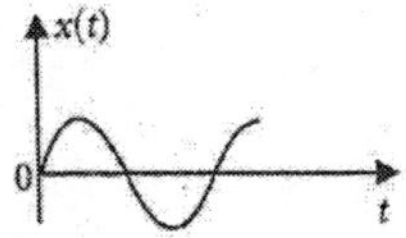

32. The particle executing simple harmonic motion has a kinetic energy $K_0\cos^2\omega t$. The maximum values of the potential energy and the total energy are respectively **(2007)**

(a) $K_0/2$ and K_0 (b) K_0 and $2K_0$

(c) K_0 and K_0 (d) 0 and $2K_0$

33. The potential energy of a simple harmonic oscillator when the particle is half way to its end point is **(2003)**

(a) $\frac{2}{3}E$ (b) $\frac{1}{8}E$

(c) $\frac{1}{4}E$ (d) $\frac{1}{2}E$

34. A particle of mass m oscillates with simple harmonic motion between points x_1 and x_2, the equilibrium position being O. Its potential energy is plotted. It will be as given below in the graph **(2003)**

(a) 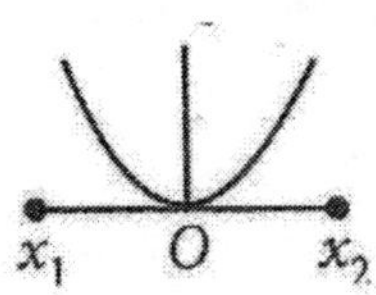

(b) 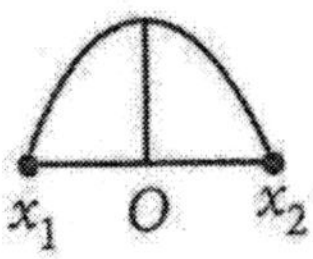

(c) 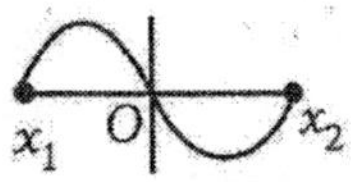

(d) 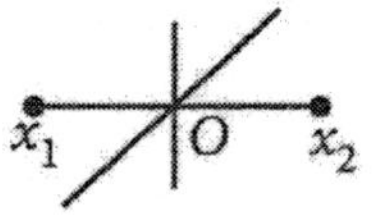

35. Displacement between maximum potential energy position and maximum kinetic energy position for a particle executing simple harmonic motion is **(2002)**

(a) $\pm a/2$ (b) $+a$

(c) $\pm a$ (d) -1

36. The total energy of particle performing SHM depends on **(2001)**

(a) k, a, m (b) k, a

(c) k, a, x (d) k, x.

37. A linear harmonic oscillator of force constant 2×10^6 N/m and displacement 0.01 m has a total mechanical energy of 160 J. Its **(1996)**

(a) P.E. is 160 J

(b) P.E. is zero

(c) P.E. is 100 J

(d) P.E. is 120 J.

38. In a simple harmonic motion, when the displacement is one-half the amplitude, what fraction of the total energy is kinetic? **(1995)**

(a) ½ (b) 3/4

(c) zero (d) 1/4.

39. A loaded vertical spring executes S.H.M. with a time period of 4sec. The difference between the kinetic energy and potential energy of this system varies with a period of **(1994)**

(a) 2sec (b) 1sec

(c) 8sec (d) 4sec

40. A body executes simple harmonic motion with an amplitude A. At what displacement from the mean position is the potential energy of the body is one fourth of its total energy? **(1993)**

(a) $A/4$

(b) A/2

(c) $3A/4$

(d) Some other fraction of A

41. The angular velocity and the amplitude of a simple pendulum is ω and a respectively. At a displacement x from the mean position if its kinetic energy is T and potential energy is V, then the ratio of T to V is **(1991)**

(a) $\frac{(a^2-x^2\omega^2)}{x^2\omega^2}$

(b) $\frac{x^2\omega^2}{(a^2-x^2\omega^2)}$

(c) $\frac{(a^2-x^2)}{x^2}$

(d) $\frac{x^2}{(a^2-x^2)}$

Some Systems Executing Simple Harmonic Motion

42. Two pendulum of length 121 cm and 100 cm start vibrating in phase. At some instant, the two are at their mean position in the same phase. The minimum number of vibrations of the shorter pendulum after which the two are again in phase at the mean position is **(2022)**

(a) 11 (b) 9

(c) 10 (d) 8

43. A spring is stretched by 5 cm by a force 10 N. The time period of the oscillations when a mass of 2 kg is suspended by it is **(2021)**

(a) 0.628 s (b) 0.0628 s

(c) 6.28 s (d) 3.14 s

44. A pendulum is hung from the roof of a sufficiently high building and is moving freely to and fro like a simple harmonic oscillator. The acceleration of the bob of the pendulum is 20 m s^{-2} at a distance of 5 m from the mean position. The time period of oscillation is **(2018)**

(a) $2\pi s$ (b) πs

(c) 2 s (d) 1 s

45. A spring of force constant k is cut into lengths of ratio $1:2:3$. They are connected in series and the new force constant is k'. Then they are connected in parallel and force constant is k''. Then $k':k''$ is **(2017)**

(a) $1:9$ (b) $1:11$

(c) $1:14$ (d) $1:6$

46. A body of mass m is attached to the lower end of a spring whose upper end is fixed. The spring has negligible mass. When the mass m is slightly pulled down and released, it oscillates with a time period of 3 s. When the mass m is increased by 1 kg, the time period of oscillations becomes 5 s. The value of m in kg is **(NEET-II 2016)**

(a) $\frac{3}{4}$ (b) $\frac{4}{3}$

(c) $\frac{16}{9}$ (d) $\frac{9}{16}$

47. The period of oscillation of a mass M suspended from a spring of negligible mass is T. If along with it another mass M is also suspended, the period of oscillation will now be **(2010)**

(a) T (b) $\frac{T}{\sqrt{2}}$

(c) $2T$ (d) $\sqrt{2}T$

48. A simple pendulum performs simple harmonic motion about $x = 0$ with an amplitude a and time period T. The speed of the pendulum at $x = a/2$ will be **(2009)**

(a) $\frac{\pi a}{T}$ (b) $\frac{3\pi^2 a}{T}$

(c) $\frac{\pi a\sqrt{3}}{T}$ (d) $\frac{\pi a\sqrt{3}}{2T}$

49. A mass of 2.0 kg is put on a flat pan attached to a vertical spring fixed on the ground as shown in the figure. The mass of the spring and the pan is negligible. When pressed slightly and released, the mass executes a simple

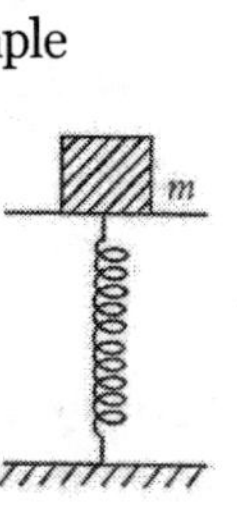

Harmonic motion. The spring constant is 200 N/m. What should be the minimum amplitude of the motion so that the mass gets detached from the pan? (take $g = 10 \text{ m/s}^2$) **(2007)**

(a) 10.0 cm

(b) any value less than 12.0 cm

(c) 4.0 cm (d) 8.0 cm

50. A rectangular block of mass m and area of crosssection A floats in a liquid of density ρ. If it is given a small vertical displacement from equilibrium it undergoes oscillation with a time period T, then **(2006)**

(a) $T \propto \frac{1}{\sqrt{m}}$ (b) $T \propto \sqrt{\rho}$

(c) $T \propto \frac{1}{\sqrt{A}}$ (d) $T \propto \frac{1}{\rho}$

51. Two springs of spring constant k_1 and k_2 are joined in series. The effective spring constant of the combination is given by **(2004)**

(a) $\sqrt{k_1 k_2}$

(b) $(k_1 + k_2)/2$

(c) $k_1 + k_2$

(d) $k_1 k_2/(k_1 + k_2)$

52. The time period of a mass suspended from a spring is T. If the spring is cut into four equal parts and the same mass is suspended from one of the parts, then the new time period will be **(2003)**

(a) $T/4$ (b) T

(c) $T/2$ (d) $2T$

53. A mass is suspendedseparately by two different springs in successive order then time periods is t_1 and t_2 respectively. If it is connected by both spring as shown in figure then time period is t_0, the correct relation is **(2002)**

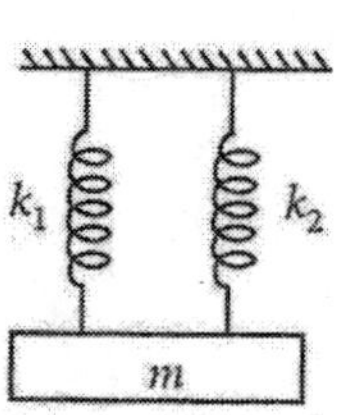

(a) $t_0^2 = t_1^2 + t_2^2$

(b) $t_0^{-2} = t_1^{-2} + t_2^{-2}$

(c) $t_0^{-1} = t_1^{-1} + t_2^{-1}$

(d) $t_0 = t_1 + t_2$

54. Two masses M_A and M_B are hung from two strings of length l_A and l_B respectively. They are executing SHM with frequency relation $f_A = 2f_B$, then relation **(2000)**

(a) $l_A = \frac{l_B}{4}$, does not depend on mass

(b) $l_A = 4l_B$, does not depend on mass

(c) $l_A = 2l_B$ and $M_A = 2M_B$

(d) $l_A = \frac{l_B}{2}$ and $M_A = \frac{M_B}{2}$

55. The bob of simple pendulum having length l, is displaced from mean position to an angular position θ with respect to vertical. If it is released, then velocity of bob at equilibrium position **(2000)**

(a) $\sqrt{2gl(1 - \cos\theta)}$

(b) $\sqrt{2gl(1 + \cos\theta)}$

(c) $\sqrt{2gl\cos\theta}$

(d) $\sqrt{2gl}$

56. Time period of a simple pendulum is 2sec. If its length is increased by 4 times, then its time period becomes **(1999)**

(a) 8sec (b) 12sec

(c) 16sec (d) 4sec

57. Two simple pendulums of length 5 m and 20 m respectively are given small linear displacement in one direction at the same time. They will again be in the phase when the pendulum of shorter length has completed oscillations. **(1998)**
(a) 2 (b) 1
(c) 5 (d) 3

58. A mass m is vertically suspended from a spring of negligible mass; the system oscillates with a frequency n. What will be the frequency of the system, if a mass $4m$ is suspended from the same spring? **(1998)**
(a) $\frac{n}{2}$ (b) $4n$
(c) $\frac{n}{4}$ (d) $2n$

59. If the length of a simple pendulum is increased by 2%, then the time period **(1997)**
(a) increase by 1%
(b) decrease by 1%
(c) increase by 2%
(d) decreases by 2%.

60. A simple pendulum with a bob of mass m oscillates from A to C and back to A such that PB is H. If the acceleration due to gravity is g, then the velocity of the bob as it passes through B is **(1995)**

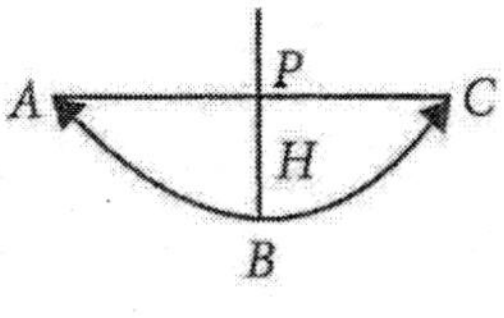

(a) mgH (b) $\sqrt{2gH}$
(c) zero (d) $2gH$.

61. A body of mass 5 kg hangs from a spring and oscillates with a time period of 2π seconds. If the ball is removed, the length of the spring will decrease by **(1994)**
(a) g/k metres (b) k/g metres
(c) 2π metres (d) g metres.

62. A seconds pendulum is mounted in a rocket. Its period of oscillation will decrease when rocket is **(1994)**
(a) moving down with uniform acceleration
(b) moving around the earth in geostationary orbit
(c) moving up with uniform velocity
(d) moving up with uniform acceleration.

63. A simple pendulum is suspended from the roof of a trolley which moves in a horizontal direction with an acceleration a, then the time period is given by $T = 2\pi\sqrt{(l/a')}$, where a' is equal to **(1991)**
(a) g (b) $g - a$
(c) $g + a$ (d) $\sqrt{(g^2 + a^2)}$

64. A mass m is suspended from the two coupled springs connected in series. The force constant for springs are k_1 and k_2. The time period of the suspended mass will be **(1990)**
(a) $T = 2\pi\sqrt{\frac{m}{k_1-k_2}}$
(b) $T = 2\pi\sqrt{\frac{mk_1k_2}{k_1+k_2}}$

(c) $T = 2\pi\sqrt{\frac{m}{k_1+k_2}}$

(d) $T = 2\pi\sqrt{\frac{m(k_1+k_2)}{k_1k_2}}$

Forced Oscillations and Resonance

65. A particle, with restoring force proportional to displacement and resisting force proportional to velocity is subjected to a force Fsin ωt. If the amplitude of the particle is maximum for $\omega = \omega_1$ and the energy of the particle is maximum for $\omega = \omega_2$, then (ω_0 is natural frequency of oscillation of the particle) **(1998, 1989)**

(a) $\omega_1 \neq \omega_0$ and $\omega_2 = \omega_0$

(b) $\omega_1 = \omega_0$ and $\omega_2 = \omega_0$

(c) $\omega_1 = \omega_0$ and $\omega_2 \neq \omega_0$

(d) $\omega_1 \neq \omega_0$ and $\omega_2 \neq \omega_0$

ANSWER KEY

1. (c)	2. (d)	3. (c)	4. (c)	5. (c)	6. (b)	7. (a)
8. (c)	9. (a)	10. (c)	11. (a)	12. (c)	13. (a)	14. (a)
15. (b)	16. (b)	17. (d)	18. (c)	19. (c)	20. (d)	21. (b)
22. (d)	23. (d)	24. (d)	25. (d)	26. (a)	27. (c)	28. (c)
29. (d)	30. (c)	31. (a)	32. (c)	33. (c)	34. (a)	35. (c)
36. (b)	37. (c)	38. (b)	39. (a)	40. (b)	41. (c)	42. (a)
43. (a)	44. (b)	45. (b)	46. (d)	47. (d)	48. (c)	49. (a)
50. (c)	51. (d)	52. (c)	53. (b)	54. (a)	55. (a)	56. (d)
57. (a)	58. (a)	59. (a)	60. (b)	61. (d)	62. (d)	63. (d)
64. (d)	65. (b)					

Hints & Explanations

1. (c) : $y = A_0 + A\sin\omega t + B\cos\omega t$.

or $(y - A_0) = A\sin\omega t + B\cos\omega t$ or $y' = A\sin\omega t + B\cos\omega t$

$$= A\cos\left(\frac{\pi}{2} - \omega t\right) + B\cos\omega t$$

Amplitude $= \sqrt{A^2 + B^2 + 2AB\cos\frac{\pi}{2}}\left[\because \phi = \frac{\pi}{2}\right]$

$= \sqrt{A^2 + B^2}$

2. (d) : for one time period it covers 4 time of amplitude length.

3. (c) : $y = \sin\omega t - \cos\omega t$

$$= \sqrt{2}\left[\frac{1}{\sqrt{2}}\sin\omega t - \frac{1}{\sqrt{2}}\cos\omega t\right]$$

$$= \sqrt{2}\sin\left(\omega t - \frac{\pi}{4}\right)$$

It represents a SHM with time period, $T = \frac{2\pi}{\omega}$.

$$y = \sin^3 \omega t = \frac{1}{4}[3\sin \omega t - \sin 3\omega t]$$

It represents a periodic motion with time period $T = \frac{2\pi}{\omega}$ but not SHM.

$$y = 5\cos\left(\frac{3\pi}{4} - 3\omega t\right) = 5\cos\left(3\omega t - \frac{3\pi}{4}\right)$$

$$[\because \cos(-\theta) = \cos\theta]$$

It represents a SHM with time period, $T = \frac{2\pi}{3\omega}$.

$$y = 1 + \omega t + \omega^2 t^2$$

It represents a non-periodic motion. Also it is not physically acceptable as $y \to \infty$ as $t \to \infty$.

4. **(c):**

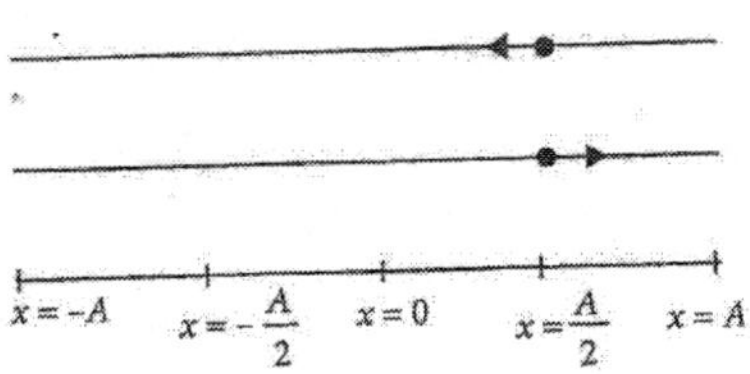

The time taken by the particle to travel from $x = 0$ to $x = \frac{A}{2}$ is $\frac{T}{12}$

The time taken by the particle to travel from $x = A$ to $x = \frac{A}{2}$ is $\frac{T}{6}$

Time difference $= \frac{T}{6} + \frac{T}{6} = \frac{T}{3}$

Phase difference, $\phi = \frac{2\pi}{T} \times$ Time difference $= \frac{2\pi}{T} \times \frac{T}{3} = \frac{2\pi}{3}$

5. **(c)** : $x = a\sin^2 \omega t = a\left(\frac{1 - \cos 2\omega t}{2}\right) = \frac{a}{2} - \frac{a\cos 2\omega t}{2}$

$$(\because \cos 2\theta = 1 - 2\sin^2\theta)$$

$\therefore$ Velocity, $v = \frac{dx}{dt} = \frac{2\omega a\sin 2\omega t}{2} = \omega a\sin 2\omega t$

Acceleration, $a = \frac{dv}{dt} = 2\omega^2 a\cos 2\omega t$

For the given displacement $x = a\sin^2 \omega t$,

$a \propto -x$ is not satisfied.

Hence, the motion of the particle is non simple harmonic motion.

The given motion is a periodic motion with a time period

$$T = \frac{2\pi}{2\omega} = \frac{\pi}{\omega}$$

6. **(b)** : $x(t) = a\sin \omega t$ (from the equilibrium position) At $x(t) = a/2$

$$\frac{a}{2} = a\sin(\omega t) \Rightarrow \sin\left(\frac{\pi}{6}\right) = \sin(\omega t) \text{ or, } \frac{\pi}{6} = \frac{2\pi t}{T}$$

or $t = T/12$

7. **(a)** : In circular motion of a particle with constant speed, particle repeats its motion after a regular interval of time but does not oscillate about a fixed point. So, motion of particle is periodic but not simple harmonic.

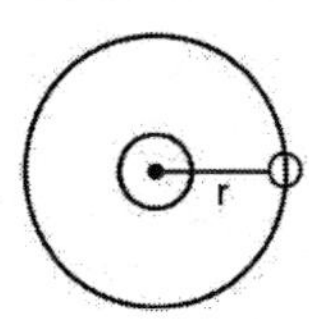

8. **(c)** : $x = a\sin \omega t; y = a\sin(\omega t + \pi/2) = a\cos \omega t$

$x^2 + y^2 = a^2$

It is an equation of a circle.

9. **(a)** :For S.H.M., $x = A\sin\left(\frac{2\pi}{T}t\right)$

when $x = A, A = A\sin\left(\frac{2\pi}{T}t\right)$

$\therefore \sin\left(\frac{2\pi}{T}\cdot t\right) = 1 \Rightarrow \sin\left(\frac{2\pi}{T}\cdot t\right)$

$= \sin\left(\frac{\pi}{2}\right)$

$\Rightarrow t = (T/4)$

When $x = \frac{A}{2}, \frac{A}{2} = A\sin\left(\frac{2\pi}{T}\cdot t\right)$

or $\sin\frac{\pi}{6} = \sin\left(\frac{2\pi}{T}t\right)$ or $t = (T/12)$

Now, time taken to travel from $x = A$ to $x = A/2$

$= T/4 - T/12 = T/6$

10. **(c)** : $x = a\sin\omega t$

and $y = b\sin(\omega t + \pi) = -b\sin\omega t.$

or $\frac{x}{a} = -\frac{y}{b}$ or $y = -\frac{b}{a}x$

It is an equation of straight line.

11. **(a)** : Here $T = 4$ s, $A = 3$ m

Time period $T = \frac{2\pi}{\omega} \Rightarrow 4 = \frac{2\pi}{\omega} \Rightarrow \omega = \frac{\pi}{2}$

As the time is noted from the extreme position,

so, $y = A\cos(\omega t) \Rightarrow y = 3\cos\left(\frac{\pi}{2}t\right)$

12. **(c)** :

$$x = A\sin(\omega t)$$

$$\frac{dx}{dt} = v = A\omega\cos(\omega t)$$

$$\frac{dv}{dt} = a = -\omega^2 A\sin(\omega t)$$

$$a = -\left(\frac{2\pi}{8}\right)^2 \times 1\sin\left(\frac{2\pi}{8}\times 2\right)$$

$$\Rightarrow a = -\frac{\pi^2}{16}\times\sin\left(\frac{\pi}{2}\right)$$

$$\therefore a = \frac{-\pi^2}{16} m/s^2$$

13. **(a)** : Displacement of the particle, $y = a\sin\omega t$, $v = \frac{dy}{dt} = a\omega\cos\omega t$

Acceleration, $a = \frac{dv}{dt} = -a\omega^2\sin\omega t$

So, phase difference between displacement and acceleration is π.

14. **(a)** : Since the displacement for a complete vibration is zero, therefore the average velocity will be zero.

15. **(b)** : Given, $A = 3$ cm, $x = 2$ cm

The velocity of a particle in simple harmonic motion is given as $v = \omega\sqrt{A^2 - x^2}$

and magnitude of its acceleration is $a = \omega^2 x$

Given $|y| = |a| \therefore \omega\sqrt{A^2 - x^2} = \omega^2 x$

$$\omega x = \sqrt{A^2 - x^2} \text{ or } \omega^2 x^2 = A^2 - x^2$$

$$\omega^2 = \frac{A^2 - x^2}{x^2} = \frac{9-4}{4} = \frac{5}{4} \text{ or } \omega = \frac{\sqrt{5}}{2}$$

Time period, $T = \frac{2\pi}{\omega} = 2\pi\cdot\frac{2}{\sqrt{5}} = \frac{4\pi}{\sqrt{5}}$ s

16. **(b)** : If A and ω be the amplitude and angular frequency of vibration, then

$\alpha = \omega^2 A \qquad$ and $\beta = \omega A$

Dividing eqn. (i) by eqn. (ii), we get

$$\frac{\alpha}{\beta} = \frac{\omega^2 A}{\omega A} = \omega$$

$\therefore$ Time period of vibration is $T = \frac{2\pi}{\omega} = \frac{2\pi}{(\alpha/\beta)} = \frac{2\pi\beta}{\alpha}$

17. **(d)** : In SHM, velocities of a particle at distances x_1 and x_2 from mean position are given by

$$V_1^2 = \omega^2(a^2 - x_1^2)$$
$$V_2^2 = \omega^2(a^2 - x_2^2)$$

From equations (i) and (ii), we get

$$V_1^2 - V_2^2 = \omega^2(x_2^2 - x_1^2)$$

$$\omega = \sqrt{\frac{V_1^2 - V_2^2}{x_2^2 - x_1^2}} \Rightarrow T = 2\pi\sqrt{\frac{x_2^2 - x_1^2}{V_1^2 - V_2^2}}$$

18. **(c)**

Here, $X = A\cos\omega t$

$\therefore$ Velocity, $v = \frac{dX}{dt} = \frac{d}{dt}(A\cos\omega t) = -A\omega\sin\omega t$

Acceleration, $a = \frac{dv}{dt} = \frac{d}{dt}(-A\omega\sin\omega t) = -A\omega^2\cos\omega t$

Hence the variation of a with t is correctly shown by graph.

19. **(c)** :

$x = a\sin\omega t$ or $\frac{x}{a} = \sin\omega t$

Velocity, $v = \frac{dx}{dt} = a\omega\cos\omega t$

$$\frac{v}{a\omega} = \cos\omega t \text{ or, } \frac{p}{ma\omega} = \cos\omega t$$

Squaring and adding (i) and (ii), we get

$$\frac{x^2}{a^2} + \frac{p^2}{m^2a^2\omega^2}$$

$$= \sin^2\omega t + \cos^2\omega t; \frac{x^2}{a^2} + \frac{p^2}{m^2a^2\omega^2} = 1$$

It is an equation of ellipse.

20. **(d)** : $\omega_1 = 100\text{rads}^{-1}; \omega_2 = 1000\text{rads}^{-1}$.

Maximum acceleration of $(1) = -\omega_1{}^2 A$

Maximum acceleration of $(2) = -\omega_2^2 A$

$$\therefore \frac{\text{Acceleration (1)}}{\text{Acceleration (2)}} = \frac{\omega_1^2}{\omega_2^2} = \frac{(100)^2}{(1000)^2} = \frac{1}{100}$$

$a(1):a(2) = 1:100$

21. **(b)** : $x = a\sin(\omega t + \pi/6)$

$$\frac{dx}{dt} = a\omega\cos(\omega t + \pi/6)$$

Max. velocity $= a\omega$

$\therefore \frac{a\omega}{2} = a\omega\cos(\omega t + \pi/6)$ or, $\cos(\omega t + \pi/6) = \frac{1}{2}$

$$\Rightarrow \frac{2\pi}{6} = \frac{2\pi}{T}\cdot t + \frac{\pi}{6} \Rightarrow \frac{2\pi}{T}\cdot t = \frac{2\pi}{6} - \frac{\pi}{6} = +\frac{\pi}{6}$$

$$\therefore t = +\frac{\pi}{6} \times \frac{T}{2\pi} = \left|+\frac{T}{12}\right|$$

22. **(d)** : Let $y = A\sin\omega t$

$$\frac{dy}{dt} = A\omega\cos\omega t = A\omega\sin\left(\omega t + \frac{\pi}{2}\right)$$

Acceleration $= -A\omega^2\sin\omega t$

The phase difference between acceleration and velocity is $\pi/2$.

23. **(d)** : $a = 5$ cm, $v_{\max} = 31.4$ cm/s

$v_{\max} = \omega a \Rightarrow 31.4 = 2\pi v \times 5$

$\Rightarrow 31.4 = 10 \times 3.14 \times v \Rightarrow v = 1$ Hz

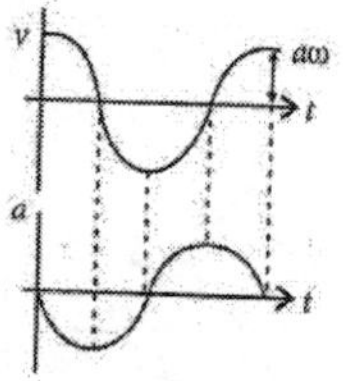

24. (d) : In SHM

$v = A\omega \sin(\omega t + \pi/2)$,

$a = A\omega^2 \sin(\omega t + \pi)$. From this we can easily find out that when v is maximum, then a is zero.

25. (d) : Maximum velocity, $v_{\max} = A\omega$

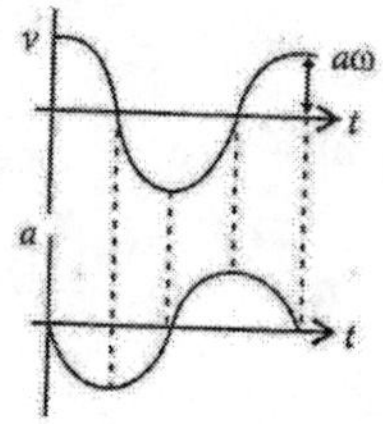

According to question, $\frac{v_{\max}}{2} = \frac{A\omega}{2} = \omega\sqrt{A^2 - y^2}$

$$\frac{A^2}{4} = A^2 - y^2 \Rightarrow y^2 = A^2 - \frac{A^2}{4} \Rightarrow y = \frac{\sqrt{3}A}{2}$$

26. (a) :

Acceleration $= -\omega^2$ displacement $\omega^2 = \frac{\text{acceleration}}{\text{displacement}} = \frac{2.0}{0.02}; \omega^2 = 100$ or $\omega = 10\text{rad/s}$

27. (c) : For simple harmonic motion velocity at displacement $x, v = \omega\sqrt{a^2 - x^2}$

$10 = \omega\sqrt{a^2 - 16}$ ...(i) ;

$8 = \omega\sqrt{a^2 - 25}$ ...(ii) ;

$\frac{100}{\omega^2} = a^2 - 16$ ...(iii) ;

$\frac{64}{\omega^2} = a^2 - 25$ ...(iv) ;

∴ Equation(iii)-(iv) gives $\frac{36}{\omega^2} = 9$

$\Rightarrow \omega = 2\text{rad/s}$ or $T = \frac{2\pi}{\omega} = \frac{2\pi}{2} = \pi\text{sec}$

28. (c) : Simple harmonic motion is defined as follows

Acceleration $\frac{d^2x}{dt^2} = -\omega^2 x$

The negative sign is very important in simple harmonic motion. Acceleration is independent of any initial displacement of equilibrium position.

Then acceleration $= -\omega^2 x$.

29. (d) : For simple harmonic motion

$$\frac{d^2x}{dt^2} \propto -x$$

Therefore force acting on the particle $= -Akx$.

30. (c) : The equation for the SHM is

$y = A\sin\omega t = A\sin(2\pi nt)$

where, A is amplitude, ω is angular frequency and y is displacement at time t.

The formula of potential energy is

$$U = \frac{1}{2}kA^2\sin^2\omega t$$

$$U = \frac{1}{2}kA^2\left(\frac{1-\cos 2\omega t}{2}\right)$$

$$= \frac{1}{2}kA^2\left[\frac{1-\cos 2\pi(2n)t}{2}\right]$$

From eqn. (i) and (ii), we get

$$\left(\because \sin^2\theta = \frac{1-\cos 2\theta}{2}\right)$$

Frequency of potential energy $= 2n$

31. (a) : We have potential energy $V = x^2$

$$\Rightarrow F=-\frac{dv}{dx}=-\frac{d}{dx}\left(x^2\right)=-2x$$

$$\Rightarrow \frac{md^2x}{dt^2}=-2x$$

$$\Rightarrow \left(\frac{d^2}{dt^2}+\frac{2}{m}x\right)=0$$

$$\frac{d^2}{dt^2}+\omega^2x=0\Rightarrow x=A\sin(\omega t+\phi)$$

At $t=0, x_{\max}\Rightarrow x_{\max}=A(\sin\phi)$

$$A=A\sin\phi\Rightarrow\phi=\frac{\pi}{2}$$

$$\Rightarrow x=A\cos\omega t$$

32. **(c)** : Kinetic energy + potential energy = total energy When kinetic energy is maximum, potential energy is zero and vice versa.

∴ Maximum potential energy = total energy $0+K_0=K_0$

33. **(c)** : Potential energy of simple harmonic oscillator

$$=\frac{1}{2}m\omega^2y^2$$

For $y=\frac{a}{2}$, P.E. $=\frac{1}{2}m\omega^2\frac{a^2}{4}\Rightarrow$ P.E. $=\frac{1}{4}\left(\frac{1}{2}m\omega^2a^2\right)=\frac{E}{4}$.

34. **(a)** : Potential energy of particle performing SHM varies parabolically in such a way that at mean position it becomes zero and maximum at extreme position.

35. **(c)** : For a simple harmonic motion between A and B, with O as the mean position, maximum kinetic energy of the particle executing SHM will be at O and maximum potential energy will be at A and B.

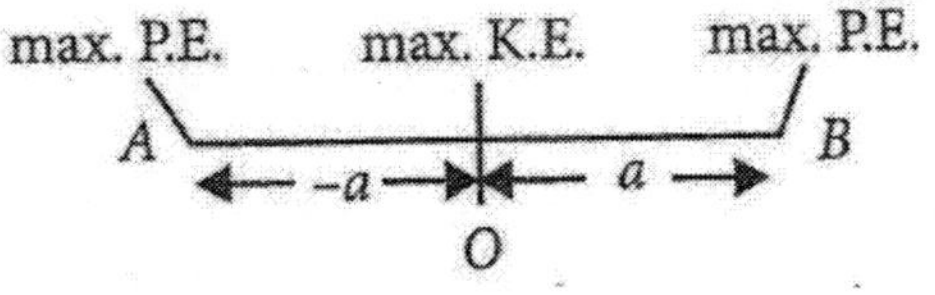

∴ Displacement between maximum potential energy and maximum kinetic energy is $\pm a$.

36. (b) : Total energy $=\frac{1}{2}m\omega^2a^2=\frac{1}{2}ka^2$

37. **(c) :** Force constant $(k)=2\times10^6$ N/m;

displacement $(x)=0.01$ m and total mechanical energy = 160 J.

Potential energy $=\frac{1}{2}kx^2=\frac{1}{2}\times(2\times10^6)(0.01)^2=100$ J

38. (b) : Displacement $(x)=\frac{a}{2}$

Total energy $=\frac{1}{2}m\omega^2a^2$ and

kinetic energy when displacement is (x)

$$=\frac{1}{2}m\omega^2(a^2-x^2)=\frac{1}{2}m\omega^2\left(a^2-\frac{a^2}{4}\right)$$
$$=\frac{3}{4}\left(\frac{1}{2}m\omega^2a^2\right)$$

Therefore fraction of the total energy at x,

$$=\frac{\frac{3}{4}\left(\frac{1}{2}m\omega^2a^2\right)}{\frac{1}{2}m\omega^2a^2}=\frac{3}{4}.$$

39. (a) : Time period $= 4\text{sec}$. In one complete oscillation, the same kinetic and potential energies are repeated two times. So the difference will vary with a period of 2 seconds.

40. (b)

$$\text{P.E} = \frac{1}{2}M\omega^2x^2 \Rightarrow \frac{1}{4}\left(\frac{1}{2}M\omega^2A^2\right) \therefore x = \frac{A}{2}$$

41. (c)

P.E., $V = \frac{1}{2}m\omega^2x^2$

and K.E., $T = \frac{1}{2}m\omega^2(a^2 - x^2) \therefore \frac{T}{V} = \frac{a^2-x^2}{x^2}$

42. (a) : Let $L_1 = 121 \text{ cm} = \frac{121}{100} = 1.21 \text{ m}$

$$L_2 = 100 \text{ cm} = \frac{100}{100} = 1 \text{ m}$$

Let $T_1 =$ longer pendulum ; $T_2 =$ shorter pendulum

We know, $T = 2\pi\sqrt{\frac{L}{g}} \Rightarrow T \propto \sqrt{L}$

$$\frac{T_1}{T_2} \propto \sqrt{\frac{L_1}{L_2}}$$

$$\frac{T_1}{T_2} \propto \sqrt{\frac{1.21}{1}} = \frac{1.1}{1}$$

$$10T_1 = 11T_2$$

10 vibration of longer pendulum $= 11$ vibration of shorter pendulum.

43. (a) : Force constant of spring, $k = \frac{F}{x}$

Here,

$$F = 10 \text{ N}, x = 5 \text{ cm}; k = \frac{10}{0.05} = 200 \text{ N/m}$$

If the mass of 2 kg is suspended by the spring, then period of oscillation is

$$T = 2\pi\sqrt{\frac{m}{k}}; T = 2\pi\sqrt{\frac{2}{200}} = 2\pi \times 0.1$$

$$T = 0.628 \text{ s}$$

44. (b) : Magnitude of acceleration of a particle moving in a SHM is, $|a| = \omega^2 y$; where y is amplitude.

$$\Rightarrow 20 = \omega^2(5) \Rightarrow \omega = 2\text{rads}^{-1}$$

$\therefore$ Time period of oscillation, $T = \frac{2\pi}{\omega} = \frac{2\pi}{2} = \pi\text{s}$

45. (b) : Let us assume, the length of spring be l.

When we cut the spring into ratio of length 1: 2: 3, we get three springs of lengths $\frac{l}{6}, \frac{2l}{6}$ and $\frac{3l}{6}$ with force constant,

$$k_1 = \frac{kl}{l_1} = \frac{kl}{l/6} = 6k, k_2 = \frac{kl}{l_2} = \frac{kl}{2l/6} = 3k$$

and $k_3 = \frac{kl}{l_3} = \frac{kl}{3l/6} = 2k$

When connected in series, $\frac{1}{k'} = \frac{1}{6k} + \frac{1}{3k} + \frac{1}{2k} = \frac{1+2+3}{6k} = \frac{1}{k}$

$\therefore k' = k$

When connected in parallel, $k'' = 6k + 3k + 2k = 11k$

$$\therefore \frac{k'}{k''} = \frac{k}{11k} = \frac{1}{11}$$

46. (d) : Time period of spring - block system, $T = 2\pi\sqrt{\frac{m}{k}}$ For given spring, $T \propto \sqrt{m}$

$$\frac{T_1}{T_2} = \sqrt{\frac{m_1}{m_2}}$$

Here, $T_1 = 3\text{ s}, m_1 = m, T_2 = 5\text{ s}, m_2 = m+1, m = ?$

$$\frac{3}{5} = \sqrt{\frac{m}{m+1}} \text{ or } \frac{9}{25} = \frac{m}{m+1}$$

$$25m = 9m + 9 \Rightarrow 16m = 9; \therefore m = \frac{9}{16}\text{ kg}$$

47. (d) : A mass M is suspended from a massless spring of spring constant k as shown in figure (a). Then, time period of oscillation is

$$T = 2\pi\sqrt{\frac{M}{k}} \quad \text{... (i)}$$

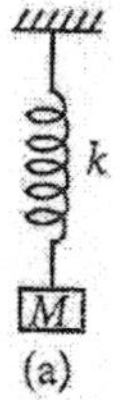

(a)

When a another mass M is also suspended with it as shown in figure (b). Then, time period of oscillation is,

$$T' = 2\pi\sqrt{\frac{M+M}{k}} = 2\pi\sqrt{\frac{2M}{k}}$$

$$= \sqrt{2}\left(2\pi\sqrt{\frac{M}{k}}\right) = \sqrt{2}T\,(\text{Using(i)})$$

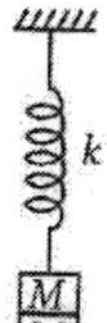

(b)

48. (c) : For simple harmonic motion,

$$v = \omega\sqrt{a^2 - x^2}.$$

When $x = \frac{a}{2}, v = \omega\sqrt{a^2 - \frac{a^2}{4}} = \omega\sqrt{\frac{3}{4}a^2}.$

As $\omega = \frac{2\pi}{T}, \therefore v = \frac{2\pi}{T}\cdot\frac{\sqrt{3}}{2}a \Rightarrow v = \frac{\pi\sqrt{3}a}{T}.$

49. (a) :

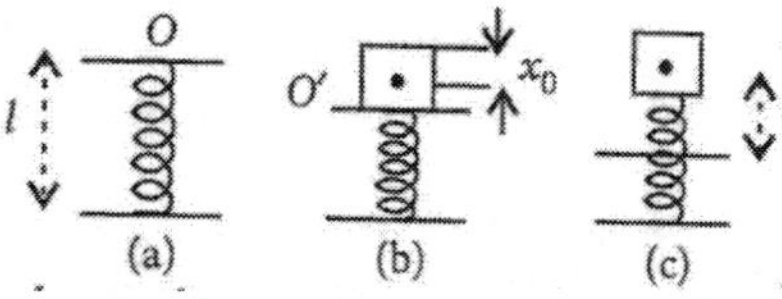

The spring has a length l. Whem m is placed over it, the equilibrium position becomes O'.

If it is pressed from O' (the equilibrium position) to O'', $O'O''$ is the amplitude.

$$\therefore\ OO' = \frac{mg}{k} = \frac{2\times 10}{200} = 0.10\text{ m}.$$
$$mg = kx_0.$$

If the restoring force $mA\omega^2 > mg$, then the mass will move up with acceleration, detached from the pan.

i.e., $> \frac{g}{k/m} \Rightarrow A > \frac{20}{200} > 0.10$ m.

The amplitude > 10 cm.

i.e. the minimum is just greater than 10 cm.

(The actual compression will include x_0 also. But when talking of amplitude, it is always from the equilibrium position with respect to which the mass is oscillating.

50. (c) : Let l be the length of block immersed in liquid as shown in the figure.

When the block is floating,

$\therefore mg = Al\rho g$

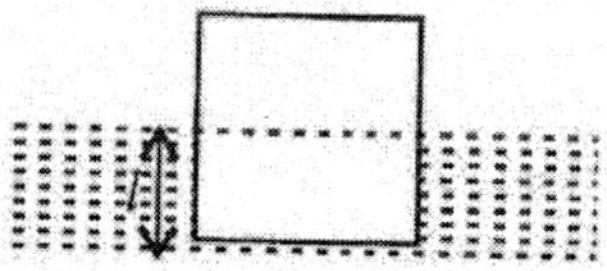

If the block is given vertical displacement y then the effective restoring force is

$F = -[A(l+y)\rho g - mg]$

$= -[A(l+y)\rho g - Al\rho g]$

$= -A\rho g y$

Restoring force $= -[A\rho g]y$. As this F is directed towards equilibrium position of block, so it will execute simple harmonic motion.

Here inertia factor = mass of block = m

Spring factor = $A\rho g$

$\therefore$ Time period, $T = 2\pi\sqrt{\frac{m}{A\rho g}}$ i.e., $T \propto \frac{1}{\sqrt{A}}$.

51. **(d):** When the spring joined in series, the total extension in spring is

$$\Rightarrow y = y_1 + y_2 = \frac{-F}{k_1} - \frac{F}{k_2} \Rightarrow y = -F\left[\frac{1}{k_1} + \frac{1}{k_2}\right]$$

Thus spring constant in this case becomes

$$k = \frac{k_1 k_2}{k_1 + k_2}$$

52. **(c)** : Let k be the force constant of spring. If k' is the force constant of each part, then

$$\frac{1}{k} = \frac{4}{k'} \Rightarrow k' = 4k$$

$\therefore$ Time period $= 2\pi\sqrt{\frac{m}{4k}} = \frac{1}{2} \times 2\pi\sqrt{\frac{m}{k}} = \frac{T}{2}$.

53. **(b)** : The time period of a spring mass system as shown in figure 1 is given by $T = 2\pi\sqrt{m/k}$, where k is the spring constant.

$\therefore t_1 = 2\pi\sqrt{m/k_1}$

and $t_2 = 2\pi\sqrt{m/k_2}$

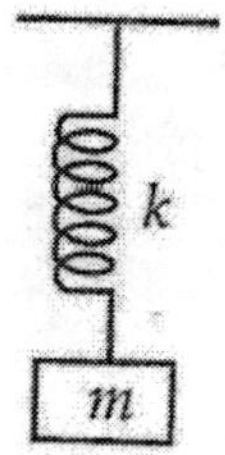

Figure 1

Now, when they are connected in parallel as shown in figure 2(a), the system can be replaced by a single spring of spring constant, $k_{eff} = k_1 + k_2$, as shown in figure 2 (b).

Since $mg = k_1x + k_2x = k_{eff}x$

$$\therefore t_0 = 2\pi\sqrt{m/k_{eff}} = 2\pi\sqrt{m/(k_1 + k_2)}$$

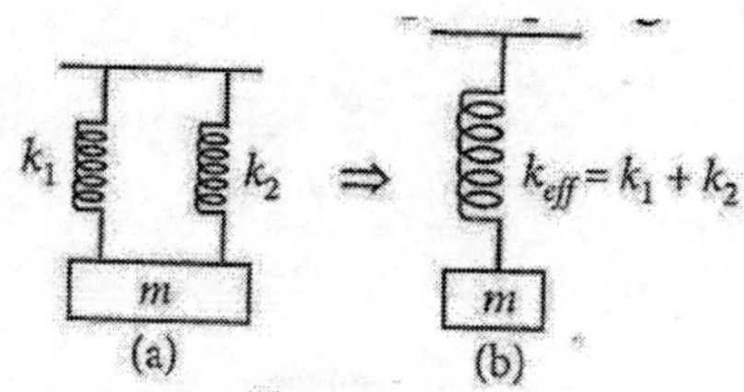

Figure 2

From (ii), $\frac{1}{t_2{}^2} = \frac{1}{4\pi^2} \times \frac{k_2}{m}$

From (iii), $\frac{1}{t_0{}^2} = \frac{1}{4\pi^2} \times \frac{k_1+k_2}{m}$

From eqns (iv), (v) and (vi)

$$=\frac{1}{t_1^2}+\frac{1}{t_2^2}=\frac{1}{t_0^2};\therefore\ t_0^{-2}=t_1^{-2}+t_2^{-2}$$

54. (a) : $f_A = 2f_B$

$\Rightarrow \frac{1}{2\pi}\sqrt{\frac{g}{l_A}} = 2\times\frac{1}{2\pi}\sqrt{\frac{g}{l_B}}$ or, $\frac{1}{l_A} = 4\times\frac{1}{l_B}$

or, $l_A = \frac{l_B}{4}$, which does not depend on mass.

55. (a) : In $\triangle\, OAC, \cos\theta = OA/l$

or, $OA = l\cos\theta$

$\therefore\ AB = l(1-\cos\theta) = h$

At point, C, the velocity of bob $= 0$.

The vertical acceleration $= g$

$\therefore\ v^2 = 2gh$

or, $v = \sqrt{2gl(1-\cos\theta)}$

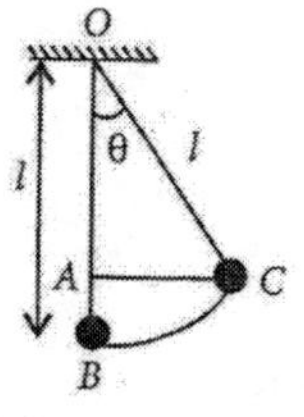

56. (d) : Time period of a simple pendulum is given by $T = 2\pi\sqrt{\frac{l}{g}} \Rightarrow T \propto \sqrt{l}$

$\therefore\ \frac{T_1}{T_2} = \sqrt{\frac{l_1}{l_2}} = \sqrt{\frac{1}{4}} = \frac{1}{2}$ or, $T_2 = 2T_1 = 4$sec.

57. (a) : Frequency of the pendulum $v_{l=5} = \frac{1}{2\pi}\sqrt{\frac{g}{5}}$,

$$v_{l=20} = \frac{1}{2\pi}\sqrt{\frac{g}{20}}$$

$$\therefore\ \frac{v_{l=5}}{v_{l=20}} = \sqrt{\frac{20}{5}} = 2 \Rightarrow v_{l=5} = 2v_{l=20}$$

As shorter length pendulum has frequency double the larger length pendulum. Therefore shorter pendulum should complete 2 oscillations before they will be again in phase.

58. (a) : $n = \frac{1}{2\pi}\sqrt{\frac{k}{m}}; n' = \frac{1}{2\pi}\sqrt{\frac{k}{4m}}$

$\therefore\ n' = n/2$

59. (a) : $l_2 = 1.02 l_1$.

Time period $(T) = 2\pi\times\sqrt{\frac{l}{g}} \propto \sqrt{l}$

Therefore $\frac{T_2}{T_1} = \sqrt{\frac{l_2}{l_1}} = \sqrt{\frac{1.02l_1}{l_1}} = 1.01$

Thus time period increased by 1%.

60. (b) : Potential energy at A or C = Kinetic energy at B.

Thus, $\frac{1}{2}mv_B^2 = mgH$ or $v_B = \sqrt{2gH}$

61. (d) : Mass $(m) = 5$ kg and time period $(T) = 2\pi$sec.

Therefore time period

$$T = 2\pi\times\sqrt{\frac{m}{k}} \Rightarrow \sqrt{\frac{5}{k}} = 1$$

or = 5 N/m.

According to Hooke's Law, $F = -kl$.

Therefore decrease in length $(l) = -\frac{F}{k} = -\frac{5g}{5} = -g$ metres

62. (d) : Period of oscillation $T = 2\pi\sqrt{\frac{l}{g}}$.

Therefore T will decrease when

acceleration (g) increases. And g will increase when the rocket moves up with a uniform acceleration.

63. (d) : The effective value of acceleration due to gravity is $\sqrt{(a^2 + g^2)}$.

64. (d) : The effective spring constant of two springs in series is $k = \frac{k_1 k_2}{k_1 + k_2}$

Time period, $T = 2\pi\sqrt{\frac{m}{k}} = 2\pi\sqrt{\frac{m(k_1+k_2)}{k_1 k_2}}$

65. (b) : The amplitude and velocity resonance occurs at the same frequency.

At resonance, i.e., $\omega_1 = \omega_0$ and $\omega_2 = \omega_0$, the amplitude and energy of the particle would be maximum.

Chapter: 14 WAVES

Transverse and Longitudinal Waves

1. Which one of the following statements is true? **(2006)**
   (a) Both light and sound waves can travel in vacuum.
   (b) Both light and sound waves in air are transverse.
   (c) The sound waves in air are longitudinal while the light waves are transverse.
   (d) Both light and sound waves in air are longitudinal.

2. With the propagation of a longitudinal wave through a material medium, the quantities transmitted in the propagation direction are **(1992)**
   (a) energy, momentum and mass
   (b) energy
   (c) energy and mass
   (d) energy and linear momentum

Displacement Relation in a Progressive Wave

3. A wave travelling in the +ve x-direction having displacement along y-direction as 1 m, wavelength 2πm and frequency of $\frac{1}{\pi}Hz$ is represented by **(2013)**
   (a) $y=\sin(10\pi x-20\pi t)$
   (b) $y=\sin(2\pi x+2\pi t)$
   (c) $y=\sin(x-2t)$
   (d) $y=\sin(2\pi x-2\pi t)$

4. Two waves are represented by the equations

   $y_1 = a\sin(\omega t + kx + 0.57)m$ and

   $y_2 = a\cos(\omega t + kx)m$, where x is in meter and t in sec. The phase difference between them is **(2011)**
   (a) 1.0 radian (b) 1.25 radian
   (c) 1.57 radian (d) 0.57 radian

5. A wave in a string has an amplitude of 2 cm. The wave travels in the +ve direction of x axis with a speed of 128 m / s and it is noted that 5 complete waves fit in 4 m length of the string. The equation describing the wave is **(2009)**
   (a) $y=(0.02)m\sin(15.7x-2010t)$
   (b) $y=(0.02)m\sin(15.7x+2010t)$
   (c) $y=(0.02)m\sin(7.85x-1005t)$
   (d) $y=(0.02)m\sin(7.85x+1005t)$

6. The wave described by $y=0.25\sin(10\pi x-2\pi t)$, where x and y

are in meters and t in seconds, is a wave travelling along the **(2008)**

(a) +ve x direction with frequency 1 Hz and wavelength $\lambda = 0.2m$.

(b) -ve x direction with amplitude 0.25 m and wavelength $\lambda = 0.2m$.

(c) -ve x direction with frequency 1 Hz.

(d) +ve x direction with frequency πHz and wavelength $\lambda = 0.2m$

7. The phase difference between two waves, represented by

$y_1 = 10^{-6}\sin[100t + (x/50) + 0.5]m$

$y_2 = 10^{-6}\cos[100t + (x/50)]m,$

where x is expressed in metres and t is expressed in seconds, is approximately **(2004)**

(a) 1.07 radians (b) 2.07 radians

(c) 0.5 radians (d) 1.5 radians

8. A wave travelling in positive X-direction with $a = 0.2ms^{-2}$, velocity $= 360ms^{-1}$ and $\lambda - 60m$, then correct expression for the wave is **(2002)**

(a) $y = 0.2\sin\left[2\pi\left(6t + \frac{x}{60}\right)\right]$

(b) $y = 0.2\sin\left[\pi\left(6t + \frac{x}{60}\right)\right]$

(c) $y = 0.2\sin\left[2\pi\left(6t - \frac{x}{60}\right)\right]$

(d) $y = 0.2\sin\left[\pi\left(6t - \frac{x}{60}\right)\right]$

9. In a sinusoidal wave, the time required for a particular point to move from maximum displacement to zero displacement is 0.170 s. The frequency of wave is **(1998)**

(a) 0.73 Hz (b) 0.36 Hz

(c) 1.47 Hz (d) 2.94 Hz

10. The equation of a sound wave is $y = 0.0015\sin(62.4x + 316t)$. **(1996)**

The wavelength of this wave is

(a) 0.3 unit

(b) 0.2 unit

(c) 0.1 unit

(d) cannot be calculated.

11. Two sound waves having a phase difference of 60° have path difference of (λ is wavelength of sound wave) **(1996)**

(a) $\frac{\lambda}{6}$ (b) $\frac{\lambda}{3}$

(c) 2λ (d) $\frac{\lambda}{2}$

12. Which one of the following represents a wave? **(1994)**

(a) $y = A\sin(\omega t - kx)$

(c) $y = A\sin kx$

(b) $y = A\cos(at - bx + c)$

(d) $y = A\sin\omega t$.

13. The frequency of sinusodial wave $y = 0.40\cos[2000t + 0.80]$ would be **(1992)**

(a) $1000\pi Hz$ (b) 2000 Hz

(c) 20 Hz (d) $\frac{1000}{\pi} Hz$

14. Equation of progressive wave is given by $y = 4\sin\left[\pi\left(\frac{t}{5} - \frac{x}{9}\right) + \frac{\pi}{6}\right]$ where y, x are in cm and t is in seconds. Then which of the following is correct ? **(1988)**

(a) v = 5 cm (b) $\lambda = 18 cm$

(c) a = 0.04 cm (d) f = 50 Hz

The Speed of a Travelling Wave

15. If the initial tension on a stretched string is doubled then the ratio of the initial and final speeds of a transverse wave along the string is **(2022)**

(a) 1 : 1 (b) $\sqrt{2} : 1$

(c) $1 : \sqrt{2}$ (d) 1 : 2

16. A uniform rope of length L and mass m_1 hangs vertically from a rigid support. A block of mass m_2 is attached to the free end of the rope. A transverse pulse of wavelength λ_1 is produced at the lower end of the rope. The wavelength of the pulse when it reaches the top of the rope is λ_2. The ratio λ_2 / λ_1 is **(NEET-I 2016)**

(a) $\sqrt{\frac{m_2}{m_1}}$ (b) $\sqrt{\frac{m_1 + m_2}{m_1}}$

(c) $\sqrt{\frac{m_1}{m_2}}$ (d) $\sqrt{\frac{m_1 + m_2}{m_2}}$

17. 4.0 g of a gas occupies 22.4 litres at NTP. The specific heat capacity of the gas at constant volume is $5.0 JK^{-1}mol^{-1}$. If the speed of sound in this gas at NTP is $952 ms^{-1}$, then the heat capacity at constant pressure is (Take gas constant $R = 8.3 JK^{-1}mol^{-1}$) **(2015)**

(a) $7.0 JK^{-1}mol^{-1}$

(b) $8.5 JK^{-1}mol^{-1}$

(c) $8.0 JK^{-1}mol^{-1}$

(d) $7.5 JK^{-1}mol^{-1}$

18. The equation of a simple harmonic wave is given by $y = 3\sin\frac{\pi}{2}(50t - x)$, where x and y are in metres and t is in seconds. The ratio of maximum particle velocity to the wave velocity is **(Mains 2012)**

(a) 2π (b) $\frac{3}{2}\pi$

(c) 3π (d) $\frac{2}{3}\pi$

19. Sound waves travel at 350 m / s through a warm air and at 3500 m / s through brass. The wavelength of a 700 Hz acoustic wave as it enters brass from warm air **(2011)**

(a) decrease by a factor 10

(b) increase by a factor 20

(c) increase by a factor 10

(d) decrease by a factor 20

20. A transverse wave is represented by $y = A\sin(\omega t - kx)$. For what value of the wavelength is the wave velocity equal to the maximum particle velocity? **(2010)**

(a) $\pi A/2$ (b) πA

(c) $2\pi A$ (d) A

21. A transverse wave propagating along x-axis is represented by

$y(x,t) = 8.0\sin(0.5\pi x - 4\pi t - \pi/4)$

where x is in metres and t is in seconds. The speed of the wave is **(2006)**

(a) $8m/s$ (b) $4\pi m/s$

(c) $0.5\pi m/s$ (d) $\pi/4m/s$.

22. A point source emits sound equally in all directions in a non-absorbing medium. Two points P and Q are at distances of 2 m and 3 m respectively from the source. The ratio of the intensities of the waves at P and Q is **(2005)**

(a) 3 : 2 (b) 2 : 3

(c) 9 : 4 (d) 4 : 9

23. The equation of a wave is represented by $y = 10^{-4}\sin\left(100t - \frac{x}{10}\right)m$, then the velocity of wave will be **(2001)**

(a) 100 m/s (b) 4 m/s

(c) 1000 m/s (d) 10 m/s

24. A transverse wave is represented by the equation $y = y_0 \sin\frac{2\pi}{\lambda}(vt - x)$

For what value of λ, is the maximum particle velocity equal to two times the wave velocity? **(1998)**

(a) $\lambda = \frac{\pi y_0}{2}$ (b) $\lambda = \frac{\pi y_0}{3}$

(c) $\lambda = 2\pi y_0$ (d) $\lambda = \pi y_0$

25. A hospital uses an ultrasonic scanner to locate tumours in a tissue. The operating frequency of the scanner is 4.2 MHz. The speed of sound in a tissue is 1.7 km/s. The wavelength of sound in the tissue is close to **(1995)**

(a) $4\times10^{-3}m$ (b) $8\times10^{-3}m$

(c) $4\times10^{-4}m$ (d) $8\times10^{-4}m$

26. The temperature at which the speed of sound becomes double as was at $27^\circ C$ is **(1993)**

(a) $273^\circ C$ (b) $0^\circ C$

(c) $927^\circ C$ (d) $1027^\circ C$

27. Velocity of sound waves in air is 330 m/s. For a particular sound wave in air, a path difference of 40 cm is equivalent to phase difference of 1.6π. The frequency of this wave is **(1990)**

(a) 165 Hz (b) 150 Hz

(c) 660 Hz (d) 330 Hz

28. A 5.5 metre length of string has a mass of 0.033 kg. If the terision in the string in 77 N, the speed of a wave on the string is

(1989)

(a) $110 ms^{-1}$ (b) $165 ms^{-1}$

(c) $77 ms^{-1}$ (d) $102 ms^{-1}$

29. If the amplitude of sound is doubled and the frequency reduced to one fourth, the intensity of sound at the same point will be **(1989)**

(a) increasing by a factor of 2
(b) decreasing by a factor of 2
(c) decreasing by a factor of 4
(d) unchanged

30. The velocity of sound in any gas depends upon **(1988)**

(a) wavelength of sound only
(b) density and elasticity of gas
(c) intensity of sound waves only
(d) amplitude and frequency of sound

The Principle of Superposition of Waves

31. Two periodic waves of intensities I_1 and I_a pass through a region at the same time in the same direction. The sum of the maximum and minimum intensities is

(2008)

(a) $\left(\sqrt{I_1}-\sqrt{I_2}\right)^2$ (b) $2\left(I_1+I_2\right)$

(c) I_1+I_2 (d) $\left(\sqrt{I_1}+\sqrt{I_2}\right)^2$

32. Two waves having equation

$$x_1 = a\sin\left(\omega t - kx + \phi_1\right),$$

$$x_a = a\sin\left(\omega t - kx + \phi_2\right)$$

If in the resultant wave the frequency and amplitude remain equal to amplitude of superimposing waves, the phase difference between them is **(2001)**

(a) $\frac{\pi}{6}$ (b) $\frac{2\pi}{3}$

(c) $\frac{\pi}{4}$ (d) $\frac{\pi}{3}$

33. The equations of two waves acting in perpendicular directions are piven as $x = a\cos(\omega t + \delta)$ and $y = a\cos(\omega t + \alpha)$, where $\delta = \alpha + \frac{\pi}{2}$, the resultant wave represents **(2000)**

(a) a parabula (b) a circle

(c) an ellipse (d) a straight line

Reflection of Waves

34. The ratio of frequencies of fundamental harmonic produced by an open pipe to that of closed pipe having the same length is

(2023)

(a) 2 : 1 (b) 1 : 3

(c) 3 : 1 (d) 1 : 2

35. A tuning fork with frequency 800 Hz produces resonance in a resonance column tube with upper end open and lower end closed by water surface. Successive resonance are observed at length 9.75 cm,

31.25 cm and 52.75 cm. The speed of sound in air is

(Odisha NEET 2019)

(a) 500 m/s (b) 156 m/s

(c) 344 m/s (d) 172 m/s

36. A tuning fork is used to produce resonance in a glass tube. The length of the air column in this tube can be adjusted by a variable piston. At room temperature of $27^{\circ}C$ two successive resonances are produced at 20 cm and 73 cm of column length. If the frequency of the tuning fork is 320 Hz, the velocity of sound in air at $27^{\circ}C$ is **(2018)**

(a) $330ms^{-1}$ (b) $339ms^{-1}$

(c) $350ms^{-1}$ (d) $300ms^{-1}$

37. The fundamental frequency in an open organ pipe is equal to the third harmonic of a closed organ pipe. If the length of the closed organ pipe is 20 cm, the length of the open organ pipe is **(2018)**

(a) 13.2 cm (b) 8 cm

(c) 12.5 cm (d) 16 cm

38. The two nearest harmonics of a tube closed at one end and open at other end are 220 Hz and 260 Hz. What is the fundamental frequency of the system?

(2017)

(a) 20 Hz (b) 30 Hz

(c) 40 Hz (d) 10 Hz

39. The second overtone of an open organ pipe has the same frequency as the first overtone of a closed pipe L metre long. The length of the open pipe will be

(NEET II 2016)

(a) L (b) 2 L

(c) $\frac{L}{2}$ (d) 4 L

40. An air column, closed at one end and open at the other, resonates with a tuning fork when the smallest length of the column is 50 cm. The next larger length of the column resonating with the same tuning fork is

(NEET-I 2016)

(a) 150 cm (b) 200 cm

(c) 66.7 cm (d) 100 cm

41. A string is stretched between fixed points separated by 75.0 cm. It is observed to have resonant frequencies of 420 Hz and 315 Hz. There are no other resonant frequencies between these two. The lowest resonant frequency for this string is **(2015)**

(a) 10.5 Hz (b) 105 Hz

(c) 155 Hz (d) 205 Hz

42. The fundamental frequency of a closed organ pipe of length 20 cm is equal to the second overtone of an organ pipe open at both the ends. The length of organ pipe open at both the ends is **(2015)**

(a) 120 cm (b)140 cm

(c) 80 cm (d) 100 cm

43. The number of possible natural oscillations of air column in a pipe closed at one end of length 85 cm whose frequencies lie below 1250 Hz are (Velocity of sound $= 340ms^{-1}$) **(2014)**

(a) 4 (b) 5

(c) 7 (d) 6

44. If we study the vibration of a pipe open at both ends, then the following statement is not true. **(2013)**

(a) All harmonics of the fundamental frequency will be generated.

(b) Pressure change will be maximum at both ends.

(c) Open end will be antinode.

(d) Odd harmonics of the fundamental frequency will be generated.

45. The length of the wire between two ends of a sonometer is 100 cm. What should be the positions of two bridges below the wire so that the three segments of the wire have their fundamental frequencies in the ratio 1 : 3 : 5. **(Karnataka NEET 2013)**

(a) $\frac{1500}{23} cm, \frac{500}{23} cm$

(b) $\frac{1500}{23} cm, \frac{300}{23} cm$

(c) $\frac{300}{23} cm, \frac{1500}{23} cm$

(d) $\frac{1500}{23} cm, \frac{2000}{23} cm$

46. When a string is divided into three segments of length l_1, l_2 and l_3 the fundamental frequencies of these three segments are v_1, v_2 and v_3 respectively. The original fundamental frequency (v) of the string is **(2012)**

(a) $\sqrt{v} = \sqrt{v_1} + \sqrt{v_2} + \sqrt{v_3}$

(b) $v = v_1 + v_2 + v_3$

(c) $\frac{1}{v} = \frac{1}{v_1} + \frac{1}{v_2} + \frac{1}{v_3}$

(d) $\frac{1}{\sqrt{v}} = \frac{1}{\sqrt{v_1}} + \frac{1}{\sqrt{v_2}} + \frac{1}{\sqrt{v_3}}$

47. The time of reverberation of a room A is one second. What will be the time (in seconds) of reverberation of a room, having all the dimensions double of those of room A ? **(2006)**

(a) 1 (b) 2

(c) 4 (d) 1 / 2

48. If the tension and diameter of a sonometer wire of fundamental frequency n is doubled and density is halved then its fundamental frequency will become **(2001)**

(a) $\frac{n}{4}$ (b) $\sqrt{2}n$

(c) n (d) $\frac{n}{\sqrt{2}}$

49. A string is cut into three parts, having fundamental frequencies n_1, n_2, n_3 respectively. Then original fundamental frequency n related by the expression as **(2000)**

(a) $\frac{1}{n} = \frac{1}{n_1} + \frac{1}{n_2} + \frac{1}{n_3}$

(b) $n = n_1 \times n_2 \times n_3$

(c) $n = n_1 + n_2 + n_3$

(d) $n = \frac{n_1 + n_2 + n_3}{3}$

50. A standing wave having 3 nodes and 2 antinodes is formed between two atoms having a distance $1.21\mathring{A}$ between them. The wavelength of the standing wave is **(1998)**

(a) $6.05\mathring{A}$ (b) $2.42\mathring{A}$
(c) $1.21\mathring{A}$ (d) $3.63\mathring{A}$

51. Standing waves are produced in 10 m long stretched string. If the string vibrates in 5 segments and wave velocity is 20 m / s, the frequency is **(1997)**

(a) 5 Hz (b) 10 Hz
(c) 2 Hz (d) 4 Hz

52. A cylindrical tube, open at both ends has fundamental frequency f in air. The tube is dipped vertically in water, so that half of it is in water. The fundamental frequency of air column is now **(1997)**

(a) f / 2 (b) 3 f / 4
(c) 2 f (d) f

53. The length of a sonometer wire A B is 110 cm. Where should the two bridges be placed from A to divide the wire in 3 segments whose fundamental frequencies are in the ratio of 1 : 2 : 3 ? **(1995)**

(a) 60 cm and 90 cm
(b) 30 cm and 60 cm
(c) 30 cm and 90 cm
(d) 40 cm and 80 cm

54. A wave of frequency 100 Hz travels along a string towards its fixed end. When this wave travels back, after reflection, a node is formed at a distance of 10 cm from the fixed end. The speed of the wave (incident and reflected) is **(1994)**

(a) 20 m / s (b) 40 m / s
(c) 5 m / s (d) 10 m / s.

55. A stationary wave is represented by $y = A\sin(100t)\cos(0.01x)$, where y and A are in millimetres, t is in seconds and x is in metres. The velocity of the wave is **(1994)**

(a) $10^4 m/s$ (b) not derivable
(c) 1 m / s (d) $10^2 m/s$

56. A stretched string resonates with tuning for k frequency 512 Hz when length of the string is 0.5 m. The length of the string required to vibrate resonantly with a tuning fork of frequency 256 Hz would be **(1993)**

(a) 0.25 m (b) 0.5 m
(c) 1 m (d) 2 m

57. A closed organ pipe (closed at one end) is excited to support the third overtone. It is found that air in the pipe has **(1991)**

(a) three nodes and three antinodes
(b) three nodes and four antinodes
(c) four nodes and three antinodes
(d) four nodes and four antinodes.

58. In a guitar, two strings A and B made of same material are slightly out of tune and produce beats of frequency 6 Hz. When tension in B is slightly decreased, the beat frequency increases to 7 Hz. If the frequency of A is 530 Hz, the original frequency of B will be **(2020)**

(a) 523 Hz (b) 524 Hz

(c) 536 Hz (d) 537 Hz

59. Three sound waves of equal amplitudes have frequencies $(n-1), n, (n+1)$. They superimpose to give beats. The number of beats produced per second will be

(NEET-II 2016)

(a) 1 (b) 4

(c) 3 (d) 2

60. A source of unknown frequency gives 4 beats/s when sounded with a source of known frequency 250 Hz. The second harmonic of the source of unknown frequency gives five beats per second, when sounded with a source of frequency 513 Hz. The unknown frequency is **(2013)**

(a) 240 Hz (b) 260 Hz

(c) 254 Hz (d) 246 Hz

61. Two sources of sound placed close to each other, are emitting progressive waves given by

$y_1 = 4\sin 600\pi t$ and $y_2 = 5\sin 608\pi t$

An observer located near these two sources of sound will hear **(2012)**

(a) 4 beats per second with intensity ratio 25 : 16 between waxing and waning.

(b) 8 beats per second with intensity ratio 25 : 16 between waxing and waning.

(c) 8 beats per second with intensity ratio 81 : 1 between waxing and waning.

(d) 4 beats per second with intensity ratio 81 : 1 between waxing and waning.

62. Two identical piano wires, kept under the same tension T have a fundamental frequency of 600 Hz. The fractional increase in the tension of one of the wires which will lead to occurrence of 6 beats/s when both the wires oscillate together would be **(Mains 2011)**

(a) 0.01 (b) 0.02

(c) 0.03 (d) 0.04

63. A tuning fork of frequency 512 Hz makes 4 beats per second with the vibrating string of a piano. The beat frequency decreases to 2 beats per second when the tension in the piano string is slightly increased. The frequency of the piano string before increasing the tension was **(2010)**

(a) 510 Hz (b) 514 Hz

(c) 516 Hz (d) 508 Hz

64. Each of the two strings of length 51.6 cm and 49.1 cm are tensioned separately by 20 N force. Mass per unit length of both the strings is same and equal to 1 g / m. When both the strings vibrate simultaneously the number of beats is **(2009)**

(a) 7 (b) 8

(c) 3 (d) 5

65. Two vibrating tuning forks produce waves given by $y_1 = 4\sin 500\pi t$ and

$y_2 = 2\sin 506\pi t$. Number of beats produced per minute is **(2006)**

(a) 360 (b) 180

(c) 60 (d) 3

66. Two sound waves with wavelengths 5.0 m and 5.5 m respectively, each propagates in a gas with velocity 330 m/s. We expect the following number of beats per second.

(2006)

(a) 6 (b) 12

(c) 0 (d) 1

67. Two waves of wavelengths 50 cm and 51 cm produced 12 beats per second. The velocity of sound is **(1999)**

(a) 340 m / s (b) 331 m / s

(c) 306 m / s (d) 360 m / s

68. A source of sound gives 5 beats per second, when sounded with another source of frequency 100 $second^{-1}$. The second harmonic of the source, together with a source of frequency 205 $second^{-1}$ gives 5 beats per second. What is the frequency of the source? **(1995)**

(a) 105 $second^{-1}$ (b) 205 $second^{-1}$

(c) 95 $second^{-1}$ (d) 100 $second^{-1}$

69. A source of frequency v gives 5 beats/second when sounded with a source of frequency 200 Hz. The second harmonic of frequency 20 of source gives 10 beats/second when sounded with a source of frequency 420 Hz. The value of v is

(1994)

(a) 205 Hz (b) 195 Hz

(c) 200 Hz (d) 210 Hz.

70. Wave has simple harmonic motion whose period is 4 seconds while another wave which also possesses simple harmonic motion has its period 3 seconds. If both are combined, then the resultant wave will have the period equal to **(1993)**

(a) 4 s (b) 5 s

(c) 12 s (d) 3 s

71. For production of beats the two sources must have **(1992)**

(a) different frequencies and same amplitude

(b) different frequencies

(c) different frequencies, same amplitude and same phase

(d) different frequencies and same phase

ANSWER KEY

1.	(c)	2.	(b)	3.	(c)	4.	(a)	5.	(c)	6.	(a)	7.	(a)
8.	(c)	9.	(c)	10.	(c)	11.	(a)	12.	(a,b)	13.	(d)	14.	(b)
15.	(c)	16.	(d)	17.	(c)	18.	(b)	19.	(c)	20.	(c)	21.	(a)
22.	(c)	23.	(c)	24.	(d)	25.	(c)	26.	(c)	27.	(c)	28.	(a)
29.	(c)	30.	(b)	31.	(b)	32.	(b)	33.	(b)	34.	(a)	35.	(c)
36.	(b)	37.	(a)	38.	(a)	39.	(b)	40.	(a)	41.	(b)	42.	(a)
43.	(d)	44.	(b)	45.	(d)	46.	(c)	47.	(b)	48.	(c)	49.	(a)
50.	(c)	51.	(a)	52.	(d)	53.	(a)	54.	(a)	55.	(a)	56.	(c)
57.	(d)	58.	(b)	59.	(d)	60.	(c)	61.	(d)	62.	(b)	63.	(d)
64.	(a)	65.	(b)	66.	(a)	67.	(c)	68.	(a)	69.	(a)	70.	(c)
71.	(b)												

Hints & Explanations

1. **(c)** : Light waves are electromagnetic waves. Light waves are transverse in nature and do not require a medium to travel, hence they can travel in vacuum. Sound waves are longitudinal waves and require a medium to travel. They do not travel in vacuum.

2. **(b)** : With the propagation of a longitudinal wave, energy alone is propagated.

3. **(c)** : The standard equation of a wave travelling along +ve x-direction is given by

$y = A\sin(kx-\omega t)$

where A = Amplitude of the wave

k = angular wave number

ω = angular frequency of the wave

Given : $A = 1m, \lambda = 2\pi m, v = \frac{1}{\pi}Hz$

As

$$k = \frac{2\pi}{\lambda} = \frac{2\pi}{2\pi} = 1; \omega = 2\pi v = 2\pi \times \frac{1}{\pi} = 2$$

$\therefore$ The equation of the given wave is

$y = 1\sin(1x-2t) = \sin(x-2t)$

4. **(a)** : $y_1 = a\sin(\omega t + kx + 0.57)$

$\therefore$ Phase, $\phi_1 = \omega t + kx + 0.57$

$$y_2 = a\cos(\omega t + kx) = a\sin\left(\omega t + kx + \frac{\pi}{2}\right)$$

$\therefore$ Phase, $\phi_2 = \omega t + kx + \frac{\pi}{2}$

Phase difference, $\Delta\phi = \phi_2 - \phi_1$

$$= \left(\omega t + kx + \frac{\pi}{2}\right) - (\omega t + kx + 0.57) = \frac{\pi}{2} - 0.57$$

$$= (1.57 - 0.57) \text{ radian } = 1 \text{ radian}$$

5. **(c) :** Amplitude = 2 cm = 0.02 m , v=128 m/s

$$\lambda = \frac{4}{5} = 0.8m; \nu = \frac{128}{0.8} = 160Hz$$

$$\omega = 2\pi\nu = 2\pi \times 160 = 1005; \quad k = \frac{2\pi}{\lambda} = \frac{2\pi}{0.8} = 7.85$$

$\therefore \quad y = (0.02)m\sin(7.85x - 1005t)$

6. **(a) :** $y = 0.25\sin(10\pi x - 2\pi t)$

$$y_{\max} = 0.25, k = \frac{2\pi}{\lambda} = 10\pi \Rightarrow \lambda = 0.2m$$

$$\omega = 2\pi f - 2\pi \Rightarrow f = 1Hz$$

The sign is negative inside the bracket. Therefore this wave travels in the positive x-direction.

7. **(a):** $y_1 = 10^{-6}\sin[100t1(x/50) + 0.5]$

$$y_2 = 10^{-6}\cos[100t + (x/50)]$$

$$= 10^{-6}\sin[100t + (x/50) + \pi/2]$$

$$= 10^{-6}\sin[100t + (x/50) + 1.57]$$

The phase difference = 1.57 – 0.5 =1.07 radians

8. **(c) :** The equation of progressive wave travelling in positive x-direction is given by

$$y = a\sin\frac{2\pi}{\lambda}(vt - x) \qquad \text{Here}$$

$$a = 0.2m, v = 360m/s, \lambda = 60m$$

$$\therefore \; y = 0.2\sin\frac{2\pi}{60}(360t - x)$$

$$= 0.2\sin\left[2\pi\left(6t - \frac{x}{60}\right)\right]$$

9. **(c) :** Displacement,

$y_{\max} = a, y_{\min} = 0$

Time taken = T / 4

$\therefore \quad T/4 = 0.170 \quad \therefore T = 0.68$

The frequency of wave = 1 / T = 1.47 Hz

10. **(c) :** Sound wave equation is

$y = 0.0015\sin(62.4x + 316t)$

Comparing it with the general equation of motion

$y = A\sin 2\pi\left[\frac{x}{\lambda} + \frac{t}{T}\right]$, we get $\frac{2\pi}{\lambda} = 62.4$

or $\lambda = \frac{2\pi}{62.4} = 0.1$ unit

11. **(a)** : Phase difference $\theta = 60^{\circ} = \frac{\pi}{3} rad$

Phase difference $(\theta) = \frac{2\pi}{\lambda} \times$ Path difference

Therefore Path difference $= \frac{\pi}{3} \times \frac{\lambda}{2\pi} = \frac{\lambda}{6}$.

12. **(a,b)** : Option (a) represents a harmonic progressive wave in the standard form whereas (b) also represents a harmonic progressive wave, both travelling in the positive x-direction. In (c), a is the angular velocity, (ω) and b is k; c is the initial phase. (d) represents only S.H.M.

13. **(d)** : Compare with the equation,

$y = a\cos(2\pi vt + \phi)$

This give $2\pi v = 2000; v = \frac{1000}{\pi} Hz$

14. **(b)** : The standard equation of a progressive wave is

$$y = a\sin\left[2\pi\left(\frac{t}{T} - \frac{x}{\lambda}\right) + \phi\right].$$

The given equation can be written as

$$y = 4\sin\left[2\pi\left(\frac{t}{10} - \frac{x}{18}\right) + \frac{\pi}{6}\right]$$

$a = 4cm, T = 10s, \lambda = 18cm$ and $\phi = \pi/6$

.

15. **(c)** : Velocity of a transverse wave in a stretched string is given by

$$v = \sqrt{\frac{T}{\mu}}$$

Where T is the tension in the string and μ is the mass per unit length of the string.

If tension T is doubled, then final speed of the wave in the string will be,

$$v' = \sqrt{\frac{2T}{\mu}}$$

From eq. (i) and (ii)

$$\frac{v}{v'} = \frac{1}{\sqrt{2}}$$

16. **(d)** : Wavelength of pulse at the lower end,

$$\lambda_1 \propto \text{velocity}(v_1) = \sqrt{\frac{T_1}{\mu}}$$

Similarly, $\lambda_2 \propto v_2 = \sqrt{\frac{T_2}{\mu}}$

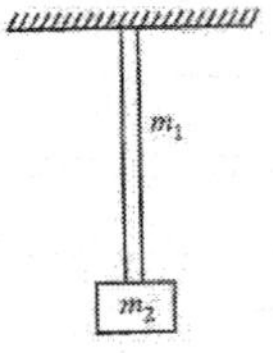

$$\therefore \frac{\lambda_2}{\lambda_1} = \sqrt{\frac{T_2}{T_1}} = \sqrt{\frac{(m_1+m_2)g}{m_2 g}} = \sqrt{\frac{m_1+m_2}{m_2}}$$

17. **(c) :** Since 4.0 g of a gas occupies 22.4 litres at NTP, so the molecular mass of the gas is $M = 4.0 gmol^{-1}$

As the speed of the sound in the gas is $v = \sqrt{\frac{\gamma RT}{M}}$ where γ is the ratio of two specific heats, R is the universal gas constant and T is the temperature of the gas.

$$\therefore \quad \gamma = \frac{Mv^2}{RT}$$

Here,

$M = 4.0 gmol^{-1} = 4.0 \times 10^{-3} kgmol^{-1}$, $v = 952 ms^{-1}$

$R = 8.3 JK^{-1}mol^{-1}$ and T = 273 K (at NTP)

$$\therefore \quad \gamma = \frac{(4.0\times10^{-3} kgmol^{-1})(952 ms^{-1})^2}{(8.3 JK^{-1}mol^{-1})(273K)}$$

=1.6

By definition, $\gamma = \frac{C_P}{C_V}$ or $C_P = \gamma C_V$

But $\gamma = 1.6$ and $C_V = 5.0 JK^{-1}mol^{-1}$

$$C_P = (1.6)(5.0 JK^{-1}mol^{-1}) = 8.0 JK^{-1}mol^{-1}$$

18. **(b) :** The given wave equation is

$$y = 3\sin\frac{\pi}{2}(50t - x)$$

$$y = 3\sin\left(25\pi t - \frac{\pi}{2}x\right)$$

The standard wave equation is

$$y = A\sin(\omega t - kx)$$

Comparing (i) and (ii), we get

$$\omega = 25\pi, k = \frac{\pi}{2}$$

Wave velocity, $v = \frac{\omega}{k} = \frac{25\pi}{(\pi/2)} = 50 ms^{-1}$

Particle velocity,

$$v_P = \frac{dy}{dt} = \frac{d}{dt}\left(3\sin\left(25\pi t - \frac{\pi}{2}x\right)\right)$$

$$= 75\pi\cos\left(25\pi t - \frac{\pi}{2}x\right)$$

Maximum particle vclocity,

$$(v_p)_{max} - 75\pi ms^{-1}$$

$$\therefore \frac{(v_p)_{max}}{v} = \frac{75\pi}{50} = \frac{3}{2}\pi$$

19. **(c) :** Here,

$v_{air} = 350 m/s, v_{brass} = 3500 m/s$

When a sound wave travels from one medium to another medium its frequency remains the same

$\because$ Frequency, $v = \frac{v}{\lambda}$

Since v remains the same in both the medium

$$\Rightarrow \frac{v_{\text{air}}}{\lambda_{\text{air}}} = \frac{v_{\text{brass}}}{\lambda_{\text{brass}}}$$

$$\lambda_{\text{brass}} = \lambda_{\text{air}} \times \frac{v_{\text{brass}}}{v_{\text{air}}} = \lambda_{\text{air}} \times \frac{3500}{350} = 10\lambda_{\text{air}}$$

20. **(c) :** The given wave equation is

$$y = A\sin(\omega t - kx)$$

Wave velocity, $v = \frac{\omega}{k}$

Particle velocity,

$$v_P = \frac{dy}{dt} = A\omega\cos(\omega t - kx)$$

Maximum particle velocity,

$$(v_P)_{\max} = A\omega$$

According to the given question

$$v = (v_P)_{\max}; \frac{\omega}{k} = A\omega$$

(Using (i) and (ii))

$$\frac{1}{k} = A \text{ or } \frac{\lambda}{2\pi} = A \quad \left(\because k = \frac{2\pi}{\lambda}\right)$$

$$\lambda = 2\pi A$$

21. **(a) :** $y(x,t) = 8.0\sin\left(0.5\pi x - 4\pi t - \frac{\pi}{4}\right)$

Compare with a standard wave equation,

$$y = a\sin\left(\frac{2\pi x}{\lambda} - \frac{2\pi t}{T} + \phi\right)$$

we get $\frac{2\pi}{\lambda} = 0.5\pi$ or,

$$\lambda = \frac{2\pi}{0.5\pi} = 4m.$$

$$\frac{2\pi}{T} = 4\pi \text{ or, } T = \frac{2\pi}{4\pi} = \frac{1}{2} sec$$

v = 1 / T = 2 Hz

Wave velocity,

$$v = \lambda \nu = 4 \times 2 = 8m/s$$

22. **(c) :** $d_1 = 2m, d_2 = 3m$

Intensity $\propto \frac{1}{(\text{distance})^2}$

$$I_1 \propto \frac{1}{2^2} \text{ and } I_2 \propto \frac{1}{3^2} \quad \therefore \quad \frac{I_1}{I_2} = \frac{9}{4}$$

23. **(c) :** Comparing the given equation with general equation,

$y = a\sin 2\pi\left(\frac{t}{T} - \frac{x}{\lambda}\right)$, we get

$$T = \frac{2\pi}{100} \text{ and } \lambda = 20\pi$$

$$\therefore \quad v = \nu\lambda = \frac{100}{2\pi} \times 20\pi = 1000m/s.$$

24. **(d) :** The given equation of wave is

$$y = y_0 \sin\frac{2\pi}{\lambda}(vt - x)$$

Particle velocity

$$= \frac{dy}{dt} = y_0 \frac{2\pi v}{\lambda} \cos \frac{2\pi}{\lambda}(vt - x)$$

$$\left(\frac{dy}{dt}\right)_{max} = y_0 \frac{2\pi}{\lambda} v$$

$$\therefore \quad y_0 \frac{2\pi}{\lambda} v = 2v \text{ or } \lambda = \pi y_0$$

25. **(c) :** Frequency (ν)

$= 4.2 MHz = 4.2 \times 10^6 Hz$

speed of sound

$(v) = 1.7 km/s = 1.7 \times 10^3 m/s$

Wavelength of sound in tissue

$$(\lambda) = \frac{v}{\nu}$$

$$= \frac{1.7 \times 10^3}{4.2 \times 10^6} = 4 \times 10^{-4} m$$

26. **(c) :** Velocity of sound, $v \propto \sqrt{T}$

$$\therefore \quad \frac{v}{2v} = \frac{\sqrt{273+27}}{\sqrt{T}} \text{ or } T = 1200K = 927^\circ C$$

27. **(c) :** From $\Delta x = \frac{\lambda}{2\pi} \Delta\phi$

$$\lambda = 2\pi \frac{\Delta x}{\Delta\phi} = \frac{2\pi(0.4)}{1.6\pi} = 0.5m$$

$$\nu = \frac{v}{\lambda} = \frac{330}{0.5} = 660Hz$$

28. **(a) :** Mass per unit length

$$\mu = \frac{0.035}{5.5} kg/m, \qquad T = 77N$$

$$v = \sqrt{\frac{T}{\mu}} = \sqrt{\frac{77 \times 5.5}{0.035}} = 110 m/s$$

29. **(c) :** Intensity $\propto$ (amplitude $)^2$ and also intensity $\propto$ (frequency) $)^2$.

Therefore original $I \propto A^2\omega^2$

$$I' \propto 4A^2 \frac{\omega^2}{16} \text{ i.e., } \frac{1}{4} I$$

30. **(b) :** Velocity of sound in any gas depends upon density and elasticity of gas.

$$v = \sqrt{\frac{\gamma P}{\rho}} \text{ or } \sqrt{\frac{B}{\rho}}$$

31. **(b) :** Other factors such as ω and v remaining the same, $I = A^2 \times$ constant (K) or $A = \sqrt{\frac{I}{K}}$

On superposition

$A_{max} = A_1 + A_2$ and $A_{min} = A_1 - A_2$

$$\therefore \quad A^2_{max} - A_1^2 + A_2^2 + 2A_1A_2$$

$$\Rightarrow \frac{I_{max}}{K} = \frac{I_1}{K} + \frac{I_2}{K} + \frac{2\sqrt{I_1I_2}}{K}$$

$$A_{min^2} = A_1^2 + A_2^2 - 2A_1A_2$$

$$\Rightarrow \frac{I_{min}}{K} = \frac{I_1}{K} + \frac{I_2}{K} - \frac{2\sqrt{I_1I_2}}{K}$$

$$\therefore \quad I_{max} + I_{min} = 2I_1 + 2I_2 = 2(I_1 + I_2)$$

32. (b) :

Resultant amplitude

$=2a(1+\cos\phi)=a$

$\therefore\ (1+\cos\phi)=1/2; \cos\phi=-\frac{1}{2};\quad \phi=\frac{2\pi}{3}.$

33. (b): Given : $x=a\cos(\omega t+\delta)$

and $y=a\cos(\omega t+\alpha)$

where, $\delta=\alpha+\pi/2$

$\therefore\ x=a\cos(\omega t+\alpha+\pi/2)=-a\sin(\omega t+\alpha)$

Given the two waves are acting in perpendicular direction with the same frequency and phase difference $\pi/2$.

From equations (i) and (ii),

$x^2+y^2=a^2$

which represents the equation of a circle.

34. (a) : $\frac{n_{oop}}{n_{cop}}=\frac{\frac{V}{2L}}{\frac{V}{4L}}$

$\Rightarrow \frac{n_{oop}}{n_{cop}}=\frac{2}{1}$

35. (c) : Frequency (v) = 800 Hz

As the pipe is closed at one end, so

$l_3-l_2=l_2-l_1=\frac{\lambda}{2}=21.5cm$

$\therefore\ \lambda=43.0cm$

As $v=\frac{v}{\lambda}\Rightarrow v=v\lambda$

$\therefore\ v=\frac{800\times43}{100}=344ms^{-1}$

36. (b): The velocity of sound in air at $27^{\circ}C$ is $v=2(v)[L_2-L_1]$; where $v=$ frequency of tuning fork and L_1, L_2 are the successive column length.

$\therefore\ v=2\times320[73-20]\times10^{-2}$

$=339.2ms^{-1}\approx339ms^{-1}$

37. (a) : For closed organ pipe, third harmonic is $\frac{3v}{4l}$.

For open organ pipe, fundamental frequency is $\frac{v}{2l'}$

Given, third harmonic for closed organ pipe = fundamental frequency for open organ pipe.

$\therefore\ \frac{3v}{4l}=\frac{v}{2l'}\Rightarrow l'=\frac{4l}{3\times2}=\frac{2l}{3};$

where l and l' are the lengths of closed and open organ pipes respectively.

$\therefore l'=\frac{2\times20}{3}=13.33cm$

38. (a) : Nearest harmonics of an organ pipe closed at one end is differ by twice of its fundamental frequency.

$\therefore\ 260-220=20, v=20Hz$

39. (b) : Second overtone of an open organ pipe

Third harmonic $=3\times v_0'=3\times\frac{v}{2L'}$

First overtone of a closed organ pipe

Third harmonic $=3\times v_0=3\times\frac{v}{4L}$

According to question,

$3v_0'=3v_0 \Rightarrow 3\times\frac{v}{2L'}=3\times\frac{v}{4L}$

$\therefore\ L'=2L$

40. (a) : From figure,

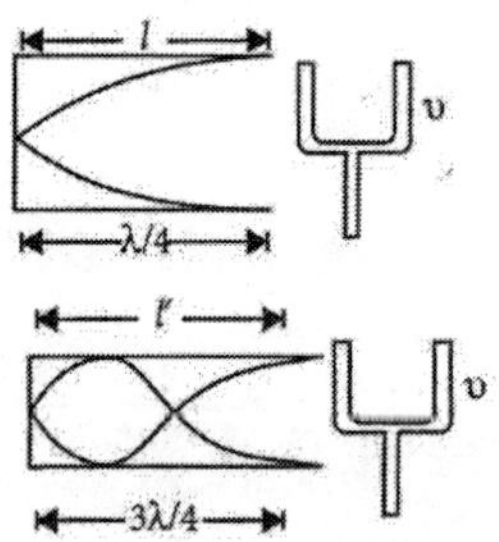

First harmonic is obtained at

$l=\frac{\lambda}{4}=50cm$

Third harmonic is obtained for resonance,

$l'=\frac{3\lambda}{4}=3\times 50=150cm.$

41. (b) : For a string fixed at both ends, the resonant frequencies are

$v_n=\frac{nv}{2L}$ where $n=1,2,3,\ldots.$

The difference between two consecutive resonant frequencies is

$\Delta v_n=v_{n+1}-v_n=\frac{(n+1)v}{2L}-\frac{nv}{2L}=\frac{v}{2L}$

which is also the lowest resonant frequency (n = 1).

Thus the lowest resonant frequency for the given string

$=420Hz-315Hz=105Hz$

42. (a): For closed organ pipe, fundamental frequency is given by $v_c=\frac{v}{4l}$

For open organ pipe, fundamental frequency is given by $v_o=\frac{v}{2l'}$

2nd overtone of open organ pipe

$v'=3v_0; v'=\frac{3v}{2l'}$

According to question, $v_c=v'$

$\frac{v}{4l}=\frac{3v}{2l'}; l'=6l$

Here, $l=20cm, l'=\ ?$

$\therefore\ l'=6\times 20=120cm$

43. (d): Fundamental frequency of the closed organ pipe is $\nu = \frac{v}{4L}$

Here,

$v = 340ms^{-1}, L = 85cm = 0.85m$

$\therefore \quad \nu = \frac{340ms^{-1}}{4 \times 0.85m} = 100Hz$

The natural frequencies of the closed organ pipe will be

$\nu_n = (2n-1)\nu = \nu, 3\nu, 5\nu, 7\nu, 9\nu, 11\nu, 13\nu, \ldots$

= 100 Hz, 300 Hz, 500 Hz, 700 Hz, 900 Hz, 1100 Hz, 1300 Hz, and so on

Thus, the number of natural frequencies lies below 1250 Hz is 6.

44. (b) : Pressure change will be minimum at both ends.

45. (d) : Let $L(=100cm)$ be the length of the wire and L_1, L_2 and L_3 are the lengths of the segments as shown in the figure.

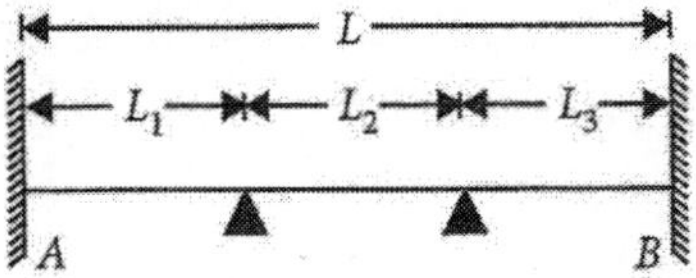

Fundamental frequency, $\nu \propto \frac{1}{L}$

As the fundamental frequencies are in the ratio of 1 : 3 : 5,

$\therefore \quad L_1 : L_2 : L_3 = \frac{1}{1} : \frac{1}{3} : \frac{1}{5} = 15:5:3$

Let x be the common factor. Then

$15x + 5x + 3x = 100$

$23x = 100 \text{ or } x = \frac{100}{23}$

$\therefore \quad L_1 = 15 \times \frac{100}{23} = \frac{1500}{23} cm$

$L_2 = 5 \times \frac{100}{23} = \frac{500}{23} cm;$

$L_3 = 3 \times \frac{100}{23} = \frac{300}{23} cm$

$\therefore$ The bridges should be placed from A at $\frac{1500}{23} cm$ and $\frac{2000}{23} cm$ respectively.

46. (c): Let l be the length of the string. Fundamental frequency is given by

$\nu = \frac{1}{2l}\sqrt{\frac{T}{\mu}}$

or $\nu \propto \frac{1}{l}$ ($\because T$ and μ are constants)

Here, $l_1 = \frac{k}{\nu_1}, l_2 = \frac{k}{\nu_2}, l_3 = \frac{k}{\nu_3}$ and $l = \frac{k}{\nu}$

But

$l = l_1 + l_2 + l_3 \therefore \quad \frac{1}{\nu} = \frac{1}{\nu_1} + \frac{1}{\nu_2} + \frac{1}{\nu_3}$

47. (b) : Reverberation time, $T = \dfrac{0.61V}{aS}$

where V is the volume of room in cubic metres, a is the average absorption coefficient of the room, S is the total surface area of room in square metres.

or, $\quad T \propto \dfrac{V}{S} \quad$ or,

$$\frac{T_1}{T_2} = \left(\frac{V_1}{V_2}\right)\left(\frac{S_2}{S_1}\right) = \left(\frac{V}{8V}\right)\left(\frac{4S}{S}\right) = \frac{1}{2}$$

or, $T_2 = 2T_1 = 2\times 1 = 2s \quad (\because T_1 = 1s)$

48. (c) : $n = \dfrac{1}{2l}\sqrt{\dfrac{T}{\pi r^2 \rho}}$

$\rho_1' = \dfrac{\rho}{2}; T' = 2T$ and $D' = 2D$ or

$r'' = 2r$

$$n' - \frac{1}{2l}\sqrt{\frac{2T}{\pi(2r)^2\frac{\rho}{2}}} - \frac{1}{2l}\sqrt{\frac{T}{\pi r^2 \rho}} = n$$

49. (a) : $n \propto \dfrac{1}{\ell}$

$\ell = \ell_1 + \ell_2 + \ell_3$

$\ell_1 = \dfrac{v}{2n_1} \qquad \ell = \dfrac{v}{2n}$

$\ell_2 = \dfrac{v}{2n_2} \quad \Rightarrow \dfrac{1}{n} = \dfrac{1}{n_1} + \dfrac{1}{n_2} + \dfrac{1}{n_3} \quad \ell_3 = \dfrac{v}{2n_3}$

50. (c) : Distance between a node and adjoining antinode $= \lambda / 4$

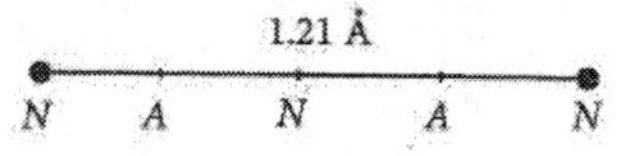

From figure, distance between two atoms

$$= 4\times\frac{\lambda}{4} = 1.21\mathring{A} \text{ or, } \lambda = 1.21\mathring{A}$$

51. (a) : The frequency of standing wave,

$$v = \frac{n}{2l}v = \frac{5\times 20}{2\times 10} = 5Hz.$$

52. (d) : For the cylindrical tube open at both ends, $f = v/2l$

When half of the tube is in water, it behaves as a closed pipe of length $l/2$.

$$\therefore \quad f' = \frac{v}{4(l/2)} = \frac{v}{2l} \Rightarrow f' = f$$

53. (a) : Length of sonometer wire $(l) = 110cm$ and ratio of frequencies $= 1:2:3$.

Frequency $(v) \propto \dfrac{1}{l}$ or $l \propto \dfrac{1}{v}$

Therefore

$$AC:CD:DB = \frac{1}{1}:\frac{1}{2}:\frac{1}{3} = 6:3:2$$

Therefore $AC = 6\times\dfrac{110}{11} = 60cm$ and

$$CD = 3\times\frac{110}{11} = 30cm$$

Thus $AD = 60 + 30 = 90cm$.

54. **(a):** Frequency $(v) = 100Hz$ and distance from fixed end $= 10cm = 0.1m$. When a stationary wave is produced, the fixed end behaves as a node.

Thus wavelength

$(\lambda) = 2 \times 0.1 = 0.2m$.

Therefore velocity

$v = v\lambda = 100 \times 0.2 = 20m/s$

55. **(a) :** $y = A\sin(100t)\cos(0.01x)$.

Comparing it with standard equation

$y = A\sin\left(\frac{2\pi}{T}t\right)\cos\left(\frac{2\pi}{\lambda}x\right)$, we get

$T = \frac{\pi}{50}$ and $\lambda = 200\pi$.

Therefore velocity,

$(v) = \frac{\lambda}{T} = \frac{200\pi}{\pi/50} = 200 \times 50$

$= 10000 = 10^4 m/s$

56. **(c) :** $f = \frac{1}{2l}\left[\frac{T}{\mu}\right]^{\frac{1}{2}}$ when f is halved, the length will be doubled.

Hence required length of string is 1 m.

57. **(d) :** Third overtone has a frequency $4n, 4^{th}$ harmonic = three full loops + one half loop, which would make four nodes and four antinodes

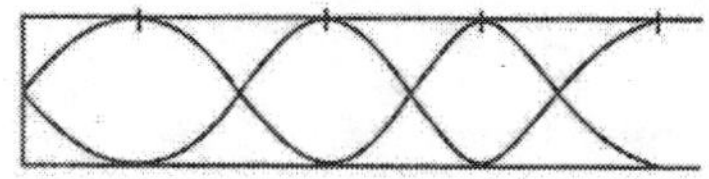

58. **(b) :** Frequency of string $A, v_A = 530Hz$ and beat frequency $\Delta v_1 = 6Hz$.

Since, $v_B = v_A \pm \Delta v_1$, we have $v_B = 536Hz$ or 524 Hz.

Now, when tension on the string is reduced, its frequency reduces.

Now, the beat frequency, $\Delta v_2 = 7Hz$.

$\therefore$ The original frequency of $B, v_B = 524Hz$.

59. **(d) :** Formula for beat frequency is

$f_b = f_2 - f_1$

where f_1 and f_2 are the frequency of two waves.

Now, $f_b = f_2 - f_1$

$f_b = (n+1) - (n-1)$

$f_b = (n + 1 - n + 1)$

$f_b = 2$

Thus the No. of beats per second will be 2.

60. **(c) :** Let v be frequency of the unknown source. As it gives 4 beats per second when sounded with a source of frequency 250 Hz,

$\therefore \quad v = 250 \pm 4 = 246Hz$ or $254Hz$

Second harmonic of this unknown source = 492 Hz or 508 Hz which gives 5 beats per second, when sounded with a source of frequency 513 Hz.

Therefore unknown frequency, v = 254 Hz

61. (d) :

Given : $y_1 = 4\sin 600\pi t, y_2 = 5\sin 608\pi t$

$\therefore \quad \omega_1 = 600\pi$ or $2\pi v_1 = 600\pi$ or $v_1 = 300Hz$

$A_1 = 4$ and $\omega_2 = 608\pi$ or

$2\pi v_2 = 608\pi$ or $v_2 = 304Hz$ $A_2 = 5$

Number of beats heard per second

$= v_2 - v_1 = 304 - 300 = 4$

$$\frac{I_{max}}{I_{min}} = \frac{(A_1 + A_2)^2}{(A_1 - A_2)^2} = \frac{(4+5)^2}{(4-5)^2} = \frac{81}{1}$$

62. (b) : As $v = \frac{1}{2L}\sqrt{\frac{T}{\mu}} \therefore \frac{\Delta v}{v} = \frac{1}{2}\frac{\Delta T}{T}$

$$\frac{\Delta T}{T} = 2\frac{\Delta v}{v} = 2 \times \frac{6}{600} = 0.02$$

63. (d) : Let the frequencies of tuning fork and piano string be v_1 and v_2 respectively.

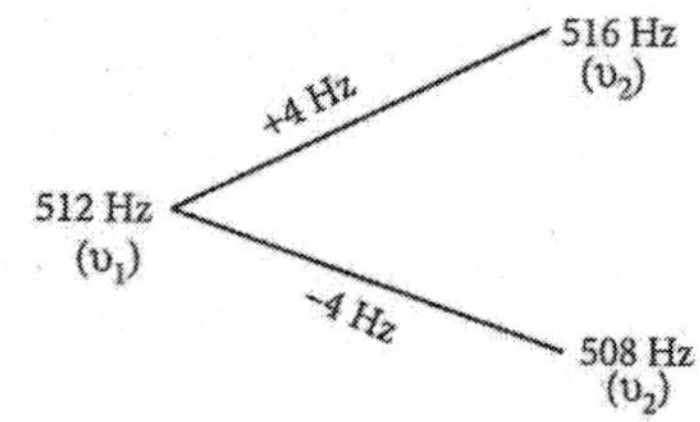

$\therefore v_2 = v_1 \pm 4 = 512Hz \pm 4 = 516Hz$ or $508Hz$

Increase in the tension of a piano string increases its frequency. If $v_2 = 516Hz$, further increase in v_2, resulted in an increase in the beat frequency. But this is not given in the question. If $v_2 = 508Hz$, further increase in v_2 resulted in decrease in the beat frequency. This is given in the question. When the beat frequency decreases to 2 beats per second. Therefore, the frequency of the piano string before increasing the tension was 508 Hz

64. (a) : $l_1 = 0.516m, l_2 = 0.491m, T = 20N$.

Mass per unit length,

$\mu = 0.001kg/m$.

Frequency, $v = \frac{1}{2l}\sqrt{\frac{T}{\mu}}$

$$v_1 = \frac{1}{2 \times 0.516}\sqrt{\frac{20}{0.001}}Hz = 137Hz$$

$$v_2 = \frac{1}{2 \times 0.491}\sqrt{\frac{20}{0.001}}Hz = 144Hz$$

$\therefore$ Number of beats $= v_1 - v_2 = 7Hz$

65. **(b) :**

$y_1 = 4\sin 500\pi t, y_2 = 2\sin 506\pi t$

$\omega_1 = 500\pi = 2\pi v_1 \Rightarrow v_1 = 250Hz$

$\omega_2 = 506\pi = 2\pi v_2 \Rightarrow v_2 = 253Hz$

$v = v_2 - v_1 = 253 - 250 = 3$ beats $/ s$

Number of beats per minute $= 3 \times 60 = 180$

66. **(a) :** Frequency $= \dfrac{\text{velocity}}{\text{wavelength}}$

$\therefore v_1 = \dfrac{v}{\lambda_1} = \dfrac{330}{5} = 66Hz$ and

$v_2 = \dfrac{v}{\lambda_2} = \dfrac{330}{5.5} = 60Hz$

Number of beats per second

$= v_1 - v_2 = 66 - 60 = 6$

67. **(c) :** Number of beats produced per second

$= v_1 - v_2 = \dfrac{v}{\lambda_1} - \dfrac{v}{\lambda_2}$

$12 = v\left[\dfrac{1}{50} - \dfrac{1}{51}\right]$ or $12 = \dfrac{v \times 1}{50 \times 51}$

or, $v = 12 \times 50 \times 51 cm/s = 306 m/s$

68. **(a) :** Frequency of first source with 5 beats $/sec = 100Hz$ and frequency of second source with 5 beats $/sec = 205$. The possible frequency of unknown sources $= 100 \pm 5 = 105$ or 95 Hz. Therefore frequency of second harmonic of unknown source = 210 Hz or 190 Hz.

As the second harmonic gives 5 beats/second with the sound of frequency 205Hz, therefore frequency of second harmonic of unknown source should be 210 Hz. The frequency of unknown source = 105 Hz.

69. **(a) :** First case: Frequency $= v$;

No. of beats/second $= 5$ and

frequency (sounded with) $= 200Hz$

Second case: Frequency $= 2v$;

No. of beats/sec and $= 10$ and

frequency (sounded with) $= 420Hz$

In the first case, frequency $(v) = 200 \pm 5 = 205$

or 195 Hz. And in the second case, frequency $(2v) = 420 \pm 10$

or $v = 210 \pm 5 = 205$ or 215. So common value of v in both the cases is 205 Hz.

70. **(c) :** Beats are produced. Frequency of beats will be $\frac{1}{3}-\frac{1}{4}=\frac{1}{12}\cdot$ per second

Hence time period =12 s

71. **(b) :** For production of beats different frequencies are essential. The different amplitudes effect the minimum and maximum amplitude of the beats. If frequencies are different, phases will be different.

Chapter: 15 ELECTRIC CHARGES AND FIELDS

Coulomb's Law

1. Two point charges A and B, having charges $+Q$ and $-Q$ respectively, are placed at certain distance apart and force acting between them is F. If 25% charge of A is transferred to B, then force between the charges becomes **(2019)**

(a) $\frac{4F}{3}$ (b) F

(c) $\frac{9F}{16}$ (d) $\frac{16F}{9}$

2. Suppose the charge of a proton and an electron differ slightly. One of them is $-e$, the other is $(e+\Delta e)$. If the net of electrostatic force and gravitational force between two hydrogen atoms placed at a distance d (much greater than atomic size) apart is zero, then Δe is of the order of

[Given: mass of hydrogen $m_h = 1.67 \times 10^{-27}$ kg] **(2017)**

(a) 10^{-23}C (b) 10^{-37}C

(c) 10^{-47}C (d) 10^{-20}C

3. Two identical charged spheres suspended from a common point by two massless strings of lengths l, are initially at a distance $d(d << l)$ apart because of their mutual repulsion. The charges begin to leak from both the spheres at a constant rate. As a result, the spheres approach each other with a velocity v. Then v varies as a function of the distance x between the spheres, as **(NEET-I 2016)**

(a) $v \propto x^{-1/2}$ (b) $v \propto x^{-1}$

(c) $v \propto x^{1/2}$ (d) $v \propto x$

4. Two pith balls carrying equal charges are suspended from a common point by strings of equal length, the equilibrium separation between them is r. Now the strings are rigidly clamped at half the height. The equilibrium separation between the balls now become **(2013)**

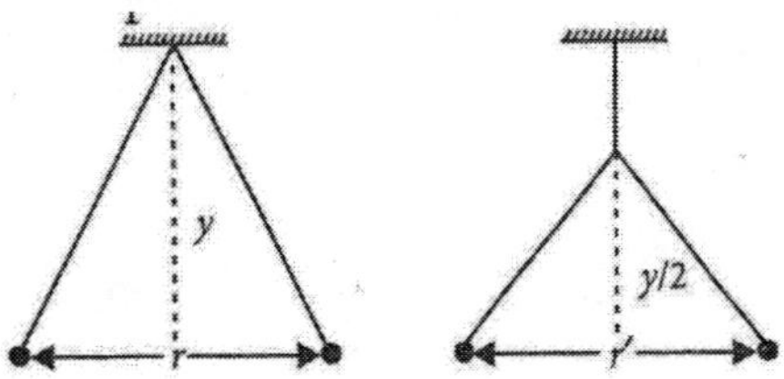

(a) $\left(\frac{2r}{\sqrt{3}}\right)$ (b) $\left(\frac{2r}{3}\right)$

(c) $\left(\frac{1}{\sqrt{2}}\right)^2$ (d) $\left(\frac{r}{\sqrt[3]{2}}\right)$

5. Two positive ions, each carrying a charge q, are separated by a distance d. If F is the force of repulsion between the ions, the number of electrons missing from each ion will be (e being the charge on an electron) **(2010)**

(a) $\frac{4\pi\varepsilon_0 F d^2}{e^2}$ (b) $\sqrt{\frac{4\pi\varepsilon_0 F e^2}{d^2}}$

(c) $\sqrt{\frac{4\pi\varepsilon_0 F d^2}{e^2}}$ (d) $\frac{4\pi\varepsilon_0 F d^2}{q^2}$

6. When air is replaced by a dielectric medium of constant K, the maximum force of attraction between two charges separated by a distance **(1999)**

(a) increases K times

(b) remains unchanged

(c) decreases K times

(d) increases K^{-1} times.

Forces between Multiple Charges

7. A charge q is placed at the centre of the line joining two equal charges Q. The system of the three charges will be in equilibrium if q is equal to

(Karnataka NEET 2013, 1995)

(a) $-Q/4$ (b) $Q/4$

(c) $-Q/2$ (d) $Q/2$

8. Point charges $+4q, -q$ and $+4q$ are kept on the X-axis at point $x = 0, x = a$ and $x = 2a$ respectively. Then **(1988)**

(a) only $-q$ is in stable equilibrium

(b) all the charges are in stable equilibrium

(c) all of the charges are in unstable equilibrium

(d) none of the charges is in equilibrium.

Electric Field

9. If $\oint_S \vec{E} \cdot \vec{dS} = 0$ over a surface, then **(2023)**

(a) The magnitude of electric field on the surface is constant

(b) All the charges must necessarily be inside the surface

(c) The electric field inside the surface is necessarily uniform

(d) The number of flux lines entering the surface must be equal to the number of flux lines leaving it

10. An electron falls from rest through a vertical distance h in a uniform and vertically upward directed electric field E. The direction of electric field is now reversed, keeping its magnitude the same. A proton is allowed to fall from rest in it through the same vertical distance h. The time of fall of the electron, in comparison to the time of fall of the proton is **(2018)**

(a) smaller

(b) 5 times greater

(c) 10 times greater

(d) equal

11. A toy car with charge q moves on a frictionless horizontal plane surface under the influence of a uniform electric field $\vec{E}$. Due to the force $q\vec{E}$, its velocity increases from 0 to 6 m s^{-1} in one second duration. At that instant the direction of the field is reversed. The car continues to move for two more seconds under the influence of this field. The average velocity and the average speed of the toy car between 0 to 3 seconds are respectively **(2018)**

(a) 2 m s^{-1}, 4 m s^{-1}

(b) 1 m s^{-1}, 3 m s^{-1}

(c) $1 \text{ m s}^{-1}, 3.5 \text{ m s}^{-1}$

(d) $1.5 \text{ m s}^{-1}, 3 \text{ m s}^{-1}$

12. A particle of mass m and charge q is placed at rest in a uniform electric field E and then released. The kinetic energy attained by the particle after moving a distance y is **(1998)**

(a) qEy (b) qE^2y

(c) qEy^2 (d) q^2Ey

Electric Field Lines

13. The given figure gives electric lines of force due to two charges q_1 and q_2. What are the signs of the two charges? **(1994)**

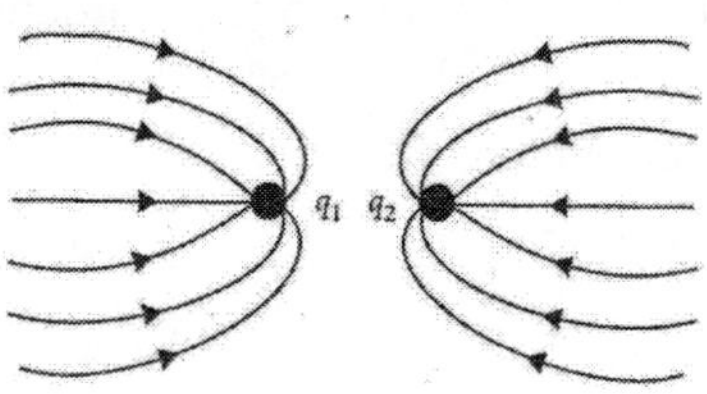

(a) q_1 is positive but q_2 is negative.

(b) q_1 is negative but q_2 is positive.

(c) both are negative.

(d) both are positive.

Electric Flux

14. A square surface of side L meter in the plane of the paper is placed in a uniform electric field E (volt /m) acting along the same plane at an angle θ with the horizontal side of the square as shown in figure. The electric flux linked to the surface, in units of volt m is **(2010)**

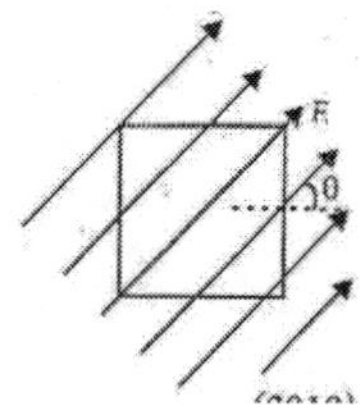

(a) EL^2 (b) $EL^2 \cos\theta$

(c) $EL^2 \sin\theta$ (d) zero

15. A square surface of side L metres is in the plane of the paper. A uniform electric field $\vec{E}$ (volt /m), also in the plane of the paper is limited only to the lower half of the square surface (see figure). The electric flux in **(2006)**

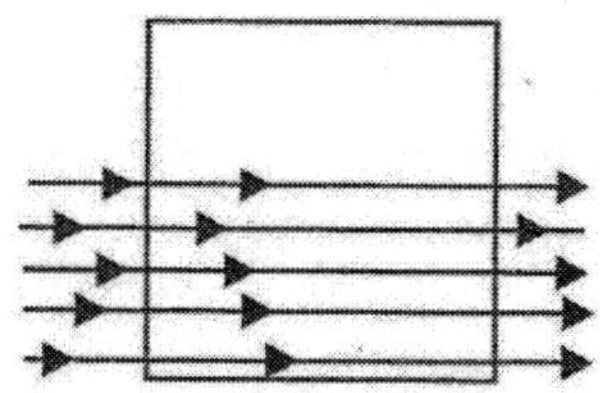

SI units associated with the surface is

(a) EL^2 (b) $EL^2/2\varepsilon_0$

(c) $EL^2/2$ (d) zero

Electric Dipole

16. Two point charges $-q$ and $+q$ are placed at a distance of L, as shown in the figure. The magnitude of electric field intensity at a distance $R(R >> L)$ varies as **(2022)**

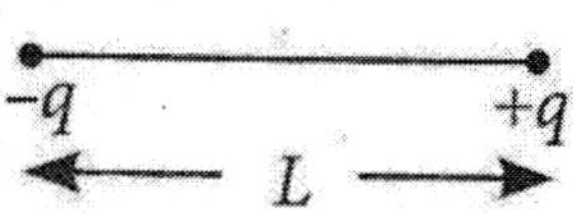

(a) $\frac{1}{R^2}$ (b) $\frac{1}{R^3}$

(c) $\frac{1}{R^4}$ (d) $\frac{1}{R^6}$

17. Polar molecular are the molecules **(2021)**

(a) having a permanent electric dipole moment.

(b) having zero dipole moment.

(c) acquire a dipole moment only in the presence of electric field due to displacement of charges.

(d) acquire a dipole moment only when magnetic field is absent.

18. Three point charges $+q, -2q$ and $+q$ are placed at points $(x = 0, y = a, z = 0), (x = 0, y = 0, z = 0)$ and $(x = a, y = 0, z = 0)$ respectively. The magnitude and direction of the electric dipole moment vector of this charge assembly are **(2007)**

(a) $\sqrt{2}qa$ along the line joining points $(x = 0, y = 0, z = 0)$ and $(x = a, y = a, z = 0)$

(b) qa along the line joining points $(x = 0, y = 0, z = 0)$ and $(x = a, y = a, z = 0)$

(c) $\sqrt{2}qa$ along $+x$ direction

(d) $\sqrt{2}qa$ along $+y$ direction.

19. A point Q lies on the perpendicular bisector of an electrical dipole of dipole moment p. If the distance of Q from the dipole is r (much larger than the size of the dipole), then the electric field at Q is proportional to **(1998)**

(a) p^2 and r^{-3} (b) p and r^{-2}

(c) p^{-1} and r^{-2} (d) p and r^{-3}

Dipole in a Uniform External Field

20. An electric dipole is placed at an angle of $30°$ with an electric field of intensity 2×10^5 N C^{-1}. It experiences a torque equal to 4 N m. Calculate the magnitude of charge on the dipole, if the dipole length is 2 cm. **(2023)**

(a) 6 mC (b) 4 mC

(c) 2 mC (d) 8 mC

21. An electric dipole is placed at an angle of $30°$ with an electric field intensity 2×10^5 NC^{-1}. It experiences a torque equal to 4 N m. The charge on the dipole, if the dipole length is 2 cm, is **(NEET-II 2016)**

(a) 8mC (b) 2Mc

(c) 5mC (d) $7\mu C$

22. A dipole of dipole moment $\vec{p}$ is placed in uniform electric field $\vec{E}$, then torque acting on it is given by **(2001)**

(a) $\vec{\tau} = \vec{p} \cdot \vec{E}$ (b) $\vec{\tau} = \vec{p} \times \vec{E}$

(c) $\vec{\tau} = \vec{p} + \vec{E}$ (d) $\vec{\tau} = \vec{p} - \vec{E}$

Continuous Charge Distribution

23. A spherical conductor of radius 10 cm has a charge of 3.2×10^{-7}C distributed uniformly. What is the magnitude of electric field at a point 15 cm from the centre of the sphere? $\left(\frac{1}{4\pi\varepsilon_0} = 9 \times 10^9 \text{ N m}^2/\text{C}^2\right)$ **(2020)**

(a) 1.28×10^4 N/C

(b) 1.28×10^5 N/C

(c) 1.28×10^6 N/C

(d) 1.28×10^7 N/C

24. A thin conducting ring of radius R is given a charge $+Q$. The electric field at the centre O of the ring due to the charge on the part AKB of the ring is E. The electric field at the centre due to the charge on the part $ACDB$ of the ring is **(2008)**

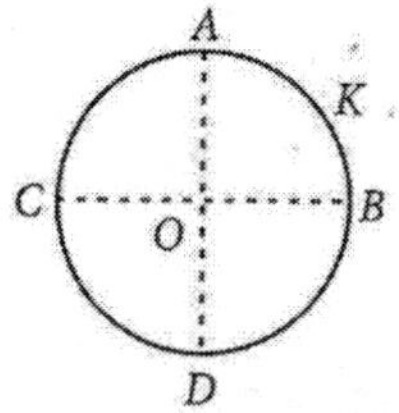

(a) E along KO (b) $3E$ along OK

(c) $3E$ along KO (d) E along OK,

25. Electric field at centre O of semicircle of radius a having linear charge density λ given as **(2000)**

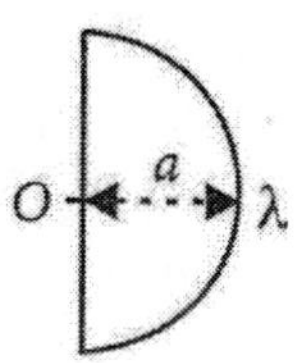

(a) $\frac{2\lambda}{\varepsilon_0 a}$ (b) $\frac{\lambda\pi}{\varepsilon_0 a}$

(c) $\frac{\lambda}{2\pi\varepsilon_0 a}$ (d) $\frac{\lambda}{\pi\varepsilon_0 a}$

Gauss's Law

26. What is the flux through a cube of side a if a point charge of q is at one of its corner? **(2012)**

(a) $\frac{2q}{\varepsilon_0}$ (b) $\frac{q}{8\varepsilon_0}$

(c) $\frac{q}{\varepsilon_0}$ (d) $\frac{q}{2\varepsilon_0}6a^2$

27. A charge Q is enclosed by a Gaussian spherical surface of radius R. If the radius is doubled, then the outward electric flux will **(2011)**

(a) increase four times

(b) be reduced to half

(c) remain the same

(d) be doubled

28. A hollow cylinder has a charge q coulomb within it. If ϕ is the electric flux in units of volt meter associated with the curved surface B, the flux linked with the plane surface A in units of V-m will be **(2007)**

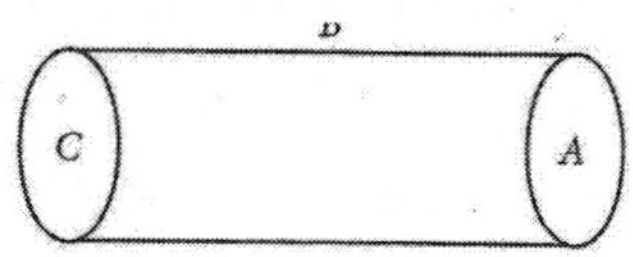

(a) $\frac{q}{2\varepsilon_0}$ (b) $\frac{\phi}{3}$

(c) $\frac{q}{\varepsilon_0} - \phi$ (d) $\frac{1}{2}\left(\frac{q}{\varepsilon_0} - \phi\right)$

29. A charge q is located at the centre of a cube. The electric flux through any face is **(2003)**

(a) $\frac{2\pi q}{6(4\pi\varepsilon_0)}$ (b) $\frac{4\pi q}{6(4\pi\varepsilon_0)}$

(c) $\frac{\pi q}{6(4\pi\varepsilon_0)}$ (d) $\frac{q}{6(4\pi\varepsilon_0)}$

30. A charge $Q\mu C$ is placed at the centre of a cube, the flux coming out from each face will be **(2001)**

(a) $\frac{Q}{6\varepsilon_0} \times 10^{-6}$ (b) $\frac{Q}{6\varepsilon_0} \times 10^{-3}$

(c) $\frac{Q}{24\varepsilon_0}$ (d) $\frac{Q}{8\varepsilon_0}$

31. A charge Q is situated at the corner of a cube, the electric flux passed through all the six faces of the cube is **(2000)**

(a) $\frac{Q}{6\varepsilon_0}$ (b) $\frac{Q}{8\varepsilon_0}$

(c) $\frac{Q}{\varepsilon_0}$ (d) $\frac{Q}{2\varepsilon_0}$

32. A point charge $+q$ is placed at the centre of a cube of side l. The electric flux emerging from the cube is **(1996)**

(a) $\frac{6ql^2}{\varepsilon_0}$ (b) $\frac{q}{6l^2\varepsilon_0}$

(c) zero (d) $\frac{q}{\varepsilon_0}$.

Applications of Gauss's Law

33. A hollow metal sphere of radius R is uniformly charged. The electric field due to the sphere at a distance r from the centre **(2019)**

(a) decreases as r increases for $r < R$ and for $r > R$

(b) increases as r increases for $r < R$ and for $r > R$

(c) zero as r increases for $r < R$, decreases as r increases for $r > R$

(d) zero as r increases for $r < R$, increases as r increases for $r > R$

34. Two parallel infinite line charges with linear charge densities $+\lambda \text{C/m}$ and $-\lambda \text{C/m}$ are placed at a distance of $2R$ in free space. What is the electric field midway between the two line charges? **(2019)**

(a) $\frac{\lambda}{2\pi\varepsilon_0 R}$ N/C (b) zero

(c) $\frac{2\lambda}{\pi\varepsilon_0 R}$ N/C (d) $\frac{\lambda}{\pi\varepsilon_0 R}$ N/C

35. The electric field at a distance $\frac{3R}{2}$ from the centre of a charged conducting spherical shell of radius R is E. The electric field at a distance $\frac{R}{2}$ from the centre of the sphere is **(Mains 2010)**

(a) zero (b) E

(c) $\frac{E}{2}$ (d) $\frac{E}{3}$

36. A hollow insulated conduction sphere is given a positive charge of $10\mu\text{C}$. What will be the electric field at the centre of the sphere if its radius is 2 metres? **(1998)**

(a) $20\mu\text{Cm}^{-2}$ (b) $5\mu\text{Cm}^{-2}$

(c) zero (d) 8mCm^{-2}

ANSWER KEY

1.	(c)	2.	(b)	3.	(a)	4.	(d)	5.	(c)	6.	(c)	7.	(a)
8.	(c)	9.	(a)	10.	(d)	11.	(b)	12.	(a)	13.	(c)	14.	(d)
15.	(d)	16.	(b)	17.	(a)	18.	(a)	19.	(d)	20.	(c)	21.	(b)
22.	(b)	23.	(b)	24.	(d)	25.	(c)	26.	(b)	27.	(c)	28.	(d)
29.	(b)	30.	(a)	31.	(b)	32.	(d)	33.	(c)	34.	(d)	35.	(a)
36.	(c)												

Hints & Explanations

1. **(c)** : In case I :

$$F = -\frac{1}{4\pi\varepsilon_0}\frac{Q^2}{r^2} \quad \text{......(i)}$$

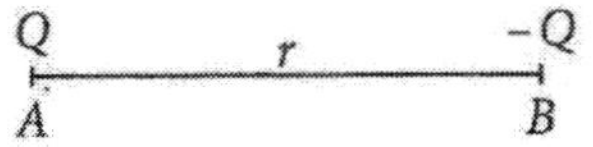

In Case II : $Q_A = Q - \frac{Q}{4}, Q_B = -Q + \frac{Q}{4}$

$$\therefore\ F' = \frac{1}{4\pi\varepsilon_0}\frac{\left(Q-\frac{Q}{4}\right)\left(-Q+\frac{Q}{4}\right)}{r^2}$$

$$= \frac{1}{4\pi\varepsilon_0}\frac{\left(\frac{3}{4}Q\right)\left(\frac{-3}{4}Q\right)}{r^2} = -\frac{1}{4\pi\varepsilon_0}\frac{9}{16}\frac{Q^2}{r^2} \quad \text{.....(ii)}$$

From equations (i) and (ii), $F' = \frac{9}{16}F$

2. **(b)** : A hydrogen atom consists of an electron and a proton. ∴ Charge on one hydrogen atom $= q_e + q_p = -e + (e + \Delta e) = \Delta e$ Since a hydrogen atom carries a net charge Δe

∴ Electrostatic force, $F_e = \frac{1}{4\pi\varepsilon_0}\frac{(\Delta e)^2}{d^2}$ ......(i)

will act between two hydrogen atoms.

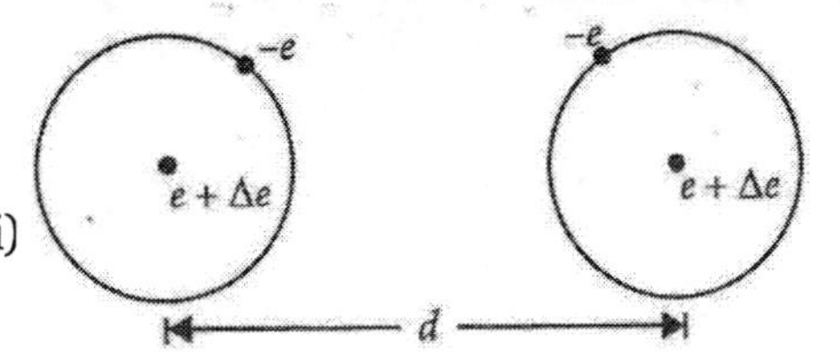

The gravitational force between two hydrogen atoms is given as

$$F_g = \frac{Gm_h m_h}{d^2} \quad \text{.....(ii)}$$

Since, the net force on the system is zero, $F_e = F_g$ Using eqns. (i) and (ii), we get

$\frac{(\Delta e)^2}{4\pi\varepsilon_0 d^2} = \frac{Gm_h^2}{d^2}$ or, $(\Delta e)^2 = 4\pi\varepsilon_0 Gm_h^2$

$= 6.67 \times 10^{-11} \times (1.67 \times 10^{-27})^2[1/(9 \times 10^9)]$

$\Delta e \approx 10^{-37}\text{C}$

3. **(a):**

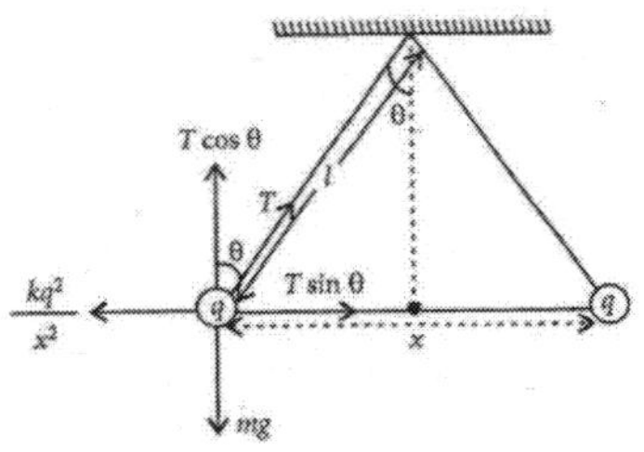

From figure, $T\cos\theta = mg$ ....(i)

$$T\sin\theta = \frac{kq^2}{x^2} \quad \text{....(ii)}$$

From eqns. (i) and (ii), $\tan\theta = \frac{kq^2}{x^2 mg}$

Since θ is small, $\therefore\ \tan\theta \approx \sin\theta = \frac{x}{2l}$

$\therefore\ \frac{x}{2l} = \frac{kq^2}{x^2 mg} \Rightarrow q^2 = x^3\frac{mg}{2lk}$ or $q \propto x^{3/2}$

$\Rightarrow \frac{dq}{dt} \propto \frac{3}{2}\sqrt{x}\frac{dx}{dt} = \frac{3}{2}\sqrt{x}v$

Since, $\frac{dq}{dt}$ = constant; $\therefore\ v \propto \frac{1}{\sqrt{x}}$

4. **(d):** Let m be mass of each ball and q be charge on each ball. Force of repulsion,

$$F = \frac{1}{4\pi\varepsilon_0}\frac{q^2}{r^2}$$

In equilibrium

$T\cos\theta = mg$ .....(i)

$T\sin\theta = F$ .....(ii)

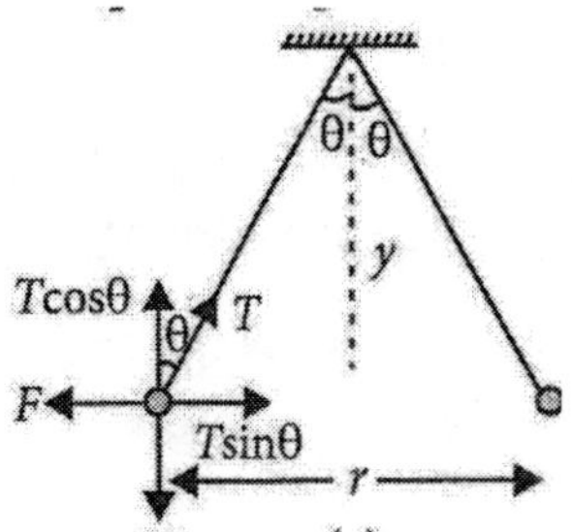

(a)

Divide (ii) by (i), we get, $\tan\theta = \frac{F}{mg}$

$$= \frac{\frac{1}{4\pi\varepsilon_0}\frac{q}{r^2}}{mg}$$

From figure (a),

$$\frac{r/2}{y} = \frac{\frac{1}{4\pi\varepsilon_0}\frac{q}{r^2}}{mg}$$

For figure (b)

$$\tan\theta' = \frac{\frac{1}{4\pi\varepsilon_0}\frac{q^2}{r'^2}}{mg} \Rightarrow \frac{r'/2}{y/2} = \frac{\frac{1}{4\pi\varepsilon_0}\frac{q^2}{r'^2}}{mg} \quad .....(iv)$$

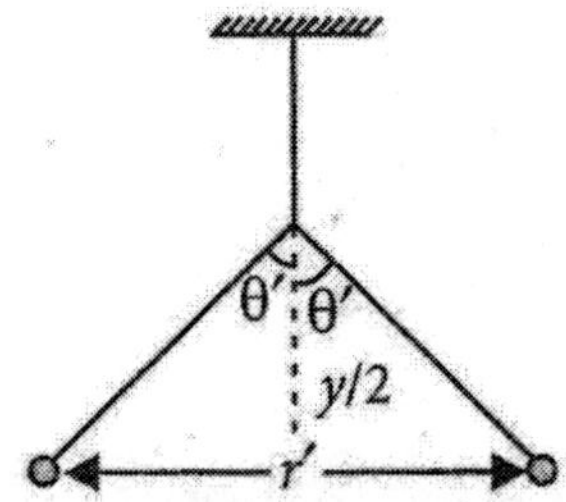

(b) Divide (iv) by (iii), we get

$$\frac{2r'}{r} = \frac{r^2}{r'^2} \Rightarrow r^3 = \frac{r^3}{2} \Rightarrow r' = \frac{r}{\sqrt[3]{2}}$$

5. **(c)** : According to Coulomb's law, the force of repulsion between the two positive ions each of charge q, separated by a distance d is given by

$$F = \frac{1}{4\pi\varepsilon_0}\frac{(q)(q)}{d^2} \text{ or } F = \frac{q^2}{4\pi\varepsilon_0 d^2}$$

$q^2 = 4\pi\varepsilon_0 F d^2$ or $q = \sqrt{4\pi\varepsilon_0 F d^2}$ ....(i)

Since, q = ne

where, n = number of electrons missing from each ion, e = magnitude of charge on electron

$\therefore n = \frac{q}{e} = \sqrt{\frac{4\pi\varepsilon_0 F d^2}{e^2}}$ (Using (i))

6. **(c):** $F_m = \frac{F_0}{K}$ i.e., decreases K times

7. **(a):** The situation is as shown in the figure.

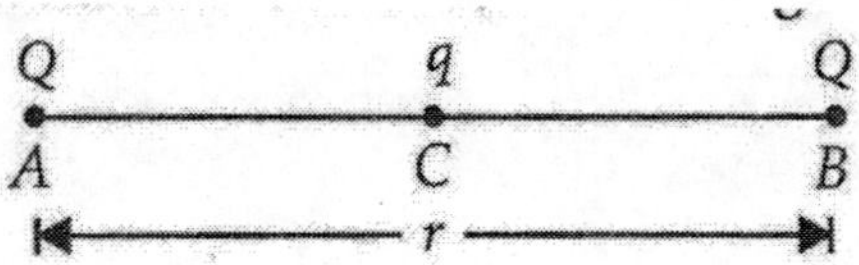

Let two equal charges Q each placed at points A and B at a distance r apart. C is the centre of AB where charge q is placed. For equilibrium, net force on charge $Q = 0$

$$\therefore \frac{1}{4\pi\varepsilon_0}\frac{QQ}{r^2} + \frac{1}{4\pi\varepsilon_0}\frac{Qq}{(r/2)^2} = 0$$

$$\frac{1}{4\pi\varepsilon_0}\frac{Q^2}{r^2} = -\frac{1}{4\pi\varepsilon_0}\frac{4Qq}{r^2} \text{ or } Q = -4q \text{ or } q = -\frac{Q}{4}$$

8. **(c)** : Net force on each of the charge due to the other charges is zero. However, disturbance in any direction other than along the line on which the charges lie, will not make the charges return.

9. **(d) :** $\phi_{\text{closed}} = 0$

So $\phi_{\text{in}} = \phi_{\text{out}}$

Number of field lines entering is equal number of field lines leaving.

10. **(a)**: Force experienced by a charged particle in an electric field, $F = qE$

As $F = ma$

$$\therefore ma = qE \Rightarrow a = \frac{qE}{m}$$

As electron and proton both fall from same height at rest. Then initial velocity = 0

From $s = ut + \frac{1}{2}at^2$ ($\because u = 0$)

$\therefore h = \frac{1}{2}at^2 \Rightarrow h = \frac{1}{2}\frac{qE}{m}t^2$ [Using (i)]

$\therefore t = \sqrt{\frac{2hm}{qE}} \Rightarrow t \propto \sqrt{m}$ as ' q ' is same for electron and proton.

As electron has smaller mass so it will take smaller time.

11. **(b)**

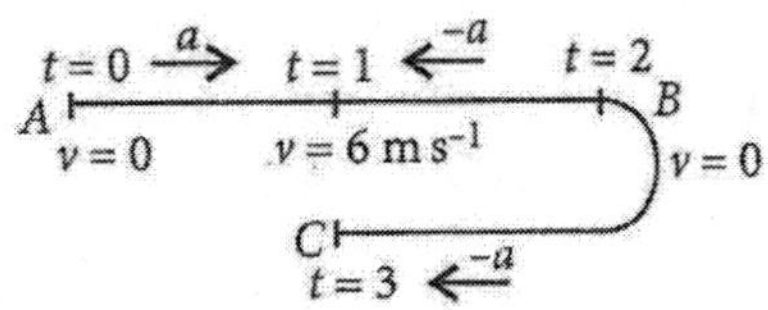

$v = -6 \text{ ms}^{-1}$

Acceleration, $a = \frac{6-0}{1} = 6 \text{ m s}^{-2}$

For $t = 0$ to $t = 1$ s, $s_1 = \frac{1}{2} \times 6(1)^2 = 3$ m

For $t = 1$ s to $t = 2$ s, $s_2 = 6 \times 1 - \frac{1}{2} \times 6(1)^2 = 3$ m

For $t = 2$ s to $t = 3$ s, $s_3 = 0 - \frac{1}{2} \times 6(1)^2 = -3$ m

Total displacement $s = s_1 + s_2 + s_3 = 3$ m

Average velocity $= \frac{3}{3} = 1 \text{ m s}^{-1}$

Total distance travelled = 9 m

Average speed $= \frac{9}{3} = 3 \text{ m s}^{-1}$

12. **(a):** As $v^2 = 0^2 + 2ay = 2(F/m)y = 2\left(\frac{qE}{m}\right)y$

K.E. $= \frac{1}{2}mv^2$

$\therefore$ K.E. $= \frac{1}{2}m\left[2\frac{(qE)}{m}y\right] \Rightarrow$ K.E. $= qEy$

13. **(c)** : Electric lines of force start from the positive charge and end at the negative charge. Since the electric lines for both the

charges are ending, therefore both q_1 and q_2 are negative charges.

14. **(d)**

15. **(d) :** Electric flux, $\phi_E = \int \vec{E} \cdot d\vec{S}$

$= \int EdS\cos\theta = \int EdS\cos 90^\circ = 0.$

The lines are parallel to the surface.

16. **(b)** : Since, $R >> L$, the given charge configuration can be treated as dipole.

Electric field due to a dipole at any arbitrary point (R, θ) is

$$E = \frac{p}{4\pi\varepsilon_0 R^3}\sqrt{3\cos^2\theta + 1}$$

Here, $E \propto \frac{1}{R^3}$.

17. **(a)**: The polar molecules are the molecules have one end slightly positive and other end is slightly negatively charged separated by some distance.

So, they have permanent electric dipole moment.

18. **(a)**: This consists of two dipoles, $-q$ and $+q$ with dipole moment along with the $+y$-direction and $-q$ and $+q$ along the x-direction.

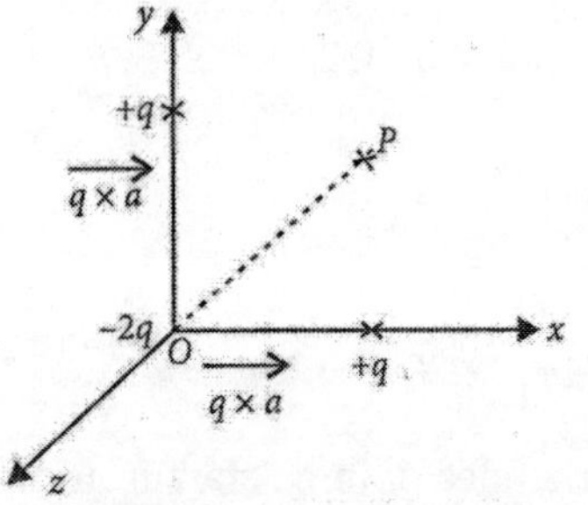

$\therefore$ The resultant moment

$= \sqrt{q^2a^2 + q^2a^2} = \sqrt{2}qa.$

Along the direction 45° that is along OP, where P is $(+a, +a, 0)$.

19. **(d)** : The electric field at a point on equatorial line (perpendicular bisector) of dipole at a distance r is given by

$$E = \frac{p}{4\pi\varepsilon_0} \cdot \frac{1}{(r^2 + a^2)^{3/2}}$$

where $2a$ = length of dipole

For $r >> a$

$\therefore E = \frac{p}{4\pi\varepsilon_0} \cdot \frac{1}{r^3}$ i.e., $E \propto p$ and $E \propto r^{-3}$

20. **(c) :** τ on a dipole $= \vec{p} \times \vec{E}$

$$\tau = pE\sin\theta$$

$$4 = q \times \ell \times E \times \sin 30^\circ$$

$$4 = q \times 2 \times 10^{-2} \times 2 \times 10^5 \times \frac{1}{2}$$

$$q = 2 \times 10^{-3}$$

q = 2 m C

21. **(b)**: Here, $\theta = 30^\circ, E = 2 \times 10^5\ \text{NC}^{-1}, \tau = 4\ \text{N m}$,

$l = 2\ \text{cm} = 0.02\ \text{m}, q = ?$

$\tau = pE\sin\theta = (ql)E\sin\theta$

$$\therefore q = \frac{\tau}{E l\sin\theta} = \frac{4}{2 \times 10^5 \times 0.02 \times \frac{1}{2}}$$

$$= \frac{4}{2 \times 10^3} = 2 \times 10^{-3}\text{C} = 2\text{mC}$$

22. (b): When an electric dipole is placed in a uniform clcctrical field $\vec{E}$, the torque on the dipole is given by $\vec{\tau} = \vec{p} \times \vec{E}$

23. (b) : Here, $r = 10$ cm, $q = 3.2 \times 10^{-7}$C

$$E = \frac{kq}{r^2} = \frac{9 \times 10^9 \times 3.2 \times 10^{-7}}{225 \times 10^{-4}}$$

$$E = 1.28 \times 10^5 \text{ N/C}$$

24. (d) :

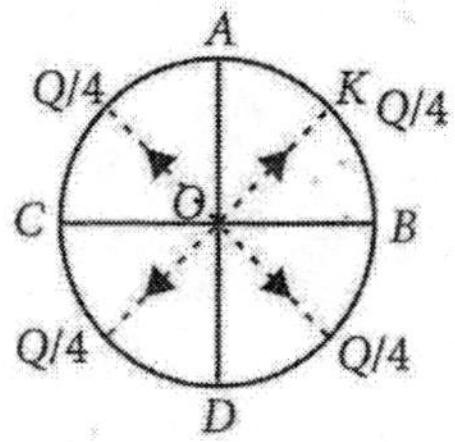

The fields at O due to AC and BD cancel each other. The field due to CD is acting in the direction OK and equal in magnitude to E due to AKB.

25. (c)

26. (b):

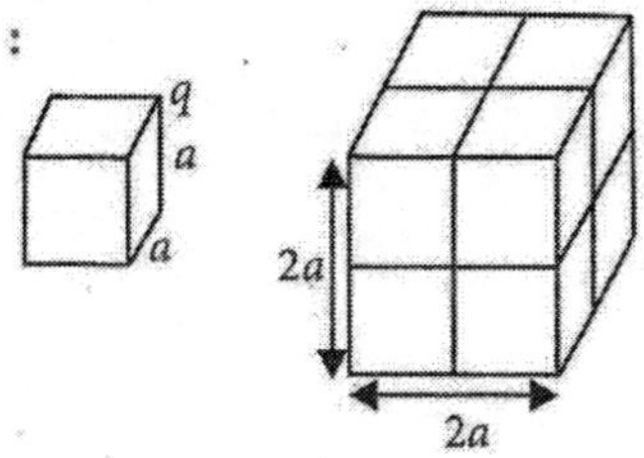

Eight identical cubes are required so that the given charge q appears at the centre of the bigger cube.

Thus, the electric flux passing through the given cube is

$$\phi = \frac{1}{8}\left(\frac{q}{\varepsilon_0}\right) = \frac{q}{8\varepsilon_0}$$

27. (c): According to Gauss's law

$$\phi_E = \frac{Q_{\text{enclosed}}}{\varepsilon_0}$$

If the radius of the Gaussian surface is doubled, the outward electric flux will remain the same. This is because electric flux depends only on the charge enclosed by the surface.

28. (d): Let ϕ_A, ϕ_B and ϕ_C are the electric flux linked with surface is A, B and C.

According to Gauss theorem,

$$\phi_A + \phi_B + \phi_C = \frac{q}{\varepsilon_0}$$

Since $\phi_A = \phi_C$,

$\therefore 2\phi_A + \phi_B = \frac{q}{\varepsilon_0}$ or $2\phi_A = \frac{q}{\varepsilon_0} - \phi_B$ or,

$2\phi_A = \frac{q}{\varepsilon_0} - \phi$

(Given : $\phi_B = \phi$)

$$\therefore \phi_A = \frac{1}{2}\left(\frac{q}{\varepsilon_0} - \phi\right)$$

29. (b): The total flux through the cube $\phi_{\text{total}} = \frac{q}{\varepsilon_0}$

$\therefore$ The electric flux through any face

$$\phi_{\text{face}} = \frac{q}{6\varepsilon_0} = \frac{4\pi q}{6(4\pi\varepsilon_0)}$$

30. (a): For complete cube, $\phi = \frac{Q}{\varepsilon_0} \times 10^{-6}$

For each face, $\phi = \frac{1}{6}\frac{Q}{\varepsilon_0} \times 10^{-6}$

31. (b) :

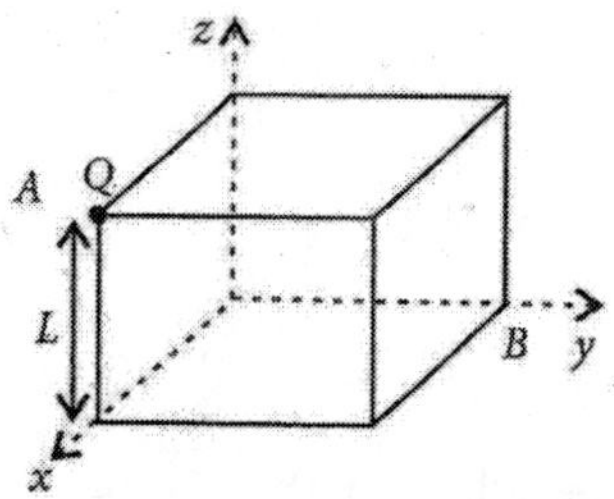

As at a corner, 8 cubes can be placed symmetrically, flux linked with each cube (due to a charge Q at the corner) will be $\frac{Q}{8\varepsilon_0}$.

Now for the faces passing through the edge A, electric field E at a face will be parallel to area of face and so flux for these three faces will be zero. Now as the cube has six faces and flux linked with three faces (through A) is zero, so flux linked with remaining three faces will be $\frac{Q}{8\varepsilon_0}$.

Hence, electric flux passed through all the six faces of the cube is $\frac{Q}{8\varepsilon_0}$.

32. **(d) :** Electric flux emerging from the cube does not depend on size of cube.

Total flux $= \frac{q}{\varepsilon_0}$

33. **(c) :** In a uniformly charged hollow conducting sphere,

(i). For $r < R, \vec{E} = 0$

(ii) For $r > R, \vec{E} = \frac{1}{4\pi\varepsilon_0}\frac{Q}{|\vec{r}^2|}\hat{r}; \vec{E}$ decreases

34. **(d) :** Electric field due to an infinite line charge, $E = \frac{\lambda}{2\pi\varepsilon_0 r}$

Net electric field at mid-point $O, \vec{E}_0 = \vec{E}_1 + \vec{E}_2$

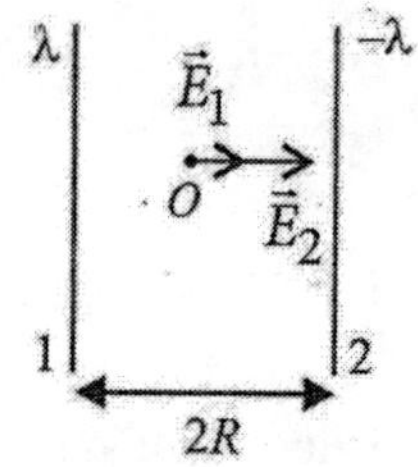

As, $E_1 = E_2 = \frac{\lambda}{2\pi\varepsilon_0 R} \therefore E_0 = 2E_1 = \frac{\lambda}{\pi\varepsilon_0 R}$ NC^{-1}

35. **(a):** Electric field inside the charged spherical shell is zero as there is no charge inside it.

36. **(c):** Field inside a conducting sphere = 0.

Chapter: 16 ELECTROSTATIC POTENTIAL

Electrostatic Potential

1. In a certain region of space with volume $0.2\ m^3$, the electric potential is found to be 5 V throughout. The magnitude of electric field in this region is **(2020)**

(a) zero (b) 0.5 N/C
(c) 1 N/C (d) 5 N/C

2. A bullet of mass 2 g is having a charge of $2\mu C$. Through what potential difference must it be accelerated, starting from rest, to acquire a speed of 10 m/s ? **(2004)**

(a) 5kV (b) 50kV
(c) 5 V (d) 50 V

Potential due to a Point Charge

3. The electric potential at a point in free space due to charge Q coulomb is $Q \times 10^{11}$ volts. The electric field at that point is **(2008)**

(a) $4\pi\varepsilon_0 Q \times 10^{20}$ volt /m
(b) $12\pi\varepsilon_0 Q \times 10^{22}$volt/m
(c) $4\pi\varepsilon_0 Q \times 10^{22}$volt/m
(d) $12\pi\varepsilon_0 Q \times 10^{20}$volt/m

4. As per the diagram a point charge $+q$ is placed at the origin O. Work done in taking another point charge $-Q$ from the point A [coordinates $(0, a)$] to another point B [coordinates $(a, 0)$] along the straight path AB is **(2005)**

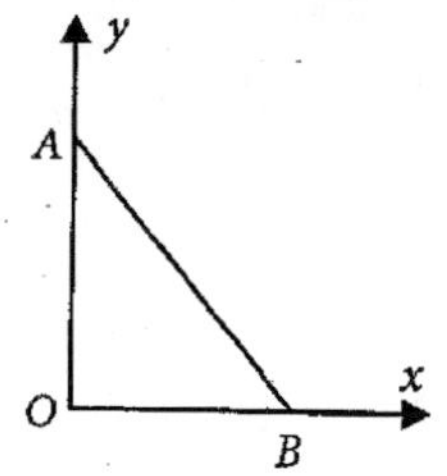

(a) zero
(b) $\left(\frac{qQ}{4\pi\varepsilon_0}\frac{1}{a^2}\right) \cdot \sqrt{2}a$
(c) $\left(\frac{-qQ}{4\pi\varepsilon_0}\frac{1}{a^2}\right) \cdot \sqrt{2}a$
(d) $\left(\frac{qQ}{4\pi\varepsilon_0}\frac{1}{a^2}\right) \cdot \frac{a}{\sqrt{2}}$

Potential due to an Electric Dipole

5. An electric dipole is placed as shown in the figure. **(2023)**

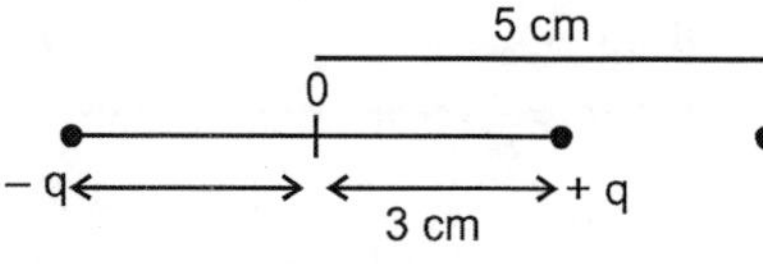

The electric potential (in 10^2 V) at point P due to the dipole is (ϵ_0 = permittivity of free space and $\frac{1}{4\pi \epsilon_0} = K$)

(a) $\left(\frac{5}{8}\right)qK$ (b) $\left(\frac{8}{5}\right)qK$

(c) $\left(\frac{8}{3}\right)qK$ (d) $\left(\frac{3}{8}\right)qK$

6. A short electric dipole has a dipole moment of 16×10^{-9}Cm. The electric potential due to the dipole at a point at a distance of 0.6 m from the centre of the dipole, situated on a line making an angle of 60° with the dipole axis is $\left(\frac{1}{4\pi\varepsilon_0} = 9 \times 10^9 \text{ N m}^2/\text{C}^2\right)$ **(2020)**

(a) 50 V (b) 200 V

(c) 400 V (d) zero

Potential due to a System of Charges

7. Two hollow conducting spheres of radii R_1 and R_2 $(R_1 >> R_2)$ have equal charges. The potential would be **(2022)**

(a) more on bigger sphere

(b) more on smaller sphere

(c) equal on both the spheres

(d) dependent on the material property of the sphere.

8. Twenty seven drops of same size are charged at 220 V each. They combine to form a bigger drop. Calculate the potential of the bigger drop. **(2021)**

(a) 1980 V (b) 660 V

(c) 1320 V (d) 1520 V

9. Two charged spherical conductors of radius R_1 and R_2 are connected by a wire. Then the ratio of surface charge densities of the spheres (σ_1/σ_2) is **(2021)**

(a) $\frac{R_1^2}{R_2^2}$ (b) $\frac{R_1}{R_2}$.

(c) $\frac{R_2}{R_1}$ (d) $\sqrt{\left(\frac{R_1}{R_2}\right)}$

10. Two metal spheres, one of radius R and the other of radius $2R$ respectively have the same surface charge density σ. They are brought in contact and separated. What will be the new surface charge densities on them?**(Odisha NEET 2019)**

(a) $\sigma_1 = \frac{5}{6}\sigma, \sigma_2 = \frac{5}{2}\sigma$

(b) $\sigma_1 = \frac{5}{2}\sigma, \sigma_2 = \frac{5}{6}\sigma$

(c) $\sigma_1 = \frac{5}{2}\sigma, \sigma_2 = \frac{5}{3}\sigma$

(d) $\sigma_1 = \frac{5}{3}\sigma, \sigma_2 = \frac{5}{6}\sigma$

11. A conducting sphere of radius R is given a charge Q. The electric potential and the electric field at the centre of the sphere respectively are **(2014)**

(a) zero and $\frac{Q}{4\pi\varepsilon_0 R^2}$

(b) $\frac{Q}{4\pi\varepsilon_0 R}$ and zero

(c) $\frac{Q}{4\pi\varepsilon_0 R}$ and $\frac{Q}{4\pi\varepsilon_0 R^2}$

(d) both are zero

12. Four point charges $-Q, -q, 2q$ and $2Q$ are placed, one at each corner of the square. The relation between Q and q for which the potential at the centre of the square is zero is **(2012)**

(a) $Q = -q$ (b) $Q = -\frac{1}{q}$

(c) $Q = q$ (d) $Q = \frac{1}{q}$

13. Four electric charges $+q, +q, -q$ and $-q$ are placed at the corners of a square of side $2L$ (see figure). The electric potential at point A, midway between the two charges $+q$ and $+q$, is **(2011)**

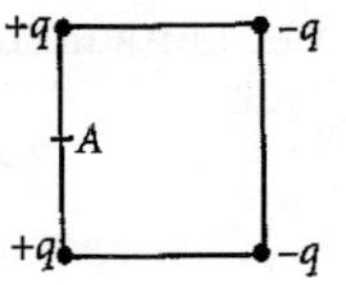

(a) $\frac{1}{4\pi\varepsilon_0}\frac{2q}{L}(1+\sqrt{5})$

(b) $\frac{1}{4\pi\varepsilon_0}\frac{2q}{L}\left(1+\frac{1}{\sqrt{5}}\right)$

(c) $\frac{1}{4\pi\varepsilon_0}\frac{2q}{L}\left(1-\frac{1}{\sqrt{5}}\right)$

(d) zero

14. Three concentric spherical shells have radii a, b and c $(a < b < c)$ and have surface charge densities $\sigma, -\sigma$ and σ respectively. If V_A, V_B and V_C denote the potentials of the three shells, then, for $c = a + b$, we have **(2009)**

(a) $V_C = V_B \neq V_A$

(b) $V_C \neq V_B \neq V_A$

(c) $V_C = V_B = V_A$

(d) $V_C = V_A \neq V_B$

15. A hollow metallic sphere of radius 10 cm is charged such that potential of its surface is 80 V. The potential at the centre of the sphere would be **(1994)**

(a) 80 V (b) 800 V

(c) zero (d) 8 V

Equipotential Surfaces

16. The angle between the electric lines of force and the equipotential surface is **(2022)**

(a) 0° (b) 45°

(c) 90° (d) 180°

17. The diagrams below show regions of equipotentials.

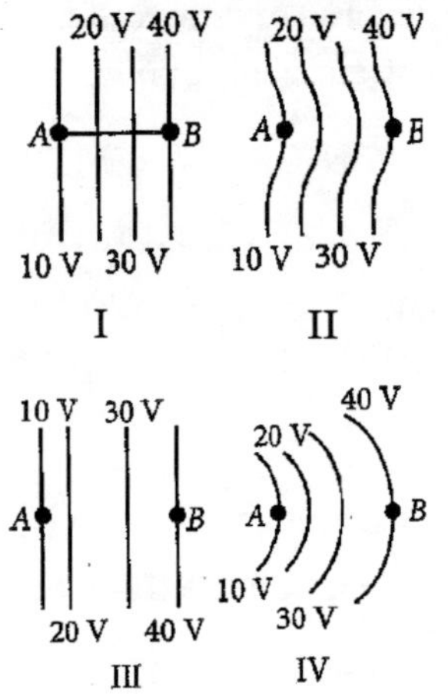

A positive charge is moved from A to B in each diagram. **(2017)**

(a) In all the four cases the work done is the same.

(b) Minimum work is required to move q in figure (I).

(c) Maximum work is required to move q in figure (II).

(d) Maximum work is required to move q in figure (III).

18. If potential (in volts) in a region is expressed as $V(x,y,z) = 6xy - y + 2yz$, the electric field (in N/C) at point (1,1,0) is **(2015)**

(a) $-(2\hat{i} + 3\hat{j} + \hat{k})$

(b) $-(6\hat{i} + 9\hat{j} + \hat{k})$

(c) $-(3\hat{i} + 5\hat{j} + 3\hat{k})$

(d) $-(6\hat{i} + 5\hat{j} + 2\hat{k})$

19. In a region, the potential is represented by $(x,y,z) = 6x - 8xy - 8y + 6yz$, where V is in volts and x, y, z are in metres. The electric force experienced by a charge of 2 coulomb situated at point (1,1,1) is

(a) $6\sqrt{5}$ N (b) 30 N

(c) 24 N (d) $4\sqrt{35}$ N(2014)

20. A, B and C are three points in a uniform electric field. The electric potential is **(2013)**

(a) maximum at C

(b) same at all the three points A, B and C

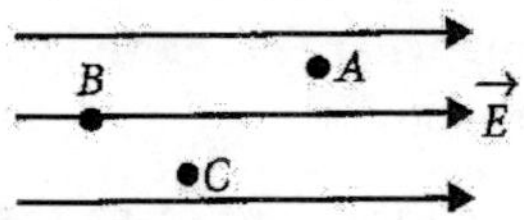

(c) maximum at A

(d) maximum at B

21. The electric potential V at any point (x, y, z), all in metres in space is given by $V = 4x^2$ volt. The electric field at the point (1,0,2) in volt/meter, is **(Mains 2011)**

(a) 8 along negative X-axis

(b) 8 along positive X-axis

(c) 16 along negative X-axis

(d) 16 along positive X-axis

22. The electric potential at a point (x, y, z) is given by $V = -x^2y - xz^3 + 4$. The electric field at that point is **(2009)**

(a) $\vec{E} = \hat{\imath}2xy + \hat{\jmath}(x^2 + y^2) + \hat{k}(3xz - y^2)$

(b) $\vec{E} = \hat{\imath}z^3 + \hat{\jmath}xyz + \hat{k}z^2$

(c) $\vec{E} = \hat{\imath}(2xy - z^3) + \hat{\jmath}xy^2 + \hat{k}3z^2x$

(d) $\vec{E} = \hat{\imath}(2xy + z^3) + \hat{\jmath}x^2 + \hat{k}3xz^2$

23. Charge q_2 is at the centre of a circular path with radius r. Work done in carrying charge q_1, once around this equipotential path, would be **(1994)**

(a) $\frac{1}{4\pi\varepsilon_0} \times \frac{q_1q_2}{r^2}$ (b) $\frac{1}{4\pi\varepsilon_0} \times \frac{q_1q_2}{r}$

(c) zero (d) infinite.

Potential Energy of a System of Charges

24. Three charges, each $+q$, are placed at the corners of an isosceles triangle ABC of sides BC and AC, $2a$. D and E are the mid points of BC and CA. The work done in taking a charge Q from D to E is **(Mains 2011)**

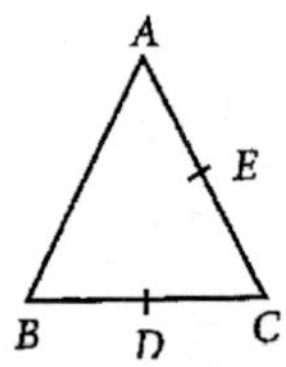

(a) $\frac{3qQ}{4\pi\varepsilon_0 a}$ (b) $\frac{3qQ}{8\pi\varepsilon_0 a}$

(c) $\frac{qQ}{4\pi\varepsilon_0 a}$ (d) zero

25. Charges $+q$ and $-q$ are placed at points A and B respectively which are a distance $2L$ apart, C is the midpoint between A and B. The work done in moving a charge $+Q$ along the semicircle CRD is **(2007)**

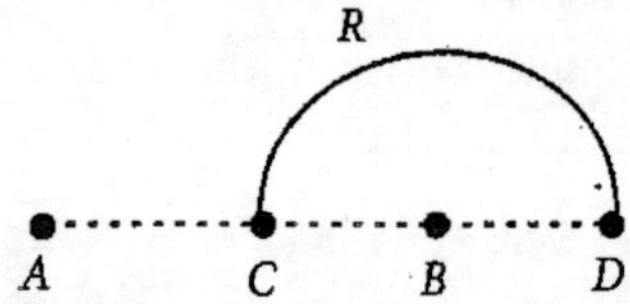

(a) $\frac{qQ}{2\pi\varepsilon_0 L}$ (b) $\frac{qQ}{6\pi\varepsilon_0 L}$

(c) $-\frac{qQ}{6\pi\varepsilon_0 L}$ (d) $\frac{qQ}{4\pi\varepsilon_0 L}$

26. Two charges q_1 and q_2 are placed 30 cm apart, as shown in the figure. A third charge q_3 is moved along the arc of a circle of radius 40 cm from C to D. The change in the potential energy of the system is $\frac{q_3}{4\pi\varepsilon_0}k$, where k is **(2005)**

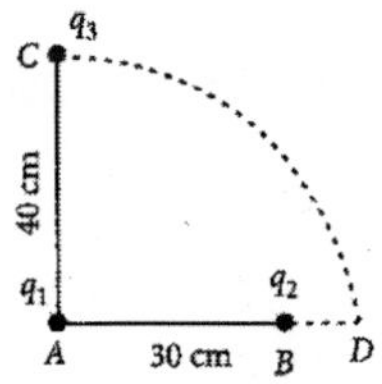

(a) $8q_1$ (b) $6q_1$

(c) $8q_2$ (d) $6q_2$

27. Identical charges $(-q)$ are placed at each corners of cube of side b, then electrostatic potential energy of charge $(+q)$ which is placed at centre of cube will be **(2002)**

(a) $\frac{-4\sqrt{2}q^2}{\pi\varepsilon_0 b}$ (b) $\frac{-8\sqrt{2}q^2}{\pi\varepsilon_0 b}$

(c) $\frac{-4q^2}{\sqrt{3}\pi\varepsilon_0 b}$ (d) $\frac{8\sqrt{2}q^2}{4\pi\varepsilon_0 b}$

28. In bringing an electron towards another electron, the electrostatic potential energy of the system **(1999)**

(a) becomes zero

(b) increases

(c) decreases

(d) remains same

Potential Energy in an External Field

29. A dipole is placed in an electric field as shown. In which direction will it move? **(2021)**

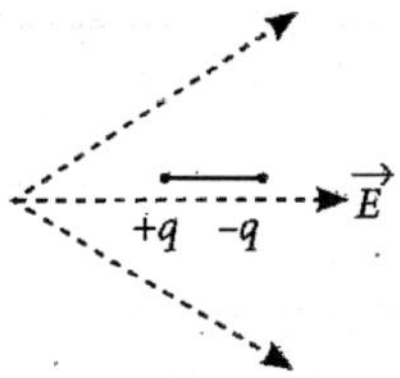

(a) towards the right as its potential energy will increase.

(b) towards the left as its potential energy will increase.

(c) towards the right as its potential energy will decrease.

(d) towards the left as its potential energy will decrease.

30. An electric dipole of dipole moment p is aligned parallel to a uniform electric field E. The energy required to rotate the dipole by 90° is **(Karnataka NEET 2013)**

(a) p^2E (b) pE

(c) infinity (d) pE^2

31. An electric dipole of moment p is placed in an electric field of intensity E. The dipole acquires a position such that the axis of the dipole makes an angle θ with the direction of the field. Assuming that the potential energy of the dipole to be zero when $\theta = 90°$, the torque and the potential energy of the dipole will respectively be **(2012)**

(a) $pE\sin\theta, -pE\cos\theta$

(b) $pE\sin\theta, -2pE\cos\theta$

(c) $pE\sin\theta, 2pE\cos\theta$

(d) $pE\cos\theta, -pE\sin\theta$

32. An electric dipole of moment $\vec{p}$ is lying along a uniform electric field $\vec{E}$. The work done in rotating the dipole by 90° is

(2006)

(a) pE (b) $\sqrt{2}pE$

(c) $pE/2$ (d) $2pE$

33. An electric dipole has the magnitude of its charge as q and its dipole moment is p. It is placed in a uniform electric field E. If its dipole moment is along the direction of the field, the force on it and its potential energy are respectively **(2004)**

(a) $2q \cdot E$ and minimum

(b) $q \cdot E$ and $p \cdot E$

(c) zero and minimum

(d) $q \cdot E$ and maximum

34. There is an electric field E in x-direction. If the work done on moving a charge of 0.2C through a distance of 2 m along a line making an angle $60°$ with x-axis is 4 J, then what is the value of E ? **(1995)**

(a) 5 N/C (b) 20 N/C

(c) $\sqrt{3}\text{ N/C}$ (d) 4 N/C

35. An electric dipole of moment p is placed in the position of stable equilibrium in uniform electric field of intensity E. This is rotated through an angle θ from the initial position. The potential energy of the electric dipole in the final position is

(1994)

(a) $-pE\cos\theta$ (b) $pE(1-\cos\theta)$

(c) $pE\cos\theta$ (d) $pE\sin\theta$

Electrostatics of Conductors

36. Some charge is being given to a conductor. Then its potential is **(2002)**

(a) maximum at surface

(b) maximum at centre

(c) remain same throughout the conductor

(d) maximum somewhere between surface and centre.

Capacitors and Capacitance

37. Two metallic spheres of radii 1 cm and 3 cm are given charges of $-1\times10^{-2}\text{C}$ and $5\times10^{-2}\text{C}$, respectively. If these are connected by a conducting wire, the final charge on the bigger sphere is

(Mains 2012)

(a) $2\times10^{-2}\text{C}$ (b) $3\times10^{-2}\text{C}$

(c) $4\times10^{-2}\text{C}$ (d) $1\times10^{-2}\text{C}$

38. Two metallic spheres of radii 1 cm and 2 cm are given charges 10^{-2}C and $5\times10^{-2}\text{C}$ respectively. If they are connected by a conducting wire, the final charge on the smaller sphere is **(1995)**

(a) $3\times10^{-2}\text{C}$ (b) $4\times10^{-2}\text{C}$

(c) $1\times10^{-2}\text{C}$ (d) $2\times10^{-2}\text{C}$

The Parallel Plate Capacitor

39. The electrostatic force between the metal plates of an isolated parallel plate capacitor C having a charge Q and area A, is

(a) independent of the distance between the plates

(b) linearly proportional to the distance between the plates

(c) proportional to the square root of the distance between the plates

(d) inversely proportional to the distance between the plates.

40. A parallel plate air capacitor has capacity C, distance of separation between plates is d and potential difference V is applied between the plates. Force of attraction between the plates of the parallel plate air capacitor is **(2015)**

(a) $\frac{CV^2}{d}$ (b) $\frac{C^2V^2}{2d^2}$

(c) $\frac{C^2V^2}{2d}$ (d) $\frac{CV^2}{2d}$

41. A parallel plate air capacitor is charged to a potential difference of V volts. After disconnecting the charging battery the distance between the plates of the capacitor is increased using an insulating handle. As a result the potential difference between the plates **(2006)**

(a) increases

(b) decreases

(c) does not change

(d) becomes zero

Effect of Dielectric on Capacitance

42. The capacitance of a parallel plate capacitor with air as medium is $6\mu F$. With the introduction of a dielectric medium, the capacitance becomes $30\mu F$. The permittivity of the medium is

$(\varepsilon_0 = 8.85 \times 10^{-12} C^2 N^{-1} m^{-2})$

(2020)

(a) $0.44 \times 10^{-13} C^2 N^{-1} m^{-2}$

(b) $1.77 \times 10^{-12} C^2 N^{-1} m^{-2}$

(c) $0.44 \times 10^{-10} C^2 N^{-1} m^{-2}$

(d) $5.00 C^2 N^{-1} m^{-2}$

43. Two thin dielectric slabs of dielectric constants K_1 and $K_2 (K_1 < K_2)$ are inserted between plates of a parallel plate capacitor, as shown in the figure. The variation of electric field E between the plates with distance d as measured from plate P is correctly shown by **(2014)**

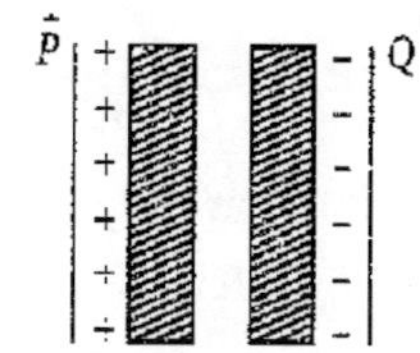

(a)
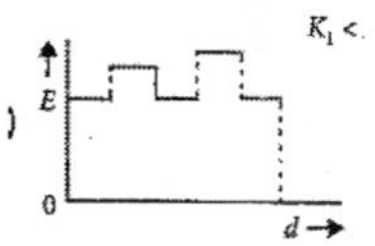

(b)
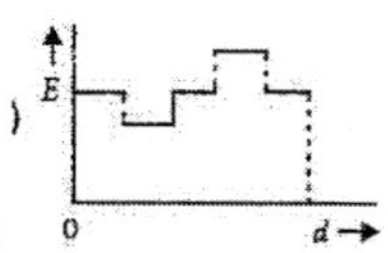

(c)
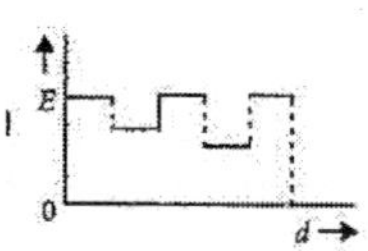

(d)
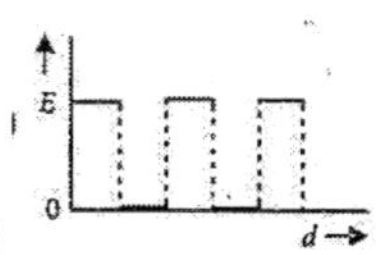

44. Two parallel metal plates having charges $+Q$ and $-Q$ face each other at a certain distance between them. If the plates are now dipped in kerosene oil tank, the electric field between the plates will

(Mains 2010)

(a) become zero (b) increase
(c) decrease (d) remain same

45. A parallel plate condenser with oil between the plates (dielectric constant of oil = 2) has a capacitance C. If the oil is removed, then capacitance of the capacitor becomes **(1999)**

(a) $\frac{C}{\sqrt{2}}$ (b) 2C
(c) $\sqrt{2}C$ (d) $\frac{C}{2}$

Combination of Capacitors

46. The equivalent capacitance of the system shown in the following circuit is **(2023)**

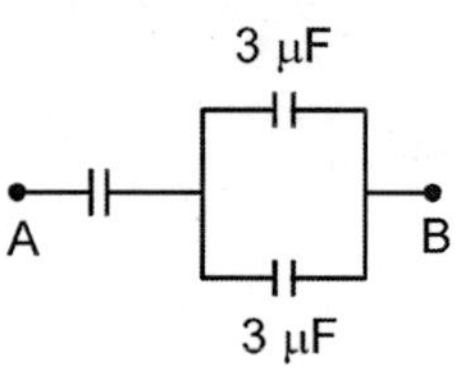

(a) 3 μF (b) 6 μF
(c) 9 μF (d) 2 μF

47. The equivalent capacitance of the combination shown in the figure is **(2021)**

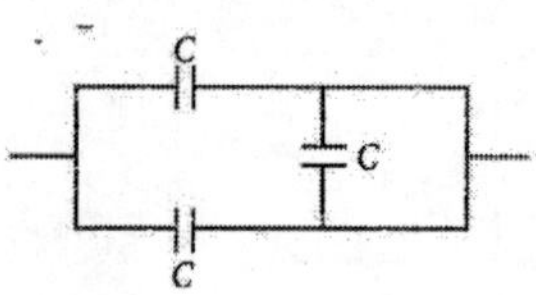

(a) $\frac{3C}{2}$ (b) $3C$
(c) $2C$ (d) $C/2$

48. A parallel-plate capacitor of area A, plate separation d and capacitance C is filled with four dielectric materials having dielectric constants k_1, k_2, k_3 and k_4 as shown in the figure. If a single dielectric material is to be used to have the same capacitance C in this capacitor, then its dielectric constant k is given by

(NEET -II 2016)

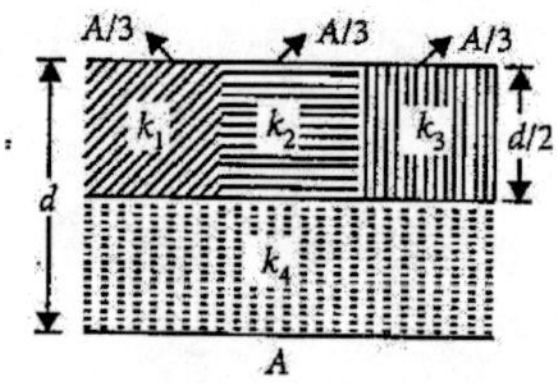

(a) $k = k_1 + k_2 + k_3 + 3k_4$
(b) $k = \frac{2}{3}(k_1 + k_2 + k_3) + 2k_4$
(c) $\frac{2}{k} = \frac{3}{k_1+k_2+k_3} + \frac{1}{k_4}$
(d) $\frac{1}{k} = \frac{1}{k_1} + \frac{1}{k_2} + \frac{1}{k_3} + \frac{3}{2k_4}$

49. Three capacitors each of capacitance C and of breakdown voltage V are joined in series. The capacitance and breakdown voltage of the combination will be **(2009)**

(a) $3C, \frac{V}{3}$ (b) $\frac{C}{3}, 3V$
(c) $3C, 3$ V (d) $\frac{C}{3}, \frac{V}{3}$

50. A network of four capacitors of capacity equal to $C_1 = C, C_2 = 2C, C_3 = 3C$ and $C_4 = 4C$ are connected to a battery as shown in the figure. The ratio of the charges on C_2 and C_4 is **(2005)**

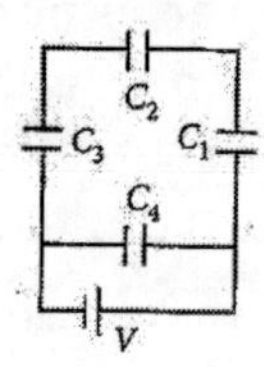

(a) $\frac{4}{7}$ (b) 3/22
(c) 7/4 (d) 22/3

51. Three capacitors each of capacity $4\mu F$ are to be connected in such a way that the effective capacitance is $6\mu F$. This can be done by **(2003)**

(a) connecting all of them in series

(b) connecting them in parallel

(c) connecting two in series and one in parallel

(d) connecting two in parallel and one in series.

52. A capacitor of capacity C_1 is charged upto V volt and then connected in parallel to an uncharged capacitor of capacity C_2. The final potential difference across each will be **(2002)**

(a) $\frac{C_2 V}{C_1+C_2}$ (b) $\frac{C_1 V}{C_1+C_2}$

(c) $\left(1+\frac{C_2}{C_1}\right)$ (d) $\left(1-\frac{C_2}{C_1}\right)V$

53. What is the effective capacitance between points X and ? **(1999)**

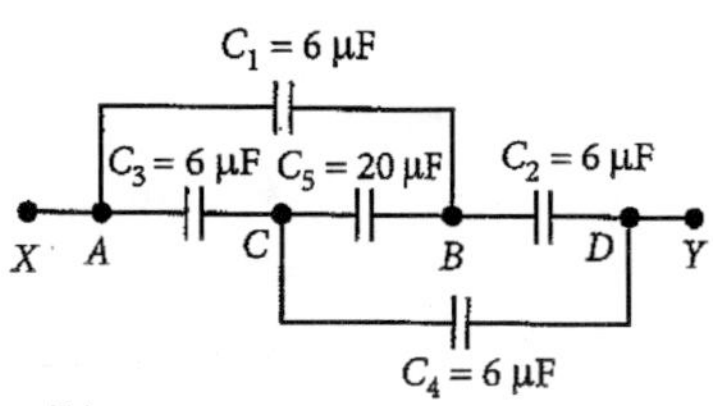

(a) $12\mu F$ (b) $18\mu F$

(c) $24\mu F$ (d) $6\mu F$

Energy Stored in a Capacitor

54. A capacitor of capacitance $C = 900pF$ is charged fully by 100 V battery B as shown in figure (a). Then it is disconnected from the battery and connected to another uncharged capacitor of capacitance $C = 900pF$ as shown in figure (b). The electrostatic energy stored by the system (b) is **(2022)**

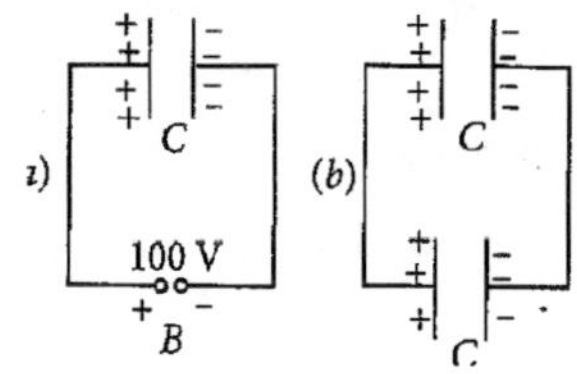

(a) 4.5×10^{-6} J (b) 3.25×10^{-6} J

(c) 2.25×10^{-6} J (d) 1.5×10^{-6} J

55. A parallel plate capacitor has a uniform electric field ' $\vec{E}$ ' in the space between the plates. If the distance between the plates is ' d ' and the area of each plate ' A ', the energy stored in the capacitor is

(ε_0 = permittivity of free space)

(2021)

(a) $\frac{E^2 Ad}{\varepsilon_0}$ (b) $\frac{1}{2}\varepsilon_0 E^2$

(c) $\varepsilon_0 EAd$ (d) $\frac{1}{2}\varepsilon_0 E^2 Ad$

56. Two identical capacitors C_1 and C_2 of equal capacitance are connected as shown in the circuit. Terminals a and b of the key k are connected to charge capacitor C_1 using battery of emf V volt. Now disconnecting a and b, the terminals b and c are connected. Due to this, what will be the percentage loss of energy?

(Odisha NEET 2019)

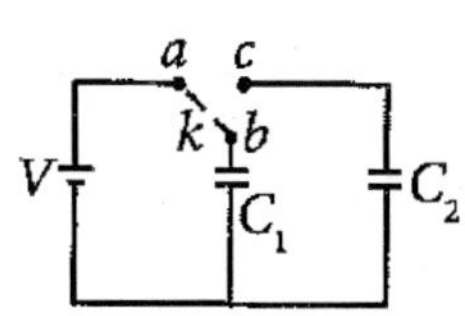

(a) 75% (b) 0%

(c) 50% (d) 25%

57. A capacitor is charged by a battery. The battery is removed and another identical uncharged capacitor is connected in parallel. The total electrostatic energy of resulting system **(2017)**

(a) decreases by a factor of 2
(b) remains the same
(c) increases by a factor of 2
(d) increases by a factor of 4.

58. A parallel plate air capacitor of capacitance C is connected to a cell of emf V and then disconnected from it. A dielectric slab of dielectric constant K, which can just fill the air gap of the capacitor, is now inserted in it. Which of the following is incorrect? **(2015 Cancelled)**

(a) The change in energy stored is $\frac{1}{2}CV^2\left(\frac{1}{K}-1\right)$.
(b) The charge on the capacitor is not conserved.
(c) The potential difference between the plates decreases K times.
(d) The energy stored in the capacitor decreases K times.

59. A parallel plate capacitor has a uniform electric field E in the space between the plates. If the distance between the plates is d and area of each plate is A, the energy stored in the capacitor is **(Mains 2012, 2011, 2008)**

(a) $\frac{1}{2}\varepsilon_0 E^2$ (b) $\frac{E^2Ad}{\varepsilon_0}$
(c) $\frac{1}{2}\varepsilon_0 E^2 Ad$ (d) $\varepsilon_0 EAd$

60. A series combination of n_1 capacitors, each of value C_1, is charged by a source of potential difference 4 V. When another parallel combination of n_2 capacitors, each of value C_2, is charged by a source of potential difference V, it has the same (total) energy stored in it, as the first combination has. The value of C_2, in terms of C_1, is then **(2010)**

(a) $\frac{2C_1}{n_1n_2}$ (b) $16\frac{n_2}{n_1}C_1$
(c) $2\frac{n_2}{n_1}C_1$ (d) $\frac{16C_1}{n_1n_2}$

61. Two condensers, one of capacity C and other of capacity $C/2$ are connected to a V-volt battery, as shown in the figure. The work done in charging fully both the condensers is **(2007)**

(a) $\frac{1}{4}CV^2$ (b) $\frac{3}{4}CV^2$
(c) $\frac{1}{2}CV^2$ (d) $2CV^2$

62. Energy per unit volume for a capacitor having area A and separation d kept at potential difference V is given by **(2001)**

(a) $\frac{1}{2}\varepsilon_0\frac{V^2}{d^2}$ (b) $\frac{1}{2\varepsilon_0}\frac{V^2}{d^2}$
(c) $\frac{1}{2}CV^2$ (d) $\frac{Q^2}{2C}$

63. A capacitor is charged with a battery and energy stored is U. After disconnecting battery another capacitor of same capacity is connected in parallel to the first capacitor. Then energy stored in each capacitor is **(2000)**

(a) $U/2$ (b) $U/4$

(c) $4U$ (d) $2U$

64. The energy stored in a capacitor of capacity C and potential V is given by

(1996)

(a) $\frac{CV}{2}$ (b) $\frac{C^2V^2}{2}$

(c) $\frac{C^2V}{2}$ (d) $\frac{CV^2}{2}$

ANSWER KEY

1. (a)	2. (b)	3. (c)	4. (a)	5. (d)	6. (b)	7. (b)
8. (a)	9. (c)	10. (d)	11. (b)	12. (a)	13. (c)	14. (d)
15. (a)	16. (c)	17. (a)	18. (d)	19. (d)	20. (d)	21. (a)
22. (d)	23. (c)	24. (d)	25. (c)	26. (c)	27. (c)	28. (b)
29. (c)	30. (b)	31. (a)	32. (a)	33. (c)	34. (b)	35. (b)
36. (c)	37. (b)	38. (d)	39. (a)	40. (d)	41. (a)	42. (c)
43. (c)	44. (c)	45. (d)	46. (d)	47. (c)	48. (c)	49. (b)
50. (b)	51. (c)	52. (b)	52. (d)	54. (c)	55. (d)	56. (c)
57. (a)	58. (b)	59. (c)	60. (d)	61. (b)	62. (a)	63. (b)
64. (d)						

Hints & Explanations

1. **(a) :** Electric field in a region, $E = -\frac{dV}{dr}$

But here electric potential is constant. Therefore electric field will be zero.

2. **(b) :** Using $\frac{1}{2}mv^2 = qV$

$$V = \frac{1}{2} \times \frac{2 \times 10^{-3} \times 10 \times 10}{2 \times 10^{-6}} = 50\text{kV}$$

3. **(c) :** $V = \frac{1}{4\pi\varepsilon_0} \cdot \frac{Q}{r} = Q.10^{11}$ volts $\therefore \frac{1}{r} = 4\pi\varepsilon_0 \times 10^{11}$

$$E = \frac{\text{potential}}{r} = Q \cdot 10^{11} \times 4\pi\varepsilon_0 \cdot 10^{11}$$

$$\Rightarrow E = 4\pi\varepsilon_0 \cdot Q \cdot 10^{22}\text{volt/m}$$

4. **(a) :** Work done is equal to zero because the potential of A and B are the same i.e., $\frac{1}{4\pi\varepsilon_0}\frac{q}{a}$.

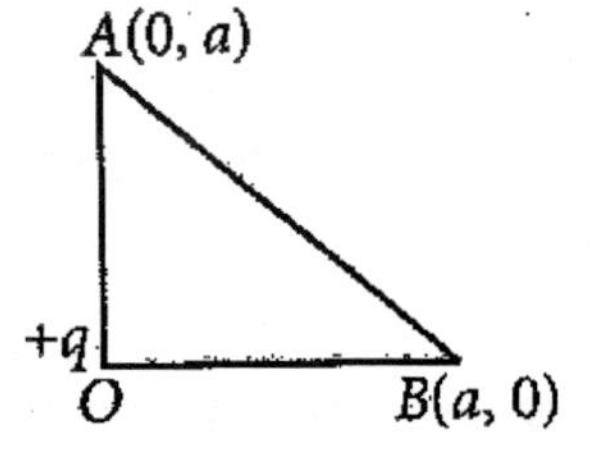

No work is done if a particle does not change its potential energy. i.e., initial potential energy = final potential energy.

5. **(d) :**

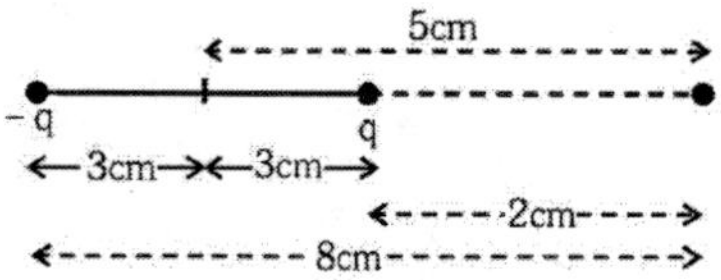

$$v=\frac{Kq}{2\times10^{-2}}-\frac{Kq}{8\times10^{-2}}$$

$$=Kq\left[\frac{3}{8}\right]\times10^{2}$$

6. **(b) :** Potential due to dipole, $V=\frac{\vec{p}\cdot\hat{r}}{4\pi\varepsilon_0 r^2}=\frac{\text{kpcos}\,\theta}{r^2}$ or $V=\frac{(9\times10^9)(16\times10^{-9})\times\cos 60^\circ}{(0.6)^2}=$ 200 V

7. **(b) :** The electrical potential at the surface of a hollow sphere is, $V=\frac{kq}{R}$

For sphere 1, $V_1=\frac{kq}{R_1}$

For sphere 2, $V_2=\frac{kq}{R_2}$

As $R_1 \gg R_2$, therefore, $V_1 < V_2$.

Hence, potential is more on smaller sphere.

8. **(a) :** Here : $n = 27$

Potential, $V = 220$ V

Potential at the surface of a solid charged sphere

$$V=\frac{1}{4\pi\varepsilon_0}\frac{q}{r}$$

$\frac{4}{3}\pi r^3\times n=\frac{4}{3}\pi r'^3$ or $r'=rn^{1/3}$

Potential of bigger drop,

$$V_n=\frac{1}{4\pi\varepsilon_0}\cdot\frac{nq}{r'}$$

$$V_n=\frac{1}{4\pi\varepsilon_0}\frac{nq}{rn^{1/3}}\ \text{(using (i))}$$

$$\therefore V_n = Vn^{2/3}$$

Putting the values of n and V in equation (ii), we get

$$V_n = 220\times(27)^{2/3}$$

or $V_n = 1980$ V

9. **(c) :** When the two spheres are connected by conducting wire, the potential of both the spheres becomes same.

$$V_1=V_2\Rightarrow\frac{kq_1}{R_1}=\frac{kq_2}{R_2}$$

$$\frac{q_1}{q_2}=\frac{R_1}{R_2}$$

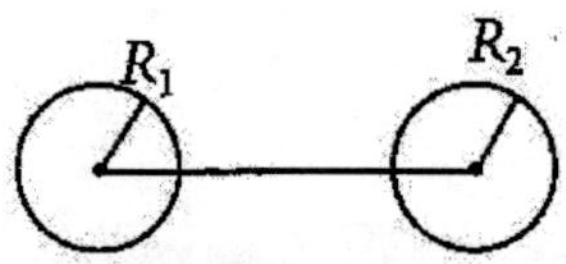

Ratio of surface charge densities

$$\frac{\sigma_1}{\sigma_2}=\frac{\frac{Q}{4\pi R_1^2}}{\frac{Q}{4\pi R_2^2}}=\frac{R_2^2}{R_1^2}\times\frac{q_1}{q_2}=\left(\frac{R_2}{R_1}\right)^2\times\frac{R_1}{R_2}$$

$$\Rightarrow\frac{\sigma_1}{\sigma_2}=\frac{R_2}{R_1}$$

10. **(d) :** Before contact, $Q_1=\sigma\cdot4\pi R^2$

and $Q_2=\sigma\cdot4\pi(2R)^2$

As, surface charge density, $\sigma=\frac{\text{Net charge }(Q)}{\text{Surface area }(A)}$

Now, after contact, $Q_1'+Q_2'=Q_1+Q_2$

$=5Q_1=5(\sigma\cdot4\pi R^2)$

They will be at equal potentials, so,

$$\frac{Q_1'}{R} = \frac{Q_2'}{2R} \Rightarrow Q_2' = 2Q_1'$$
$$\therefore\ 3Q_1' = 5(\sigma \cdot 4\pi R^2)$$
$$\text{and } Q_2' = \frac{10}{3}(\sigma \cdot 4\pi R^2)$$
$$\therefore\ \sigma_1 = \frac{5}{3}\sigma \text{ and } \sigma_2 = \frac{5}{6}\sigma.$$

(From equation (i))

11. **(b) :** For the conducting sphere, Potential at the centre = Potential on the sphere = $\frac{1}{4\pi\varepsilon_0}\frac{Q}{R}$

12. **(a) :** Let a be the side of the square $ABCD$.

$$\therefore\ AC = BD = \sqrt{a^2 + a^2} = a\sqrt{2}$$

$$OA = OB = OC = OD = \frac{a\sqrt{2}}{2} = \frac{a}{\sqrt{2}}$$

Potential at the centre O due to given charge configuration is

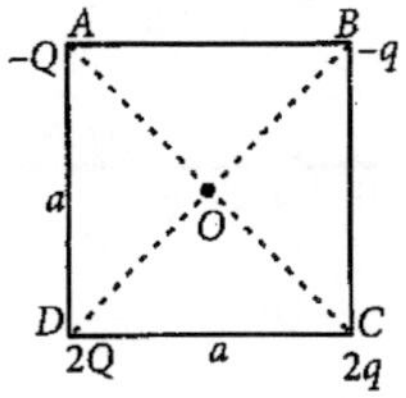

$$V = \frac{1}{4\pi\varepsilon_0}\left[\frac{(-Q)}{\left(\frac{a}{\sqrt{2}}\right)} + \frac{(-q)}{\left(\frac{a}{\sqrt{2}}\right)} + \frac{(2q)}{\left(\frac{a}{\sqrt{2}}\right)} + \frac{2Q}{\left(\frac{a}{\sqrt{2}}\right)}\right] = 0$$

$\Rightarrow -Q - q + 2q + 2Q = 0$ or $Q + q = 0$ or $Q = -q$

13. **(c) :** A is the midpoint of PS

$$\therefore\ PA = AS = L$$

$$AR = AQ = \sqrt{(SR)^2 + (AS)^2}$$

$$= \sqrt{(2L)^2 + (L)^2} = L\sqrt{5}$$

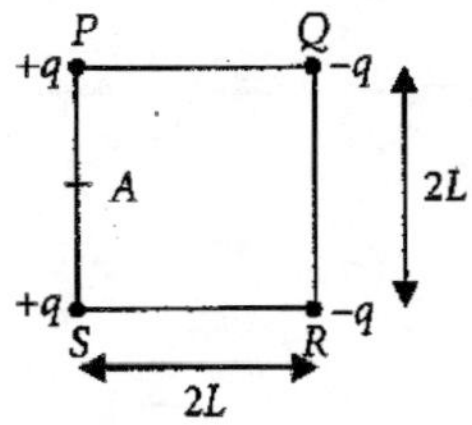

Electric potential at point A due to the given charge configuration is

$$V_A = \frac{1}{4\pi\varepsilon_0}\left[\frac{q}{PA} + \frac{q}{AS} + \frac{(-q)}{AQ} + \frac{(-q)}{AR}\right]$$
$$= \frac{1}{4\pi\varepsilon_0}\left[\frac{q}{L} + \frac{q}{L} - \frac{q}{L\sqrt{5}} - \frac{q}{L\sqrt{5}}\right]$$
$$= \frac{1}{4\pi\varepsilon_0}\left[\frac{2q}{L} - \frac{2q}{L\sqrt{5}}\right] = \frac{1}{4\pi\varepsilon_0}\frac{2q}{L}\left[1 - \frac{1}{\sqrt{5}}\right]$$

14. **(d) :** $V_A = \frac{1}{4\pi\varepsilon_0}\left\{\frac{q_A}{a} + \frac{q_B}{b} + \frac{q_C}{c}\right\}$

$$= \frac{4\pi}{4\pi\varepsilon_0}\left\{\frac{a^2\sigma}{a} - \frac{b^2\sigma}{b} + \frac{c^2\sigma}{c}\right\}$$

$$V_A = \frac{1}{\varepsilon_0}\left\{\frac{a^2\sigma}{a} - \frac{b^2\sigma}{b} + \frac{c^2\sigma}{c}\right\}$$

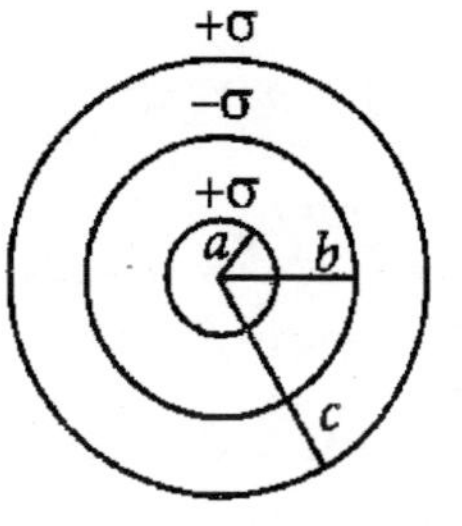

$$V_B = \frac{1}{\varepsilon_0}\left\{\frac{a^2\sigma}{b} - \frac{b^2\sigma}{b} + \frac{c^2\sigma}{c}\right\}, V_C$$
$$= \frac{1}{\varepsilon_0}\left\{\frac{a^2\sigma}{c} - \frac{b^2\sigma}{c} + \frac{c^2\sigma}{c}\right\}$$

Using $c = a + b, V_A = \frac{2a\sigma}{\varepsilon_0}$

$$V_B = \frac{\sigma}{\varepsilon_0}\left(\frac{a^2}{b} + a\right) = \frac{\sigma}{\varepsilon_0}\frac{ac}{b}$$

$$V_C = \frac{\sigma}{\varepsilon_0}\left[\frac{(a+b)(a-b)}{c} + c\right]$$

$$= \frac{\sigma}{\varepsilon_0}(a - b + c) = \frac{2a\sigma}{\varepsilon_0}$$

$$\therefore V_A = V_C \neq V_B$$

15. (a) : Potential inside the sphere is the same as that on the surface i.e., 80 V.

16. (c) : The equipotential surface is always perpendicular to the electric field lines. so, the angle between the electric lines of force and the equipotential surface is 90°.

17. (a) : Work done is given as $W = q\Delta V$

In all the four cases the potential difference from A to B is same.

$\therefore$ In all the four cases the work done is same.

18. (d) : The electric field $\vec{E}$ and potential V in a region are related as $\vec{E} = -\left[\frac{\partial V}{\partial x}\hat{\imath} + \frac{\partial V}{\partial y}\hat{\jmath} + \frac{\partial V}{\partial z}\hat{k}\right]$

Here, $V(x,y,z) = 6xy - y + 2yz$

$$\therefore \vec{E} = -\left[\frac{\partial}{\partial x}(6xy - y + 2yz)\hat{\imath} + \frac{\partial}{\partial y}(6xy - y + 2yz)\hat{\jmath} + \frac{\partial}{\partial z}(6xy - y + 2yz)\hat{k}\right]$$

$$= -[(6y)\hat{\imath} + (6x - 1 + 2z)\hat{\jmath} + (2y)\hat{k}]$$

At point (1,1,0),

$$\vec{E} = -[(6(1))\hat{\imath} + (6(1) - 1 + 2(0))\hat{\jmath} + (2(1))\hat{k}]$$

$$= -(6\hat{\imath} + 5\hat{\jmath} + 2\hat{k})$$

19. (d) :

Here, $V(x,y,z) = 6x - 8xy - 8y + 6yz$

The x, y and z components of electric field are

$$E_x = -\frac{\partial V}{\partial x} = -\frac{\partial}{\partial x}(6x - 8xy - 8y + 6yz)$$

$$= -(6 - 8y) = -6 + 8y$$

$$E_y = -\frac{\partial V}{\partial y} = -\frac{\partial}{\partial y}(6x - 8xy - 8y + 6yz)$$

$$= -(-8x - 8 + 6z) = 8x + 8 - 6z$$

$$E_z = -\frac{\partial V}{\partial z} = -\frac{\partial}{\partial z}(6x - 8xy - 8y + 6yz) = -6y$$

$$\vec{E} = E_x\hat{\imath} + E_y\hat{\jmath} + E_z\hat{k}$$

$$= (-6 + 8y)\hat{\imath} + (8x + 8 - 6z)\hat{\jmath} - 6y\hat{k}$$

At point (1,1,1)

$$\vec{E} = (-6 + 8)\hat{\imath} + (8 + 8 - 6)\hat{\jmath} - 6\hat{k} = 2\hat{\imath} + 10\hat{\jmath} - 6\hat{k}$$

The magnitude of electric field $\vec{E}$ is

$$\vec{E} = \sqrt{E_x^2 + E_y^2 + E_z^2}$$

$$= \sqrt{(2)^2 + (10)^2 + (-6)^2}$$

$$= \sqrt{140} = 2\sqrt{35}\ \text{NC}^{-1}$$

Electric force experienced by the charge

$$F = qE = 2\text{C} \times 2\sqrt{35}\ \text{NC}^{-1} = 4\sqrt{35}\ \text{N}$$

20. (d) : In the direction of electric field, electric potential decreases.

$$\therefore V_B > V_C > V_A$$

21. (a) : $\vec{E} = -\left[\hat{\imath}\frac{\partial V}{\partial x} + \hat{\jmath}\frac{\partial V}{\partial y} + \hat{k}\frac{\partial V}{\partial z}\right]$

Here, $V = 4x^2 \therefore \vec{E} = -8x\hat{\imath}$

The electric field at point (1,0,2) is

$$\vec{E}_{(1,0,2)} = -8\hat{\imath}\text{Vm}^{-1}$$

So electric field is along the negative X-axis.

22. **(d) :** The electric potential at a point,

$$V = -x^2y - xz^3 + 4$$

The field $\vec{E} = -\vec{\nabla}V = -\left(\frac{\partial V}{\partial x}\hat{\imath} + \frac{\partial V}{\partial y}\hat{\jmath} + \frac{\partial V}{\partial z}\hat{k}\right)$

$$\therefore\ \vec{E} = \hat{\imath}(2xy + z^3) + \hat{\jmath}x^2 + \hat{k}(3xz^2)$$

23. **(c) :** Work done on carrying a charge from one place to another on an equipotential surface is zero.

24. **(d)**

Here, $AC = BC = 2a$

D and E are the midpoints of BC and AC.

$\therefore\ AE = EC = a$ and $BD = DC = a$

In $\triangle ADC, (AD)^2 = (AC)^2 - (DC)^2$

$= (2a)^2 - (a)^2 = 4a^2 - a^2 = 3a^2$

$\Rightarrow AD = a\sqrt{3}$

Similarly, potential at point D due to the given charge configuration is

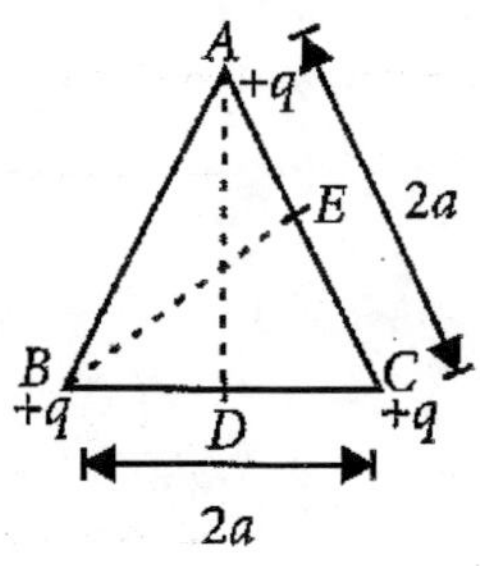

$$V_D = \frac{1}{4\pi\varepsilon_0}\left[\frac{q}{BD} + \frac{q}{DC} + \frac{q}{AD}\right]$$

$$= \frac{q}{4\pi\varepsilon_0}\left[\frac{1}{a} + \frac{1}{a} + \frac{1}{\sqrt{3}a}\right] = \frac{q}{4\pi\varepsilon_0 a}\left[2 + \frac{1}{\sqrt{3}}\right]$$

Potential at point E due to the given charge configuration is

$$V_E = \frac{1}{4\pi\varepsilon_0}\left[\frac{q}{AE} + \frac{q}{EC} + \frac{q}{BE}\right]$$

$$= \frac{q}{4\pi\varepsilon_0}\left[\frac{1}{a} + \frac{1}{a} + \frac{1}{a\sqrt{3}}\right] = \frac{q}{4\pi\varepsilon_0 a}\left[2 + \frac{1}{\sqrt{3}}\right]$$

From (i) and (ii), it is clear that

$$V_D = V_E$$

The work done in taking a charge Q from D to E is

$$W = Q(V_E - V_D) = 0$$

25. **(c) :**

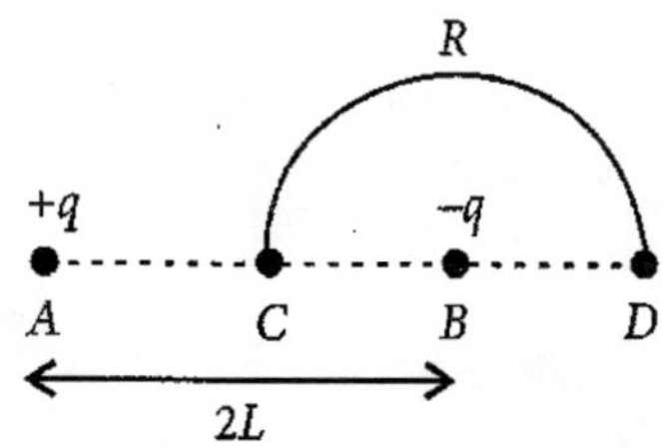

From figure, $AC = L, BC = L, BD = BC = L$

$$AD = AB + BD = 2L + L = 3L$$

Potential at C is given by

$$V_C = \frac{1}{4\pi\varepsilon_0}\left[\frac{q}{AC} + \frac{(-q)}{BC}\right] = \frac{1}{4\pi\varepsilon_0}\left[\frac{q}{L} - \frac{q}{L}\right] = 0$$

Potential at D is given by

$$V_D = \frac{1}{4\pi\varepsilon_0}\left[\frac{q}{AD} + \frac{(-q)}{BD}\right] = \frac{1}{4\pi\varepsilon_0}\left[\frac{q}{3L} - \frac{q}{L}\right]$$

$$= \frac{1}{4\pi\varepsilon_0}\frac{q}{L}\left[\frac{1}{3} - 1\right] = \frac{-q}{6\pi\varepsilon_0}.$$

Work done in moving charge $+Q$ along the semicircle CRD is given by

$$W = [V_D - V_C](+Q) = \left[\frac{-q}{6\pi\varepsilon_0} - 0\right](Q)$$

$$= \frac{-qQ}{6\pi\varepsilon_0 L}$$

Comments : Potential at C is zero because the charges are equal and opposite and the distances are the same.

Potential at D due to $-q$ is greater than that at $A(+q)$, because D is closer to B. Therefore it is negative.

26. **(c)** : The potential energy when q_3 is at point C

$$U_1 = \frac{1}{4\pi\varepsilon_0}\left[\frac{q_1q_3}{0.40} + \frac{q_2q_3}{\sqrt{(0:40)^2 + (0.30)^2}}\right]$$

The potential energy when q_3 is at point D

$$U_2 = \frac{1}{4\pi\varepsilon_0}\left[\frac{q_1q_3}{0.40} + \frac{q_2q_3}{0.10}\right]$$

Thus change in potential energy is $\Delta U = U_2 - U_1$

$$\Rightarrow \frac{q_3}{4\pi\varepsilon_0}k = \frac{1}{4\pi\varepsilon_0}\left[\frac{q_1q_3}{0.40} + \frac{q_2q_3}{0.10} - \frac{q_1q_3}{0.40} - \frac{q_2q_3}{0.50}\right]$$

$$\Rightarrow k = \frac{5q_2 - q_2}{0.50} = \frac{4q_2}{0.50} = 8q_2.$$

27. **(c)** : There are eight corners of a cube and in each corner there is a charge of $(-q)$. At the centre of the corner there is a charge of $(+q)$. Each corner is equidistant from the centres of the cube and the distance (d) is half of the diagonals of the cube.

Diagonal of the cube $= \sqrt{b^2 + b^2 + b^2} = \sqrt{3}b$

$$\therefore d = \sqrt{3}b/2$$

Now, electric potential energy of the charge $(+q)$ due to a charge $(-q)$ at one corner $= U$

$$= \frac{q_1q_2}{4\pi\varepsilon_0 r} = \frac{(+q)\times(-q)}{4\pi\varepsilon_0(\sqrt{3}b/2)} = -\frac{q^2}{2\pi\varepsilon_0(\sqrt{3}b)}$$

$\therefore$ Total electric potential energy due to all the eight identical charges

$$= 8U = -\frac{8q^2}{2\pi\varepsilon_0\sqrt{3}b} = \frac{-4q^2}{\sqrt{3}\pi\varepsilon_0 b}$$

28. **(b)** : In bringing an electron towards another electron, work has to be done (since same charges repel each other). The work done stored as electrostatic potential energy, and hence, electrostatic potential energy of the system increases.

29. **(c)** : Electric field is always direct from high potential to low potential. For the given situation the electric potential is decreasing from left to right therefore, potential energy of the dipole will also decrease. Thus dipole will move from towards the right.

30. **(b)** : Potential energy of dipole,

$$U = -pE(\cos\theta_2 - \cos\theta_1)$$

Here, $\theta_1 = 0°, \theta_2 = 90°$

$$\therefore U = -pE(\cos 90° - \cos 0°)$$
$$= -pE(0 - 1) = pE$$

31. **(a)** : Torque, $\tau = pE\sin\theta$

Potential energy, $U = -pE\cos\theta$

32. **(a)** : Work done in deflecting a dipole through an angle θ is given by

$$W = \int_0^\theta pE\sin\theta d\theta = pE(1-\cos\theta)$$

Since $\theta = 90°$

$\therefore W = pE(1-\cos 90°)$ or, $W = pE$.

33. (c) : The total force on dipole is zero because $F = qE$ is applied on each charge but in opposite direction. The potential energy is $U = -\vec{p}\cdot\vec{E}$, which is minimum when $\vec{p}$ and $\vec{E}$ are parallel.

34. (b) : Charge (q) = 0.2C; Distance (d) = 2 m;

Angle $\theta = 60°$ and work done $(W) = 4$ J

Work done in moving the charge (W)

$= F\cdot d\cos\theta = qEd\cos\theta$

$$E = \frac{W}{qd\cos\theta} = \frac{4}{0.2\times 2\times\cos 60°} = \frac{4}{0.4\times 0.5}$$

$= 20$ N/C

35. (b) : To orient the dipole at any angle θ from its initial position, work has to be done on the dipole from $\theta = 0°$ to θ.

$\therefore$ Potential energy $= pE(1-\cos\theta)$

36. (c) : Electric field intensity E is zero within a conductor due to charge given to it.

Also, $E = -\frac{dV}{dx}$ or $\frac{dV}{dx} = 0$

(inside the conductor)

$\therefore V =$ constant.

So potential remains same throughout the conductor.

37. (b)

38. (d) : Radii of spheres $R_1 = 1\text{ cm} = 1\times 10^{-2}$ m;

$R_2 = 2\text{ cm} = 2\times 10^{-2}$ m and charges on sphere;

$Q_1 = 10^{-2}$C and $Q_2 = 5\times 10^{-2}$C

Common potential $(V) = \frac{\text{Total charge}}{\text{Total capacity}} = \frac{Q_1+Q_2}{C_1+C_2}$

$$= \frac{(1\times 10^{-2})+(5\times 10^{-2})}{4\pi\varepsilon_0 10^{-2} + 4\pi\varepsilon_0(2\times 10^{-2})}$$

$$= \frac{6\times 10^{-2}}{4\pi\varepsilon_0(3\times 10^{-2})}$$

Therefore final charge on smaller sphere = C_1V

$= 4\pi\varepsilon_0\times 10^{-2}\times\frac{6\times 10^{-2}}{4\pi\varepsilon_0\times 3\times 10^{-2}} = 2\times 10^{-2}$C.

39. (a) : Electrostatic force,

$$F_{\text{plate}} = QE = Q\times\frac{Q}{2\varepsilon_0 A} = \frac{Q^2}{2A\varepsilon_0}$$

F is independent of the distance between plates.

40. (d) : Force of attraction between the plates of the parallel plate air capacitor is $F = \frac{Q^2}{2\varepsilon_0 A}$

where Q is the charge on the capacitor, ε_0 is the permittivity of free space and A is the area of each plate.

But $Q = CV$ and $C = \frac{\varepsilon_0 A}{d}$ or $\varepsilon_0 A = Cd$

$$\therefore F = \frac{C^2V^2}{2Cd} = \frac{CV^2}{2d}$$

41. (a) : Capacitance of a parallel plate capacitor

$$C = \frac{\varepsilon_0 A}{d}$$

When battery is disconnected and the distance between the plates of the capacitor is increased then capacitance decreases and charge remains constant.

Since, Charge = Capacitance × Potential difference

∴ Potential difference increases.

42. (c) : Given : capacitance without dielectric, $C = 6\mu\text{F}$ and capacitance with dielectric, $C' = 30\mu\text{F}$.

∴ Dielectric constant, $K = \frac{C'}{C} = \frac{30}{6} = 5.$

Now, permittivity of the medium, $\varepsilon = K\varepsilon_0$

$= 5 \times 8.85 \times 10^{-12}$

$= 0.44 \times 10^{-10} \text{C}^2 \text{ N}^{-1} \text{ m}^{-2}$

43. (c) : $E_{\text{medium}} = \frac{E_{\text{vacuum}}}{K}$

The electric field inside the dielectrics will be less than the electric field in vacuum. The electric field inside the dielectric could not be zero. As $K_2 > K_1$ the drop in electric field for K_2 dielectric must be more than K_1.

44. (c) : Electric field between two parallel plates placed in vacuum is given by $E = \frac{\sigma}{\varepsilon_0}$

In a medium of dielectric constant

$K, E' = \frac{\sigma}{\varepsilon_0 K}$

For kerosene oil $K > 1 \Rightarrow E' < E$

45. (d) : Capacitance of capacitor with oil between the plate, $C = \frac{K\varepsilon_0 A}{d}$

If oil is removed capacitance,

$$C' = \frac{\varepsilon_0 A}{d} = \frac{C}{K} = \frac{C}{2}$$

46. (d) : $C_{AB} = \frac{3 \times 6}{3 + 6} = 2\mu F$

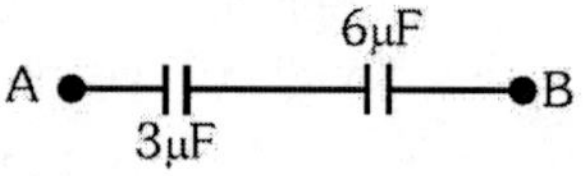

47. (c) :

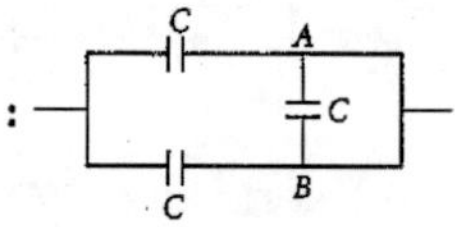

Here, AB arm is short, so the two capacitors C and C in parallel

$$C_{eq} = C + C = 2C$$

48. (c) : Here, $C_1 = \frac{2\varepsilon_0 k_1 A}{3d}, C_2 = \frac{2\varepsilon_0 k_2 A}{3d}$

$$C_3 = \frac{2\varepsilon_0 k_3 A}{3d}, C_4 = \frac{2\varepsilon_0 k_4 A}{d}$$

Given system of C_1, C_2, C_3 and C_4 can be simplified as

$$\therefore \frac{1}{C_{AB}} = \frac{1}{C_1 + C_2 + C_3} + \frac{1}{C_4}$$

Suppose, $C_{AB} = \frac{k\varepsilon_0 A}{d}$

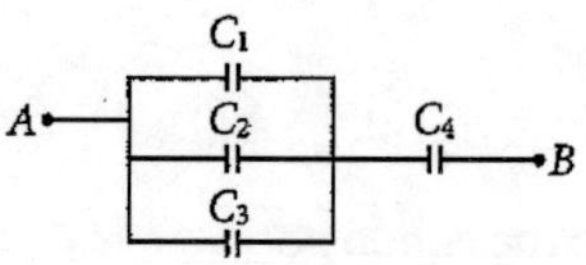

$$\frac{1}{k\left(\frac{\varepsilon_0 A}{d}\right)} = \frac{1}{\frac{2}{3}\frac{\varepsilon_0 A}{d}(k_1 + k_2 + k_3)} + \frac{1}{\frac{2\varepsilon_0 A}{d}k_4}$$

$$\Rightarrow \frac{1}{k} = \frac{3}{2(k_1 + k_2 + k_3)} + \frac{1}{2k_4}$$

$$\therefore \frac{2}{k} = \frac{3}{k_1 + k_2 + k_3} + \frac{1}{k_4}$$

49. (b) : Three capacitors of capacitance C each are in series.

$\therefore$ Total capacitance, $C_{\text{total}} = \frac{C}{3}$.

The charge is the same, Q, when capacitors are in series.

$$V_{\text{total}} = \frac{Q}{C} = \frac{Q}{C/3} = 3V.$$

50. (b) : C_1, C_2 and C_3 are in series

$$\frac{1}{C'} = \frac{1}{C} + \frac{1}{2C} + \frac{1}{3C}$$

$$\text{or, } \frac{1}{C'} = \frac{6+3+2}{6C} = \frac{11}{6C} \text{ or, } C' = \frac{6C}{11}$$

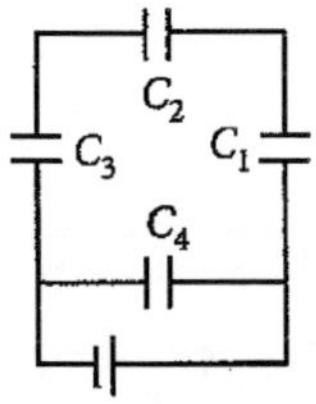

As the capacitors C_1, C_2 and C_3 are in series so the charge on each capacitor is

$Q' = \frac{6}{11}CV$

Also charge on capacitor C_4 is $Q = 4CV$

$\therefore$ Ratio $= \frac{Q'}{Q} = \frac{6CV}{11 \times 4CV} = \frac{3}{22}$.

51. (c) : To get equivalent capacitance 6μF. Out of the 4μF capacitance, two are connected in series and third one is connected in parallel.

$C_{\text{eq}} = \frac{4 \times 4}{4+4} + 4 = 2 + 4 = 6\mu$F.

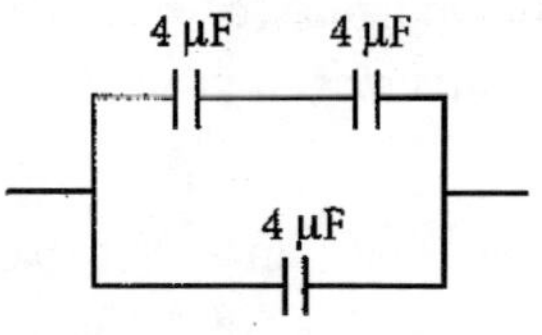

52. (b) : Charge on first capacitor $= q_1 = C_1V$

Charge on second capacitor $= q_2 = 0$

When they are connected, in parallel the total charge $q = q_1 + q_2 \therefore q = C_1V$ and capacitance, $C = C_1 + C_2$

Let V' be the common potential difference across each capacitor, then $q = CV'$.

$$\therefore V' = \frac{q}{C} = \frac{C_1}{C_1 + C_2}V$$

53. (d) : The given circuit can be simplified as

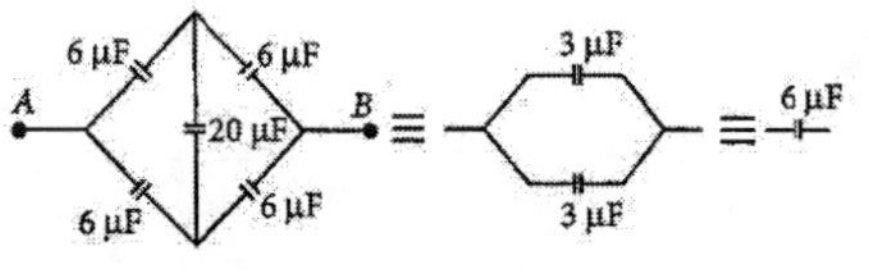

54. (c) : Here, $C_1 = C_2 = 900$pF

$V_1 = 100$ V, $V_2 = 0$ V

When C_1 and C_2 are joined, their common potential is given as,

$V = \frac{C_1V_1 + C_2V_2}{C_1 + C_2} = \frac{900 \times 100 + 900 \times 0}{1800}$

$V = 50$ V

Electrostatic energy stored in system (b) is

$U = \frac{1}{2}(C_1 + C_2)V^2$

$U = \frac{1}{2} \times 1800 \times 10^{-12} \times 50 \times 50$

$U = 2.25 \times 10^{-6}$ J

According to figure (b), charge on both the plate of capacitor is positive which is not possible.

55. **(d)** : The capacitance of a parallel plate capacitor of plate area A and separation d is given by

$$C = \frac{\varepsilon_0 A}{d}$$

The potential is given by $V = Ed$

where E is electric field.

Energy, $U = \frac{1}{2}CV^2 = \frac{1}{2} \times \frac{\varepsilon_0 A}{d} \times E^2 d^2; U = \frac{1}{2}\varepsilon_0 E^2 Ad$

56. **(c)** : As we know that, loss of electrostatic energy,

$$E_{\text{loss}} = \frac{1}{2}\frac{C_1 C_2}{(C_1 + C_2)}V^2 = \frac{1}{2} \times \frac{C^2}{2C}V^2$$

$$= \frac{1}{2}\left(\frac{1}{2}CV^2\right) = \frac{1}{2}E$$

$$[\because C_1 = C_2 = C]$$

$\therefore$ Percentage of loss of energy $= \frac{\frac{1}{2}E}{E} \times 100\%$

$$= \frac{1}{2} \times 100\% = 50\%$$

57. **(a)** : When the capacitor is charged by a battery of potential V, then energy stored in the capacitor,

$$U_i = \frac{1}{2}CV^2$$

When the battery is removed and another identical uncharged capacitor is connected in parallel

Common potential, $V' = \frac{CV}{C+C} = \frac{V}{2}$

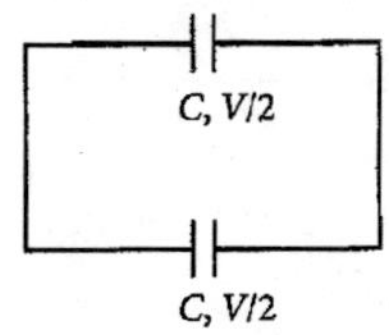

Then the energy stored in the capacitor,

$$U_f = \frac{1}{2}(2C)\left(\frac{V}{2}\right)^2 = \frac{1}{4}CV^2$$

$\therefore$ From eqns. (i) and (ii)

$$U_f = \frac{U_i}{2}$$

It means the total electrostatic energy of resulting system will decreases by a factor of 2 .

58. **(b)** :

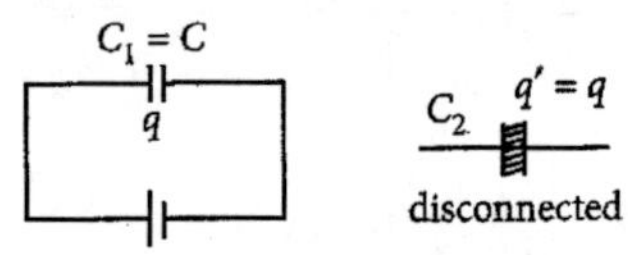

$$q = CV \Rightarrow V = q/C$$

Due to dielectric insertion, new capacitance

$$C_2 = CK$$

disconnected

$C_2 = CK$

Initial energy stored in capacitor, $U_1 = \frac{q^2}{2C}$

Final energy stored in capacitor, $U_2 = \frac{q^2}{2KC}$

Change in energy stored, $\Delta U = U_2 - U_1$

$$\Delta U = \frac{q^2}{2C}\left(\frac{1}{K} - 1\right) = \frac{1}{2}CV^2\left(\frac{1}{K} - 1\right)$$

New potential difference between plates $V' = \frac{q}{CK} = \frac{V}{K}$

59. **(c) :** Capacitance of a parallel plate capacitor is

$$C = \frac{\varepsilon_0 A}{d}$$

Potential difference between the plates is

$$V = Ed$$

The energy stored in the capacitor is

$$U = \frac{1}{2}CV^2 = \frac{1}{2}\left(\frac{\varepsilon_0 A}{d}\right)(Ed)^2 \text{ (Using (i) and (ii))}$$

$$= \frac{1}{2}\varepsilon_0 E^2 Ad$$

60. **(d) :** A series combination of n_1 capacitors each of capacitance C_1 are connected to $4V$ source as shown in the figure.

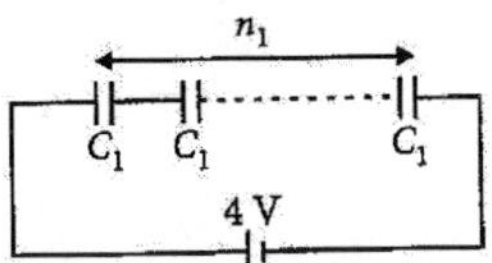

of the series combination

Total capacitance of the series combination of the capacitors is $\frac{1}{C_s} = \frac{1}{C_1} + \frac{1}{C_1} + \frac{1}{C_1} + \cdots \ldots\ldots$ upto n_1 terms $= \frac{n_1}{C_1}$ or $C_s = \frac{C_1}{n_1}$

Total energy stored in a series combination of the capacitors is

$$U_s = \frac{1}{2}C_s(4V)^2 = \frac{1}{2}\left(\frac{C_1}{n_1}\right)(4V)^2 \text{ (Using(i))}$$

A parallel combination of n_2 capacitors each of capacitance C_2 are connected to V source as shown in the figure.

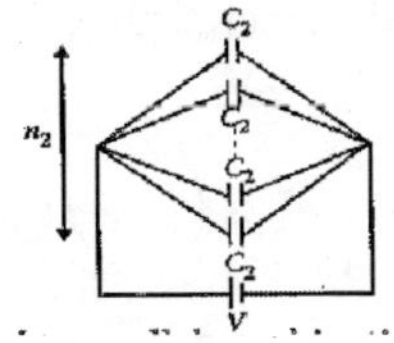

Total capacitance of the parallel combination of capacitors is $C_p = C_2 + C_2 + +$ upto n_2 terms $= n_2C_2$ or $C_p = n_2C_2$

Total energy stored in a parallel combination of capacitors is

$$U_p = \frac{1}{2}C_pV^2 = \frac{1}{2}(n_2C_2)(V)^2 \text{ (Using(iii))}$$

According to the given problem,

$$U_s = U_p$$

Substituting the values of U_s and U_p from equations (ii) and (iv), we get

$$\frac{1}{2}\frac{C_1}{n_1}(4V)^2 = \frac{1}{2}(n_2C_2)(V)^2$$

or $\frac{16C_1}{n_1} = n_2C_2$ or $C_2 = \frac{16C_1}{n_1n_2}$

61. **(b) :** As the capacitors are connected in parallel, therefore potential difference across both the condensers remains the same:

$\therefore\ Q_1 = CV;$

$$Q_2 = \frac{C}{2}V.$$

Also, $Q = Q_1 + Q_2$

$$= CV + \frac{C}{2}V = \frac{3}{2}CV$$

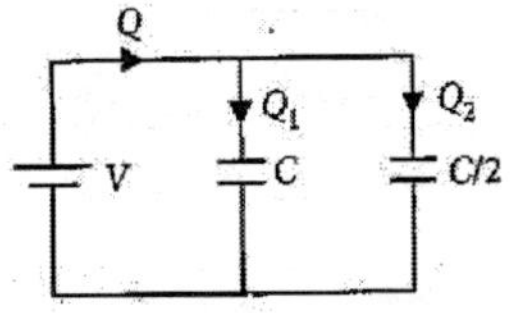

Work done in charging fully both the condensers is given

by $W = \frac{1}{2}QV = \frac{1}{2} \times \left(\frac{3}{2}CV\right)V = \frac{3}{4}CV^2$.

62. (a) : Energy density $= \frac{1}{2}\varepsilon_0 \frac{V^2}{d^2}$

63. (b) : Let q be the charge on each capacitor.

$\therefore$ Energy stored, $U = \frac{1}{2}CV^2 = \frac{1}{2}\frac{q^2}{C}$

Now, when battery is disconnected and another capacitor of same capacity is

connected in parallel to the first capacitor, then voltage across each capacitor, $V = \frac{q}{2C}$

$\therefore$ Energy stored $= \frac{1}{2}C\left(\frac{q}{2C}\right)^2 = \frac{1}{4}\cdot\frac{1}{2}\cdot\frac{q^2}{C} = \frac{1}{4}U$.

64. (d)

Chapter: 17 CURRENT ELECTRICITY

Electric Current

1. A flow of 10^7 electrons per second in a conducting wire constitutes a current of **(1994)**

(a) 1.6×10^{-12} A (b) 1.6×10^{26} A
(c) 1.6×10^{-26} A (d) 1.6×10^{12} A

Ohm's Law

2. The resistance of a wire is ' R ' ohm. If it is melted and stretched to ' n ' times its original length, its new resistance will be **(2017)**

(a) $\frac{R}{n}$ (b) n^2R
(c) $\frac{R}{n^2}$ (d) nR

3. A wire of resistance 4Ω is stretched to twice its original length. The resistance of stretched wire would be **(2013)**

(a) 8Ω (b) 16Ω
(c) 2Ω (d) 4Ω

4. A wire of a certain material is stretched slowly by ten percent. Its new resistance and specific resistance become respectively **(2008)**

(a) both remain the same
(b) 1.1 times, 1.1 times
(c) 1.2 times, 1.1 times
(d) 1.21 times, same

5. The electric resistance of a certain wire of iron is R. If its length and radius are both doubled, then **(2004)**

(a) The resistance will be doubled and the specific resistance will be halved
(b) The resistance will be halved and the specific resistance will remain unchanged
(c) The resistance will be halved and the specific resistance will be doubled
(d) The resistance and the specific resistance, will both remain unchanged.

6. A 6 volt battery is connected to the terminals of a three metre long wire of uniform thickness and resistance of 100ohm. The difference of potential between two points on the wire separated by a distance of 50 cm will be **(2004)**

(a) 2 volt (b) 3 volt
(c) 1 volt (d) 1.5 volt

7. Three copper wires of lengths and cross-sectional areas are $(l, A), (2l, A/2)$ and $(l/2, 2A)$. Resistance is minimum in **(1997)**

(a) wire of cross-sectional area 2 A
(b) wire of cross-sectional area $\frac{A}{2}$
(c) wire of cross-sectional area A
(d) same in all three cases.

8. A wire 50 cm long and $1\ mm^2$ in cross-section carries a current of 4 A when connected to a 2 V battery. The resistivity of the wire is **(1994)**

(a) $4 \times 10^{-6} \Omega m$ (c) $2 \times 10^{-7} \Omega m$

(b) $1 \times 10^{-6} \Omega m$ (d) $5 \times 10^{-7} \Omega m$

9. The masses of the wires of copper is in the ratio of 1: 3: 5 and their lengths are in the ratio of 5: 3: 1. The ratio of their electrical resistance is **(1988)**

(a) 1: 3: 5 (b) 5: 3: 1

(c) 1: 25: 125 (d) 125: 15: 1

Drift of Electrons and the Origin of Resistivity

10. A copper wire of length 10 m and radius $(10^{-2}/\sqrt{\pi})$m has electrical resistance of 10Ω. The current density in the wire for an electric field strength of 10(V/m) is

(2022)

(a) $10^4\ A/m^2$ (b) $10^6\ A/m^2$

(c) $10^{-5}\ A/m^2$ (d) $10^5\ A/m^2$

11. Column-I gives certain physical terms associated with flow of current through a metallic conductor. Column-II gives some mathematical relations involving electrical quantities. Match column-I and column-II with appropriate relations. **(2021)**

Column-I	Column-II
(A) Drift velocity	(P) $\frac{m}{ne^2\rho}$
(B) Electrical Resistivity	(Q) nev $_d$
(C) Relaxation Period	(R) $\frac{eE}{m}\tau$
(D) Current Density	(S) $\frac{E}{J}$

(a) (A)-(R), (B)-(Q), (C)-(S), (D)-(P)

(b) (A)-(R), (B)-(S), (C)-(P), (D)-(Q)

(c) (A)-(R), (B)-(S), (C)-(Q), (D)-(P)

(d) (A)-(R), (B)-(P), (C)-(S), (D)-(Q)

12. A charged particle having drift velocity of $7.5 \times 10^{-4}\ m\ s^{-1}$ in an electric field of $3 \times 10^{-10}\ V\ m^{-1}$, has a mobility in $m^2\ V^{-1}\ s^{-1}$ of **(2020)**

(a) 2.25×10^{15} (b) 2.5×10^6

(c) 2.5×10^{-6} (d) 2.25×10^{-15}

13. The mean free path of electrons in a metal is 4×10^{-8} m. The electric field which can give on an average 2eV energy to an electron in the metal will be in units V/m

(2009)

(a) 5×10^{-11} (b) 8×10^{-11}

(c) 5×10^7 (d) 8×10^7

14. The velocity of charge carriers of current (about 1 ampere) in a metal under normal conditions is of the order of **(1991)**

(a) a fraction of mm/sec

(b) velocity of light

(c) several thousand metres/second

(d) a few hundred metres per second

Limitations of Ohm's Law

15. The resistance of a discharge tube is

(1999)

(a) non-ohmic

(b) ohmic

(c) zero

(d) both (b) and (c)

16. From the graph between current (I) and voltage (V) is shown. Identify the portion corresponding to negative resistance

(1997)

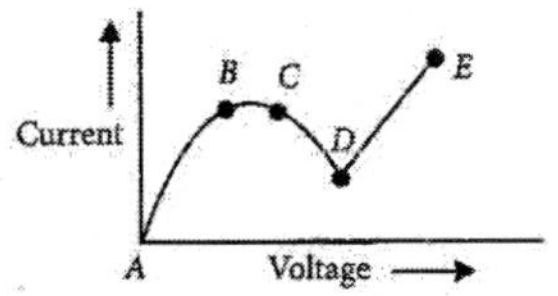

(a) CD (b) DE

(c) AB (d) BC

Temperature Dependence of Resistivity

17. As the temperature increases, the electrical resistance **(2022)**

(a) increase for both conductors and semiconductors

(b) decreases for both conductors and semiconductors

(c) increases for conductors but decrease for semiconductors

(d) decreases for conductors but increases for semiconductors.

18. Which of the following graph represents the variation of resistivity (ρ) with temperature (T) for copper? **(2020)**

(a)
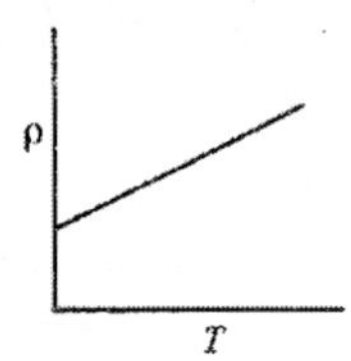

(b)
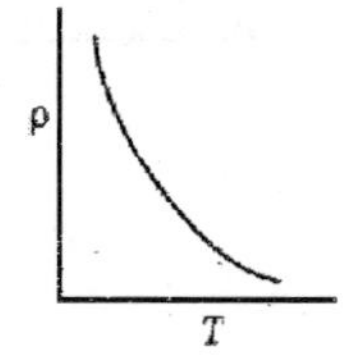

(c)
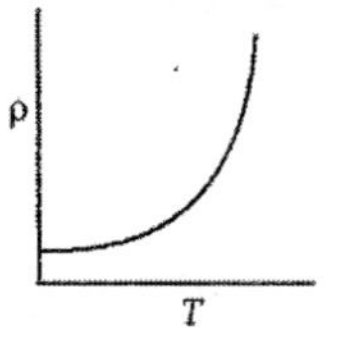

(d)
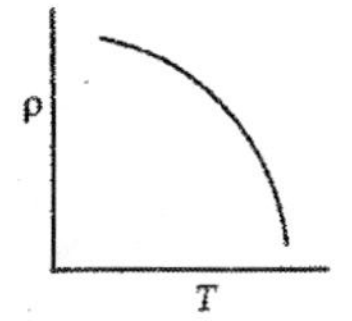

19. The solids which have the negative temperature coefficient of resistance are

(2020)

(a) metals

(b) insulators only

(c) semiconductors only

(d) insulators and semiconductors.

20. Specific resistance of a conductor increases with **(2002)**

(a) increase in temperature

(b) increase in cross-section area

(c) increase in cross-section and decrease in length

(d) decrease in cross-section area.

21. Copper and silicon is cooled from 300 K to 60 K, the specific resistance **(2001)**

(a) decreases in copper but increases in silicon

(b) increases in copper but decreases in silicon

(c) increase in both

(d) decreases in both.

Electrical Energy, Power

22. Two resistors of resistance, 100Ω and 200Ω are connected in parallel in an electrical circuit. The ratio of the thermal energy by developed in 100Ω to that in 200Ω in a given time is **(2022)**

(a) 1: 2 (b) 2: 1

(c) 1: 4 (d) 4: 1

23. Which of the following acts as a circuit protection device? **(2019)**

(a) fuse (b) conductor

(c) inductor (d) switch

24. The charge flowing through a resistance R varies with time t as $Q = at - bt^2$, where a and b are positive constants. The total heat produced in R is **(NEET-I 2016)**

(a) $\frac{a^3R}{2b}$ (b) $\frac{a^3R}{b}$

(c) $\frac{a^3R}{6b}$ (d) $\frac{a^3R}{3b}$

25. Two cities are 150 km apart. Electric power is sent from one city to another city through copper wires. The fall of potential per km is 8 volt and the average resistance per km is 0.5Ω. The power loss in the wire is **(2014)**

(a) 19.2 W (b) 19.2 kW

(c) 19.2 J (d) 12.2 kW

26. If voltage across a bulb rated 220 volt- 100 watt drops by 2.5% of its rated value, the percentage of the rated value by which the power would decrease is **(2012)**

(a) 20% (b) 2.5%

(c) 5% (d) 10%

27. An electric kettle takes 4 A current at 220 V. How much time will it take to boil 1 kg of water from temperature 20°C ? The temperature of boiling water is 100°C. **(2008)**

(a) 12.6 min (b) 4.2 min

(c) 6.3 min (d) 8.4 min

28. A 5 ampere fuse wire can withstand a maximum power of 1 watt in the circuit. The resistance of the fuse wire is **(2005)**

(a) 0.04ohm (b) 0.2ohm

(c) 5ohm (d) 0.4ohm

29. In India electricity is supplied for domestic use at 220 V. It is supplied at 110 V in USA. If the resistance of a 60 W bulb for use in India is R, the resistance of a 60 W bulb for use in USA will be **(2004)**

(a) R (b) $2R$

(c) $R/4$ (d) $R/2$

30. Fuse wire is a wire of **(2003)**

(a) high resistance and high melting point

(b) high resistance and low melting point

(c) low resistance and low melting point

(d) low resistance and high melting point

31. Two bulbs are of (40 W, 200 V), and (100 W, 200 V). Then correct relation for their resistances is **(2000)**

(a) $R_{40} < R_{100}$

(b) $R_{40} > R_{100}$

(c) $R_{40} = R_{100}$

(d) no relation can be predicted.

32. A 5°C rise in temperature is observed in a conductor by passing a current. When the current is doubled the rise in temperature will be approximately **(1998)**

(a) 20°C (b) 16°C

(c) 10°C (d) 12°C

33. A (100 W, 200 V) bulb is connected to a 160 volts supply. The power consumption would be **(1997)**

(a) 100 W (b) 125 W

(c) 64 W (d) 80 W

34. One kilowatt hour is equal to **(1997)**

(a) 36×10^{-5} J (b) 36×10^{-4} J

(c) 36×10^{5} J (d) 36×10^{3} J

35. A 4μF capacitor is charged to 400 V. If its plates are joined through a resistance of 2kΩ, then heat produced in the resistance is **(1995)**

(a) 0.64 J (b) 1.28 J

(c) 0.16 J (d) 0.32 J

36. An electric bulb is rated 60 W, 220 V. The resistance of its filament is **(1994)**

(a) 870Ω (b) 780Ω

(c) 708Ω (d) 807Ω

37. A current of 2 A, passing through a conductor produces 80 J of heat in 10 seconds. The resistance of the conductor in ohm is **(1989)**

(a) 0.5 (b) 2

(c) 4 (d) 20

Combination of Resistors-Series & Parallel

38. Three resistors having resistances r_1, r_2 and r_3 are connected as shown in the given circuit. The ratio $\frac{i_3}{i_1}$ of currents in terms of resistances used in the circuit is **(2021)**

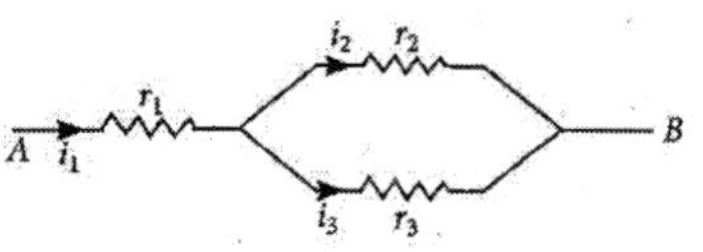

(a) $\frac{r_2}{r_1+r_3}$ (b) $\frac{r_1}{r_2+r_3}$

(c) $\frac{r_2}{r_2+r_3}$ (d) $\frac{r_1}{r_1+r_2}$

39. The effective resistance of a parallel connection that consists of four wires of equal length, equal area of cross-section and same material is 0.25Ω. What will be the effective resistance if they are connected in series? **(2021)**

(a) 4Ω (b) 0.25Ω

(c) 0.5Ω (d) 1Ω

Hence, the equivalent resistance in series will be 4ohm.

40. In the circuits shown below, the readings of the voltmeters and the ammeters will be **(2019)**

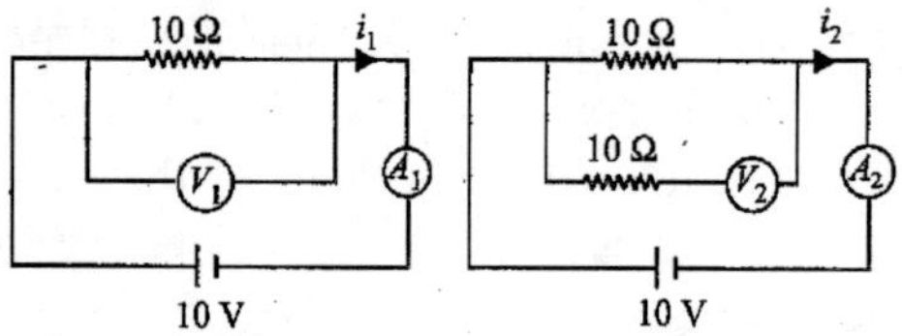

Circuit 1 Circuit 2

(a) $V_2 > V_1$ and $i_1 > i_2$

(b) $V_2 > V_1$ and $i_1 = i_2$

(c) $V_1 = V_2$ and $i_1 > i_2$

(d) $V_1 = V_2$ and $i_1 = i_2$

41. Six similar bulbs are connected as shown in the figure with a DC source of emf E, and zero internal resistance. The ratio of power consumption by the bulbs when (i) all are glowing and (ii) in the situation when two from section A and one from section B are glowing, will be **(2019)**

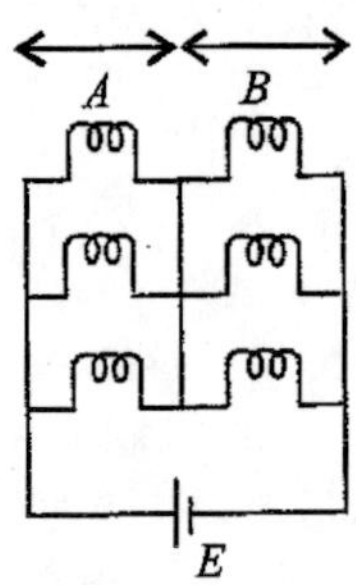

(a) $2:1$ (b) $4:9$

(c) $9:4$ (d) $1:2$

42. A filament bulb $(500\text{ W}, 100\text{ V})$ is to be used in a 230 V main supply. When a resistance R is connected in series, it works perfectly and the bulb consumes 500 W. The value of R is

(NEET-II 2016)

(a) 230Ω (b) 46Ω

(c) 26Ω (d) 13Ω

43. Two metal wires of identical dimensions are connected in series. If σ_1 and σ_2 are the conductivities of the metal wires respectively, the effective conductivity of the combination is **(2015)**

(a) $\frac{\sigma_1+\sigma_2}{\sigma_1\sigma_2}$ (b) $\frac{\sigma_1\sigma_2}{\sigma_1+\sigma_2}$

(c) $\frac{2\sigma_1\sigma_2}{\sigma_1+\sigma_2}$ (d) $\frac{\sigma_1+\sigma_2}{2\sigma_1\sigma_2}$

44. A circuit contains an ammeter, a battery of 30 V and a resistance 40.8ohm all connected in series. If the ammeter has a coil of resistance 480ohm and a shunt of 20ohm, the reading in the ammeter will be

(2015)

(a) 2 A (b) 1 A

(c) 0.5 A (d) 0.25 A

45. A, B and C are voltmeters of resistance $R, 1.5R$ and $3R$ respectively as shown in the figure. When some potential difference is applied between X and Y, the voltmeter readings are V_A, V_B and V_C respectively. Then **(2015 Cancelled)**

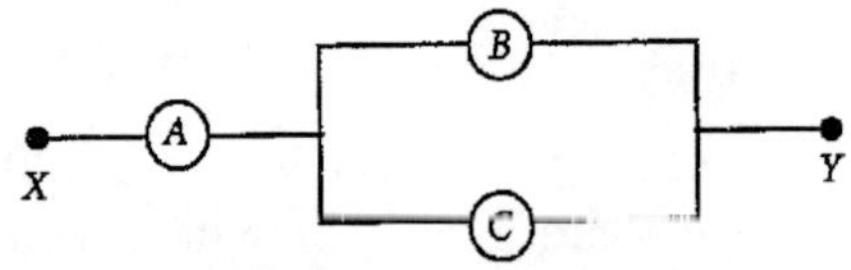

(a) $V_A = V_B \neq V_C$

(b) $V_A \neq V_B \neq V_C$

(c) $V_A = V_B = V_C$

(d) $V_A \neq V_B = V_C$

46. Two rods are joined end to end, as shown. Both have a cross-sectional area of 0.01 cm^2. Each is 1 meter long. One rod is of copper with a resistivity of 1.7×10^{-6} ohm-centimeter, the other is of iron with a resistivity of 10^{-5}ohm-centimeter. How much voltage is required to produce a current of 1 ampere in the rods?

(Karnataka NEET 2013)

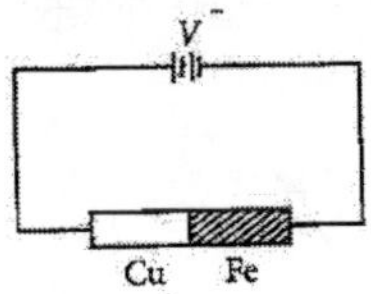

(a) 0.00145 V (b) 0.0145 V

(c) 1.7×10^{-6} V (d) 0.117 V

47. A 12 cm wire is given a shape of a right angled triangle ABC having sides 3 cm, 4 cm and 5 cm as shown in the figure. The resistance between two ends (AB, BC, CA) of the respective sides are measured one by one by a multimeter. The resistances will be in the ratio

(Karnataka NEET 2013)

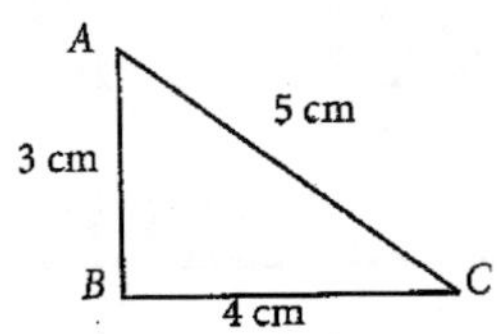

(a) 9: 16: 25 (b) 27: 32: 35

(c) 21: 24: 25 (d) 3: 4: 5

48. A ring is made of a wire having a resistance $R_0 = 12\Omega$. Find the points A and B, as shown in the figure, at which a current carrying conductor should be connected so that the resistance R of the sub circuit between these points is equal to $\frac{8}{3}\Omega$ **(2012)**

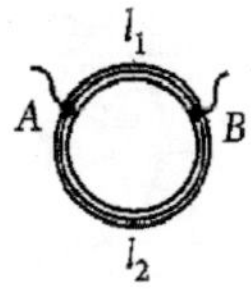

(a) $\frac{l_1}{l_2} = \frac{5}{8}$ (b) $\frac{l_1}{l_2} = \frac{1}{3}$

(c) $\frac{l_1}{l_2} = \frac{3}{8}$ (d) $\frac{l_1}{l_2} = \frac{1}{2}$

49. The power dissipated in the circuit shown in the figure is 30 watts. The value of R is

(Mains 2012)

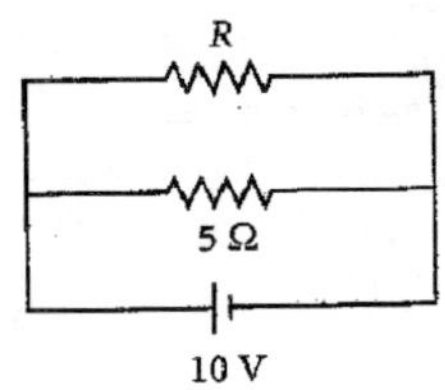

(a) 20Ω (b) 15Ω

(c) 10Ω (d) 30Ω

50. If power dissipated in the 9Ω resistor in the circuit shown is 36watt, the potential difference across the 2Ω resistor is **(2011)**

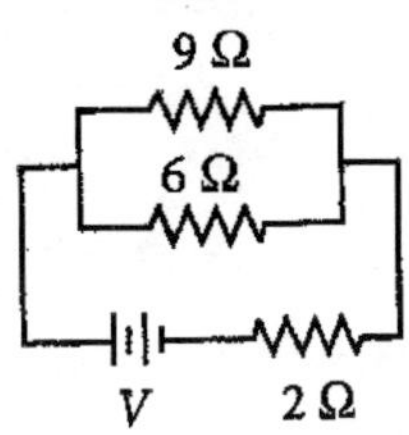

(a) 4 volt (b) 8 volt

(c) 10 volt (d) 2 volt

51. A wire of resistance 12ohms per meter is bent to form a complete circle of radius 10 cm. The resistance between its two diametrically opposite points, A and B as shown in the figure is **(2009)**

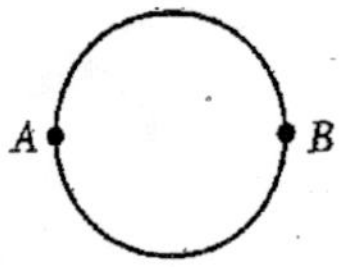

(a) 3Ω (b) 6πΩ

(c) 6Ω (d) 0.6πΩ

52. In the circuit shown, the current through the 4 Ω resistor is 1amp when the points P and M are connected to a d.c. voltage source. The potential difference between the points M and N is **(2008)**

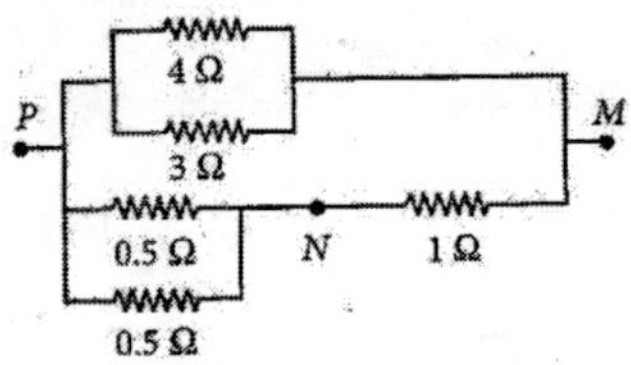

(a) 0.5 volt (b) 3.2 volt

(c) 1.5 volt (d) 1.0 volt

53. A current of 3amp. flows through the 2Ω resistor shown in the circuit. The power dissipated in the 5Ω resistor is **(2008)**

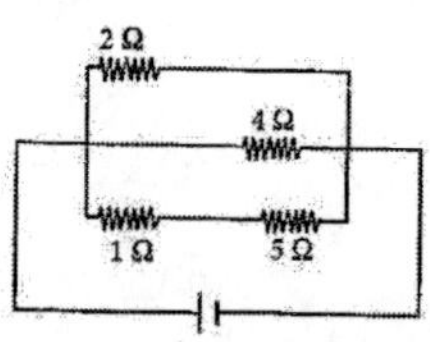

(a) 1 watt (b) 5 watt

(c) 4 watt (d) 2 watt

54. The total power dissipated in watt in the circuit shown here is **(2007)**

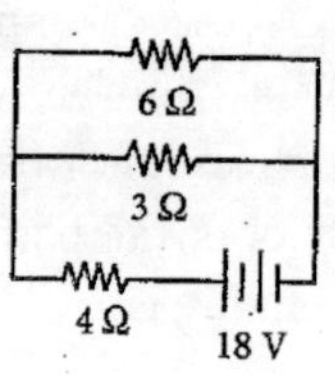

(a) 40 (b) 54

(c) 4 (d) 16

55. Power dissipated across the 8Ω resistor in the circuit shown here is 2 watt. The power dissipated in watt units across the 3Ω resistor is **(2006)**

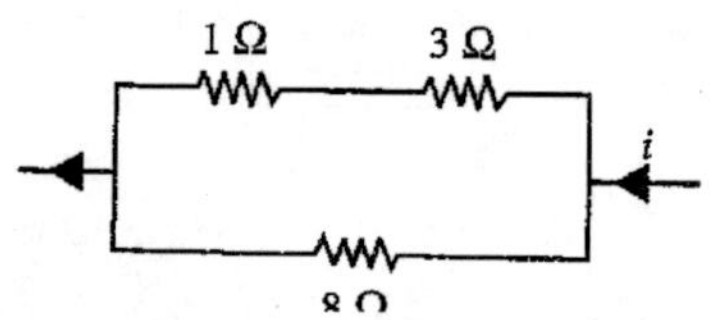

(a) 3.0 (b) 2.0

(c) 1.0 (d) 0.5

56. When a wire of uniform cross-section a, length l and resistance R is bent into a complete circle, resistance between any two of diametrically opposite points will be **(2005)**

(a) $R/4$ (b) $4R$

(c) $R/8$ (d) $R/2$

57. Resistance n, each of $r$ohm, when connected in parallel give an equivalent resistance of Rohm. If these resistances were connected in series, the combination would have a resistance in ohms, equal to **(2004)**

(a) n^2R (b) R/n^2

(c) R/n (d) nR

58. When three identical bulbs of 60 watt, 200 volt rating are connected in series to a 200 volt supply, the power drawn by them will be **(2004)**

(a) 60 watt (b) 180 watt

(c) 10 watt (d) 20 watt

59. Two 220 volt, 100 watt bulbs are connected first in series and then in parallel. Each time the combination is connected to a 220 volt a.c. supply line. The power drawn by the combination in each case respectively will be **(2003)**

(a) 50 watt, 100 watt

(b) 100 watt, 50 watt

(c) 200 watt, 150 watt

(d) 50 watt, 200 watt

60. An electric kettle has two heating coils. When one of the coils is connected to an a.c. source, the water in the kettle boils in 10 minutes. When the other coil is used the water boils in 40 minutes. If both the coils are connected in parallel, the time taken by the same quantity of water to boil will be **(2003)**

(a) 8 minutes (b) 4 minutes

(c) 25 minutes (d) 15 minutes

61. The current in the given circuit is **(1999)**

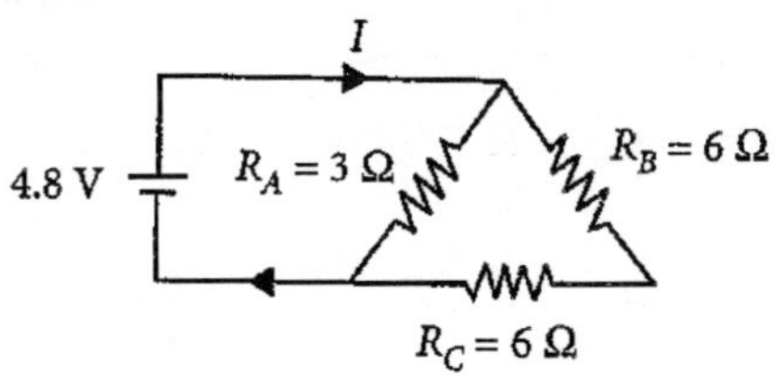

(a) 4.9 A (b) 6.8 A

(c) 8.3 A (d) 2.0 A

62. Three equal resistors connected in series across a source of e.m.f. together dissipate 10 watt of power. What will be the power dissipated in watt if the same resistors are connected in parallel across the same source of e.m.f.? **(1998)**

(a) 30 (b) $\frac{10}{3}$

(c) 10 (d) 90

63. The current in the following circuit is **(1997)**

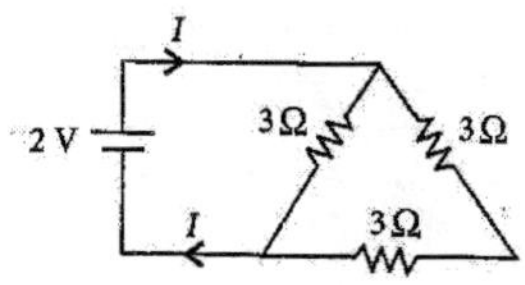

(a) 2/3 A (b) 1 A

(c) 1/8 A (d) 2/9 A

64. If two bulbs, whose resistances are in the ratio of 1: 2 are connected in series, the power dissipated in them has the ratio of **(1997)**

(a) 2: 1 (b) 1: 4

(c) 1: 1 (d) 1: 2.

65. What will be the equivalent resistance between the two points A and ? **(1996)**

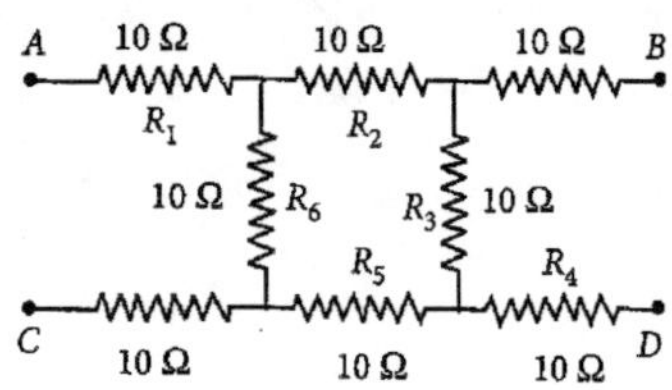

(a) 30Ω (b) 40Ω

(c) 20Ω (d) 10Ω.

66. Two wires of the same metal have same length, but their cross-sections are in the ratio 3: 1. They are joined in series. The resistance of thicker wire is 10Ω. The total resistance of the combination will be

(1995)

(a) 40Ω (b) 100Ω

(c) $(5/2)\Omega$ (d) $(40/3)\Omega$.

67. A heating coil is labelled $100\ W, 220\ V$. The coil is cut in half and the two pieces are joined in parallel to the same source. The energy now liberated per second is

(1995)

(a) 200 W (b) 400 W

(c) 25 W (d) 50 W

68. Six resistors of 3Ω each are connected along the sides of a hexagon and three resistors of 6Ω each are connected along AC, AD and AE as shown in the figure. The equivalent resistance between A and B is equal to **(1994)**

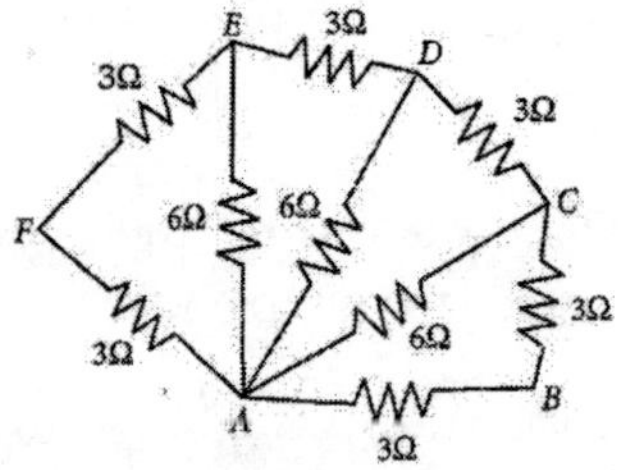

(a) 2Ω (b) 6Ω

(c) 3Ω (d) 9Ω

69. Three resistances each of 4Ω are connected to form a triangle. The resistance between any two terminals is

(1993)

(a) 12Ω (b) 2Ω

(c) 6Ω (d) $8/3\Omega$

70. Current through 3Ω resistor is 0.8 ampere, then potential drop through 4Ω resistor is

(1993)

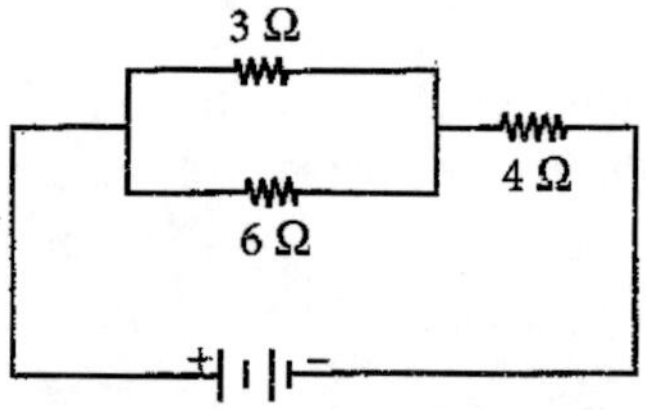

(a) 9.6 V (b) 2.6 V

(c) 4.8 V (d) 1.2 V

71. In the network shown in figure each resistance is 1Ω. The effective resistance between A and B is

(1990)

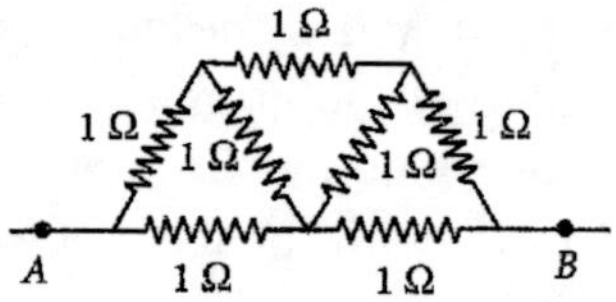

(a) $\frac{4}{3}\Omega$ (b) $\frac{3}{2}\Omega$

(c) 7Ω (d) $\frac{8}{7}\Omega$

72. You are given several identical resistances each of value $R = 10\Omega$ and each capable of carrying a maximum current of one ampere. It is required to make a suitable combination of these resistances of 5Ω which can carry a current of 4 ampere. The minimum number of resistances of the type R that will be required for this job is

(1990)

(a) 4 (b) 10

(c) 8 (d) 20

73. 40 electric bulbs are connected in series across a 220 V supply. After one bulb is fused the remaining 39 are connected again in series across the same supply. The illumination will be **(1989)**

(a) more with 40 bulbs than with 39

(b) more with 39 bulbs than with 40

(c). equal in both the cases

(d) in the ratio $40^2 : 39^2$.

74. n equal resistors are first connected in series and then connected in parallel. What is the ratio of the maximum to the minimum resistance? **(1989)**

(a) n (b) $1/n^2$

(c) n^2 (d) $1/n$

Cells, EMF, Internal Resistance

75. A set of n equal resistors, of value R each, are connected in series to a battery of emf E and internal resistance R. The current drawn is I. Now, the n resistors are connected in parallel to the same battery. Then the current drawn from battery becomes $10I$. The value of n is **(2018)**

(a) 10 (b) 11

(c) 20 (d) 9

76. The internal resistance of a 2.1 V cell which gives a current of 0.2 A through a resistance of 10Ω is **(2013)**

(a) 0.8Ω (b) 1.0Ω

(c) 0.2Ω (d) 0.5Ω

77. A cell having an emf ε and internal resistance r is connected across a variable external resistance R. As the resistance R is increased, the plot of potential difference V across R is given by

(Mains 2012)

(a) 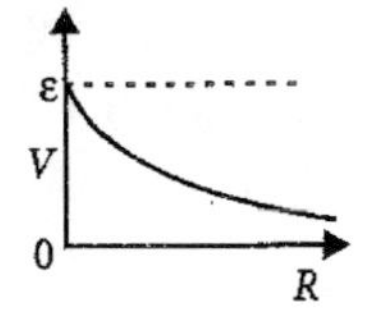

(b) 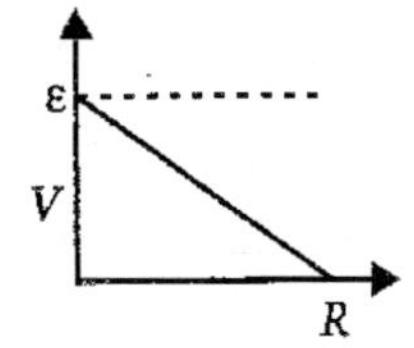

(c) 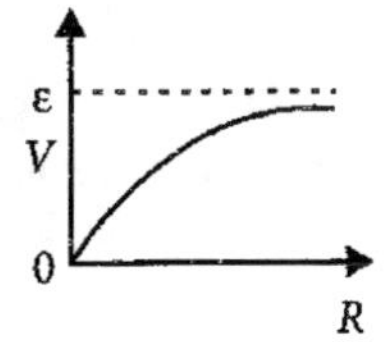

(d) 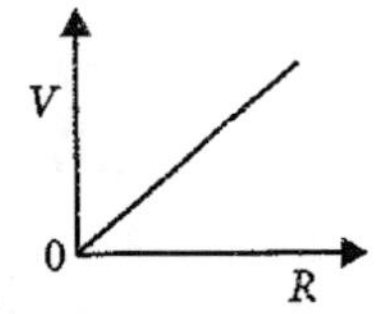

78. A current of 2 A flows through a 2Ω resistor when connected across a battery. The same battery supplies a current of 0.5 A when connected across a 9Ω resistor. The internal resistance of the battery is

(2011)

(a) 0.5Ω (b) $1/3\Omega$

(c) $1/4\Omega$ (d) 1Ω

79. A student measures the terminal potential difference (V) of a cell (of emf ε and internal resistance) as a function of the current (I) flowing through it. The slope,

and intercept, of the graph between V and I, then, respectively, equal **(2009)**

(a) $-r$ and ε (b) r and $-\varepsilon$

(c) $-\varepsilon$ and r (d) ε and $-r$

80. For a cell terminal potential difference is 2.2 V when circuit is open and reduces to 1.8 V when cell is connected to a resistance of $R = 5\Omega$. Determine internal resistance of cell (r). **(2002)**

(a) $\frac{10}{9}\Omega$ (b) $\frac{9}{10}\Omega$

(c) $\frac{11}{9}\Omega$ (d) $\frac{5}{9}\Omega$

81. A car battery of emf 12 V and internal resistance $5 \times 10^{-2}\Omega$, receives a current of 60amp from external source, then terminal potential difference of battery is

(2000)

(a) 12 V (b) 9 V

(c) 15 V (d) 20 V

82. The internal resistance of a cell of e.m.f. 2 V is 0.1Ω. It is connected to a resistance of 3.9Ω. The voltage across the cell will be

(1999)

(a) 1.95 V (b) 1.9 V

(c) 0.5 V (d) 2 V

83. A battery of e.m.f 10 V and internal resistance 0.5Ω is connected across a variable resistance R. The value of R for which the power delivered in it is maximum is given by **(1992)**

(a) 0.5Ω (b) 1.0Ω

(c) 2.0Ω (d) 0.25Ω

Cells in Series and in Parallel

84. The magnitude and direction of the current in the following circuit is **(2023)**

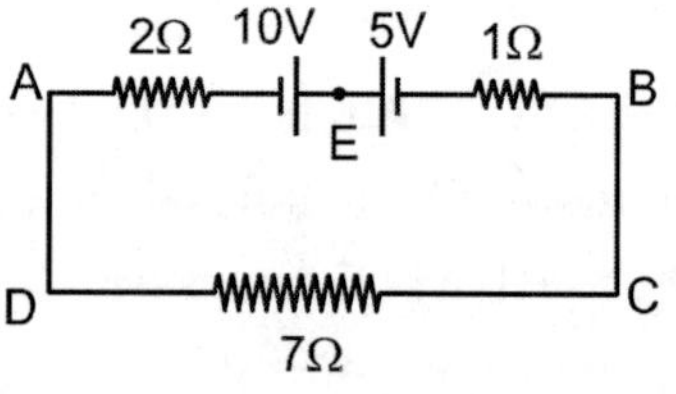

(a) 0.5 A from A to B through E

(b) $\frac{5}{9}$ A from A to B through E

(c) 1.5 A from B to A through E

(d) 0.2 A from B to A through E

85. If the galvanometer G does not show any deflection in the circuit shown, the value of R is given by **(2023)**

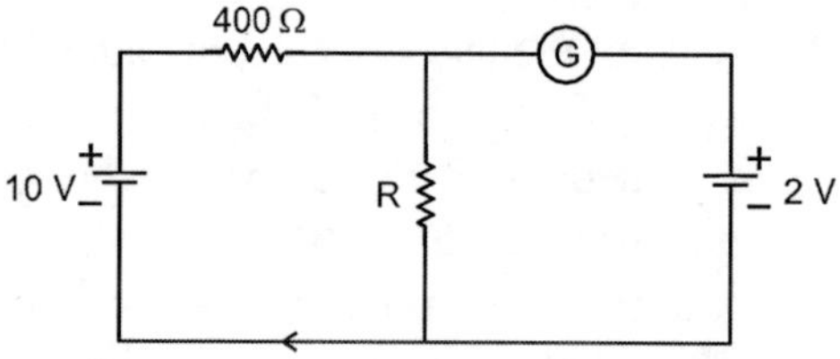

(a) 50 Ω (b) 100 Ω

(c) 400 Ω (d) 200 Ω

86. 10 resistors, each of resistance R are connected in series to a battery of emf E and negligible internal resistance. Then those are connected in parallel to the same battery, the current is increased n times. The value of n is **(2023)**

(a) 100 (b) 1

(c) 1000 (d) 10

87. A battery consists of a variable number n of identical cells (having internal resistance r each) which are connected in series. The terminals of the battery are short-circuited and the current I is measured. Which of the graphs shows the correct relationship between I and ?

(2018)

(a) 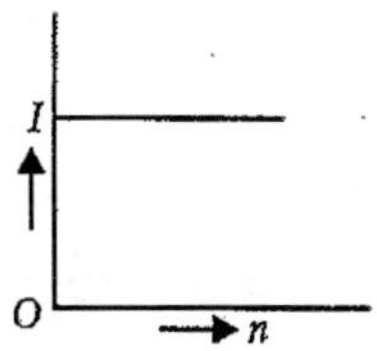

(b) 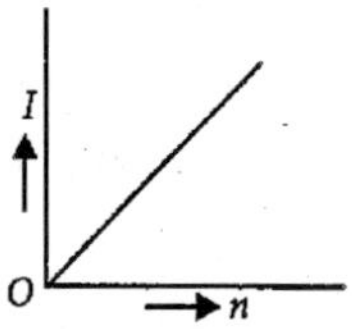

(c) 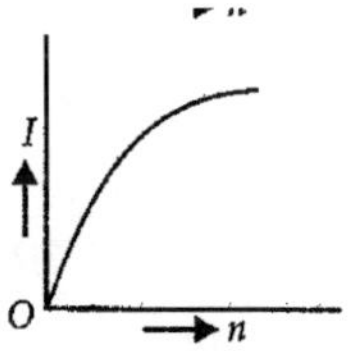

(d) 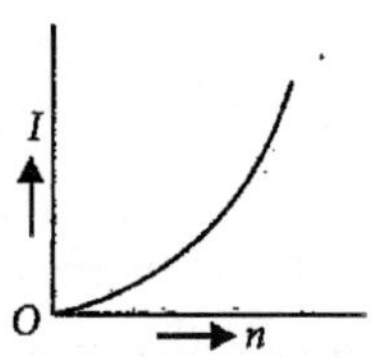

88. Ten identical cells connected in series are needed to heat a wire of length one meter and radius ' r ' by 10°C in time ' t '. How many cells will be required to heat the wire of length two meter of the same radius by the same temperature in time ' t '?

(Karnataka NEET 2013)

(a) 20 (b) 30
(c) 40 (d) 10

89. Two cells, having the same e.m.f. are connected in series through an external resistance R. Cells have internal resistances r_1 and $r_2 (r_1 > r_2)$ respectively. When the circuit is closed, the potential difference across the first cell is zero. The value of R is **(2006)**

(a) $r_1 + r_2$ (b) $r_1 - r_2$
(c) $\frac{r_1+r_2}{2}$ (d) $\frac{r_1-r_2}{2}$

90. Two batteries, one of emf 18 volts and internal resistance 2Ω and the other of emf 12 volts and internal resistance 1Ω, are connected as shown. The voltmeter V will record a reading of **(2005)**

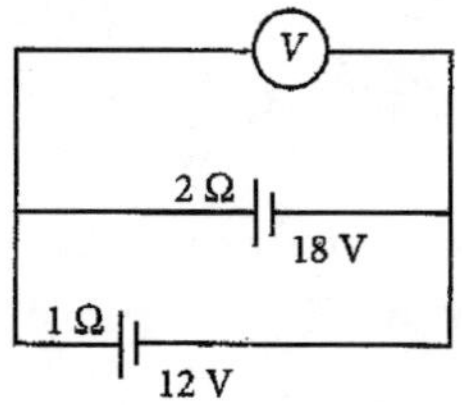

(a) 30 volt (b) 18 volt
(c) 15 volt (d) 14 volt

91. Two identical batteries each of e.m.f 2 V and internal resistance 1Ω are available to produce heat in an external resistance by passing a current through it. The maximum power that can be developed across R using these batteries is **(1990)**

(a) 3.2 W (b) 2.0 W
(c) 1.28 W (d) $\frac{8}{9}$ W

92. Two batteries of emf 4 V and 8 V with internal resistance 1Ω and 2Ω are connected in a circuit with resistance of 9Ω as shown in figure.

The current and potential difference between the points P and Q are **(1988)**

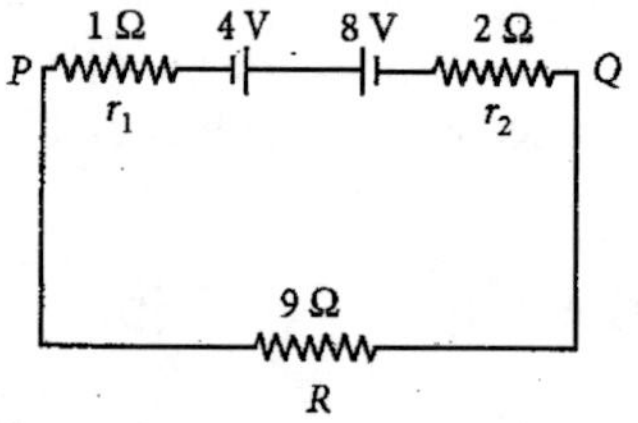

(a) $\frac{1}{3}$ A and 3 V

(b) $\frac{1}{6}$ A and 4 V

(c) $\frac{1}{9}$ A and 9 V

(d) $\frac{1}{12}$ A and 12 V

Kirchhoff's Rules

93. The potential difference $(V_A - V_B)$ between the points A and B in the given figure is **(NEET-II 2016)**

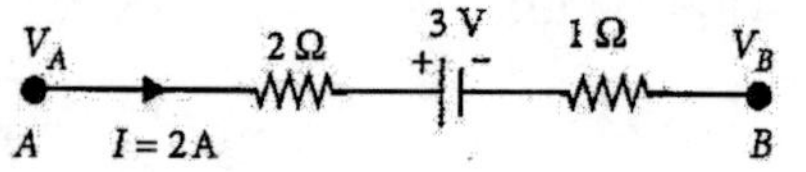

(a) -3 V (b) $+3$ V

(c) $+6$ V (d) $+9$ V

94. In the circuit shown the cells A and B have negligible resistances. For $V_A = 12$ V, $R_1 = 500\Omega$ and $R = 100\Omega$ the galvanometer (G) shows no deflection. The value of V_B is **(2012)**

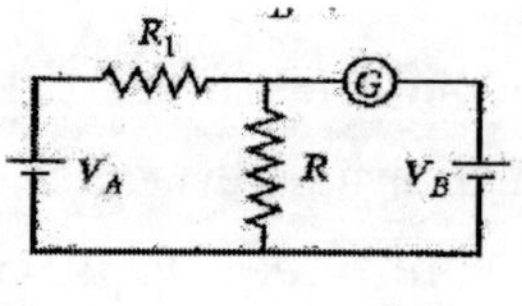

(a) 4 V (b) 2 V

(c) 12 V (d) 6 V

95. In the circuit shown in the figure, if the potential at point A is taken to be zero, the potential at point B is **(Mains 2011)**

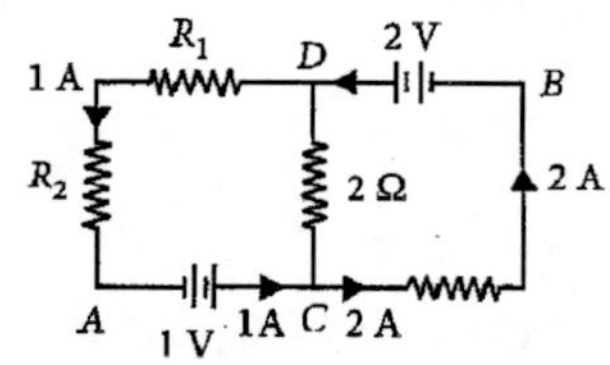

(a) $+1$ V (b) -1 V

(c) $+2$ V (d) -2 V

96. Consider the following two statements.

(A) Kirchhoff's junction law follows from the conservation of charge.

(B) Kirchhoff's loop law follows from the conservation of energy.

Which of the following is correct? **(2010)**

(a) Both (A) and (B) are wrong.

(b) (A) is correct and (B) is wrong.

(c) (A) is wrong and (B) is correct.

(d) Both (A) and (B) are correct.

97. See the electrical circuit shown in this figure. Which of the following equations is a correct equation for it? **(2009)**

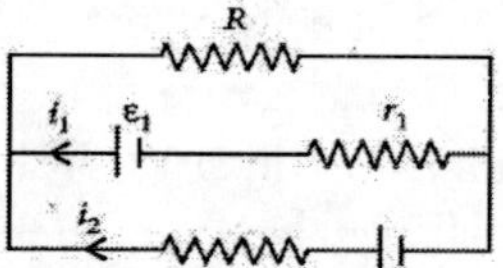

(a) $\varepsilon_2 - i_2 r_2 - \varepsilon_1 - i_1 r_1 = 0$

(b) $-\varepsilon_2 - (i_1 + i_2)R + i_2 r_2 = 0$

(c) $\varepsilon_1 - (i_1 + i_2)R + i_1 r_1 = 0$

(d) $\varepsilon_1 - (i_1 + i_2)R - i_1 r_1 = 0$

98. Kirchhoff's first and second laws of electrical circuits are consequences of **(2006)**

(a) conservation of energy and electric charge respectively

(b) conservation of energy

(c) conservation of electric charge and energy respectively

(d) conservation of electric charge.

99. Kirchhoff's first law, i.e. $\Sigma i = 0$ at a junction, deals with the conservation of **(1997, 1992)**

(a) momentum

(b) angular momentum

(c) charge

(d) energy

Wheatstone Bridge

100. A wheatstone bridge is used to determine the value of unknown resistance X by adjusting the variable resistance Y as shown in the figure. For the most precise measurement of X, the resistances P and Q **(2022)**

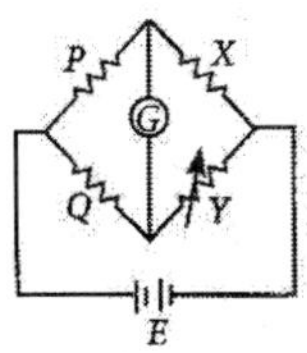

(a) should be approximately equal to $2X$.

(b) should be approximately equal and are small

(c) should be very large and unequal

(d) do not play any significant role

101. The resistances of the four arms P, Q, R and S in a Wheatstone's bridge are 10ohm, 30ohm, 30ohm and 90ohm, respectively. The e.m.f. and internal resistance of the cell are 7 volt and 5ohm respectively. If the galvanometer resistance is 50ohm, the current drawn from the cell will be **(2013)**

(a) 0.1 A (b) 2.0 A

(c) 1.0 A (d) 0.2 A

102. Three resistances P, Q, R each of 2Ω and an unknown resistance S form the four arms of a Wheatstone bridge circuit. When a resistance of 6Ω is connected in parallel to S the bridge gets balanced. What is the value of ? **(2007)**

(a) 3Ω (b) 6Ω

(c) 1Ω (d) 2Ω

103. In the circuit shown, if a conducting wire is connected between points A and B, the current in this wire will **(2006)**

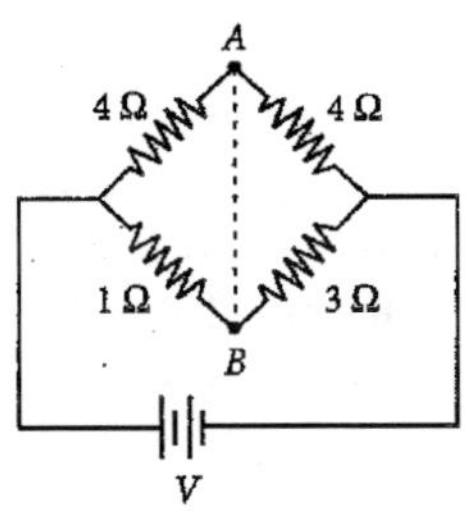

(a) flow from B to A

(b) flow from A to B

(c) flow in the direction which will be decided by the value of V

(d) be zero.

104. For the network shown in the figure the value of the current i is **(2005)**

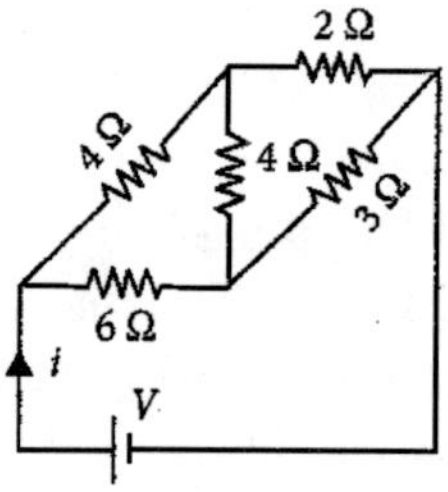

(a) $\frac{9V}{35}$ (b) $\frac{18V}{5}$

(c) $\frac{5V}{9}$ (d) $\frac{5V}{18}$

105. Five equal resistances each of resistance R are connected as shown in the figure. A battery of V volts is connected between A and B. The current flowing in AFCEB will be **(2004)**

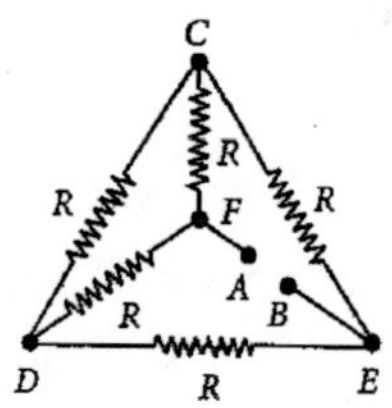

(a) $\frac{3V}{R}$ (b) $\frac{V}{R}$

(c) $\frac{V}{2R}$ (d) $\frac{2V}{R}$

106. In a Wheatstone's bridge all the four arms have equal resistance R. If the resistance of the galvanometer arm is also R, the equivalent resistance of the combination as seen by the battery is **(2003)**

(a) $R/4$ (b) $R/2$

(c) R (d) $2R$

107. The resistance of each arm of the Wheatstone's bridge is 10ohm. A resistance of 10ohm is connected in series with a galvanometer then the equivalent resistance across the battery will be **(2001)**

(a) 10ohm (b) 15ohm

(c) 20ohm (d) 40ohm

108. The net resistance of the circuit between A and B is **(2000)**

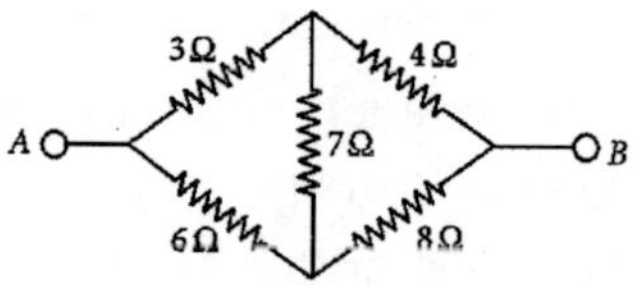

(a) $\frac{8}{3}\Omega$ (b) $\frac{14}{3}\Omega$

(c) $\frac{16}{3}\Omega$ (d) $\frac{22}{3}\Omega$

109. In the network shown in the figure, each of the resistance is equal to 2Ω. The resistance between the points A and B is **(1995)**

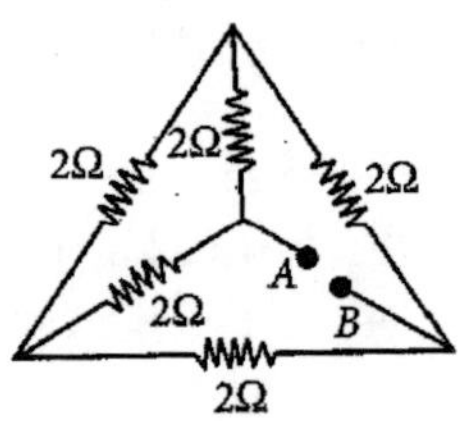

(a) 3Ω (b) 4Ω

(c) 1Ω (d) 2Ω

Metre Bridge

110. A resistance wire connected in the left gap of a metre bridge balances a 10Ω resistance in the right gap at a point which divides the bridge wire in the ratio 3: 2. If the length of the resistance wire is 1.5 m, then the length of 1Ω of the resistance wire is **(2020)**

(a) 1.0×10^{-2} m (b) 1.0×10^{-1} m

(c) 1.5×10^{-1} m (d) 1.5×10^{-2} m

111. The metre bridge shown is in balance position with $\frac{P}{Q} = \frac{l_1}{l_2}$. If we now interchangc the positions of galvanometer and cell, will the bridge work? If yes, what will be balanced condition?

(Odisha NEET 2019)

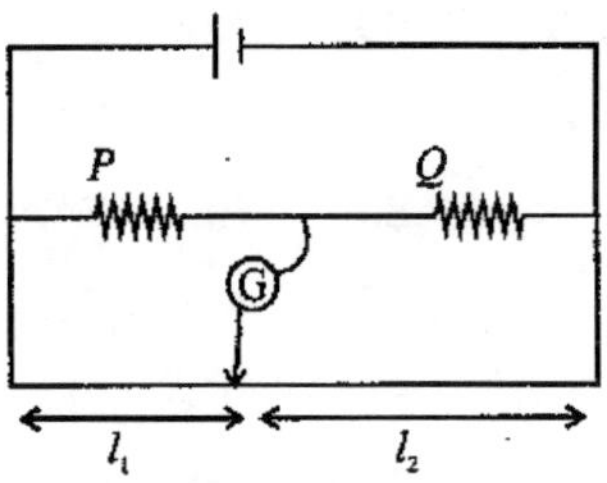

(a) yes, $\frac{P}{Q} = \frac{l_2 - l_1}{l_2 + l_1}$

(b) no, no null point

(c) yes, $\frac{P}{Q} = \frac{l_2}{l_1}$

(d) yes, $\frac{P}{Q} = \frac{l_1}{l_2}$

112. The resistances in the two arms of the meter bridge are 5Ω and RΩ respectively. When the resistance R is shunted with an equal resistance, the new balance point is at $1.6l_1$. The resistance R is **(2014)**

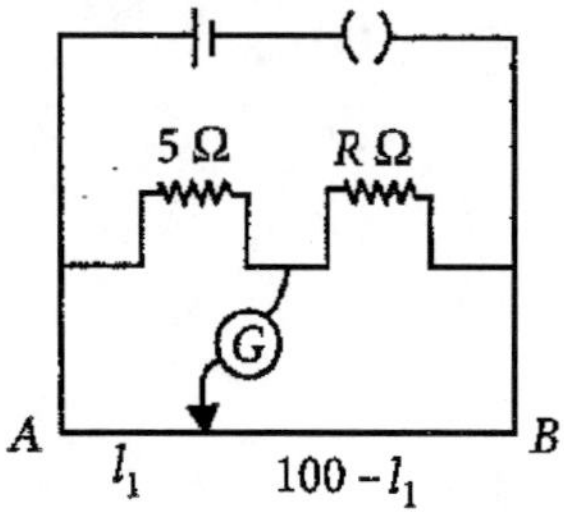

(a) 10Ω (b) 15Ω

(c) 20Ω (d) 25Ω

113. In a metre bridge, the balancing length from the left end (standard resistance of one ohm is in the right gap) is found to be 20 cm. The value of the unknown resistance is **(1999)**

(a) 0.8Ω (b) 0.5Ω

(c) 0.4Ω (d) 0.25Ω

ANSWER KEY

1.	(a)	2.	(b)	3.	(b)	4.	(d)	5.	(b)	6.	(c)	7.	(a)
8.	(b)	9.	(d)	10.	(d)	11.	(b)	12.	(b)	13.	(c)	14.	(a)
15.	(a)	16.	(a)	17.	(c)	18.	(c)	19.	(d)	20.	(a)	21.	(a)
22.	(b)	23.	(a)	24.	(c)	25.	(b)	26.	(c)	27.	(c)	28.	(a)
29.	(c)	30.	(b)	31.	(b)	32.	(a)	33.	(c)	34.	(c)	35.	(d)
36.	(d)	37.	(b)	38.	(c)	39.	(a)	40.	(d)	41.	(c)	42.	(c)
43.	(c)	44.	(c)	45.	(c)	46.	(d)	47.	(b)	48.	(d)	49.	(c)
50.	(c)	51.	(d)	52.	(b)	53.	(b)	54.	(b)	55.	(a)	56.	(a)
57.	(a)	58.	(d)	59.	(d)	60.	(a)	61.	(d)	62.	(d)	63.	(b)
64.	(d)	65.	(a)	66.	(a)	67.	(b)	68.	(a)	69.	(d)	70.	(c)
71.	(d)	72.	(c)	73.	(b)	74.	(c)	75.	(a)	76.	(d)	77.	(c)
78.	(b)	79.	(a)	80.	(a)	81.	(c)	82.	(a)	83.	(a)	84.	(a)
85.	(2)	86.	(1)	87.	(a)	88.	(a)	89.	(b)	90.	(d)	91.	(b)
92.	(a)	93.	(d)	94.	(b)	95.	(a)	96.	(d)	97.	(d)	98.	(c)
99.	(c)	100.	(b)	101.	(d)	102.	(a)	103.	(a)	104.	(d)	105.	(c)
106.	(c)	107.	(a)	108.	(b)	109.	(d)	110.	(b)	111.	(d)	112.	(b)
113.	(d)												

Hints & Explanations

1. **(a) :** Flow of electrons, $\frac{n}{t} = 10^7/$ second

Therefore, current$(I) = \frac{q}{t} = \frac{ne}{t} = \frac{n}{t} \times e$

$= 10^7 \times (1.6 \times 10^{-19}) = 1.6 \times 10^{-12}$ A

2. **(b) :** The resistance of a wire of length l and area A and resistivity ρ is given as

$$R = \frac{\rho l}{A}$$

Given, $l' = nl$

As the volume of the wire remains constant

$\therefore A'l' = Al$ or $A' = \frac{Al}{l'} = \frac{Al}{nl}$ or $A' = \frac{A}{n}$

$\therefore R' = \frac{\rho l'}{A'}$ or $R' = \frac{\rho nl}{\frac{A}{n}} = \frac{n^2 \rho l}{A} = n^2 R$

3. **(b) :** Resistance of a wire, $R = \rho \frac{l}{A} = 4\Omega$

When wire is stretched twice, its new length be l'. Then

$$l' = 2l$$

On stretching volume of the wire remains constant.

$\therefore lA = l'A'$ where A' is the new cross-sectional area

or $A' = \frac{l}{l'}A = \frac{l}{2l}A = \frac{A}{2}$

$\therefore$ Resistance of the stretched wire is

$$R' = \rho\frac{l'}{A'} = \rho\frac{2l}{(A/2)} = 4\rho\frac{l}{A}$$
$$= 4(4\Omega) = 16\Omega \text{ (Using (i))}$$

4. **(d) :** $\frac{\Delta l}{l} = 0.1 \therefore l = 1.1$

But the area also decreases by 0.1 .

Mass $= \rho lA = V\rho, \ln l + \ln A = \ln$ mass.

$$\therefore \frac{\Delta l}{l} + \frac{\Delta A}{A} = 0 \Rightarrow \frac{\Delta l}{l} = \frac{-\Delta A}{A}$$

Length increases by 0.1 , resistance increases, area decreases by 0.1 , then also resistance will increase. Total increase in resistance is approximately 1.2 times, due to increase in length and decrease in area. But specific resistance does not change.

5. **(b) :** Resistance of wire $= \rho\frac{l}{A}$

$$R \propto \frac{l}{A} = \frac{l}{\pi r^2}$$

When length and radius are both doubled

$$R_1 \propto \frac{2l}{\pi(2r)^2} \Rightarrow R_1 \propto \frac{1}{2}R$$

The specific resistance of wire is independent of geometry of the wire, it only depends on the material of the wire.

6. **(c)** : According to given parameters in question

$$R = \rho\frac{l}{A} \Rightarrow 100\Omega = \rho\frac{3}{A} \Rightarrow \frac{\rho}{A} = \frac{100}{3}.$$

Thus total resistance of 50 cm wire is

$$R_1 = \frac{\rho}{A}l = \frac{100}{3} \times 0.5 = \frac{50}{3}\Omega$$

The total current in the wire is $= \frac{6}{100}$ A.

Therefore potential difference across the two points on the wire separated by a distance of 50 m is

$$V = IR_1 = \frac{50}{3} \times \frac{6}{100} = 1 \text{ V}$$

7. **(a)** : Three wires of lengths and cross-sectional areas $= (l, A)$, $(2l, A/2)$ and $(l/2, 2A)$.

Resistance of a wire $R \propto \frac{l}{A}$

For Ist wire, $R_1 \propto l/A = R$

For II nd wire, $R_2 \propto \frac{2l}{A/2} = 4R$

For III rd wire, $R_3 \propto \frac{l/2}{2A} = \frac{R}{4}$

Therefore resistance of the wire will be minimum for IIIrd wire.

8. **(b) :** Length $(l) = 50$ cm $= 0.5$ m;

Area $(A) = 1 \text{ mm}^2 = 1 \times 10^{-6} \text{ m}^2$;

Current $(I) = 4$ A and voltage $(V) = 2$ volts.

Resistance $(R) = \frac{V}{I} = \frac{2}{4} = 0.5\Omega$

$$\text{Resistivity}(\rho) = R \times \frac{A}{l} = 0.5 \times \frac{1 \times 10^{-6}}{0.5}$$
$$= 1 \times 10^{-6}\Omega\text{m}$$

9. **(d) :** $m = l \times \text{area} \times \text{density}$

Area $\propto \frac{m}{l}$

$$R \propto \frac{l}{\text{Area}} \propto \frac{l^2}{m}$$

$$R_1 : R_2 : R_3 = \frac{l_1^2}{m_1} : \frac{l_2^2}{m_2} : \frac{l_3^2}{m_3}$$

$$R_1 : R_2 : R_3 = \frac{25}{1} : \frac{9}{3} : \frac{1}{5} = 125 : 15 : 1$$

10. (d) : length, $l = 10$ m

radius, $r = \frac{10^{-2}}{\sqrt{\pi}} m$

Resistance, $R = 10\Omega$

Electric field, $E = 10$ V/m

The current density, $j = \sigma E = \frac{E}{\rho}$

So, $\rho = \frac{RA}{l} = \frac{10 \times \pi \times \frac{10^{-4}}{\pi}}{10} = 10^{-4}\Omega\text{m}$

From equation (i),

$$V = \frac{10}{10^{-4}} = 10^5 \text{ A/m}^2$$

11. (b) : The formula of drift velocity is

$v_d = \frac{eE}{m}\tau$

Current density $J = \frac{I}{A} = \frac{neAv_d}{A} = nev_d$

Resistivity is $\rho = \frac{m}{ne^2\tau} \Rightarrow \tau = \frac{m}{ne^2\rho}$

Resistance is $R = \frac{V}{I}$

$$\rho\frac{l}{A} = \frac{El}{I} \Rightarrow \rho = \frac{EA}{I} = \frac{E}{J}$$

where, E = electric field, A = area of cross section e = electronic charge, n = number of density of electrons, τ = relaxation time.

12. (b) : Here, $v_d = 7.5 \times 10^{-4}$ m/s, $E = 3 \times 10^{-10}$ V/m

Mobility, $\mu = \frac{v_d}{E} = \frac{7.5 \times 10^{-4}}{3 \times 10^{-10}}$

$$\mu = 2.5 \times 10^6$$

13. (c) : Energy = 2eV = $eE\lambda$

$$\therefore E = \frac{2}{\lambda} = \frac{2}{4 \times 10^{-8}} = 5 \times 10^7 \text{ V/m}$$

14. (a) **15. (a)**

16. (a) : For the negative resistance, when we increase the voltage, the current will decrease. Therefore from the graph, we find that the current in CD is decreased when voltage is increased.

17. (c) : The temperature coefficient of resistance (α) is positive for conductors and negative for insulators.

So, as the temperature increases, the resistance of conductor increases and for semi conductors decreases.

18. (c) : For metals, resistivity versus time graph is

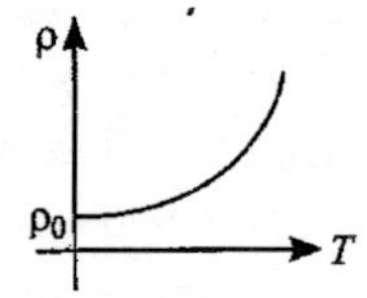

19. (d)

20. (a) : Specific resistance is a property of a material and it increases with the increase of temperature, but not vary with the dimensions (length, cross-section) of the conductor.

21. (a) : For metal specific resistance decreases with decrease in temperature whereas for semiconductor specific resistance increases with decrease in temperature.

22. **(b)** : The two resistances are connected in parallel, so, they both have same potential difference as V.

Heat energy is given by:

$$H = \frac{V^2}{R}t$$

o, $H_1 = \frac{V^2}{100}t$

$$H_2 = \frac{V^2}{200}t$$

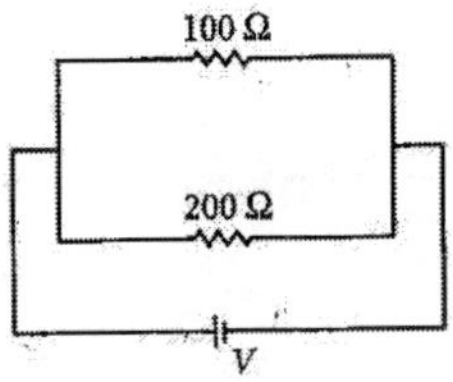

So, $\frac{H_1}{H_2} = \frac{200}{100} = 2:1$

23. **(a) :** Fuse is an electrical safety device that operates to provide over current protection to an electrical circuit.

24. **(c)** : Given, $Q = at - bt^2$

$$\therefore I = \frac{dQ}{dt} = a - 2bt$$

At $t = 0, Q = 0 \Rightarrow I = 0$

Also, $I = 0$ at $t = a/2b$

$\therefore$ Total heat produced in resistance R,

$$H = \int_0^{a/2b} I^2 R dt = R\int_0^{a/2b} (a - 2bt)^2 dt$$

$$= R\int_0^{a/2b} (a^2 + 4b^2t^2 - 4abt)dt$$

$$= R\left[a^2t + 4b^2\frac{t^3}{3} - 4ab\frac{t^2}{2}\right]_0^{a/2b}$$

$$= R\left[a^2 \times \frac{a}{2b} + \frac{4b^2}{3} \times \frac{a^3}{8b^3} - \frac{4ab}{2} \times \frac{a^2}{4b^2}\right]$$

$$= \frac{a^3R}{b}\left[\frac{1}{2} + \frac{1}{6} - \frac{1}{2}\right] = \frac{a^3R}{6b}$$

25. **(b)** : Here,

Distance between two cities = 150 km

Resistance of the wire, $R = (0.5\Omega\text{km}^{-1})(150 \text{ km}) = 75\Omega$

Voltage drop across the wire, $V = (8 \text{ V km}^{-1})(150 \text{ km}) = 1200 \text{ V}$

Power loss in the wire is

$$P = \frac{V^2}{R} = \frac{(1200 \text{ V})^2}{75\Omega} = 19200 \text{ W}$$
$$= 19.2 \text{ kW}$$

26. **(c) :** Power, $P = \frac{V^2}{R}$

As the resistance of the bulb is constant

$$\therefore \frac{\Delta P}{P} = \frac{2\Delta V}{V}$$

% decrease in power

$$= \frac{\Delta P}{P} \times 100 = \frac{2\Delta V}{V} \times 100$$

$$= 2 \times 2.5\% = 5\%$$

27. **(c) :** Power = 220 V × 4 A = 880 watts.

Heat needed to raise the temperature of 1 kg water through 80°C $= ms.\Delta T = 1 \times 4200 \times 80 \text{ J} = 336 \times 10^3 \text{ J}$

$\therefore$ Time taken $= \frac{336\times10^3}{880} = 382 \text{ s} = 6.3 \text{ min}$

28. **(a) :** $P = i^2R$ or $1 = 25 \times R$

$$R = \frac{1}{25} = 0.04\Omega$$

29. (c) : In India, $P_I = \frac{(220)^2}{R}$; In USA, $P_U = \frac{(110)^2}{R_U}$

As $P_I = P_U \Rightarrow \frac{(220)^2}{R} = \frac{(110)^2}{R_U} \Rightarrow R_U = \frac{R}{4}$

30. (b) : Fuse wire should have high resistance and low melting point.

31. (b) : $P = \frac{V^2}{R}$ or, $R \propto \frac{1}{P}$ $\therefore R_{40} > R_{100}$

32. (a) : $H = I^2Rt = ms\Delta T$

$\frac{I_1^2}{I_2^2} = \frac{\Delta T_1}{\Delta T_2}$ or, $\Delta T_2 = \frac{\Delta T_1 I_2^2}{I_1^2}$

$$\Delta T_2 = 5 \times \frac{(2I_1)^2}{I_1^2} = 20°\text{C}$$

33. (c) : Power = 100 W; Voltage of bulb = 200 V and supply voltage (V_s) = 160 V

Therefore resistance of bulb (R)

$$= \frac{V^2}{P} = \frac{(200)^2}{100} = 400\Omega$$

and power consumption (P)

$$= \frac{V_s^2}{R} = \frac{(160)^2}{400} \doteq 64 \text{ W}.$$

34. (c) : 1kWh = 1000Wh = (1000 W) × (3600 s) = 36×10^5 J

35. (d) : Capacitance $(C) = 4\mu\text{F} = 4 \times 10^{-6}$ F; Voltage $(V) = 400$ volts and resistance $(R) = 2\text{k}\Omega = 2 \times 10^3\Omega$

Heat produced = Electrical energy stored $= \frac{1}{2}\text{CV}^2$

$$= \frac{1}{2} \times (4 \times 10^{-6}) \times (400)^2 = 0.32 \text{ J}$$

36. (d) : Power (P) = 60 W and voltage (V) = 220 V

Resistance of the filament,

$$R = \frac{V^2}{P} = \frac{(220)^2}{60} = 807\Omega$$

37. (b) : $H = I^2Rt$ or $R = \frac{H}{(I^2t)} = \frac{80}{(2^2 \times 10)} = 2\Omega$

38. (c) : By KCL

$$i_1 = i_2 + i_3$$

Voltage is same in r_2 and r_3 as they are in parallel

$$i_2 r_2 = i_3 r_3$$
$$i_2 = \frac{i_3 r_3}{r_2}$$

From eqn. (i) and (ii),

$$i_1 = \frac{i_3 r_3}{r_2} + i_3$$

or $i_1 = \frac{i_3 r_3 + i_3 r_2}{r_2} = i_3\left(\frac{r_2 + r_3}{r_2}\right)$

$$\frac{i_3}{i_1} = \frac{r_2}{r_2 + r_3}$$

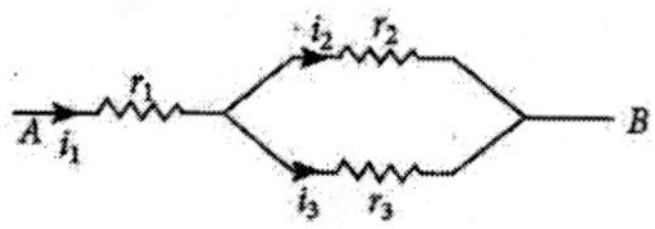

39. (a) : Given that, four wires of same material, equal area of cross-section and equal length.

Resistance of each wire is ' R '.

For parallel combination, $R_{eq} = 0.25\Omega$

When wires are connected in parallel,

$$\frac{1}{R_{eq}} = \frac{1}{R_1} + \frac{1}{R_2} + \frac{1}{R_3} + \frac{1}{R_4}$$
$$\frac{1}{R_{eq}} = \frac{1}{R} + \frac{1}{R} + \frac{1}{R} + \frac{1}{R}$$
$$\frac{1}{0.25} = \frac{4}{R} \Rightarrow R = 1\Omega$$

So, resistance of each wire is 1Ω.

Now, wires are connected in series. Then, equivalent resistance is

$R_{eq} = R_1 + R_2 + R_3 + R_4$

$R_{eq} = 1\Omega + 1\Omega + 1\Omega + 1\Omega = 4\Omega$

Hence, the equivalent resistance in series will be 4ohm.

40. (d)

41. (c)

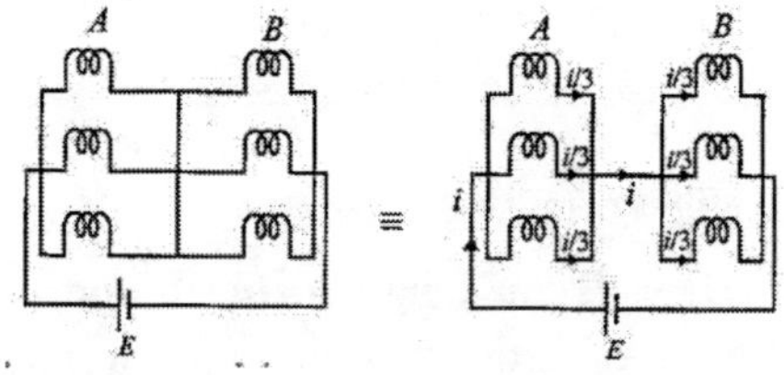

Let R be the resistance of the each bulb.

Case (i)

Net resistance of the circuit; $R_1 = \frac{R}{3} + \frac{R}{3} = \frac{2R}{3}$

Power consumption by the bulbs = Power supply by the sources ⇒ $P_1 = \frac{E^2}{(2R/3)} = \frac{3E^2}{2R}$

Case (ii)

Net resistance of the circuit,

$$R_2 = \frac{R}{2} + R = \frac{3R}{2}$$

Power consumption by the bulbs,

$$P_2 = \frac{E^2}{(3R/2)} = \frac{2}{3}\left(\frac{E^2}{R}\right); \frac{P_1}{P_2} = \frac{3}{2} \times \frac{3}{2} = \frac{9}{4}$$

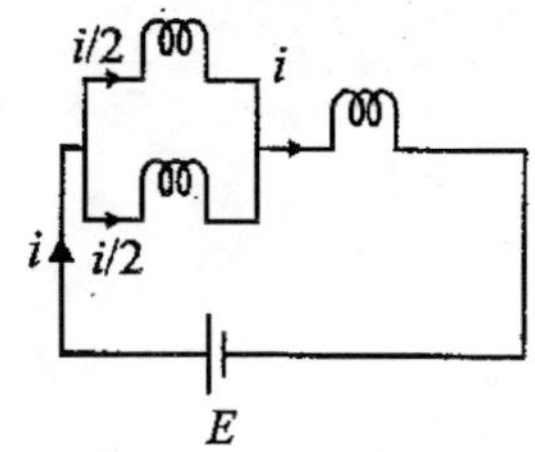

42. (c) : Resistance of bulb, $R_B = \frac{V^2}{P} = \frac{(100)^2}{500} = 20\Omega$

Power of the bulb in the circuit,

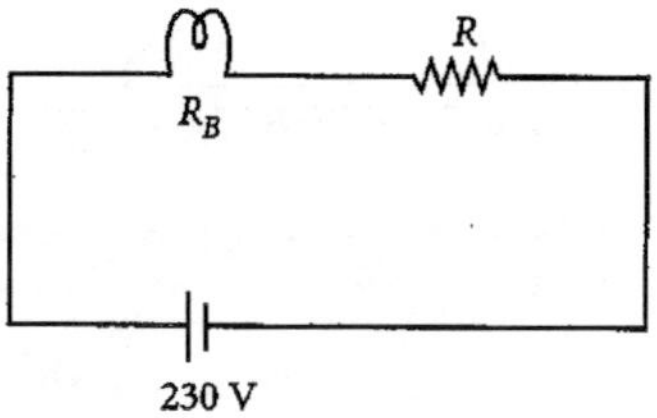

$$P = VI; I = \frac{P}{V_B}; I = \frac{500}{100} = 5\text{ A}$$
$$V_R = IR \Rightarrow (230 - 100) = 5 \times R \therefore R = 26\Omega$$

43. (c) : As both metal wires are of identical dimensions, so their length and area of cross-section will be same. Let them be l and A respectively. Then the resistance of the first wire is

$$R_1 = \frac{l}{\sigma_1 A}$$

and that of the second wire is $R_2 = \frac{l}{\sigma_2 A}$

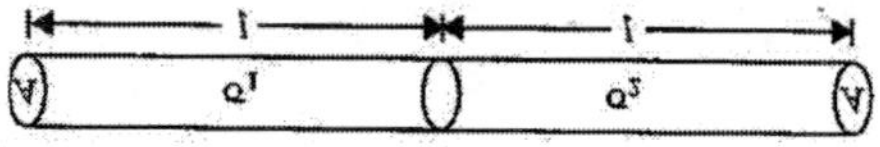

As they are connected in series, so their effective resistance is

$$R_s = R_1 + R_2 = \frac{l}{\sigma_1 A} + \frac{l}{\sigma_2 A}$$
$$= \frac{l}{A}\left(\frac{1}{\sigma_1} + \frac{1}{\sigma_2}\right)$$

(using (i) and (ii))

If σ_{eff} is the effective conductivity of the combination, then

$$R_s = \frac{2l}{\sigma_{\text{eff}} A}$$

Equating eqns. (iii) and (iv), we get

$$\frac{2l}{\sigma_{\text{eff}} A} = \frac{l}{A}\left(\frac{1}{\sigma_1} + \frac{1}{\sigma_2}\right)$$
$$\frac{2}{\sigma_{\text{eff}}} = \frac{\sigma_2 + \sigma_1}{\sigma_1 \sigma_2} \text{ or } \sigma_{\text{eff}} = \frac{2\sigma_1\sigma_2}{\sigma_1 + \sigma_2}$$

44. **(c) :** The circuit is shown in the figure

Resistance of the ammeter is

$$R_A = \frac{(480\Omega)(20\Omega)}{(480\Omega + 20\Omega)} = 19.2\Omega$$

(As 480Ω and 20Ω are in parallel) As ammeter is in series with 40.8Ω,

∴ Total resistance of the circuit is

$R = 40.8\Omega + R_A = 40.8\Omega + 19.2$

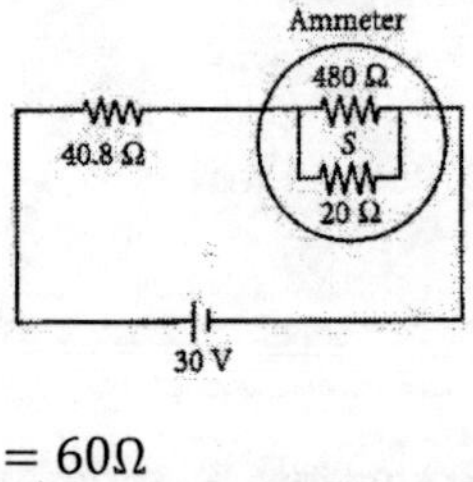

$\Omega = 60\Omega$

By Ohm's law, current in the circuit is

$$I = \frac{V}{R} = \frac{30\text{ V}}{60\Omega} = \frac{1}{2}\text{ A} = 0.5\text{ A}$$

Thus the reading in the ammeter will be 0.5 A.

45. **(c) :** The current flowing in the different branches of circuit is indicated in the figure.

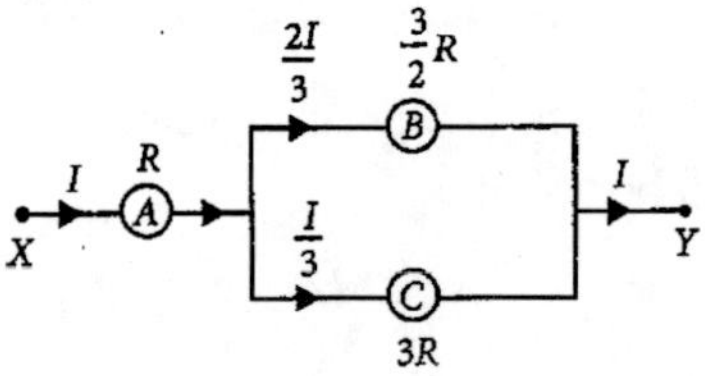

$$V_A = IR, V_B = \frac{2I}{3} \times \frac{3}{2}R = IR, V_C = \frac{I}{3} \times 3R$$
$$= IR$$

Thus, $V_A = V_B = V_C$

46. **(d) :** Here, length of each rod, $l = 1$ m Area of cross-section of each rod, $A = 0.01\text{ cm}^2 = 0.01 \times 10^{-4}\text{ m}^2$ Resistivity of copper rod,

$$\rho_{\text{cu}} = 1.7 \times 10^{-6}\Omega\text{cm}$$
$$= 1.7 \times 10^{-6} \times \mathbf{10^{-2}}\Omega\text{m}$$
$$= 1.7 \times 10^{-8}\Omega\text{m}$$

Resistivity of iron rod, $\rho_{\text{Fe}} = 10^{-5}\Omega\text{cm} = 10^{-5} \times 10^{-2}\Omega\text{m} = 10^{-7}\Omega\text{m}$

∴ Resistance of copper rod, $R_{\text{Cu}} = \rho_{\text{Cu}}\frac{l}{A}$

and resistance of iron rod, $R_{\text{Fe}} = \rho_{\text{Fe}}\frac{l}{A}$

As copper and iron rods are connected in series, therefore equivalent resistance is

$$R = R_{\text{Cu}} + R_{\text{Fe}} = \rho_{\text{Cu}}\frac{l}{A} + \rho_{\text{Fe}}\frac{l}{A}$$
$$= (\rho_{\text{Cu}} + \rho_{\text{Fe}})\frac{l}{A}$$

Voltage required to produce

1 A current in the rods is

$V = IR = (1)(R_{Cu} + R_{Fe})$

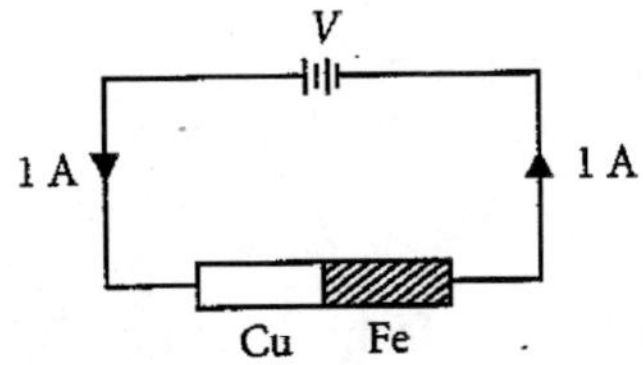

$= (\rho_{Cu} + \rho_{Fe})\left(\frac{l}{A}\right)$

$= (1.7 \times 10^{-8} + 10^{-7})\left(\frac{1}{0.01\times10^{-4}}\right)$ V

$= 10^{-7}(0.17 + 1)(10^6)\text{V} = 1.17 \times 10^{-1}$ V

$= 0.117$ V

47. (b) : Let ρ and A be resistivity and area of cross-section of the wire respectively.

The wire is bent in the form of right triangle as shown in figure.

Resistance of side AB is $R_1 = \frac{3\rho}{A}$

Resistance of side BC is $R_2 = \frac{4\rho}{A}$

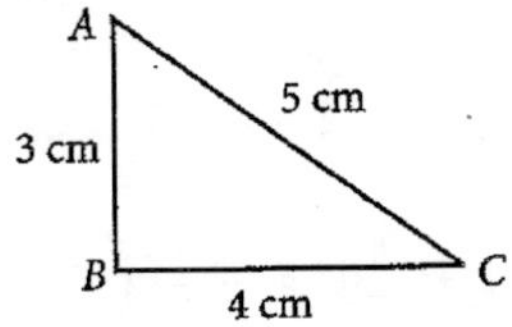

Resistance of side AC is $R_3 = \frac{5\rho}{A}$

$\therefore$ The resistance between the ends A and B is

$$R_{AB} = \frac{R_1(R_2 + R_3)}{R_1 + R_2 + R_3} = \frac{\frac{3\rho}{A}\left(\frac{4\rho}{A} + \frac{5\rho}{A}\right)}{\frac{3\rho}{A} + \left(\frac{4\rho}{A} + \frac{5\rho}{A}\right)} = \frac{27}{12}\frac{\rho}{A}$$

The resistance between the ends B and C is

$$R_{BC} = \frac{R_2(R_1 + R_3)}{R_2 + R_1 + R_3} = \frac{\frac{4\rho}{A}\left(\frac{3\rho}{A} + \frac{5\rho}{A}\right)}{\frac{4\rho}{A} + \frac{3\rho}{A} + \frac{5\rho}{A}} = \frac{32}{12}\frac{\rho}{A}$$

The resistance between the ends A and C is

$$R_{AC} = \frac{R_3(R_1 + R_2)}{R_3 + R_1 + R_2} = \frac{\frac{5\rho}{A}\left(\frac{3\rho}{A} + \frac{4\rho}{A}\right)}{\frac{5\rho}{A} + \frac{3\rho}{A} + \frac{4\rho}{A}} = \frac{35}{12}\frac{\rho}{A}$$

$$\therefore R_{AB}:R_{BC}:R_{AC} = \frac{27}{12}:\frac{32}{12}:\frac{35}{12} = 27:32:35$$

48. (d) : Let x be resistance per unit length of the wire. Then, the resistance of the upper portion is, $R_1 = xl_1$ the resistance of the lower portion is, $R_2 = xl_2$

Equivalent resistance between A and B is

$$R = \frac{R_1R_2}{R_1 + R_2} = \frac{(xl_1)(xl_2)}{xl_1 + xl_2}$$

$$\frac{8}{3} = \frac{xl_1l_2}{l_1+l_2} \text{ or } \frac{8}{3} = \frac{xl_1l_2}{l_2\left(\frac{l_1}{l_2}+1\right)} \text{ or } \frac{8}{3} = \frac{xl_1}{\left(\frac{l_1}{l_2}+1\right)}$$

Also $R_0 = xl_1 + xl_2$

$$12 = x(l_1 + l_2)$$

$$12 = xl_2\left(\frac{l_1}{l_2} + 1\right)$$

Divide (i) by (ii), we get

$$\frac{\frac{8}{3}}{12} = \frac{\frac{xl_1}{\left(\frac{l_1}{l_2}+1\right)}}{xl_2\left(\frac{l_1}{l_2}+1\right)} \text{ or } \frac{8}{36} = \frac{l_1}{l_2\left(\frac{l_1}{l_2}+1\right)^2}$$

$$\left(\frac{l_1}{l_2} + 1\right)^2 \frac{8}{36} = \frac{l_1}{l_2} \text{ or } \left(\frac{l_1}{l_2} + 1\right)^2 \frac{2}{9} = \frac{l_1}{l_2}$$

Let $y = \frac{l_1}{l_2}$

$\therefore\ 2(y+1)^2 = 9y$ or $2y^2 + 2 + 4y = 9y$ or $2y^2 - 5y + 2 = 0$ Solving this quadratic equation, we get

$$y = \frac{1}{2} \text{ or } 2 \therefore \frac{l_1}{l_2} = \frac{1}{2}$$

49. (c) : The equivalent resistance of the given circuit is

$$R_{eq} = \frac{5R}{5+R}$$

Power dissipated in the given circuit is

$$P = \frac{V^2}{R_{eq}} \text{ or } 30 = \frac{(10)^2}{\left(\frac{5R}{5+R}\right)}$$

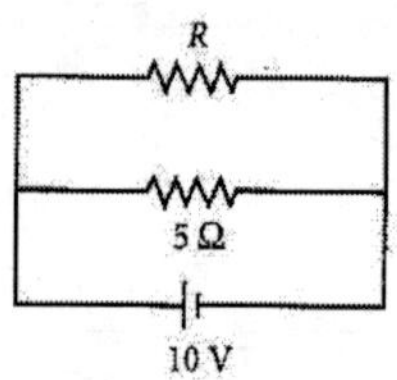

$150R = 100(5+R)$ or $150R = 500 + 100R$ or $50R = 500$

$$R = \frac{500}{50} = 10\Omega$$

50. (c) : As $P = I^2R$

Current flows through the 9Ω resistor is $I_1^2 = \frac{36}{9} = 4$

$I_1 = 2\text{ A}$

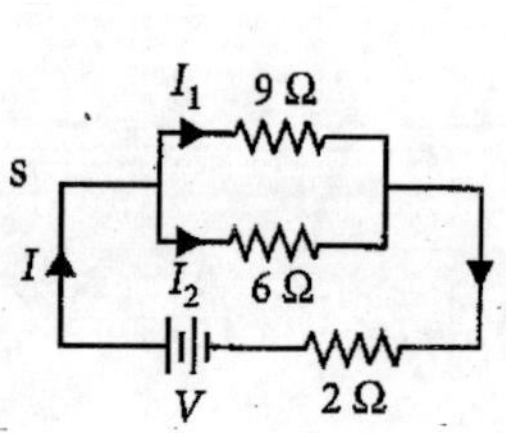

As the resistors 9Ω and 6Ω are connected in parallel, therefore potential difference across them is same.

$$\therefore\ 9I_1 = 6I_2; I_2 = \frac{9\times 2}{6} = 3\text{ A}$$

Current drawn from the battery is $I = I_1 + I_2 = (2+3)\text{A} = 5\text{ A}$ The potential difference across the 2Ω resistor

$$= (5\text{ A})(2\Omega) = 10\text{ V}$$

51. (d) : Wire of length $2\pi \times 0.1$ m of resistance $12\Omega/\text{m}$ is bent to form a circle.

Resistance of each part

$$= 12 \times \pi \times 0.1 = 1.2\pi\Omega$$

$\therefore$ Resistance between A and $B = 0.6\pi\Omega$

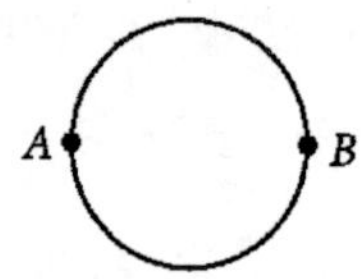

52. (b) : As the P.D. across 4Ω and 3Ω (in parallel), are the same,

$$V = 4 \times 1\text{ A} = 4\text{ V}$$

$\therefore$ P.D.across points P and $M = 4$ V

Current in $MNP = \frac{1}{1.25} = \frac{1\times 1}{5} = \frac{16}{5}$ A $\therefore$ P.D. across $1\Omega = \frac{16}{5}\text{ A} \times 1\Omega = \frac{16}{5}$ volt = 3.2 volt

53. (b)

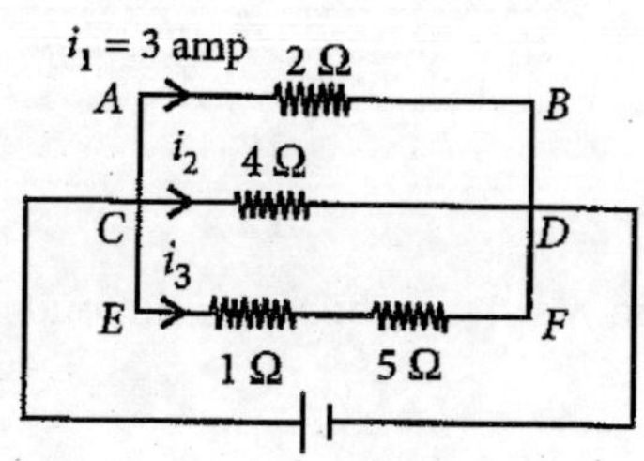

$2\Omega, 4\Omega$ and $(1\Omega + 5\Omega)$ are in parallel. So potential difference is the same.

$$V = 2\Omega \cdot i_1 = 4\Omega \cdot i_2 = 6\Omega \cdot i_3$$
$$2 \cdot 3 = 6\Omega \cdot i_3 \Rightarrow i_3 = 1\text{amp}.$$

$\therefore$ Power dissipated in 5Ω resistance

$= i_3^2 R = 1^2 \times 5 = 5$ W

54. **(b) :** In the given circuit 6Ω and 3Ω are in parallel, and hence its equivalent resistance is given by

$\frac{1}{R_p} = \frac{1}{6} + \frac{1}{3}$ or $R_p = 2\Omega$

The equivalent circuit diagram is given in figure. Total current in the circuit,

$$I = \frac{18}{2+4} = 3 \text{ A}$$

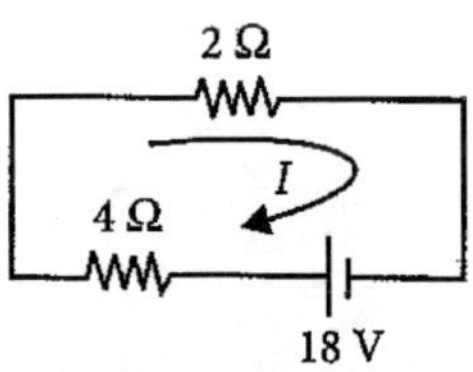

Power in the circuit $= VI = 18 \times 3 = 54$ watt

55. **(a) :** Resistance of series combination of 3Ω and 1Ω is $R_1 = 3 + 1 = 4\Omega, R_2 = 8\Omega$

Let i be the total current in the circuit.

Current through R_1 is

$$i_1 = \frac{i \times R_2}{R_1 + R_2} = \frac{i \times 8}{12} = \frac{2i}{3}$$

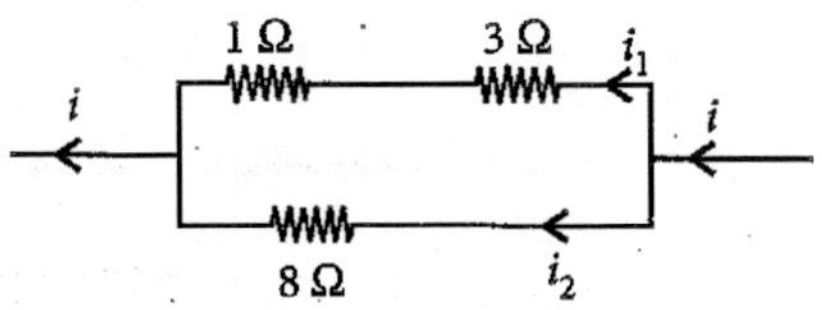

Current through R_2 is $i_2 = \frac{i \times R_1}{R_1 + R_2} = \frac{i \times 4}{12} = \frac{i}{3}$

Power dissipated in 3Ω resistor is

$$P_1 = i_1^2 \times 3$$

Power dissipated in 8Ω resistor is

$$P_2 = i_2^2 \times 8$$

$\therefore \frac{P_1}{P_2} = \frac{i_1^2 \times 3}{i_2^2 \times 8}$ or, $\frac{P_1}{P_2} = \frac{(2i/3)^2 \times 3}{(i/3)^2 \times 8} = \frac{12}{8} = \frac{3}{2}$

$$P_1 = \frac{3}{2} \times P_2 = \frac{3}{2} \times 2 = 3\text{watt}$$

$\therefore$ Power dissipated across 3Ω resistor is 3 watt.

56. **(a) :** Both are in parallel.

$$\frac{1}{R'} = \frac{2}{R} + \frac{2}{R} = \frac{4}{R} \Rightarrow R' = \frac{R}{4}$$

57. **(a) :** When n resistance of r ohm connected in parallel then their equivalent resistance is

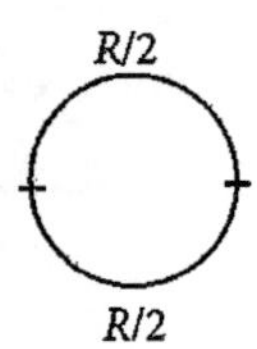

$$\frac{1}{R} = \frac{1}{r} + \frac{1}{r} + \frac{1}{r} + \cdots \ldots\ldots\ldots\ldots n \text{ times}$$

$$\therefore \frac{1}{R} = \frac{n}{r} \Rightarrow R = \frac{r}{n} \Rightarrow r = nR$$

When these resistance connected in series

$$R_s = r + r + \cdots \ldots\ldots\ldots\ldots n \text{ times}$$
$$= nr = n \times nR = n^2 R$$

58. **(d) :** The resistance of each bulb $= \frac{V^2}{P} = \frac{(200)^2}{60}\Omega$

When three bulbs are connected in series their resultant resistance = $\frac{3\times(200)^2}{60}\Omega$

Thus power drawn by bulb when connected across 200 V supply

$$P = \frac{V^2}{R_{re}} = \frac{(200)^2}{3\times(200)^2/60} = 20\text{ W}$$

59. (d) : $R = \frac{V^2}{P} = \frac{220\times220}{100} = 484\Omega$

In series, $R_{eq} = 484 + 484 = 968\Omega$

$\therefore P_{eq} = \frac{V^2}{968} = \frac{220\times220}{968} = 50$ watt

In parallel, $R_{eq} = 242\Omega$

$\therefore P_{eq} = \frac{V^2}{242} = \frac{220\times220}{242} = 200$ watt.

60. (a) : Let R_1 and R_2 be the resistance of the two coils and V be the voltage supplied.

Effective resistance of two coils in parallel $= \frac{R_1R_2}{R_1+R_2}$

Let H be the heat required to begin boiling in kettle.

Then H = Power × time $= \frac{V^2t_1}{R_1} = \frac{V^2t_2}{R_2}$

For parallel combination, $H = \frac{V^2(R_1+R_2)t_p}{R_1R_2}$

$$\Rightarrow \frac{1}{t_p} = \left(\frac{t_2+t_1}{t_2t_1}\right)$$

$\therefore t_p = \frac{t_1t_2}{t_1+t_2} = \frac{10\times40}{10+40} = 8$ minutes

61. (d) : In given circuit R_B and R_C are in series.

$\therefore R_{BC} = 6 + 6 = 12\Omega$.

Now, R_A and R_{BC} are in parallel.

Therefore, equivalent resistance of circuit,

$$R_{eq} = \frac{12\times3}{12+3} = \frac{36}{15}\Omega$$

Using Ohm's law, $= \frac{V}{R_{eq}} = \frac{4.8}{36/15} = 2$ A.

62. (d) : For series, $R_{eq} = 3r$

Power $= \frac{V^2}{3r} = 10 \Rightarrow \frac{V^2}{r} = 30$

For parallel $R_{eq} = r/3$

Power $= \frac{V^2}{r/3} = \frac{3V^2}{r} = 3\times30 = 90$ watt.

63. (b) : Applied voltage $(V) = 2$ V and resistances $= 3\Omega, 3\Omega, 3\Omega$.

From the given circuit, we find that two resistances are in series and third resistance is in parallel. Therefore equivalent resistance for series resistances $= 3 + 3 = 6\Omega$. Now it is connected parallel with 3Ω resistance. Therefore

$$\frac{1}{R} = \frac{1}{3} + \frac{1}{6} = \frac{3}{6} = \frac{1}{2} \text{ or } R = 2\Omega$$

And current flowing in the circuit

$(I) = \frac{V}{R} = \frac{2}{2} = 1$ A

64. (d) : Ratio of resistance $R_1 : R_2 = 1:2$ or $\frac{R_1}{R_2} = \frac{1}{2}$.

In series combination, power dissipated $(P) = I^2R$

Therefore $\frac{P_1}{P_2} = \frac{R_1}{R_2} = \frac{1}{2}$ or $P_1 : P_2 = 1:2$

65. (a) : Lower resistance on extreme left and upper resistance on extreme right are ineffective.

The resistance R_2 and R_3 are in series combination. Therefore their equivalent resistance,

$$R' = R_2 + R_3 = 10 + 10 = 20\Omega$$

Similarly, the resistance R_5 and R_6 are in series combination.

Therefore their equivalent resistance,

$$R'' = R_5 + R_6 = 10 + 10 = 20\Omega$$

Now the equivalent resistances R' and R'' are in parallel combination. Therefore their equivalent resistance,

$$R''' = \frac{R'R''}{R' + R''} = \frac{20 \times 20}{20 + 20} = \frac{400}{40} = 10\Omega$$

Thus equivalent resistance between A and D,

$$R = R_1 + R''' + R_4 = 10 + 10 + 10 = 30\Omega$$

66. (a) : Ratio of cross-sectional areas of the wires $= 3:1$

and resistance of thick wire $(R_1) = 10\Omega$

Resistance $(R) = \rho\frac{l}{A} \propto \frac{1}{A}$.

Therefore $\frac{R_1}{R_2} = \frac{A_2}{A_1} = \frac{1}{3}$ or $R_2 = 3R_1 = 3 \times 10 = 30\Omega$ and equivalent resistance of these two resistances in series combination

$$= R_1 + R_2 = 30 + 10 = 40\Omega$$

67. (b) : Power of heating coil $= 100$ W and voltage $(V) = 220$ volts. When the heating coil is cut into two equal parts and these parts are joined in parallel, the resistance of the coil is reduced to one-fourth of the previous value. Therefore energy liberated per second becomes 4 times. i.e. $4 \times 100 = 400$ W.

68. (a) : Resistances R_{AF} and R_{FE} are in series combination. Therefore their equivalent resistance $R' = R_{AF} + R_{FE} = 3 + 3 = 6\Omega$. Now the resistance R_{AE} and equivalent resistance R' are in parallel combination. Therefore relation for their equivalent resistance

$$\frac{1}{R''} = \frac{1}{R'} + \frac{1}{R_{AE}} = \frac{1}{6} + \frac{1}{6} = \frac{2}{6} = \frac{1}{3} \Rightarrow R'' = 3\Omega$$

We can reduce the circuit in similar way and finally the circuit reduces as shown in the figure.

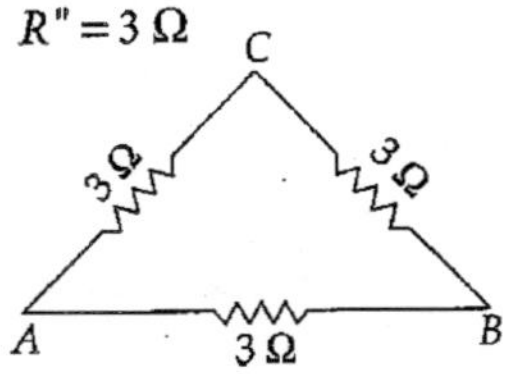

Therefore, the equivalent resistance between A and B

$$= \frac{(3+3) \times 3}{(3+3)+3} = \frac{18}{9} = 2\Omega$$

69. (d) : The two resistances are connected in series and the resultant is connected in parallel with the third resistance.

$\therefore R = 4\Omega + 4\Omega = 8\Omega$ and $\frac{1}{R''} = \frac{1}{8} + \frac{1}{4} = \frac{3}{8}$

or $R'' = \frac{8}{3}\Omega$

70. (c) : Current across $3\Omega = 0.8$ A

6Ω is in parallel, current across $6\Omega = 0.4$ A

Total current $= 1.2$ A

$\therefore$ Potential difference across 4Ω resistor $= 1.2\text{ A} \times 4\Omega = 4.8$ V

71. (d) :

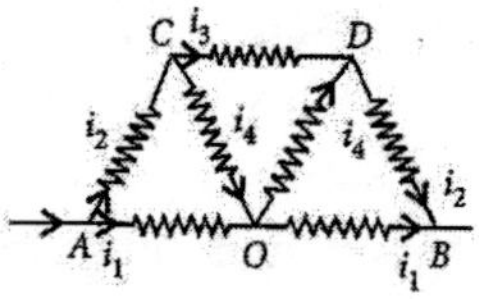

By symmetry, currents i_1 and i_2 from A is the same as i_1 and i_2 reaching B.

As the same current is flowing from A to O and O to B, O can be treated as detached from AB.

Now CO and OD will be in series hence its total resistance = 2Ω It is in parallel with CD so equivalent resistance = $\frac{2\times1}{2+1} = \frac{2}{3}\Omega$

This equivalent resistance is in series with AC and DB. So total resistance $= \frac{2}{3} + 1 + 1 = \frac{8}{3}\Omega$

Now $\frac{8}{3}\Omega$ is parallel to AB that is 2Ω. So total resistance

$$= \frac{(8/3)\times 2}{(8/3)+2} = \frac{16/3}{14/3} = \frac{16}{14} = \frac{8}{7}\Omega$$

72. **(c) :** To carry a current of 4 ampere, we need four paths, each carrying a current of one ampere. Let r be the resistance of each path. These are connected in parallel. Hence their equivalent resistance will be $r/4$. According to the given problem $\frac{r}{4} = 5$ or $r = 20\Omega$

For this purpose two resistances should be connected in series. There are four such combinations that are connected in parallel. Hence, the total number of resistance = $4 \times 2 = 8$.

73. **(b) :** Since, the supply voltage is same for the two combinations, the net resistance is less for 39 bulbs. Hence the combination of 39 bulbs will glow more as current is more.

74. **(c) :** In series $R_s = nR$

In parallel $\frac{1}{R_P} = \frac{1}{R} + \frac{1}{R} + \cdots..n \text{ terms} = \frac{n}{R}$

$$\Rightarrow R_P = \frac{R}{n} \ \therefore\ R_s/R_p = n^2/1$$

75. **(a) :** Current drawn from a battery when n resistors are connected in series is

$$I = \frac{E}{nR + R}$$

Current drawn from same battery when n resistors are connected in parallel is

$$10I = \frac{E}{R/n + R}$$

On dividing eqn. (ii) by (i), $10 = \frac{(n+1)R}{(1/n+1)R}$

After solving the equation, $n = 10$

76. **(d) :** $I = \frac{\varepsilon}{R+r}$ or $IR + Ir = \varepsilon$

Here, $= 10\Omega, r = ?,$

$$\varepsilon = 2.1\text{ V}, I = 0.2\text{ A}$$

$$\therefore\ 0.2\times 10 + 0.2\times r = 2.1$$

$$2 + 0.2r = 2.1$$

$$0.2r = 0.1 \text{ or } r = \frac{1}{2} = 0.5\Omega$$

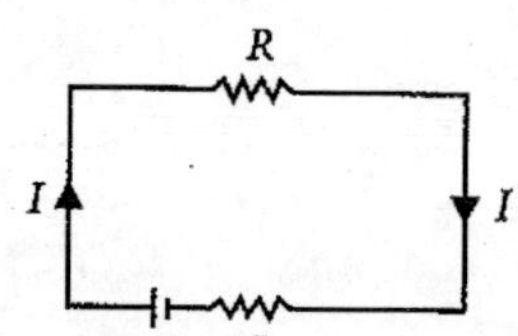

77. **(c) :** Current in the circuit, $I = \frac{\varepsilon}{R+r}$

Potential difference across R,

$$V = IR = \left(\frac{\varepsilon}{R+r}\right)R$$

$$V = \frac{\varepsilon}{1+\frac{r}{R}}$$

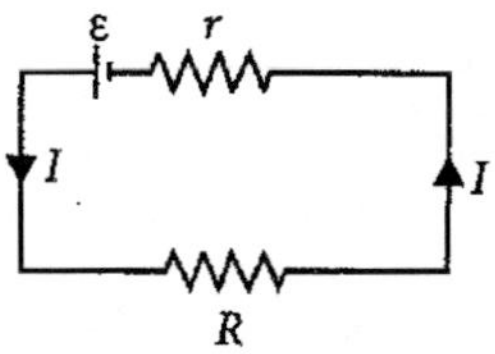

When $R = 0, V = 0; R = \infty, V = \varepsilon$

Hence, option (c) represents the correct graph.

78. **(b)** : Let ε be the emf and r be internal resistance of the battery.

In the first case,

$$2 = \frac{\varepsilon}{2+r}$$

In the second case,

$$0.5 = \frac{\varepsilon}{9+r}$$

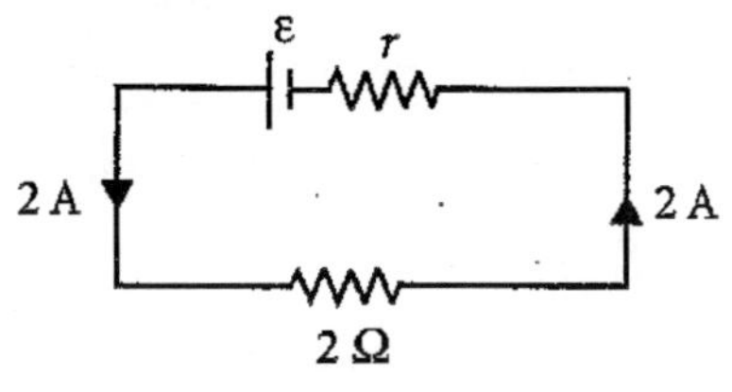

Divide (i) by (ii), we get

$$\frac{2}{0.5} = \frac{9+r}{2+r} \Rightarrow 4 + 2r = 4.5 + 0.5r$$

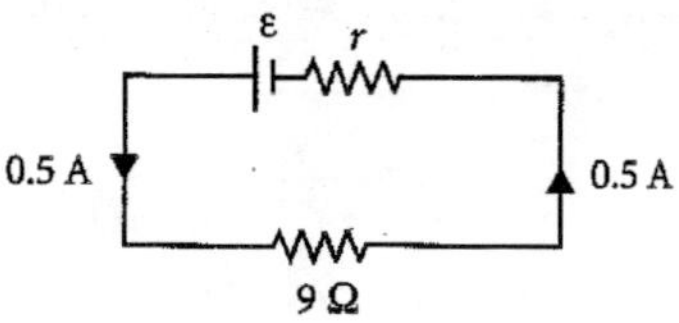

$$1.5r = 0.5 \Rightarrow r = \frac{0.5}{1.5} = \frac{1}{3}\Omega$$

79. **(a) :**

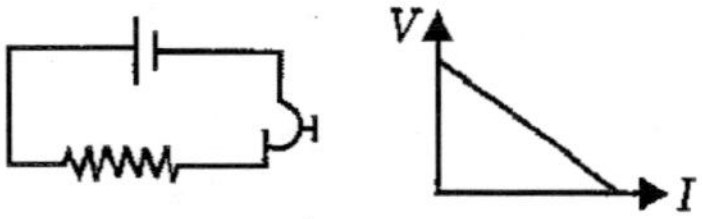

$V = \varepsilon - Ir$, comparing with $y = c - mx$

$\therefore$ Slope $= -r$, internal resistance

V_{max} = emf ε. This is intercept on the y-axis.

As I decreases as R increases, so slope is negative.

80. **(a) :** Terminal potential difference is 2.2 V when circuit is open.

$\therefore$ e.m.f. of the cell = E = 2.2 volt

Now, when the cell is connected to the external resistance, current in the circuit I is given by

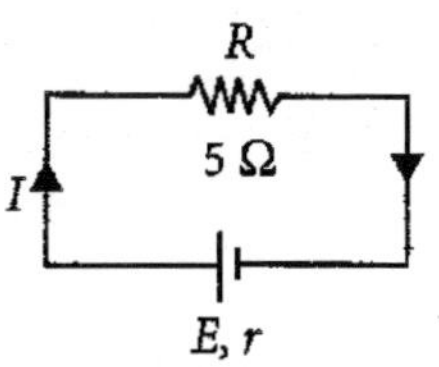

$I = \frac{E}{R+r} = \frac{2.2}{5+r}$ ampere, where r is the internal resistance of the cell.

Potential difference across the cell = IR

or, $= \frac{2.2}{5+r} \times 5 = 1.8$ or, $5 + r = 11/1.8$

$$\therefore\ r = \frac{11}{1.8} - 5 = \frac{110-90}{18} = \frac{10}{9}\Omega$$

81. **(c) :** $\frac{V-E}{r} = I \Rightarrow \frac{V-12}{5\times10^{-2}} = 60$

$$\Rightarrow V = 15\text{ V}$$

82. **(a) :** $i = \frac{2}{4} = 0.5$ Ampere

$$V = \varepsilon - ir = 2 - 0.5 \times 0.1 = 1.95\text{ V}$$

83. **(a) :** The output power of a cell is given by

$$P = \frac{V^2}{(r+R)^2}R$$

Maximum power is delivered to the load only when the internal resistance of the source is equal to the load resistance (R). Then

$$P_{\max} = \frac{V^2}{4R} = \frac{V^2}{4r}$$

(where = R)

84. **(a) :** $i = \frac{10-5}{10} = \frac{5}{10}A$

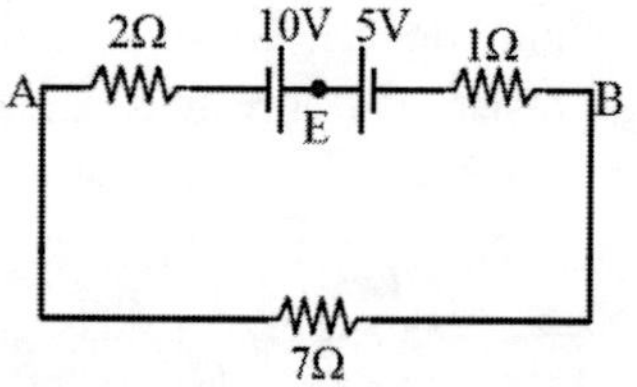

= 0.5 A

from A to B through E.

85. **(b)** **:** For no reading galvanometer. Potential across it is same.

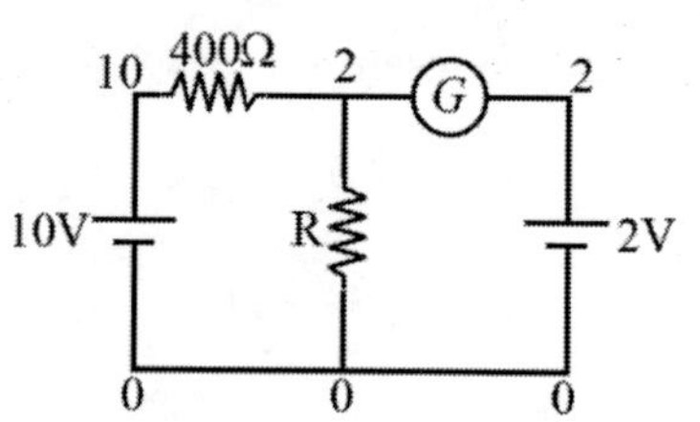

$$i_{400\Omega} \Rightarrow \frac{10-2}{400} = \frac{8}{400} = \frac{1}{50} = i_R$$

$$i_R \Rightarrow \frac{V_R}{R} \Rightarrow \frac{2}{R} = \frac{1}{50} \Rightarrow R = 100\Omega$$

86. **(a) :** $I_S = \frac{E}{10R}$

$$I_P = \frac{E}{R/10} = \frac{10E}{R}$$

$$n = \frac{I_P}{I_S} = 100 \Rightarrow n = 100$$

87. **(a) :** Current drawn from the cell is

$$I = \frac{n\varepsilon}{nr} = \frac{\varepsilon}{r}$$

So, I is independent of n and I is constant.

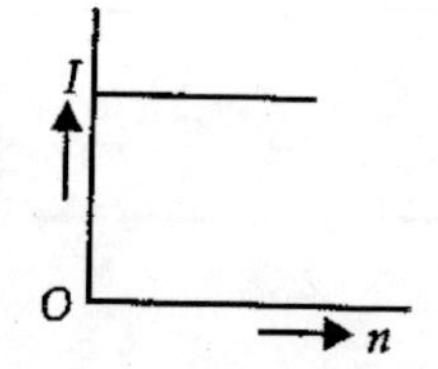

88. **(a)** : Let ρ be resistivity of the material of the wire and r be radius of the wire.

Therefore, resistance of 1 m wire is

$$R = \frac{\rho(1)}{\pi r^2} = \frac{\rho}{\pi r^2}$$

$\left(\because R = \frac{\rho l}{A}\right)$

Let ε be emf of each cell. In first case, 10 cells each of emf ε are connected in series to heat the wire of length 1 m by $\Delta T(= 10°C)$ in time t.

$$\therefore \quad \frac{(10\varepsilon)^2}{R}t = ms\Delta T$$

In second case, resistance of same wire of length 2 m is

$$R' = \frac{\rho(2)}{\pi r^2} = \frac{2\rho}{\pi r^2} = 2R$$

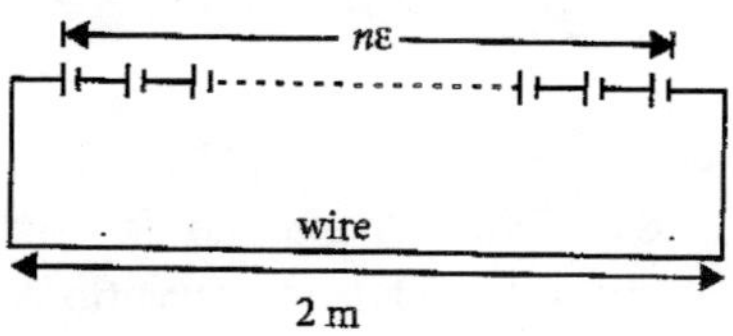

Let n cells each of emf ε are connected in series to heat the same wire of length 2 m, by the same temperature $\Delta T(= 10°C)$ in the same time t.

$$\therefore \quad \frac{(n\varepsilon)^2 t}{2R} = (2m)s\Delta T$$

Divide (ii) by (i), we get

$$\frac{n^2}{200} = 2 \Rightarrow n^2 = 400 \ \therefore \ n = 20$$

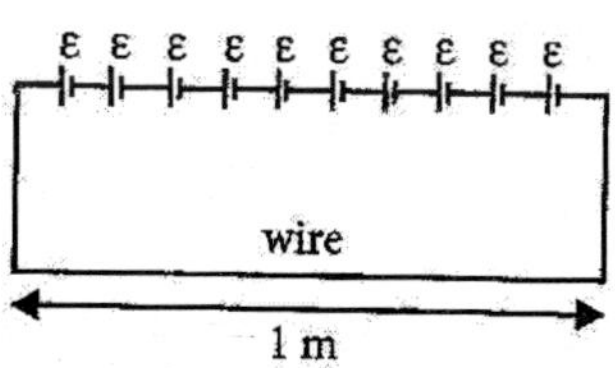

89. (b) : Current in the circuit,

$$i = \frac{2E}{(r_1+r_2+R)}.$$

As per question, $E - ir_1 = 0$

$$i = \frac{E}{r_1} \text{ or, } \frac{2E}{r_1+r_2+R} = \frac{E}{r_1}$$

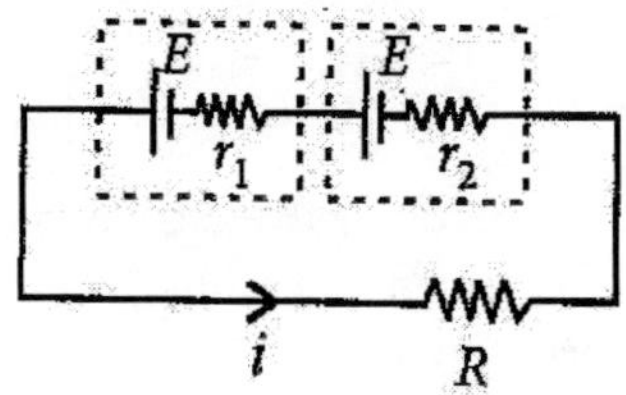

or, $2r_1 = r_1 + r_2 + R$ or, $R = r_1 - r_2$

90. (d) : Current in the circuit,

$$I = \frac{V}{R} = \frac{6}{3} = 2 \text{ A}$$

Voltage drop across 2Ω,

$$V_1 = 2 \times 2 = 4 \text{ V}$$

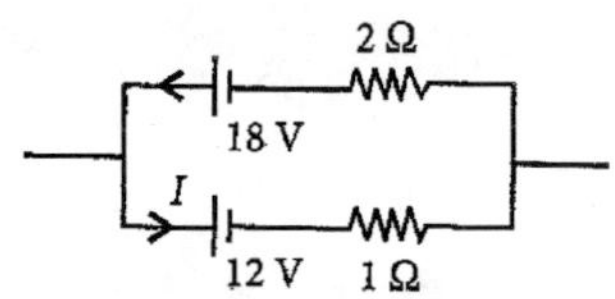

Voltmeter reading = 18 – 4 = 14 V

91. (b) : For maximum current, the two batteries should be connected in series. The current will be maximum when external resistance is equal to the total internal resistance of cells i.e. 2Ω. Hence power developed across the resistance R will be

$$I^2R = \left(\frac{2E}{R+2r}\right)^2 R = \left(\frac{2\times 2}{2+2}\right)^2 \times 2 = 2 \text{ W}$$

92. (a) : $I = \frac{8-4}{1+2+9} = \frac{4}{12} = \frac{1}{3}$ A

$$V_P - V_Q = 4 - \frac{1}{3} \times 3 = 3 \text{ volt}$$

93. (d) :

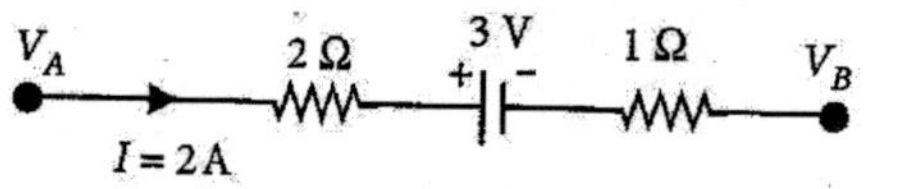

$$V_{AB} = V_A - V_B = 2 \times 2 + 3 + 1 \times 2 = 9\ \text{V}$$

94. (b) : Since the galvanometer shows no deflection so current will flow as shown in the figure.

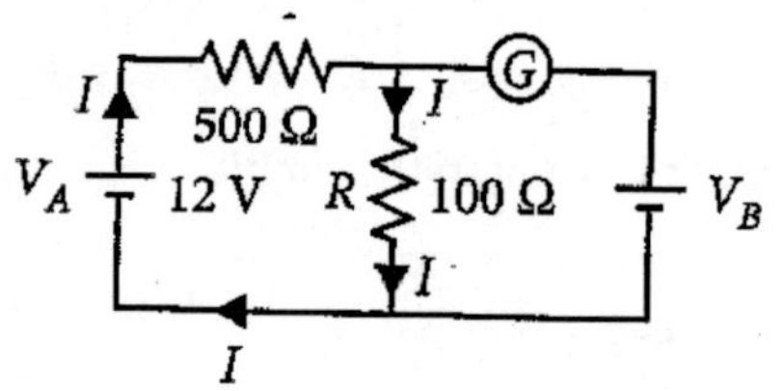

Current, $I = \frac{V_A}{R_1+R} = \frac{12\ \text{V}}{(500+100)\Omega} = \frac{12}{600}$ A

$$V_B = IR = \left(\frac{12}{600}\ \text{A}\right)(100\Omega) = 2\ \text{V}$$

95. (a) :

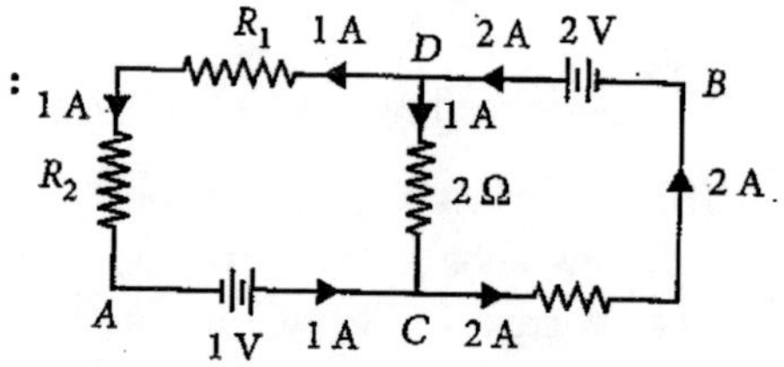

Applying Kirchhoff's voltage law a long path $ACDB$ as shown in the figure.

$\therefore\ V_A + 1 + 2(1) - 2 = V_B$

$0 + 1 = V_B$

$V_B = +1$ V

$\because V_A = 0\text{V}$(Given)

96. (d) : Kirchhoff's junction law or Kirchhoff's first law is based on the conservation of charge.

Kirchhoff's loop law or Kirchhoff's second law is based on the conservation of energy.

Hence both statements (A) and (B) are correct.

97. (d) :

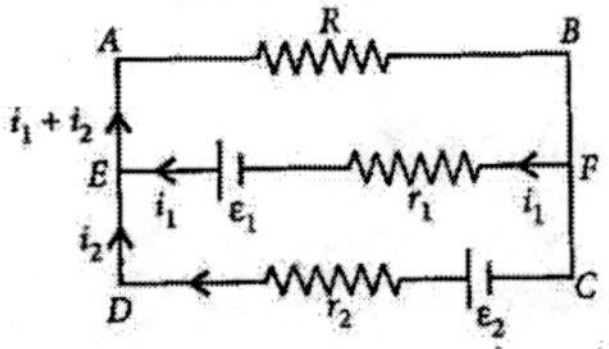

Applying Kirchhoff's equation to the loop $ABFE$,

$$-(i_1 + i_2)R - i_1 r_1 + \varepsilon_1 = 0$$

or $\varepsilon_1 - (i_1 + i_2)R - i_1 r_1 = 0$

98. (c) : Kirchhoff's first law of electrical circuit is based on conservation of charge and Kirchhoff's second law of electrical circuit is based on conservation of energy.

99. (c)

100. (b) : For a balanced wheat stone bridge, current through a galvanometer is zero.

$$\therefore \frac{P}{Q} = \frac{X}{Y}$$

Here resistances P and Q should be approximately equal and small, as it decreases error in experiment.

101. (d) : The situation is as shown in the figure. For a balanced Wheatstone's bridge

$$\frac{P}{Q} = \frac{R}{S}$$

$$\therefore \frac{10\Omega}{30\Omega} = \frac{30\Omega}{90\Omega} \text{ or } \frac{1}{3} = \frac{1}{3}$$

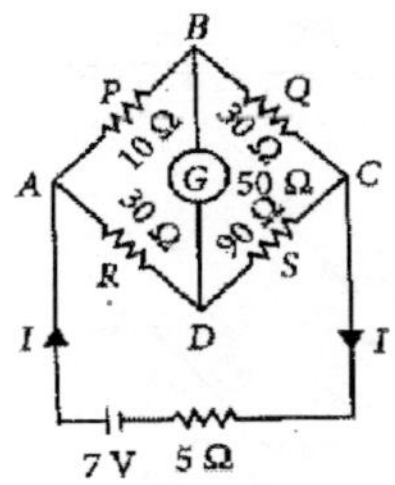

It is a balanced Wheatstone's bridge. Hence no current flows in the galvanometer arm. Hence, resistance 50Ω becomes ineffective.

∴ The equivalent resistance of the circuit is

$$R_{eq} = 5\Omega + \frac{(10\Omega + 30\Omega)(30\Omega + 90\Omega)}{(10\Omega + 30\Omega) + (30\Omega + 90\Omega)}$$

$$= 5\Omega + \frac{(40\Omega)(120\Omega)}{40\Omega + 120\Omega} = 5\Omega + 30\Omega = 35\Omega$$

Current drawn from the cell is

$$I = \frac{7\text{ V}}{35\Omega} = \frac{1}{5}\text{ A} = 0.2\text{ A}$$

102. (a) :

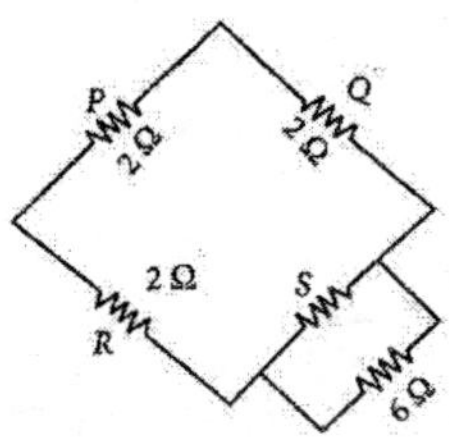

Let X be the equivalent resistance between S and 6Ω.

$$\therefore\ \frac{1}{X} = \frac{1}{S} + \frac{1}{6}$$

Therefore, the equivalent circuit diagram drawn here

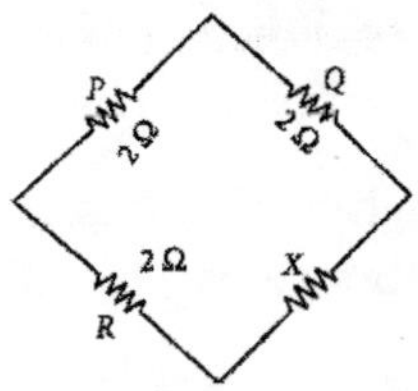

For a balanced Wheatstone's bridge, we get

$\frac{P}{Q} = \frac{R}{X}$ or $\frac{2}{2} = \frac{2}{X} \Rightarrow X = 2\Omega$.

From eqn. (i), we get

$\frac{1}{2} = \frac{1}{S} + \frac{1}{6}$ or, $\frac{1}{S} = \frac{2}{6}$ or, $S = 3\Omega$.

103. (a) :

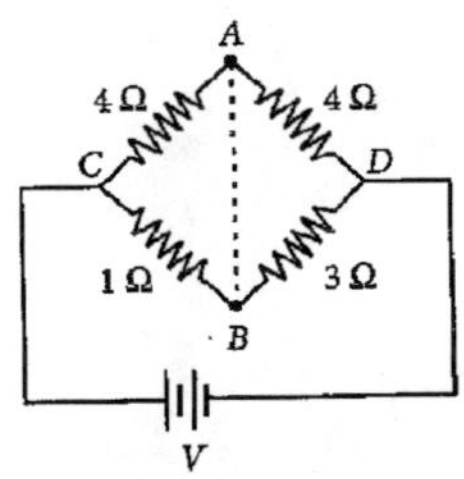

Current through arm $CAD, I = \frac{V}{8}$ amp

Potential difference between C and A = $V_C - V_A = \frac{V}{8} \times 4 = \frac{V}{2}$ volt

Current through $CBD, I' = \frac{V}{4}$ amp

Potential difference between C and B = $V_C - V_B$

$$= \frac{V}{4} \times 1 = \frac{V}{4}\text{ volt.}$$

Potential between A and $B = V_A - V_B$

$\therefore V_A - V_B = V_C - V_B - (V_C - V_A) = \frac{V}{4} - \frac{V}{2} = -\frac{V}{4}$.

$\Rightarrow V_A - V_B < 0$ or, $V_A < V_B$

As $V_A < V_B$, so direction of current will be from B to A.

104. (d) : Since given circuit is in the form of Wheatstone bridge,

$$\frac{1}{R_{eq}} = \frac{1}{(4+2)} + \frac{1}{(6+3)}; R_{eq} = 18/5\Omega$$

$$V = iR_{eq} \Rightarrow i = \frac{V}{R_{eq}} = \frac{5\text{ V}}{18}.$$

105. (c) : Equivalent circuit of given circuit is shown in figure (i).

Also this is equivalent to a balanced Wheatstone bridge C and D are at equal potential, no current will flow in this resistance therefore this resistance can be neglected.

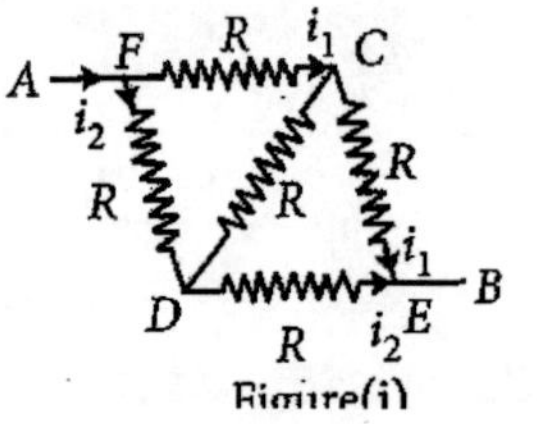

Figure(i)

Thus equivalent resistance of this remaining circuit shown in figure (ii) is R.

Then current in AFCEB branch is

$$i_1 = \frac{V}{R} \times \frac{2R}{2R+2R} = \frac{V}{2R}$$

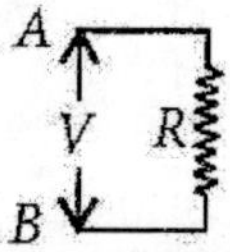

Figure(ii)

106. (c) : In balance Wheatstone bridge, the galvanometer arm can be neglected. So equivalent resistance will be

$$\frac{2R \times 2R}{2R+2R} = \frac{4R^2}{4R} = R$$

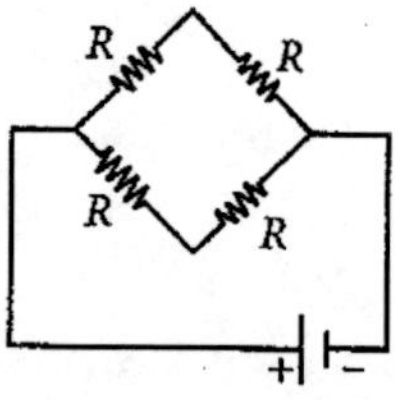

107. (a)

108. (b) : This is a balanced Wheatstone's bridge so no current flows through the 7Ω resistor.

$$\therefore \frac{1}{R_{eq}} = \frac{1}{4+3} + \frac{1}{6+8} \text{ or } R_{eq} = \frac{14}{3}\Omega$$

109. (d) : The circuit is equivalent to a balanced Wheatstone bridge. Therefore resistance between A and B is 2Ω.

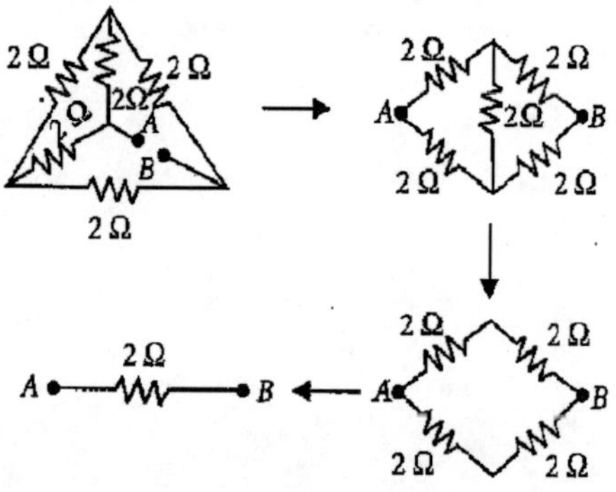

110. (b) : Unknown is $X, R = 10\Omega$.

Here, $\frac{l_1}{l_2} = \frac{3}{2}; \frac{X}{R} = \frac{l_1}{l_2}$

$$\Rightarrow X = \frac{3}{2} \times 10 \Rightarrow X = 15\Omega$$

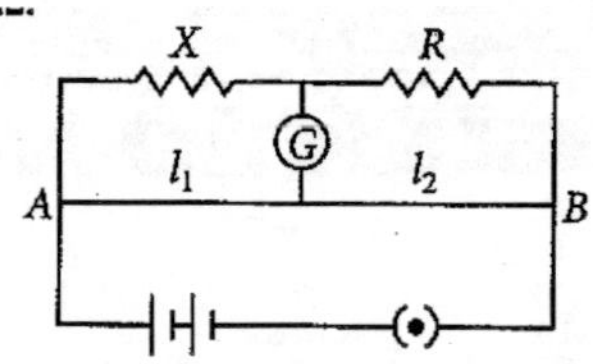

Thus, 1.5 m length has resistance 15Ω hence, length of 1Ω of the resistance wire $= \frac{1.5}{15} = 0.1 \text{ m} = 1.0 \times 10^{-1} \text{ m}$

111. (d) : Yes, the bridge will work. For a balanced condition, the current drawn from the battery will be zero. Also, $P \propto l_1$ and $Q \propto l_2$ Therefore, the condition $\frac{P}{Q} = \frac{l_1}{l_2}$ will remain same after interchanging the cell and galvanometer.

112. (b) : In the first case,

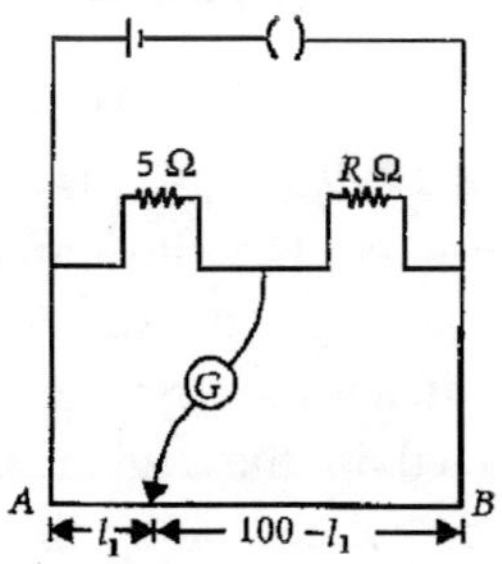

At balance point

$$\frac{5}{R} = \frac{l_1}{100 - l_1} \quad \text{...(i)}$$

In the second case,

At balance point

$$\frac{5}{(R/2)} = \frac{1.6 l_1}{100 - 1.6 l_1} \quad \text{..(ii)}$$

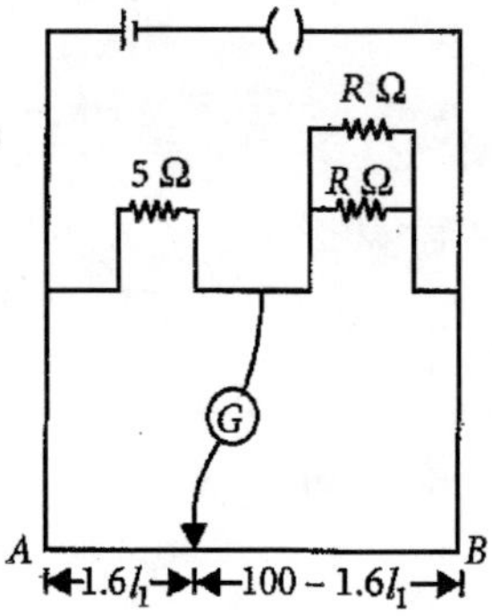

Divide eqn. (i) by eqn. (ii), we get

$$\frac{1}{2} = \frac{100 - 1.6 l_1}{1.6(100 - l_1)}$$

or $160 - 1.6 l_1 = 200 - 3.2 l_1$

$$1.6 l_1 = 40 \text{ or } l_1 = \frac{40}{1.6} = 25 \text{ cm}$$

Substituting this value in eqn. (i), we get

$$\frac{5}{R} = \frac{25}{75} \text{ or } R = \frac{375}{25} \Omega = 15\Omega$$

113. (d) : Metre bridge works on the principle of Wheatstone's bridge.

$\therefore \frac{P}{Q} = \frac{l}{100 - l}$ or, $P = \frac{l}{100 - l} \times Q = \frac{20}{80} \times 1 =$ 0.25Ω.

Chapter: 18 MOVING CHARGES AND MAGNETISM

Magnetic Force

1. In the product

$\vec{F} = q(\vec{v} \times \vec{B}) = q\vec{v} \times (B\hat{\imath} + B\hat{\jmath} + B_0\hat{k})$

For $q = 1$ and $\vec{v} = 2\hat{\imath} + 4\hat{\jmath} + 6\hat{k}$ and

$\vec{F} = 4\hat{\imath} - 20\hat{\jmath} + 12\hat{k}$

What will be the complete expression for $\vec{B}$? **(2021)**

(a) $6\hat{\imath} + 6\hat{\jmath} - 8\hat{k}$ (b) $-8\hat{\imath} - 8\hat{\jmath} - 6\hat{k}$

(c) $-6\hat{\imath} - 6\hat{\jmath} - 8\hat{k}$ (d) $8\hat{\imath} + 8\hat{\jmath} - 6\hat{k}$

2. A metallic rod of mass per unit length 0.5 kg m^{-1} is lying horizontally on a smooth inclined plane which makes an angle of $30°$ with the horizontal. The rod is not allowed to slide down by flowing a current through it when a magnetic field of induction 0.25 T is acting on it in the vertical direction. The current flowing in the rod to keep it stationary is **(2018)**

(a) 7.14 A (b) 5.98 A

(c) 14.76 A (d) 11.32 A

3. When a proton is released from rest in a room, it starts with an initial acceleration a_0 towards west. When it is projected towards north with a speed v_0 it moves with an initial acceleration $3a_0$ toward west. The electric and magnetic fields in the room are **(2013)**

(a) $\frac{ma_0}{e}$ east, $\frac{3ma_0}{ev_0}$ up

(b) $\frac{ma_0}{e}$ east, $\frac{3ma_0}{ev_0}$ down

(c) $\frac{ma_0}{e}$ west, $\frac{2ma_0}{ev_0}$ up

(d) $\frac{ma_0}{e}$ west, $\frac{2ma_0}{ev_0}$ down

4. A long straight wire carries a certain current and produces a magnetic field $2 \times 10^{-4} \text{ Wb m}^{-2}$ at a perpendicular distance of 5 cm from the wire. An electron situated at 5 cm from the wire moves with a velocity 10^7 m/s towards the wire along perpendicular to it. The force experienced by the electron will be (charge on electron $1.6 \times 10^{-19}\text{C}$)

(Karnataka NEET 2013)

(a) 3.2 N (b) 3.2×10^{-16} N

(c) 1.6×10^{-16} N (d) zero

5. A uniform electric field and a uniform magnetic field are acting along the same direction in a certain region. If an electron is projected in the region such that its velocity is pointed along the direction of fields, then the electron **(2011)**

(a) will turn towards right of direction of motion

(b) speed will decrease

(c) speed will increase

(d) will turn towards left of direction of motion.

6. The magnetic force acting on a charged particle of charge $-2\mu\text{C}$ in a magnetic field of 2 T acting in y direction, when the particle velocity is $(2\hat{\imath} + 3\hat{\jmath}) \times 10^6 \text{ m s}^{-1}$ is

(2009)

(a) 4 N in z direction

(b) 8 N in y direction

(c) 8 N in z direction

(d) 8 N in $-z$ direction.

7. When a charged particle moving with velocity $\vec{v}$ is subjected to a magnetic field of induction $\vec{B}$, the force on it is non-zero. This implies that **(2006)**

(a) angle between is either zero or 180°

(b) angle between is necessarily 90°

(c) angle between can have any value other than 90°

(d) angle between can have any value other than zero and 180°.

8. A very long straight wire carries a current I. At the instant when a charge $+Q$ at point P has velocity $\vec{v}$, as shown, the force on the charge is **(2005)**

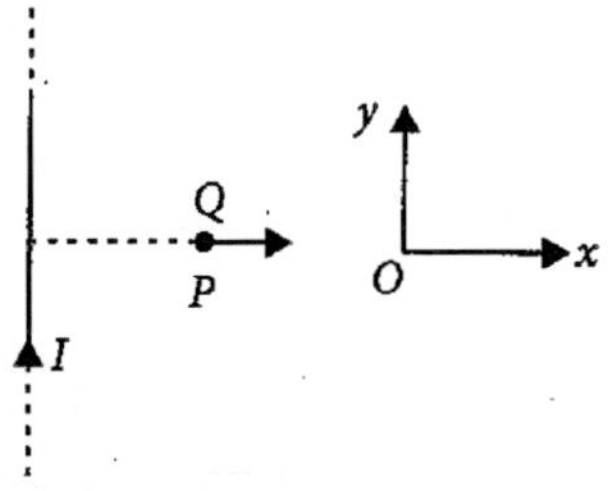

(a) along Oy

(b) opposite to Oy

(c) along Ox

(d) opposite to Ox.

9. A charge q moves in a region where electric field and magnetic field both exist, then force on it is **(2002)**

(a) $q(\vec{v} \times \vec{B})$ (b) $q\vec{E} + q(\vec{v} \times \vec{B})$

(c) $q\vec{E} + \vec{q}(\vec{B} \times \vec{v})$ (d) $q\vec{B} + q(\vec{E} \times \vec{v})$

10. Tesla is the unit of **(1997, 1988)**

(a) electric field (b) magnetic field

(c) electric flux (d) magnetic flux

11. A charge moving with velocity v in X-direction is subjected to a field of magnetic induction in negative X-direction. As a result, the charge will **(1993)**

(a) remain unaffected

(b) start moving in a circular path Y - Z plane

(c) retard along X-axis

(d) moving along a helical path around X-axis.

12. A straight wire of length 0.5 metre and carrying a current of 1.2 ampere is placed in uniform magnetic field of induction 2 tesla. The magnetic field is perpendicular to the length of the wire. The force on the wire is **(1992)**

(a) 2.4 N (b) 1.2 N

(c) 3.0 N (d) 2.0 N.

Motion in a Magnetic Field

13. Ionized hydrogen atoms and α-particles with same momenta enters perpendicular to a constant magnetic field, B. The ratio of their radii of their paths $r_H : r_\alpha$ will be **(2019)**

(a) 1: 4 (b) 2: 1

(c) 1: 2 (d) 4: 1

14. A proton and an alpha particle both enter a region of uniform magnetic field B,

moving at right angles to the field B. If the radius of circular orbits for both the particles is equal and the kinetic energy acquired by proton is 1MeV, the energy acquired by the alpha particle will be

(2015)

(a) 1.5MeV (b) 1MeV

(c) 4MeV (d) 0.5MeV

15. A proton carrying 1MeV kinetic energy is moving in a circular path of radius R in uniform magnetic field. What should be the energy of an α-particle to describe a circle of same radius in the same field?

(Mains 2012)

(a) 2MeV (b) 1MeV

(c) 0.5MeV (d) 4MeV

16. Under the influence of a uniform magnetic field, a charged particle moves with a constant speed v in a circle of radius R. The time period of rotation of the particle

(2009, 2007)

(a) depends on R and not on v.

(b) is independent of both v and R

(c) depends on both v and R

(d) depends on v and not on R.

17. A particle of mass m, charge Q and kinetic energy T enters in a transverse uniform magnetic field of induction $\vec{B}$. After 3 seconds the kinetic energy of the particle will be **(2008)**

(a) T (b) $4T$

(c) $3T$ (d) $2T$

18. A charged particle moves through a magnetic field in a direction perpendicular to it. Then the **(2003)**

(a) speed of the particle remains unchanged

(b) direction of the particle remains unchanged

(c) acceleration remains unchanged

(d) velocity remains unchanged.

19. An electron having mass m and kinetic energy E enter in uniform magnetic field B perpendicularly, then its frequency will be

(2001)

(a) $\frac{eE}{qvB}$ (b) $\frac{2\pi m}{eB}$

(c) $\frac{eB}{2\pi m}$ (d) $\frac{2m}{eBE}$

20. A charge having e/m equal to 10^8 C/kg and with velocity 3×10^5 m/s enters into a uniform magnetic field $B = 0.3$ tesla at an angle 30° with direction of field. The radius of curvature will be **(1999)**

(a) 0.01 cm (b) 0.5 cm

(c) 1 cm (d) 2 cm

21. A positively charged particle moving due East enters a region of uniform magnetic field directed vertically upwards. This particle will **(1997)**

(a) move in a circular path with a decreased speed

(b) move in a circular path with a uniform speed

(c) get deflected in vertically upward direction

(d) move in circular path with an increased speed.

22. A 10eV electron is circulating in a plane at right angles to a uniform field at magnetic induction 10^{-4} Wb/m^2 (= 1.0 gauss), the orbital radius of electron is **(1996)**

(a) 11 cm (b) 18 cm
(c) 12 cm (d) 16 cm

23. A uniform magnetic field acts right angles to the direction of motion of electrons. As a result, the electron moves in a circular path of radius 2 cm. If the speed of electrons is doubled, then the radius of the circular path will be **(1991)**

(a) 2.0 cm (b) 0.5 cm
(c) 4.0 cm (d) 1.0 cm

24. A deuteron of kinetic energy 50keV is describing a circular orbit of radius 0.5 metre in a plane perpendicular to magnetic field B. The kinetic energy of the proton that describes a circular orbit of radius 0.5 metre in the same plane with the same B is **(1991)**

(a) 25keV (b) 50keV
(c) 200keV (d) 100keV

Motion in Combined Electric and Magnetic Fields

25. An alternating electric field, of frequency v, is applied across the dees (radius $= R$) of a cyclotron that is being used to accelerate protons (mass $= m$). The operating magnetic field (B) used in the cyclotron and the kinetic energy (K) of the proton beam, produced by it, are given by **(2012)**

(a) $B = \frac{mv}{e}$ and $K = 2m\pi^2v^2R^2$
(b) $B = \frac{2\pi mv}{e}$ and $K = m^2\pi vR^2$
(c) $B = \frac{2\pi mv}{e}$ and $K = 2m\pi^2v^2R^2$
(d) $B = \frac{mv}{e}$ and $K = m^2\pi vR^2$.

26. A particle having a mass of 10^{-2} kg carries a charge of 5×10^{-8}C. The particle is given an initial horizontal velocity of 10^5 m s^{-1} in the presence of electric field $\vec{E}$ and magnetic field $\vec{B}$. To keep the particle moving in a horizontal direction, it is necessary that

(1) $\vec{B}$ should be perpendicular to the direction of velocity and $\vec{E}$ should be along the direction of velocity
(2) Both $\vec{B}$ and $\vec{E}$ should be along the direction of velocity
(3) Both $\vec{B}$ and $\vec{E}$ are mutually perpendicular and perpendicular to the direction of velocity.
(4) $\vec{B}$ should be along the direction of velocity and $\vec{E}$ should be perpendicular to the direction of velocity

Which one of the following pairs of statements is possible? **(Mains 2010)**

(a) (1) and (3) (b) (3) and (4)
(c) (2) and (3) (d) (2) and (4)

27. A beam of electron passes undeflected through mutually perpendicular electric and magnetic fields. If the electric field is switched off, and the same magnetic field is maintained, the electrons move **(2007)**

(a) in a circular orbit
(b) along a parabolic path
(c) along a straight line
(d) in an elliptical orbit.

28. In a mass spectrometer used for measuring the masses of ions, the ions are initially accelerated by an electric potential V and then made to describe semicircular paths of radius R using a magnetic field B. If V and B are kept constant, the ratio $\left(\frac{\text{charge on the ion}}{\text{mass of the ion}}\right)$ will be proportional to

(2007)

(a) $1/R^2$ (b) R^2
(c) R (d) $1/R$

29. In Thomson mass spectrograph $\vec{E} \perp \vec{B}$ then the velocity of electron beam will be

(2001)

(a) $\frac{|\vec{E}|}{|\vec{B}|}$ (b) $\vec{E} \times \vec{B}$
(c) $\frac{|\vec{B}|}{|\vec{E}|}$ (d) $\frac{\vec{E}^2}{\vec{B}^2}$

30. A beam of electrons is moving with constant velocity in a region having electric and magnetic fields of strength 20 V m^{-1} and 0.5 T at right angles to the direction of motion of the electrons. What is the velocity of the electrons? **(1996)**

(a) 8 m s^{-1} (b) 5.5 m s^{-1}
(c) 20 m s^{-1} (d) 40 m s^{-1}

Magnetic Field due to a Current Element, Biot-Savart Law

31. Given below are two statements :

Statement I: Biot-Savart's law gives us the expression for the magnetic field strength of an infinitesimal current element (Idl) of a current carrying conductor only.

Statement II : Biot-Savart's law is analogous to Coulomb's inverse square law of charge q, with the former being related to the field produced by a scalar source, Idl while the latter being produced by a vector source, q.

In light of above statements choose the most appropriate answer from the options given below. **(2022)**

(a) Both Statement I and Statement II are correct.
(b) Both Statement I and Statement II are incorrect.
(c) Statement I is correct and Statement II is incorrect.
(d) Statement I is incorrect and Statement II is correct.

32. The magnetic field $d\vec{B}$ due to a small current element $d\vec{l}$ at a distance $\vec{r}$ and element carrying current i is **(1996)**

(a) $d\vec{B} = \frac{\mu_0}{4\pi} i^2 \left(\frac{d\vec{l} \times \vec{r}}{r}\right)$

(b) $d\vec{B} = \frac{\mu_0}{4\pi} i \left(\frac{d\vec{l} \times \vec{r}}{r^3}\right)$

(c) $d\vec{B} = \frac{\mu_0}{4\pi} i \left(\frac{d\vec{l} \times \vec{r}}{r}\right)$

(d) $d\vec{B} = \frac{\mu_0}{4\pi} i^2 \left(\frac{d\vec{l} \times \vec{r}}{r^2}\right)$

Magnetic Field on the Axis of a Circular Current Loop

33. A very long conducting wire is bent in a semi-circular shape from A to B as shown in figure. The magnetic field at point P for steady current configuration is given by

(2023)

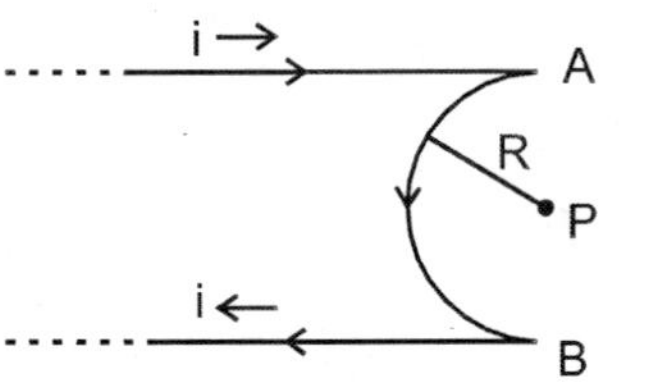

(a) $\frac{\mu_0 i}{4R}$ pointed away from the page

(b) $\frac{\mu_0 i}{4R}\left[1-\frac{2}{\pi}\right]$ pointed away from page

(c) $\frac{\mu_0 i}{4R}\left[1-\frac{2}{\pi}\right]$ pointed into the page

(d) $\frac{\mu_0 i}{4R}$ pointed into the page

34. A straight conductor carrying current i splits into two parts as shown in the figure. The radius of the circular loop is R. The total magnetic field at the centre P at the loop is **(Odisha NEET 2019)**

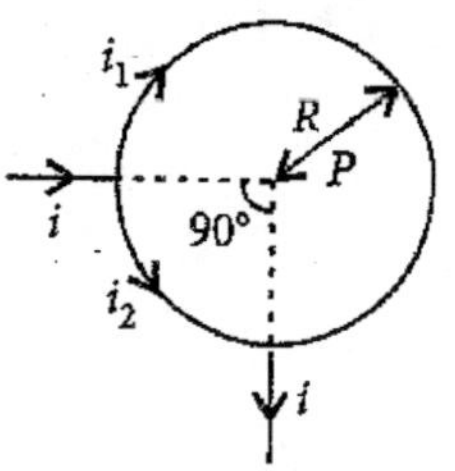

(a) Zero

(b) $3\mu_0 i/32R$, outward

(c) $3\mu_0 i/32R$, inward

(d) $\frac{\mu_0 i}{2R}$, inward

35. A long wire carrying a steady current is bent into a circular loop of one turn. The magnetic field at the centre of the loop is B. It is then bent into a circular coil of n turns. The magnetic field at the centre of this coil of n turns will be

(NEET-II 2016)

(a) nB (b) n^2B

(c) $2nB$ (d) $2n^2B$.

36. A wire carrying current I has the shape as shown in adjoining figure.

Linear parts of the wire are very long and parallel to X-axis while semicircular portion of radius R is lying in $Y-Z$ plane. Magnetic field at point O is

(2015 Cancelled)

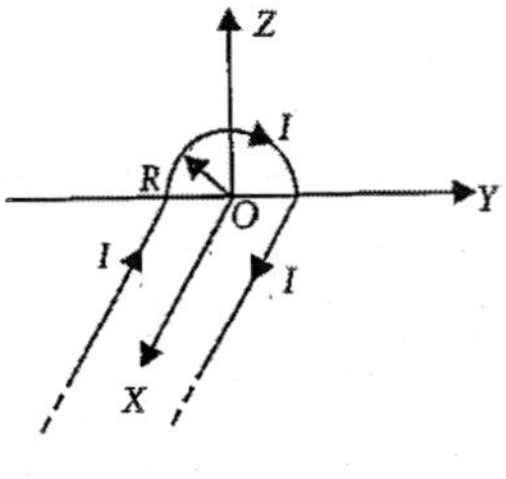

(a) $\vec{B} = -\frac{\mu_0}{4\pi}\frac{I}{R}(\pi\hat{\imath} + 2\hat{k})$

(b) $\vec{B} = \frac{\mu_0}{4\pi}\frac{I}{R}(\pi\hat{\imath} - 2\hat{k})$

(c) $\vec{B} = \frac{\mu_0}{4\pi}\frac{I}{R}(\pi\hat{\imath} + 2\hat{k})$

(d) $\vec{B} = -\frac{\mu_0}{4\pi}\frac{I}{R}(\pi\hat{\imath} - 2\hat{k})$.

37. Two similar coils of radius R are lying concentrically with their planes at right angles to each other. The currents flowing in them are I and $2I$, respectively. The resultant magnetic field induction at the centre will be **(2012)**

(a) $\frac{\sqrt{5}\mu_0 I}{2R}$ (b) $\frac{\sqrt{5}\mu_0 I}{R}$

(c) $\frac{\mu_0 I}{2R}$ (d) $\frac{\mu_0 I}{R}$

38. Charge q is uniformly spread on a thin ring of radius R. The ring rotates about its axis with a uniform frequency Hz. The magnitude of magnetic induction at the center of the ring is **(Mains 2011, 2010)**

(a) $\frac{\mu_0 qf}{2\pi R}$ (b) $\frac{\mu_0 qf}{2R}$

(c) $\frac{\mu_0 q}{2fR}$ (d) $\frac{\mu_0 q}{2\pi fR}$

39. A current loop consists of two identical semicircular parts each of radius R, one lying in the $x-y$ plane and the other in $x-z$ plane. If the current in the loop is i. The resultant magnetic field due to the two semicircular parts at their common centre is **(Mains 2010)**

(a) $\frac{\mu_0 i}{2\sqrt{2}R}$ (b) $\frac{\mu_0 i}{2R}$

(c) $\frac{\mu_0 i}{4R}$ (d) $\frac{\mu_0 i}{\sqrt{2}R}$

40. Two circular coils 1 and 2 are made from the same wire but the radius of the 1st coil is twice that of the 2nd coil. What potential difference in volts should be applied across them so that the magnetic field at their centres is the same? **(2006)**

(a) 2 (b) 3

(c) 4 (d) 6

41. An electron moves in a circular orbit with a uniform speed v. It produces a magnetic field B at the centre of the circle. The radius of the circle is proportional to **(2005)**

(a) $\sqrt{B/v}$ (b) B/v

(c) $\sqrt{v/B}$ (d) v/B

42. The magnetic field of given length of wire for single turn coil at its centre is B then its value for two turns coil for the same wire is **(2002)**

(a) $B/4$ (b) $B/2$

(c) $4B$ (d) $2B$

43. Magnetic field due to 0.1 A current flowing through a circular coil of radius 0.1 m and 1000 turns at the centre of the coil is **(1999)**

(a) 6.28×10^{-4} T

(b) 4.31×10^{-2} T

(c) 2×10^{-1} T

(d) 9.81×10^{-4} T

44. Magnetic field intensity at the centre of the coil of 50 turns, radius 0.5 m and carrying a current of 2 A, is **(1999)**

(a) 3×10^{-5} T

(b) 1.25×10^{-4} T

(c) 0.5×10^{-5} T

(d) 4×10^{6} T

45. A coil of one turn is made of a wire of certain length and then from the same length a coil of two turns is made. If the same current is passed in both the cases, then the ratio of the magnetic inductions at their centres will be **(1998)**

(a) $4:1$ (b) $1:4$

(c) $2:1$ (d) $1:2$

Ampere's Circuital Law

46. A wire carrying a current I along the positive x-axis has length L. It is kept in a magnetic field $\vec{B} = (2\hat{i} + 3\hat{j} - 4\hat{k})$T. The magnitude of the magnetic force acting on the wire is **(2023)**

(a) $\sqrt{5}$IL (b) 5 IL

(c) $\sqrt{3}$IL (d) 3 IL

47. From Ampere's circuital law for a long straight wire of circular cross-section carrying a steady current, the variation of magnetic field in the inside and outside region of the wire is **(2022)**

(a) uniform and remains constant for both the regions

(b) a linearly increasing function of distance upto the boundary of the wire and then linearly decreasing for the outside region

(c) a linearly increasing function of distance r upto the boundry of the wire and then decreasing one with $1/r$ dependence for the outside region

(d) a linearly decreasing function of distance upto the boundary of the wire and then a linearly increasing one for the outside region.

48. A thick current carrying cable of radius 'R' carries current 'I' uniformaly distributed across its crosssection. The variation of magnetic field $B(r)$ due to the cable with the distance 'r' from the axis of the cable is represented by **(2021)**

(a) 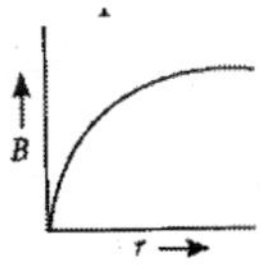

(b) 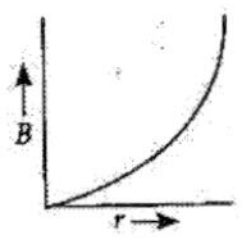

(c) 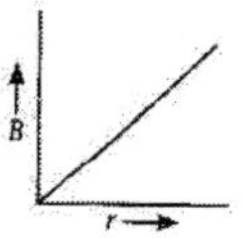

(d) 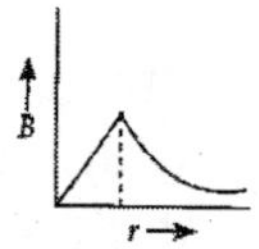

49. An infinitely long straight conductor carries a current of 5 A as shown. An electron is moving with a speed of 10^5 m/s parallel to the conductor. The perpendicular distance between the electron and the conductor is 20 cm at an instant. Calculate the magnitude of the force experienced by the electron at that instant. **(2021)**

Electron $v = 10^5$ m/s

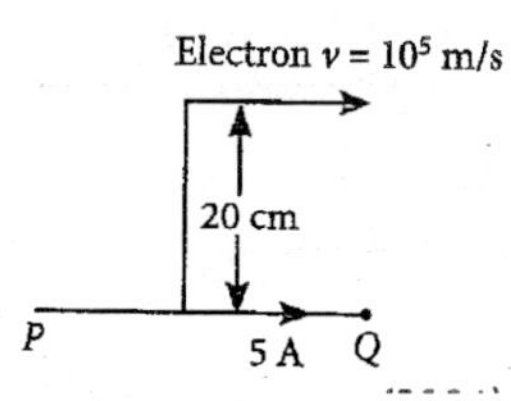

(a) 8×10^{-20} N (b) 4×10^{-20} N

(c) $8\pi \times 10^{-20}$ N (d) $4\pi \times 10^{-20}$ N

50. A cylindrical conductor of radius R is carrying a constant current. The plot of the magnitude of the magnetic field, B with the distance, d from the centre of the conductor, is correctly represented by the figure **(2019)**

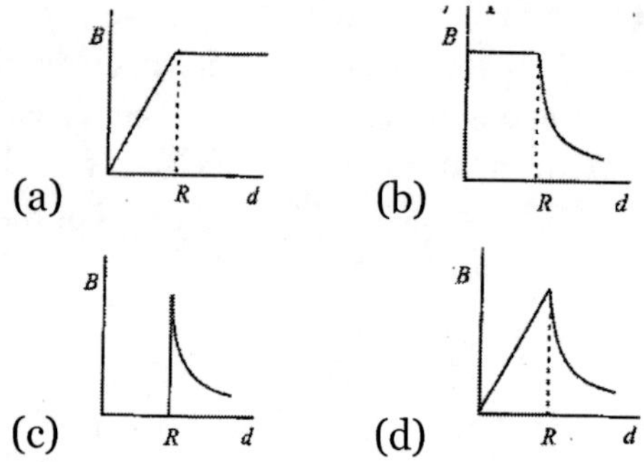

51. A long straight wire of radius a carries a steady current I. The current is uniformly distributed over its cross-section. The ratio of the magnetic fields B and B', at radial distances $a/2$ and $2a$ respectively, from the axis of the wire is **(NEET-I 2016)**

(a) 1 (b) 4

(c) $\frac{1}{4}$ (d) $\frac{1}{2}$

52. Two identical long conducting wires AOB and COD are placed at right angle to each other, with one above other such that O is their common point for the two. The wires carry I_1 and I_2 currents, respectively. Point P is lying at distance d from O along a direction perpendicular to the plane containing the wires. The magnetic field at the point P will be **(2014)**

(a) $\frac{\mu_0}{2\pi d}\left(\frac{I_1}{I_2}\right)$

(b) $\frac{\mu_0}{2\pi d}(I_1 + I_2)$

(c) $\frac{\mu_0}{2\pi d}(I_1^2 - I_2^2)$

(d) $\frac{\mu_0}{2\pi d}(I_1^2 + I_2^2)^{1/2}$.

53. The magnetic field at centre, P will be **(2000)**

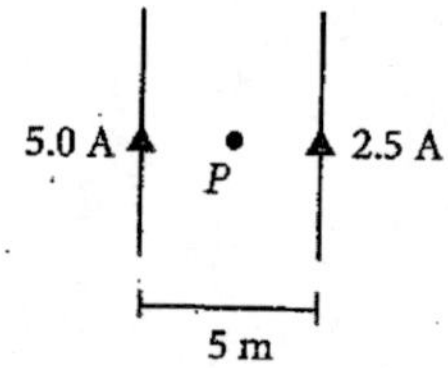

(a) $\frac{\mu_0}{4\pi}$ (b) $\frac{\mu_0}{\pi}$

(c) $\frac{\mu_0}{2\pi}$ (d) $4\mu_0\pi$

54. A straight wire of diameter 0.5 mm carrying a current of 1 A is replaced by the another wire of 1 mm diameter carrying the same current. The strength of the magnetic field far away is **(1999, 1997)**

(a) one-quarter of the earlier value

(b) one-half of the earlier value

(c) twice the earlier value

(d) same as the earlier value.

55. If a long hollow copper pipe carries a current, then produced magnetic field will be **(1999)**

(a) both inside and outside the pipe

(b) outside the pipe only

(c) inside the pipe only

(d) neither inside nor outside the pipe.

56. Two equal electric currents are flowing perpendicular to each other as shown in the figure. AB and CD are perpendicular to each other and symmetrically placed with respect to the currents.

Where do we expect the resultant magnetic field to be zero? **(1996)**

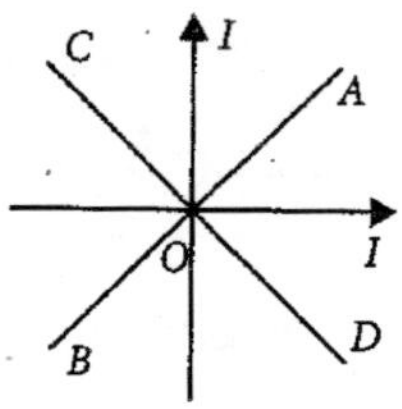

(a) On CD (b) On AB

(c) On both OD and BO

(d) On both AB and CD

57. The magnetic field at a distance r from a long wire carrying current i is 0.4 tesla. The magnetic field at a distance $2r$ is

(1992)

(a) 0.2 tesla (b) 0.8 tesla

(c) 0.1 tesla (d) 1.6 tesla

58. The magnetic induction at a point P which is at the distance of 4 cm from a long current carrying wire is 10^{-3} T. The field of induction at a distance 12 cm from the current will be **(1990)**

(a) 3.33×10^{-4} T (c) 33×10^{-3} T

(b) 1.11×10^{-4} T (d) 9×10^{-3} T

The Solenoid and the Toroid

59. A long solenoid of radius 1 mm has 100 turns per mm. If 1 A current flows in the solenoid, the magnetic field strength at the centre of the solenoid is **(2022)**

(a) 6.28×10^{-2} T (b) 12.56×10^{-2} T

(c) 12.56×10^{-4} T

(d) 6.28×10^{-4} T

60. A long solenoid of 50 cm length having 100 turns carries a current of 2.5 A. The magnetic field at the centre of the solenoid is ($\mu_0 = 4\pi \times 10^{-7}$ T m A^{-1}) **(2020)**

(a) 6.28×10^{-4} T

(b) 3.14×10^{-4} T

(c) 6.28×10^{-5} T

(d) 3.14×10^{-5} T

61. Two toroids 1 and 2 have total number of turns 200 and 100 respectively with average radii 40 cm and 20 cm respectively. If they carry same current i, the radio of the magnetic fields along the two loops is

(Odisha NEET 2019)

(a) 1: 1 (b) 4: 1

(c) 2: 1 (d) 1: 2

62. A long solenoid carrying a current produces a magnetic field B along its axis. If the current is doubled and the number of turns per cm is halved, the new value of the magnetic field is **(2003)**

(a) $B/2$ (b) B

(c) $2B$ (d) $4B$

Force between Two Parallel Currents, the Ampere

63. An arrangement of three parallel straight wires placed perpendicular to plane of paper carrying same current ' I ' along the same direction as shown in figure.

Magnitude of force per unit length on the middle wire ' B ' is given by **(2017)**

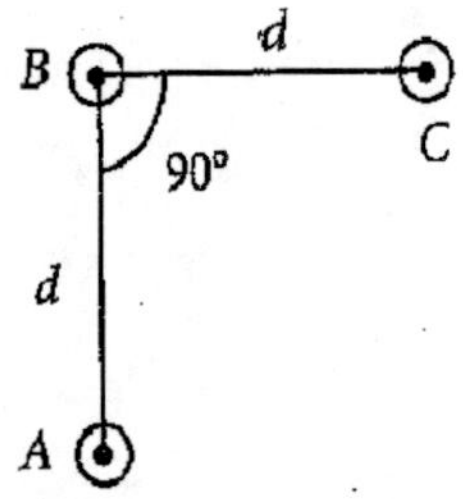

(a) $\frac{2\mu_0 I^2}{\pi d}$ (b) $\frac{\sqrt{2}\mu_0 I^2}{\pi d}$

(c) $\frac{\mu_0 I^2}{\sqrt{2}\pi d}$ (d) $\frac{\mu_0 I^2}{2\pi d}$

64. A square loop $ABCD$ carrying a current i, is placed near and coplanar with a long straight conductor XY carrying a current I, the net force on the loop will be

(NEET-I 2016)

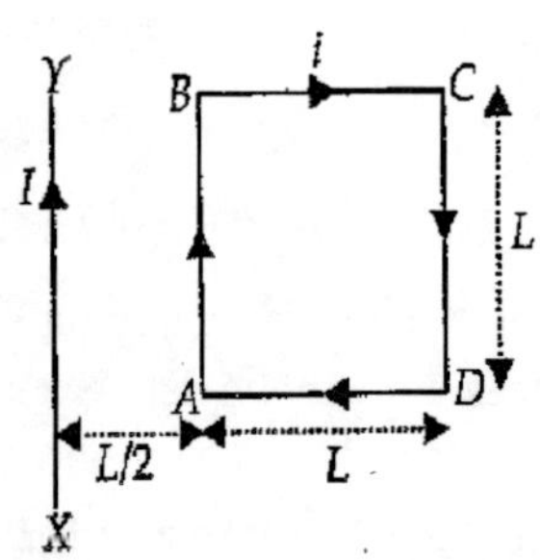

(a) $\frac{2\mu_0 IiL}{3\pi}$ (b) $\frac{\mu_0 IiL}{2\pi}$

(c) $\frac{2\mu_0 Ii}{3\pi}$ (d) $\frac{\mu_0 Ii}{2\pi}$

65. A square loop, carrying a steady current I, is placed in a horizontal plane near a long straight conductor carrying a steady current I_1 at a distance d from the conductor as shown in figure. The loop will experience **(Mains 2011)**

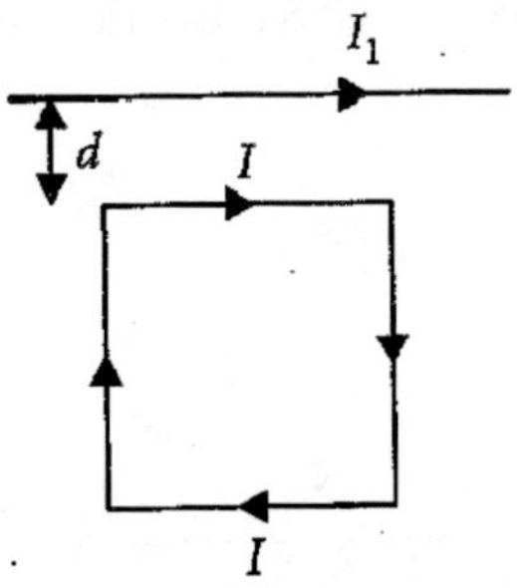

(a) a net attractive force towards the conductor

(b) a net repulsive force away from the conductor

(c) a net torque acting upward perpendicular to the horizontal plane

(d) a net torque acting downward normal to the horizontal plane.

66. Two long parallel wires are at a distance of 1 metre. Both of them carry one ampere of current. The force of attraction per unit length between the two wires is **(1998)**

(a) 5×10^{-8} N/m (b) 2×10^{-8} N/m

(c) 2×10^{-7} N/m (d) 10^{-7} N/m

67. Two parallel wires in free space are 10 cm apart and each carries a current of 10 A in the same direction. The force exerted by one wire on the other, per metre length is

(1997)

(a) 2×10^{-4} N, repulsive

(b) 2×10^{-7} N, repulsive

(c) 2×10^{-4} N, attractive

(d) 2×10^{-7} N, attractive.

Torque on Current Loop, Magnetic Dipole

68. A uniform conducting wire of length $12a$ and resistance ' R ' is wound up as a current carrying coil in the shape of

(i) an equilateral triangle of side ' a '.

(ii) a square of side ' a '.

The magnetic dipole moment of the coil in each case respectively are **(2021)**

(a) $4Ia^2$ and $3Ia^2$

(b) $\sqrt{3}Ia^2$ and $3Ia^2$

(c) $3Ia^2$ and Ia^2

(d) $3Ia^2$ and $4Ia^2$

69. A rectangular coil of length 0.12 m and width 0.1 m having 50 turns of wire is suspended vertically in a uniform magnetic field of strength 0.2Weber/m^2. The coil carries a current of 2 A. If the plane of the coil is inclined at an angle of $30°$ with the direction of the field, the torque required to keep the coil in stable equilibrium will be **(2015)**

(a) 0.24 N m (b) 0.12 N m

(c) 0.15 N m (d) 0.20 N m

70. A current loop in a magnetic field **(2013)**

(a) can be in equilibrium in two orientations, both the equilibrium states are unstable.

(b) can be in equilibrium in two orientations, one stable while the other is unstable.

(c) experiences a torque whether the field is uniform or non uniform in all orientations.

(d) can be in equilibrium in one orientation.

71. A circular coil $ABCD$ carrying a current ' i ' is placed in a uniform magnetic field. If the magnetic force on the segment AB is $\vec{F}$, the force on the remaining segment $BCDA$ is

(Karnataka NEET 2013)

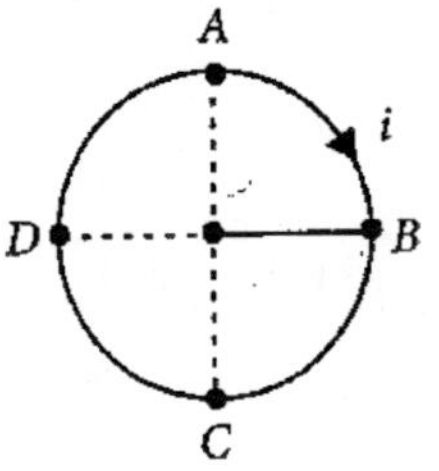

(a) $-\vec{F}$ (b) $3\vec{F}$

(c) $-3\vec{F}$ (d) $\vec{F}$

72. A current carrying closed loop in the form of a right angle isosceles triangle ABC is placed in a uniform magnetic field acting along AB. If the magnetic force on the arm BC is $\vec{F}$ the force on the arm AC is **(2011)**

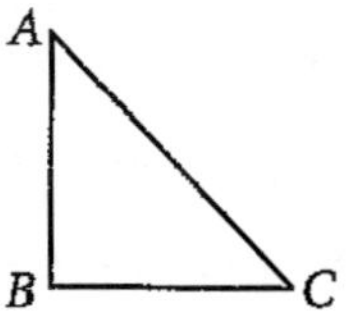

(a) $-\sqrt{2}\vec{F}$ (b) $-\vec{F}$

(c) $\vec{F}$ (d) $\sqrt{2}\vec{F}$

73. A square current carrying loop is suspended in a uniform magnetic field acting in the plane of the loop. If the force on one arm of the loop is $\vec{F}$ the net force on the remaining three arms of the loop is **(2010)**

(a) $3\vec{F}$ (b) $-\vec{F}$

(c) $-3\vec{F}$ (d) $\vec{F}$

74. A closed loop $PQRS$ carrying a current is placed in a uniform magnetic field. If the magnetic forces on segments PS, SR and RQ are F_1, F_2 and F_3 respectively and are in the plane of the paper and along the directions shown, the force on the segment QP is **(2008)**

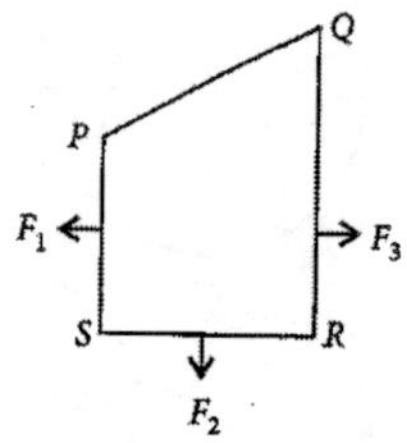

(a) $\sqrt{(F_3 - F_1)^2 - F_2^2}$

(b) $F_3 - F_1 + F_2$

(c) $F_3 - F_1 - F_2$

(d) $\sqrt{(F_3 - F_1)^2 + F_2^2}$.

75. A charged particle (charge) is moving in a circle of radius R with uniform speed v. The associated magnetic moment μ is given by **(2007)**

(a) qvR^2 (b) $qvR^2/2$

(c) qvR (d) $qvR/2$

76. A coil in the shape of an equilateral triangle of side l is suspended between the pole pieces of a permanent magnet such that $\vec{B}$ is in plane of the coil. If due to a current i in the triangle a torque τ acts on it, the side l of the triangle is **(2005)**

(a) $\frac{2}{\sqrt{3}}\left(\frac{\tau}{Bi}\right)$ (b) $2\left(\frac{\tau}{\sqrt{3}Bi}\right)^{1/2}$

(c) $\frac{2}{\sqrt{3}}\left(\frac{\tau}{Bi}\right)^{1/2}$ (d) $\frac{1}{\sqrt{3}}\frac{\tau}{Bi}$

77. If number of turns, area and current through a coil is given by n, A and i respectively then its magnetic moment will be **(2001)**

(a) niA (b) n^2iA

(c) niA^2 (d) $\frac{ni}{\sqrt{A}}$.

78. A circular loop of area $0.01\ \text{m}^2$ carrying a current of 10 A, is held perpendicular to a magnetic field of intensity 0.1 T. The torque acting on the loop is **(1994)**

(a) 0.001 N m (b) 0.8 N m

(c) zero (d) 0.01 N m.

79. A coil carrying electric current is placed in uniform magnetic field **(1993)**

(a) torque is formed

(b) e.m.f is induced

(c) both (a) and (b) are correct

(d) none of these

80. A current carrying coil is subjected to a uniform magnetic field. The coil will orient so that its plane becomes **(1988)**

(a) inclined at 45° to the magnetic field

(b) inclined at any arbitrary angle to the magnetic field

(c) parallel to the magnetic field

(d) perpendicular to magnetic field.

The Moving Coil Galvanometer

81. Current sensitivity of a moving coil galvanometer is 5 div/mA and its voltage sensitivity (angular deflection per unit voltage applied) is 20div/V. The resistance of the galvanometer is **(2018)**

(a) 40Ω (b) 25Ω

(c) 250Ω (d) 500Ω

82. In an ammeter 0.2% of main current passes through the galvanometer. If resistance of galvanometer is G, the resistance of ammeter will be **(2014)**

(a) $\frac{1}{499}G$ (b) $\frac{499}{500}G$

(c) $\frac{1}{500}G$ (d) $\frac{500}{499}G$

83. A milli voltmeter of 25 milli volt range is to be converted into an ammeter of 25 ampere range. The value (in ohm) of necessary shunt will be **(2012)**

(a) 0.001 (b) 0.01

(c) 1 (d) 0.05

84. A galvanometer of resistance, G, is shunted by a resistance S ohm. To keep the main current in the circuit unchanged, the resistance to be put in series with the galvanometer is **(Mains 2011)**

(a) $\frac{G}{(S+G)}$ (b) $\frac{S^2}{(S+G)}$

(c) $\frac{SG}{(S+G)}$ (d) $\frac{G^2}{(S+G)}$

85. A galvanometer has a coil of resistance 100ohm and gives a full scale deflection for 30 mA current. If it is work as a voltmeter of 30 volt range, the resistance required to be added will bc **(2010)**

(a) 900Ω (b) 1800Ω

(c) 500Ω (d) 1000Ω.

86. A galvanometer having a coil of resistance 60Ω shows full scale deflection when a current of 1.0amp passes through it. It can be converted into an ammeter to read currents upto 5.0amp by **(2009)**

(a) putting in series a resistance of 15Ω

(b) putting in series a resistance of 240Ω

(c) putting in parallel a resistance of 15Ω

(d) putting in parallel a resistance of 240Ω.

87. A galvanometer of resistance 50Ω is connected to a battery of 3 V along with a resistance of 2950Ω in series. A full scale deflection of 30 divisions is obtained in the galvanometer. In order to reduce this deflection to 20 divisions, the resistance in series should be **(2008)**

(a) 6050Ω (b) 4450Ω

(c) 5050Ω (d) 5550Ω

88. The resistance of an ammeter is 13Ω and its scale is graduated for a current upto 100 amps. After an additional shunt has been connected to this ammeter it becomes possible to measure currents upto 750 amperes by this meter. The value of shunt resistance is **(2007)**

(a) 2Ω (b) 0.2Ω

(c) $2k\Omega$ (d) 20Ω

89. A galvanometer of 50ohm resistance has 25 divisions. A current of 4×10^{-4} ampere gives a deflection of one division. To convert this galvanometer into a voltmeter having a range of 25 volts, it should be connected with a resistance of **(2004)**

(a) 2500Ω as a shunt

(b) 2450Ω as a shunt

(c) 2550Ω in series

(d) 2450Ω in series.

90. To convert a galvanometer into a voltmeter one should connect a **(2004 2002)**

(a) high resistance in series with galvanometer

(b) low resistance in series with galvanometer

(c) high resistance in parallel with galvanometer

(d) low resistance in parallel with galvanometer.

91. A galvanometer having a resistance of 9ohm is shunted by a wire of resistance 2ohm. If the total current is 1amp, the part of it passing through the shunt will be **(1998)**

(a) 0.2amp (b) 0.8amp

(c) 0.25amp (d) 0.5amp

92. To convert a galvanometer into a ammeter, one needs to connect a **(1992)**

(a) low resistance in parallel

(b) high resistance in parallel

(c) low resistance in series

(d) high resistance in series.

ANSWER KEY

1.	(c)	2.	(d)	3.	(d)	4.	(b)	5.	(b)	6.	(d)	7.	(d)
8.	(a)	9.	(b)	10.	(b)	11.	(a)	12.	(b)	13.	(b)	14.	(b)
15.	(b)	16.	(b)	17.	(a)	18.	(a)	19.	(c)	20.	(d)	21.	(b)
22.	(a)	23.	(c)	24.	(d)	25.	(c)	26.	(c)	27.	(a)	28.	(a)
29.	(a)	30.	(d)	31.	(c)	32.	(b)	33.	(b)	34.	(a)	35.	(b)
36.	(a)	37.	(a)	38.	(b)	39.	(a)	40.	(*)	41.	(c)	42.	(c)
43.	(a)	44.	(b)	45.	(b)	46.	(b)	47.	(c)	48.	(d)	49.	(a)
50.	(d)	51.	(a)	52.	(d)	53.	(c)	54.	(d)	55.	(b)	56.	(b)
57.	(a)	58.	(a)	59.	(b)	60.	(a)	61.	(a)	62.	(b)	63.	(c)
64.	(c)	65.	(a)	66.	(c)	67.	(c)	68.	(b)	69.	(d)	70.	(b)
71.	(a)	72.	(b)	73.	(b)	74.	(d)	75.	(d)	76.	(b)	77.	(a)
78.	(c)	79.	(a)	80.	(d)	81.	(c)	82.	(c)	83.	(a)	84.	(d)
85.	(a)	86.	(c)	87.	(b)	88.	(a)	89.	(d)	90.	(a)	91.	(b)
92.	(a)												

Hints & Explanations

1. **(c)** : Given: $\vec{v} = 2\hat{\imath} + 4\hat{\jmath} + 6\hat{k}$ and $q = 1; \vec{B} = B\hat{\imath} + B\hat{\jmath} + B_0\hat{k}$

$\vec{F} = 4\hat{\imath} - 20\hat{\jmath} + 12\hat{k}$

Now, $\vec{v} \times \vec{B} = \begin{vmatrix} \hat{\imath} & \hat{\jmath} & \hat{k} \\ 2 & 4 & 6 \\ B & B & B_0 \end{vmatrix}$

$= \hat{\imath}(4B_0 - 6B) - \hat{\jmath}(2B_0 - 6B) + \hat{k}(2B - 4B).$

Force $\vec{F} = q(\vec{v} \times \vec{B})$

$4\hat{\imath} - 20\hat{\jmath} + 12\hat{k} = 1\left[(4B_0 - 6B)\hat{\imath} - (2B_0 - 6B)\hat{\jmath} - 2B\hat{k}\right]$

By comparison

$$4B_0 - 6B = 4$$
$$-2B = 12$$
$$\Rightarrow B = -6$$

From eqn. (i) and (ii), $4B_0 - 6(-6) = 4$

$\Rightarrow 4B_0 + 36 = 4 \Rightarrow 4B_0 = -32 \Rightarrow B_0 = -8$

So, $\vec{B} = -6\hat{\imath} - 6\hat{\jmath} - 8\hat{k}$

2. **(d)** : Mass per unit length of a metallic rod is $\frac{m}{l} = 0.5 \text{ kg m}^{-1}$.

Let I be the current flowing.

For equilibrium, $mg\sin 30° = IlB\cos 30°$

$$I = \frac{mg}{lB}\tan 30° = \frac{0.5 \times 9.8}{0.25 \times \sqrt{3}} = 11.32 \text{ A}$$

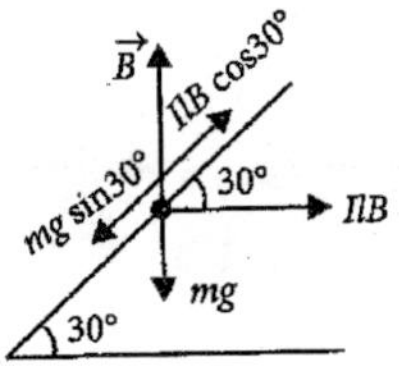

3. **(d)**

4. **(b)** : The situation is as shown in the figure.

Here, $v = 10^7$ m/s, $B = 2 \times 10^{-4}$ Wb/m^2

The magnitude of the force experienced by the electron is $F = evB\sin\theta$

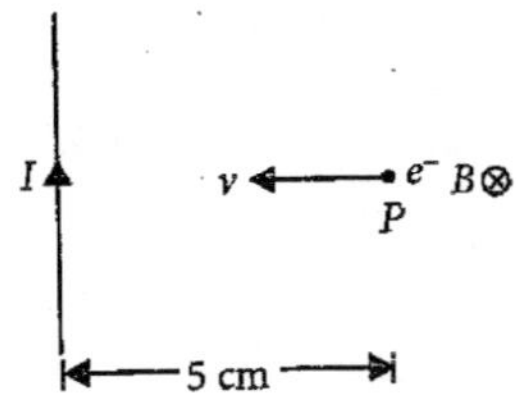

($\because \vec{v}$ and $\vec{B}$ are perpendicular to each other)

$= evB\sin 90° = 1.6 \times 10^{-19} \times 10^7 \times 2 \times 10^{-4} \times 1$
$= 3.2 \times 10^{-16}$ N

5. **(b)** : Force on electron due to electric field, $\vec{F}_E = -e\vec{E}$ Force on electron due to magnetic field, $\vec{F}_B = -e(\vec{v} \times \vec{B}) = 0$ Since $\vec{v}$ and $\vec{B}$ are in the same direction.

Total force on the electron,

$\vec{F} = \vec{F}_E + \vec{F}_B = -e\vec{E}$

Electric field opposes the motion of the electron, hence speed of the electron will decrease.

6. **(d)** : Lorentz force $= q(\vec{v} \times \vec{B})$

$= (-2 \times 10^{-6})[(2\hat{\imath} + 3\hat{\jmath})10^6 \times 2\hat{\jmath}]$

$= -8\hat{k}$ N

$= 8$ N in $-z$ direction.

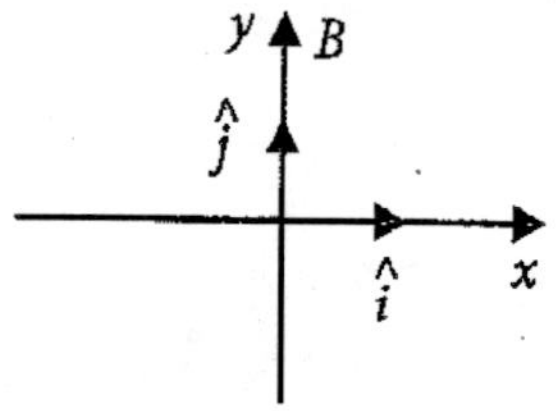

7. **(d) :** Force acting on a charged particle moving with velocity $\vec{v}$ is subjected to magnetic field $\vec{B}$ is given by

$$\vec{F} = q(\vec{v} \times \vec{B});\ F = qvB\sin\theta$$

(i) When $\theta = 0°, F = qvB\sin 0° = 0$

(ii) When $\theta = 90°, F = qvB\sin 90° = qvB$

(iii) When $\theta = 180°, F = qvB\sin 180° = 0$

This implies force acting on a charged particle is non-zero, when angle between $\vec{v}$ and $\vec{B}$ can have any value other than zero and 180°

8. **(a) :** According to Fleming's left hand rule direction of force is along Oy axis.

$\vec{F} = e(\vec{v} \times \vec{B})$.

B due to i is acting inwards i.e., into the paper. v is along Ox.

$\Rightarrow F = Q[v\hat{\imath} \times B(-\hat{k})]$

$\therefore\ \vec{F} = +QvB\hat{\jmath}$ i.e., in Oy direction.

9. **(b) :** The force experienced by a charged particle moving in space where electric and magnetic field exists is called Lorentz force.

When a charged particle carrying charge q is subjected to an electric field of strength $\vec{E}$, it experiences a force given by $\vec{F_e} = q\vec{E}$ whose direction is same as $\vec{E}$ or opposite of $\vec{E}$ depending on the nature of charge, positive or negative.

If a charged particle is moving in a magnetic field of strength $\vec{B}$ with a velocity $\vec{v}$ it experiences a force given by $\vec{F_m} = q(\vec{v} \times \vec{B})$.

The direction of this force is in the direction of $\vec{v} \times \vec{B}$ i.e., perpendicular to the plane containing $\vec{v}$ and $\vec{B}$ is directed as given by right hand screw rule.

Due to both the electric and magnetic fields, the total force experienced by the charge q is given by

$$\vec{F} = \vec{F_e} + \vec{F_m} = q\vec{E} + q(\vec{v} \times \vec{B})$$

10. **(b)**

11. **(a) :** The force acting on a charged particle in magnetic field is given by $\vec{F} = q(\vec{v} \times \vec{B}); F = qvB\sin\theta$

$\therefore F = 0$

when angle between $\vec{v}$ and $\vec{B}$ is 180°.

12. **(b) :** From, $F = il \times B = 1.2 \times 0.5 \times 2 = 1.2$ N

13. **(b) :** As, $r = \frac{mv}{qB} = \frac{p}{qB}$

For given p and $B, r \propto \frac{1}{q} \Rightarrow \frac{r_H}{r_\alpha} = \frac{q_\alpha}{q_H} = \frac{2}{1}$

14. **(b) :** The kinetic energy acquired by a charged particle in a uniform magnetic field B is

$$K = \frac{q^2B^2R^2}{2m}\ \left(\text{as } R = \frac{mv}{qB} = \frac{\sqrt{2mK}}{qB}\right)$$

where q and m are the charge and mass of the particle and R is the radius of circular orbit.

$\therefore$ The kinetic energy acquired by proton is $K_p = \frac{q_p^2 B^2 R_p^2}{2m_p}$

and that by the alpha particle is $K_\alpha = \frac{q_\alpha^2 B^2 R_\alpha^2}{2m_\alpha}$

Thus, $\frac{K_\alpha}{K_p} = \left(\frac{q_\alpha}{q_p}\right)^2 \left(\frac{m_p}{m_\alpha}\right) \left(\frac{R_\alpha}{R_p}\right)^2$

or $K_\alpha = K_p \left(\frac{q_\alpha}{q_p}\right)^2 \left(\frac{m_p}{m_\alpha}\right) \left(\frac{R_\alpha}{R_p}\right)^2$

Here, $K_p = 1\text{MeV}, \frac{q_\alpha}{q_p} = 2, \frac{m_p}{m_\alpha} = \frac{1}{4}$ and $\frac{R_\alpha}{R_p} = 1$

$$\therefore K_\alpha = (1\text{MeV})(2)^2\left(\frac{1}{4}\right)(1)^2 = 1\text{MeV}$$

15. (b) :

16. (b) : For the circular motion of a charged particle in a uniform magnetic field

$$qvB = \frac{mv^2}{R} \Rightarrow qB = m\omega = \frac{m \times 2\pi}{T}$$

$\therefore T = \frac{2\pi m}{qB}$ is independent of v and R.

17. (a) : When a charged particle having K.E., T enters in a field of magnetic induction, which is perpendicular to its velocity, it takes a circular trajectory. It does not increase in energy, therefore T is the K.E.

18. (a) : If a moving charged particle is subjected to a perpendicular uniform magnetic field, then according to $F = qvB\sin\theta$, it will experience a maximum force which will provide the centripetal force to particle and it will describe a circular path with uniform speed.

19. (c) : The frequency of revolution of a charged particle in a perpendicular magnetic field is

$$\nu = \frac{1}{T} = \frac{1}{2\pi r/v} = \frac{v}{2\pi r} = \frac{v}{2\pi} \times \frac{eB}{mv} = \frac{eB}{2\pi m}$$

20. (b) :

$$R = \frac{mv_\perp}{qB}$$

$$R = \frac{mv\sin\theta}{qB} = \frac{3 \times 10^5 \times \frac{1}{2}}{10^8 \times 0.3} = 0.05 \text{ m}$$
$$= 0.5 \text{ cm}$$

21. (b) : When a positively charged particle enters in a region of uniform magnetic field, directed perpendicular to the velocity it experiences a centripetal force which will move it in circular path with a uniform speed.

22. (a) :

Kinetic energy of electron $\left(\frac{1}{2} \times mv^2\right) = 10\text{eV}$ and magnetic induction $(B) = 10^{-4}$ Wb/m^2

Therefore, $\frac{1}{2}(9.1 \times 10^{-31})v^2 = 10 \times (1.6 \times 10^{-19})$

or, $v^2 = \frac{2 \times 10 \times (1.6 \times 10^{-19})}{9.1 \times 10^{-31}} = 3.52 \times 10^{12}$

or, $\boldsymbol{v} = 1.876 \times 10^6$ m/s

Centripetal force, $\frac{mv^2}{r} = Bev$

Therefore, $r = \frac{mv}{Be} = \frac{(9.1 \times 10^{-31}) \times (1.876 \times 10^6)}{10^{-4} \times (1.6 \times 10^{-19})}$

$$= 11 \times 10^{-2} \text{ m} = 11 \text{ cm}$$

23. (c) : $r = \frac{mv}{qB}$ or $r \propto v$

As v is doubled, the radius also becomes doubled. Hence new radius $= 2 \times 2 =$ 4 cm.

24. (d) : For a charged particle orbiting in a circular path in a magnetic field

$\frac{mv^2}{r} = Bvq \Rightarrow v = \frac{Bqr}{m}$

$$E_K = \frac{1}{2}mv^2 = \frac{1}{2}Bqvr = Bq\frac{r}{2} \cdot \frac{Bqr}{m} = \frac{B^2q^2r^2}{2m}$$

For deuteron, $E_1 = \frac{B^2q^2 \times r^2}{2 \times 2m}$

For proton, $E_2 = \frac{B^2q^2r^2}{2m}$

$$\frac{E_1}{E_2} = \frac{1}{2} \Rightarrow \frac{50\text{keV}}{E_2} = \frac{1}{2} \Rightarrow E_2 = 100\text{keV}$$

25. (c) : Frequency, $v = \frac{eB}{2\pi m}$ or $B = \frac{2\pi m v}{e}$

As $\frac{mv^2}{R} = evB$ or $v = \frac{eBR}{m} = 2\pi v R$

Kinetic energy, $K = \frac{1}{2}mv^2 = \frac{1}{2}m(2\pi v R)^2 = 2m\pi^2 v^2 R^2$

26. (c)

27. (a) : Electron travelling in a magnetic field perpendicular to its velocity follows a circular path.

28. (a) : In mass spectrometer when ions are accelerated through potential V,

$$\frac{1}{2}mv^2 = qV$$

where m is the mass of ion, q is the charge of the ion.

As the magnetic field curves the path of the ions in a semicircular orbit

$$\therefore\ Bqv = \frac{mv^2}{R} \Rightarrow v = \frac{BqR}{m}$$

Substituting (ii) in (i), we get

$$\frac{1}{2}m\left[\frac{BqR}{m}\right]^2 = qV$$

$$\text{or, } \frac{q}{m} = \frac{2V}{B^2R^2}$$

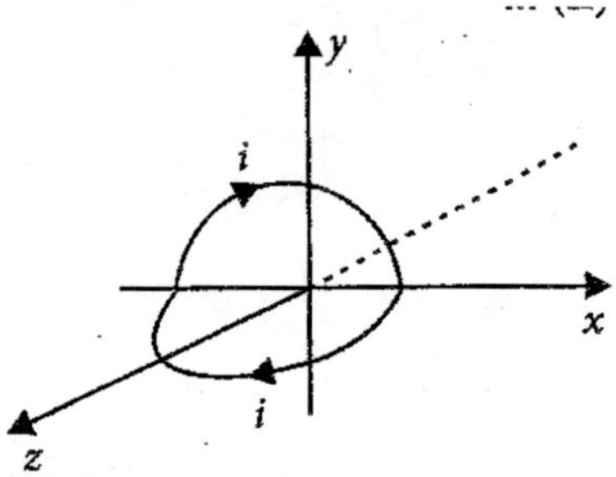

Since V, B are constants,

$\frac{q}{m} \propto \frac{1}{R^2}$ or, $\frac{\text{charge on the ion}}{\text{mass of the ion}} \propto \frac{1}{R^2}$

29. (a) : $eE = evB \ \therefore v = \frac{|\vec{E}|}{|\vec{B}|}$

30. (d) :

Electric field $(E) = 20$ V/m and magnetic field $(B) = 0.5$ T.

The force on electron in a magnetic field $= evB$

Force on electron in an electric field $= eE$

Since the electron is moving with constant velocity, therefore the resultant force on electron is zero. i.e., $eE = evB \Rightarrow v = E/B = 20/0.5 = 40 \text{ m s}^{-1}$

31. **(c) :** Statement I is correct, but statement II is incorrect because, the magnetic field is produced by vector source Idl and the coulomb's force is produced by scalar source q.

32. **(b) :** According to Biot-Savart's law,

$$d\vec{B} \propto i\left(\frac{d\vec{l} \times \vec{r}}{r^3}\right) \text{ or } d\vec{B} = \frac{\mu_0}{4\pi} i\left(\frac{d\vec{l} \times \vec{r}}{r^3}\right)$$

33. **(b) :** $B = \frac{\mu_0}{4\pi}\frac{I}{R}(\pi) - \frac{\mu_0}{4\pi}\frac{2I}{R}$

$= \frac{\mu_0 I}{4R}\left[1 - \frac{2}{\pi}\right]$ outward i.e away from page.

34. **(a) :** Magnetic field due to $i_1 = \frac{\mu_0 i_1}{2R}\frac{\theta_1}{2\pi}$

Magnetic field due to $i_2 = \frac{\mu_0 i_2}{2R}\frac{\theta_2}{2\pi}$

(Into the plane)

For parallel combination

Now, $\frac{i_1}{i_2} = \frac{\rho l_2}{A} \times \frac{A}{\rho l_1} = \frac{l_2}{l_1}$

$$\Rightarrow \frac{i_1}{i_2} = \frac{\frac{1}{4}(2\pi R)}{\frac{3}{4}(2\pi R)} = \frac{1}{3} \Rightarrow i_1 = \frac{i_2}{3} \Rightarrow i_2 = 3i_1$$

(Out of the plane)

$\therefore$ Net magnetic field, $= \frac{\mu_0 i_1}{2R}\left(\frac{\theta_1}{2\pi}\right) - \frac{\mu_0 i_2}{2R}\left(\frac{\theta_2}{2\pi}\right)$

$$= \frac{\mu_0 i_1}{2R}\left(\frac{3\pi}{2 \times 2\pi}\right) - \frac{\mu_0 i_2}{2R}\left(\frac{\pi}{2 \times 2\pi}\right)$$

$$= \frac{\mu_0}{2R}\left[\frac{3i_1}{4} - \frac{i_2}{4}\right] = \frac{\mu_0}{2R}\left[\frac{3i_1}{4} - \frac{3i_1}{4}\right] = 0$$

35. **(b) :** Let l be the length of the wire. Magnetic field at the centre of the loop is

$$B = \frac{\mu_0 I}{2R} \therefore B = \frac{\mu_0 \pi I}{l} \quad (\because l = 2\pi R)$$

$$B' = \frac{\mu_0 nI}{2r} = \frac{\mu_0 nI}{2\left(\frac{l}{2n\pi}\right)} \text{ or, } B' = \frac{\mu_0 n^2 \pi I}{l}$$

From eqns. (i) and (ii), we get $B' = n^2 B$

36. **(a) :** Given situation is shown in the figure.

Parallel wires 1 and 3 are semiinfinite, so magnetic field at O due to them

$$\vec{B}_1 = \vec{B}_3 = -\frac{\mu_0 I}{4\pi R}\hat{k}$$

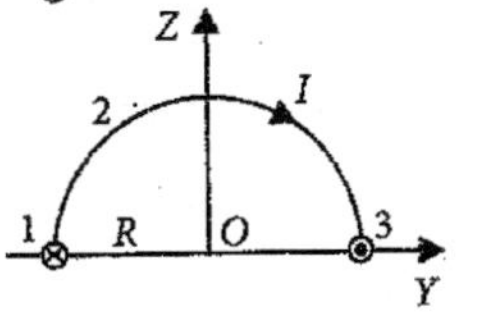

Magnetic field at O due to semi-circular arc in

YZ-plane is given by $\vec{B}_2 = -\frac{\mu_0 I}{4R}\hat{i}$

Net magnetic field at point O is given by

$$\vec{B} = \vec{B}_1 + \vec{B}_2 + \vec{B}_3$$

$$= -\frac{\mu_0 I}{4\pi R}\hat{k} - \frac{\mu_0 I}{4R}\hat{i} - \frac{\mu_0 I}{4\pi R}\hat{k} = -\frac{\mu_0 I}{4\pi R}(\pi\hat{i} + 2\hat{k})$$

37. **(a) :** Magnetic field induction due to vertical loop at the centre O is

$$B_1 = \frac{\mu_0 I}{2R}$$

It acts in horizontal direction.

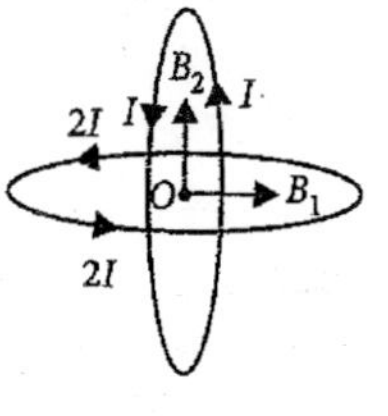

Magnetic field induction due to horizontal loop at the centre O is

$$B_2 = \frac{\mu_0 2I}{2R}$$

It acts in vertically upward direction.

As B_1 and B_2 are perpendicular to each other, therefore the resultant magnetic field induction at the centre O is

$$B_{\text{net}} = \sqrt{B_1^2 + B_2^2} = \sqrt{\left(\frac{\mu_0 I}{2R}\right)^2 + \left(\frac{\mu_0 2I}{2R}\right)^2}$$

$$B_{\text{net}} = \frac{\mu_0 I}{2R}\sqrt{(1)^2 + (2)^2} = \frac{\sqrt{5}\mu_0 I}{2R}$$

38. **(b) :** The current flowing in the ring is

$$I = qf$$

The magnetic induction at the centre of the ring is

$$B = \frac{\mu_0 I}{2R} = \frac{\mu_0 qf}{2R}$$

39. **(a) :** The loop mentioned in the question must look like one as shown in the figure.

Magnetic field at the centre due to semicircular loop lying in $x - y$ plane, $B_{xy} - \frac{1}{2}\left(\frac{\mu_0 i}{2R}\right)$ negative z direction.

Similarly field due to loop in $x - z$ plane, $B_{xz} = \frac{1}{2}\left(\frac{\mu_0 i}{2R}\right)$ in negative y direction.

∴ Magnitude of resultant magnetic field,

$$B = \sqrt{B_{xy}^2 + B_{xz}^2} = \sqrt{\left(\frac{\mu_0 i}{4R}\right)^2 + \left(\frac{\mu_0 i}{4R}\right)^2}$$

$$= \frac{\mu_0 i}{4R}\sqrt{2} = \frac{\mu_0 i}{2\sqrt{2}R}$$

40. **(*) :** The magnetic field at the centre of the coil,

$$B = \frac{\mu_0 ni}{2r}; \text{ where } r \text{ is the radius.}$$

$$E/R = i$$

∴ $R \propto 2\pi r \Rightarrow R = cr$, where c is a constant.

∴ In the first coil, $B_1 = \frac{\mu_0 ni_1}{2r_1} = \frac{\mu_0 nE}{2r_1(cr_1)} = \frac{\mu_0 nE}{2cr_1^2}$

If $r_1 = 2r_2, B_1 = \frac{\mu_0 nE_1}{2c(2r_2)^2} = \frac{\mu_0 nE_1}{2c\cdot 4r_2^2}$

$$B_2 = \frac{\mu_0 nE_2}{2cr_2^2}$$

As B_1 will not be equal to B_2 unless E_1 is different from E_2, E_1 and E_2 will not be the same.

It is wrong to ask what potential difference should be applied across them. It should be perhaps the ratio of potential differences.

In that case, $B_1 = B_2, \frac{E_1}{4} = E_2 \Rightarrow E_1 = 4E_2$

∴ $\frac{E_1}{E_2} = 4.$

* Question is not correct.

41. **(c) :** The magnetic field is produced by moving electron in circular path $B = \frac{\mu_0 i}{2r}$

where $i = \frac{q}{t} = \frac{q}{2\pi r} \times v$

$$\therefore B = \frac{\mu_0 qv}{4\pi r^2} \Rightarrow r \propto \sqrt{\frac{v}{B}}$$

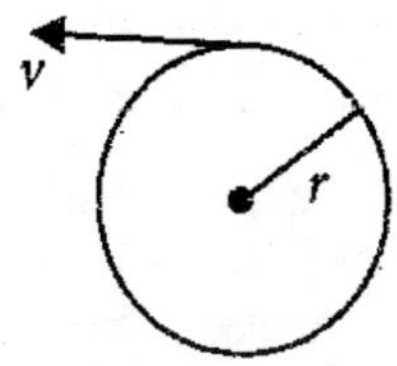

42. **(c) :** The magnetic field B produced at the centre of a circular coil due to current I flowing through this is given by $B = \frac{\mu_0 NI}{2r}$, N is number of turns and r is radius of the coil. Here $B = \frac{\mu_0 I}{2r}$ $[N = 1]$

Here, $2 \times 2\pi r' = 2\pi r \therefore r' = r/2$

$\therefore$ Magnetic field at the centre for two turns $(N = 2)$ is given by $B' = \frac{\mu_0 \times 2I}{2r'} = \frac{\mu_0 \times 2I}{2r/2} = \frac{4\mu_0 I}{2r} = 4B$.

43. **(a) :**

$B = \frac{\mu_0 Ni}{2r} = \frac{4\pi \times 10^{-7} \times 1000 \times 0.1}{2 \times 0.1} = 6.28 \times 10^{-4}$ T

44. **(b) :**

$B = \frac{\mu_0 (Ni)}{2r} = \frac{4\pi \times 10^{-7} \times 50 \times 2}{2 \times 0.5} = 1.256 \times 10^{-4}$ T

45. **(b) :** Magnetic field at the centre of the coil, $B = \frac{\mu_0}{2\pi}\frac{NI}{a}$

Let l be the length of the wire, then

$$B_1 = \frac{\mu_0}{2\pi} \cdot \frac{1 \times I}{l/2\pi} = \frac{\mu_0 I}{l} \text{ and } B_2 = \frac{\mu_0}{2\pi} \cdot \frac{2 \times I}{l/4\pi} = \frac{4\mu_0 I}{l}$$

Therefore, $\frac{B_1}{B_2} = \frac{1}{4}$ or, $B_1 : B_2 = 1 : 4$

46. **(b) :** $\vec{F} = I(\vec{\ell} \times \vec{B})$

$$= I[(L\hat{i}) \times (2\hat{i} + 3\hat{j} - 4\hat{k})]$$

$$= I(4L\hat{j} + 3L\hat{k})$$

$$|\vec{F}| = 5IL$$

47. **(c) :** Using Ampere's circuital law

$$B_{in} = \frac{\mu_0 Ir}{2\pi a^2}, \text{ or } B_{in} \propto r$$

$$B_{out} = \frac{\mu_0 I}{2\pi r}, \text{ or } B_{out} \propto \frac{1}{r}$$

48. **(d) :** By Ampere's circuital law,

$$\oint \vec{B} \cdot d\vec{l} = \mu_0 \times \text{current losed by path}$$

$$\Rightarrow B \cdot 2\pi r = \mu_0 \times \frac{Ir^2}{a^2} (\because R = a)$$

$$\Rightarrow B = \frac{\mu_0 Ir}{2\pi a^2} (\text{ for } r < a)$$

At surface $r = a$, so $B = \frac{\mu_0 I}{2\pi a}$

$\therefore B = \frac{\mu_0 I}{2\pi r} (\text{ for } r > a)$

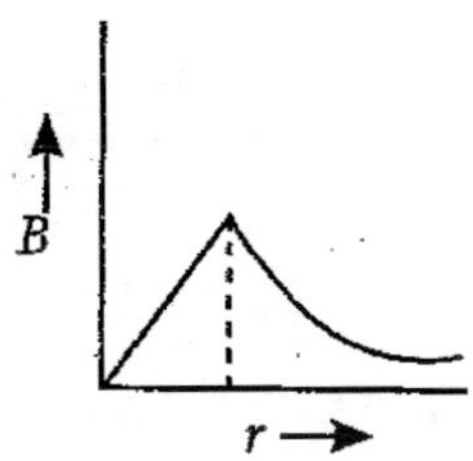

The variation of magnetic field with distance 'r' from the axis is given by the above figure.

49. **(a) :** The magnetic field due to a straight wire at the location of electron is

$$B = \frac{\mu_0}{4\pi} \cdot \frac{2I}{r}$$

$$B = 10^{-7} \times \frac{2 \times 5}{0.2} = 50 \times 10^{-7} \text{ T}(\hat{k})$$

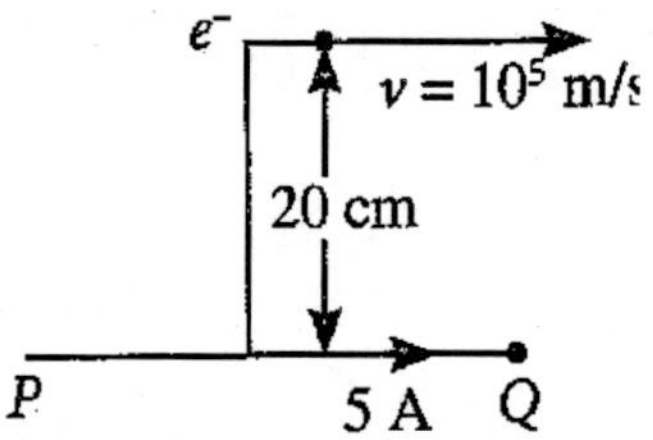

The direction is given by right hand thumb rule.

The force on charged particle moving in magnetic field is

$\vec{F} = q(\vec{v} \times \vec{B})$
$\vec{F} = -1.6 \times 10^{-19} \times \left(10^5\hat{\imath} \times 50 \times 10^{-7}\hat{k}\right)$
$\vec{F} = 8 \times 10^{-20}\ \text{N}\hat{\jmath}$

50. (d) : Magnetic field due to long solid cylindrical conductor of radius R,

(i) For $d < R, I' = \frac{Id^2}{R^2}$

$$\int \vec{B} \cdot d\vec{l} = \mu_0 I' \Rightarrow B(2\pi d) = \frac{\mu_0 I d^2}{R^2} \Rightarrow B = \frac{\mu_0 I d}{2\pi R^2}$$

$\therefore B \propto d$

(ii) For $d = R, B = \mu_0 I/2\pi R$ (maximum)

(iii) For $d > R, B = \mu_0 I/2\pi d \Rightarrow B \propto 1/d$

51. (a) : Magnetic field at a point inside the wire at distance $r\left(=\frac{a}{2}\right)$ from the axis of wire is

$$B = \frac{\mu_0 I}{2\pi a^2} r = \frac{\mu_0 I}{2\pi a^2} \times \frac{a}{2} = \frac{\mu_0 I}{4\pi a}$$

Magnetic field at a point outside the wire at a distance $r(= 2a)$. from the axis of wire is

$$B' = \frac{\mu_0 I}{2\pi r} = \frac{\mu_0 I}{2\pi} \times \frac{1}{2a} = \frac{\mu_0 I}{4\pi a} \quad \therefore \frac{B}{B'} = 1$$

52. (d) : The magnetic field at the point P, at a perpendicular distance d from O in a direction perpendicular to the plane $ABCD$ due to currents through AOB and COD are perpendicular to each other. Hence,

$$B = (B_1^2 + B_2^2)^{1/2}$$

$$= \left[\left(\frac{\mu_0}{4\pi}\frac{2I_1}{d}\right)^2 + \left(\frac{\mu_0}{4\pi}\frac{2I_2}{d}\right)^2\right]^{1/2}$$

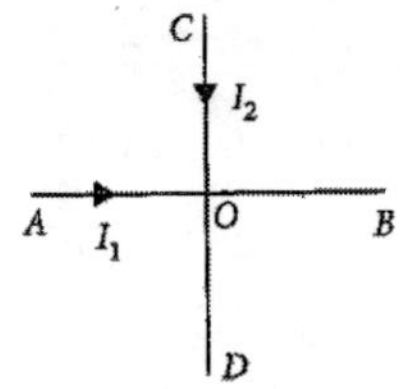

$$= \frac{\mu_0}{2\pi d}(I_1^2 + I_2^2)^{1/2}$$

53. (c) :

$$B = \frac{\mu_0}{4\pi}\frac{2i_2}{(r/2)} - \frac{\mu_0}{4\pi}\frac{2i_1}{(r/2)} = \frac{\mu_0}{4\pi}\frac{4}{r}(i_2 - i_1)$$

$$= \frac{\mu_0}{4\pi}\frac{4}{5}(2.5 - 5.0) = -\frac{\mu_0}{2\pi}$$

Negative sign shows that B is acting inwards i.e., into the plane.

54. (d) : Diameter of first wire $(d_1) =$ 0.5 mm;

Current in first wire $(I_1) = 1$ A; Diameter of second wire $(d_2) = 1$ mm and current in second wire $(I_2) = 1$ A

Strength of magnetic field due to current flowing in a conductor,

$(B) = \frac{\mu_0}{4\pi} \times \frac{2I}{a}$ or $B \propto I$

Since the current in both the wires is same, therefore there is no change in the strength of the magnetic field.

55. (b) : Use Ampère's law $\oint B \cdot dl = \mu_0 i_{\text{enclosed}}$.

Outside : $i_{\text{enclosed}} \neq 0$ (some value) $\Rightarrow B \neq 0$

Inside = $i_{\text{enclosed}} = 0 \Rightarrow B = 0$

56. (b) : The direction of the magnetic field, due to current, is given by the right-hand rule. At axis AB, the components of magnetic field will cancel each other and the resultant magnetic field will be zero.

57. (a) : $B = \frac{\mu_0 i}{2\pi r}$ or $B \propto \frac{1}{r}$

When r is doubled, the magnetic field becomes halved i.e.,now the magnetic field will be 0.2 T.

58. (a) : $B \propto 1/r$, for given current.

As the distance is increased to three times, the magnetic induction reduces to one third.

Hence $B = \frac{1}{3} \times 10^{-3}\ \text{T} = 3.33 \times 10^{-4}\ \text{T}$

59. (b) : Here, number of turns in the solenoid,

$n = 100/1\ \text{mm} = 100 \times 10^3/\text{m}$

Current in the solenoid, $I = 1$ A

Magnetic field strength at the centre of the solenoid,

$B = \mu_0 nI$

$= 4\pi \times 10^{-7} \times 10^5 \times 1 = 12.56 \times 10^{-2}$ T

60. (a) : Here, $l = 50$ cm, $N = 100$, $i = 2.5$ A

Magnetic field inside the solenoid,

$$B = \mu_0 ni = \frac{\mu_0 NI}{l}$$

$$B = \frac{4\pi \times 10^{-7} \times 100 \times 2.5}{0.5}$$
$$= 6.28 \times 10^{-4}\ \text{T}$$

61. (a) : For a toroid magnetic field, $B = \mu_0 ni$

Where, n = number of turns per unit length $= \frac{N}{2\pi r}$

Now, $\frac{B_1}{B_2} = \frac{\mu_0 n_1 i}{\mu_0 n_2 i} = \frac{n_1}{n_2} = \frac{N_1}{2\pi r_1} \times \frac{2\pi r_2}{N_2}$

$$\Rightarrow \frac{B_1}{B_2} = \frac{200}{2\pi \times 40 \times 10^{-2}} \times \frac{2\pi \times 20 \times 10^{-2}}{100}$$

$$\Rightarrow \frac{B_1}{B_2} = \frac{1}{1} \Rightarrow B_1 : B_2 = 1:1$$

62. (b) : Magnetic field induction at point inside a long solenoid l, having n turns per unit length carrying current i is given by $B = \mu_0 ni$. If $i \to$ doubled, $n \to$ halved then $B \to$ remains same.

63. (c) : Force between wires A and B = force between wires B and C

$$\therefore F_{BC} = F_{AB} = \frac{\mu_0 I^2 l}{2\pi d}$$

As, $\vec{F}_{AB} \perp \vec{F}_{BC}$ net force on wire B,

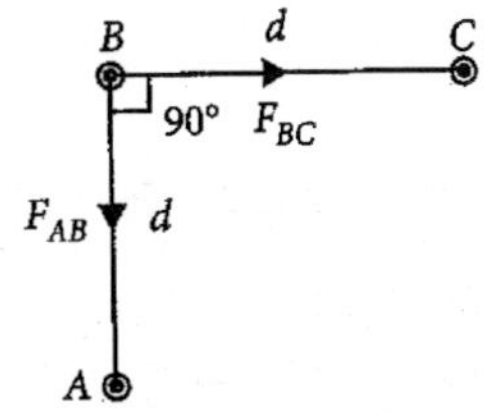

$$F_{\text{net}} = \sqrt{2} F_{BC} = \frac{\sqrt{2}\mu_0 I^2 l}{2\pi d} \text{ or } \frac{F_{\text{net}}}{l} = \frac{\mu_0 I^2}{\sqrt{2}\pi d}$$

64. (c) : Force on arm AB due to current in conductor XY is

$$F_1 = \frac{\mu_0}{4\pi}\frac{2IiL}{(L/2)} = \frac{\mu_0 Ii}{\pi}$$

acting towards XY in the plane of loop.

Force on arm CD due to current in conductor XY is

$$F_2 = \frac{\mu_0}{4\pi}\frac{2ILL}{3(L/2)} = \frac{\mu_0 Ii}{3\pi}$$

acting away from XY in the plane of loop.

$\therefore$ Net force on the loop $= F_1 - F_2$

$$= \frac{\mu_0 Ii}{\pi}\left[1 - \frac{1}{3}\right] = \frac{2}{3}\frac{\mu_0 Ii}{\pi}$$

65. (a)

66. (c) :

$F = \frac{\mu_0}{4\pi}\frac{2I_1 I_2}{r} = \frac{10^{-7} \times 2(1) \times (1)}{1} = 2 \times 10^{-7}$ N/m

67. (c) : Distance between two parallel wires,

$x = 10$ cm $= 0.1$ m;

Current in each wire $= I_1 = I_2 = 10$ A and

length of wire $(l) = 1$ m

Force on the wire $(F) = \frac{\mu_0 I_1 \cdot I_2 \times l}{2\pi x}$

$$= \frac{(4\pi \times 10^{-7}) \times 10 \times 10 \times 1}{2\pi \times 0.1} = 2 \times 10^{-4}\ \text{N}$$

Since the current is flowing in the same direction, therefore the force will be attractive.

68. (b) : For an equilateral triangle of side :

As total length of the wire $= 12a$

So, number of loops, $n = \frac{12a}{3a} = 4$

Magnetic moment of coil, $m = nIA$

Area of triangle, $A = \frac{\sqrt{3}}{4}a^2$

From equation (i), $m = 4I\frac{\sqrt{3}}{4}a^2$

$\therefore m = \sqrt{3}Ia^2$

For an square of side : Area, $A = a^2$

Number of loops, $n = \frac{12a}{4a} = 3$

Magnetic moment, $m = nIA = 3I(a^2) = 3Ia^2$

69. (d) : The required torque is $\tau = NIAB\sin\theta$

where N is the number of turns in the coil, I is the current through the coil, B is the uniform magnetic field, A is the area of the coil and θ is the angle between the direction of the magnetic field and normal to the plane of the coil.

Here, $N = 50, I = 2\text{ A}, A = 0.12\text{ m} \times 0.1\text{ m} = 0.012\text{ m}^2$

$B = 0.2\text{ Wb/m}^2$ and $\theta = 90° - 30° = 60°$

$\therefore \tau = (50)(2\text{ A})(0.012\text{ m}^2)(0.2\text{ Wb/m}^2)\sin 60° = 0.20$ N m

70. (b) : When a current loop is placed in a magnetic field it experiences a torque. It is given by $\vec{\tau} = \vec{M} \times \vec{B}$

where, $\vec{M}$ is the magnetic moment of the loop and $\vec{B}$ is the magnetic field.

$\tau = MB\sin\theta$ where θ is angle between $\vec{M}$ and $\vec{B}$

When $\vec{M}$ and $\vec{B}$ and are parallel (i.e., $\theta = 0°$) the equilibrium is stable and when they are antiparallel (i.e., $\theta = \pi$) the equilibrium is unstable.

71. **(a)** : The net magnetic force on a current loop in a uniform magnetic field is always zero.

$\therefore \vec{F}_{AB} + \vec{F}_{BCDA} = 0$

$$\vec{F}_{BCDA} = -\vec{F}_{AB} = -\vec{F}$$

72. **(b)** : Here, $\vec{F}_{BC} = \vec{F}$ and $\vec{F}_{AB} = I(\vec{l} \times \vec{B}) = 0$

The net magnetic force on a current carrying closed loop in a uniform magnetic field is zero.

$\therefore \vec{F}_{AB} + \vec{F}_{BC} + \vec{F}_{AC} = 0$

$$\Rightarrow \vec{F}_{AC} = -\vec{F}_{BC} \left(\because \vec{F}_{AB} = 0\right)$$

73. **(b)**

74. **(d)** :

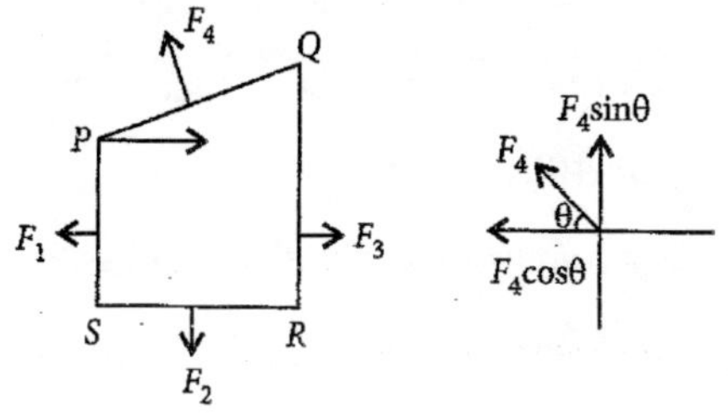

$F_4 \sin\theta = F_2$

$$F_4 \cos\theta = (F_3 - F_1)$$

$\therefore F_4 = \sqrt{(F_3 - F_1)^2 + F_2^2}$

For a closed loop there is no translation.

75. **(d)** : Magnetic moment $\mu = IA$

Since $T = \frac{2\pi R}{v}$ Also, $r = \frac{q}{T} = \frac{qv}{2\pi R}$

$\therefore \mu = \left(\frac{qv}{2\pi R}\right)(\pi R^2) = \frac{qvR}{2}$.

76. **(b)** : The current flowing clockwise in the equilateral triangle has a magnetic field in the direction $\hat{k}$

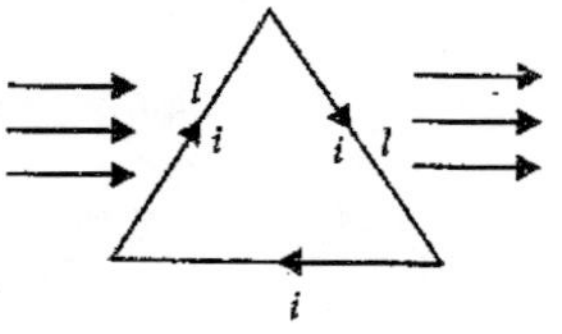

$\tau = BiNA\sin\theta = BiA\sin 90°$

(as it appears that $N = 1$)

$$\tau = Bi \times \frac{\sqrt{3}}{4} l^2 \Rightarrow l = 2\left(\frac{\tau}{Bi\sqrt{3}}\right)^{1/2}$$

77. **(a)** : Magnetic moment $M = niA$

78. **(c)** : Area $(A) = 0.01 \text{ m}^2$; Current $(I) = 10 \text{ A}$;

Angle $(\phi) = 90°$ and magnetic field $(B) = 0.1 \text{ T}$

Therefore actual angle

$\theta = (90° - \phi) = (90° - 90°) = 0°$

Torque acting on the loop $(\tau) = IAB\sin\theta$

$$= 10 \times 0.01 \times 0.1 \times \sin 0° = 0$$

79. **(a)** : A current carrying coil has magnetic dipole moment. Hence a torque $\vec{m} \times \vec{B}$ acts on it in a magnetic field.

80. **(d)** : The plane of coil will orient itself so that area vector aligns itself along the magnetic field.

81. (c) : Let $N =$ number of turns in galvanometer, $A =$ Area, $B =$ magnetic field

$k =$ the restoring torque per unit twist.

Current sensitivity, $I_S = \frac{NBA}{k}$

Voltage sensitivity, $V_S = \frac{NBA}{kR_G}$

So, resistance of galvanometer

$$R_G = \frac{I_S}{V_S} = \frac{5 \times 1}{20 \times 10^{-3}} = \frac{5000}{20} = 250\Omega$$

82. (c) : Here, resistance of the galvanometer $= G$

Current through the galvanometer,

$I_G = 0.2\%$ of $I = \frac{0.2}{100} I = \frac{1}{500} I$

$\therefore$ Current through the shunt,

$$I_S = I - I_G = I - \frac{1}{500} I = \frac{499}{500} I$$

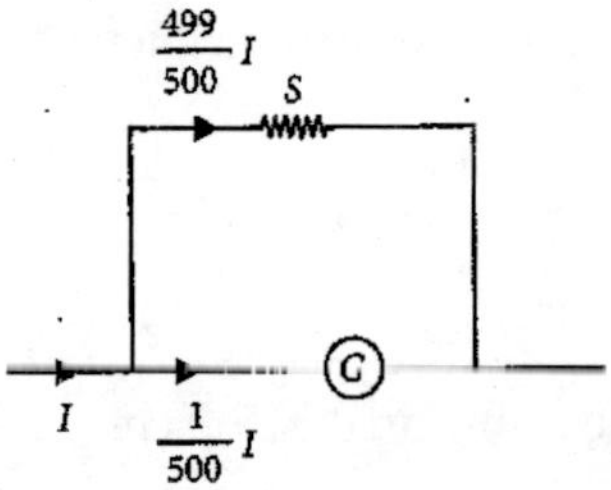

As shunt and galvanometer are in parallel

$\therefore I_G G = I_S S$

$$\left(\frac{1}{500} I\right) G = \left(\frac{499}{500}\right) S \text{ or } S = \frac{G}{499}$$

Resistance of the ammeter R_A is

$$\frac{1}{R_A} = \frac{1}{G} + \frac{1}{S} = \frac{1}{G} + \frac{1}{\frac{G}{499}} = \frac{500}{G}$$

$$R_A = \frac{1}{500} G$$

83. (a) : $S = \frac{V_g}{(I - I_g)}$

Neglecting I_g

$$\therefore S = \frac{V_g}{I} = \frac{25 \times 10^{-3}\text{ V}}{25\text{ A}} = 0.001\Omega$$

84. (d) : Let resistance R is to be put in series with galvanometer G to keep the main current in the circuit unchanged.

$$\therefore \frac{GS}{G+S} + R = G$$

$$R = G - \frac{GS}{G+S} \Rightarrow R = \frac{G^2 + GS - GS}{G+S}$$

$$= \frac{G^2}{G+S}$$

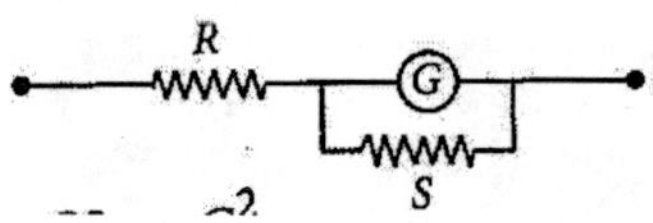

85. (a) : Here, Resistance of galvanometer,

$G = 100\Omega$

Current for full scale deflection, $I_g =$ 30 mA

$$= 30 \times 10^{-3}\text{ A}$$

Range of voltmeter, $V = 30$ V

To convert the galvanometer into an voltmeter of a given range, a resistance R is connected in series with it as shown in the figure. From figure, $V = I_g(G + R)$

or $R = \frac{V}{I_g} - G$

$= \frac{30}{30 \times 10^{-3}} - 100\Omega = 1000 - 100 = 900\Omega$

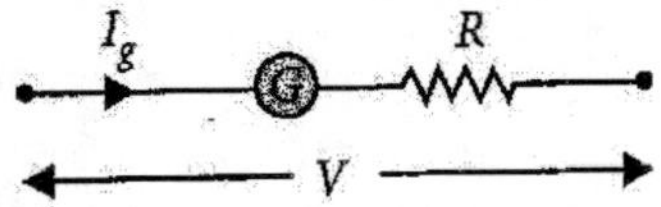

86. (c) : $iG = (I - i)S$ where G is the galvanometer resistance and S is the shunt used with the ammeter.

$1.0 \times 60 = (5 - 1)S$ where S is the shunt used to read a 5 A current when the galvanometer can stand by 1 A.

$$S = \frac{1.0 \times 60}{4} = 15\Omega \text{ in parallel.}$$

87. (b) : Total initial resistance

$= R_G + R_1 = (50 + 2950)\Omega = 3000\Omega$

$\varepsilon = 3\text{ V}$

$\therefore$ Current $= \frac{3\text{ V}}{3000\Omega} = 1 \times 10^{-3}\text{ A} = 1\text{ mA}$

If the deflection has to be reduced to 20 divisions, current $i = 1\text{ mA} \times \frac{2}{3}$ as the full deflection scale for 1 mA = 30 divisions.

$3\text{ V} = 3000\Omega \times 1\text{ mA} = x\Omega \times \frac{2}{3}\text{ mA}$

$\Rightarrow x = 3000 \times 1 \times \frac{3}{2} = 4500\Omega$

But the galvanometer resistance $= 50\Omega$

Therefore the resistance to be added

$= (4500 - 50)\Omega = 4450\Omega.$

88. (a) : Let the shunt resistance be S.

Given: = 750 A,

$I_g = 100\text{ A}, R_G = 13\Omega$

From the figure, $I_g R_G = (I - I_g)S$

or $100 \times 13 = [750 - 100]S$

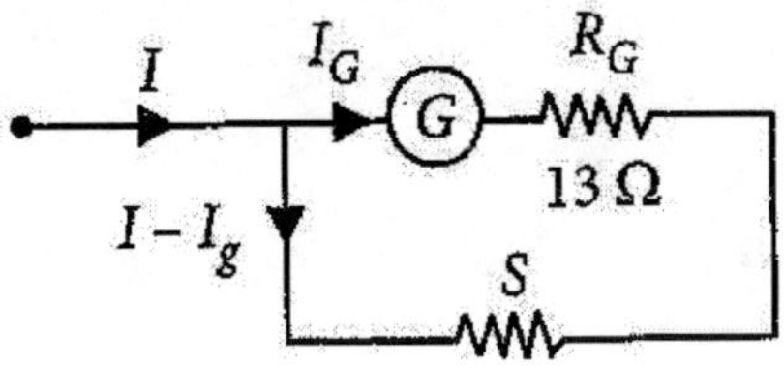

or $1300 = 650\text{ S}$

$\therefore S = 1300/650 = 2\Omega$

89. (d) : The total current shown by the galvanometer is $25 \times 4 \times 10^{-4}$ A.

$\therefore I_g = 10^{-2}\text{ A}$

The value of resistance connected in series to convert galvanometer into voltmeter of 25 V is

$$R = \frac{V}{I_g} - G = \frac{25}{10^{-2}} - 50 = 2450\Omega$$

90. (a) : Voltmeter is used to measure the potential difference across a resistance and it is connected in parallel with the circuit. A high resistance is connected to the galvanometer in series so that only a small fraction (I_g) of the main circuit current (I) passes through it. If a considerable amount of current is allowed to pass through the voltmeter, then the reading obtained by this voltmeter will not be close to the actual potential difference between the same two points.

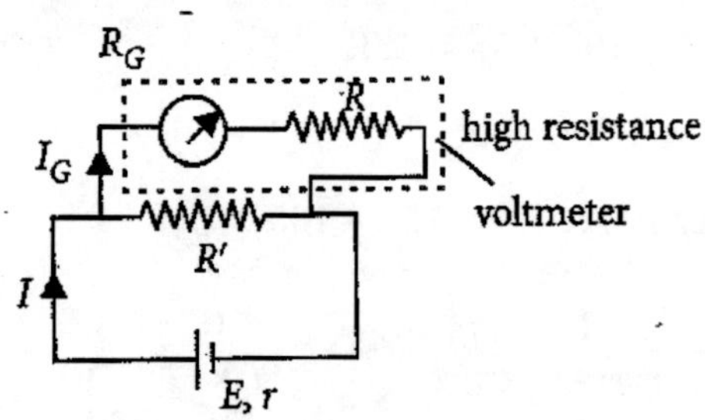

91. **(b)** : The shunt and galvanometer are in parallel.

Therefore, $\frac{1}{R_{eq}} = \frac{1}{9} + \frac{1}{2}$ or $R_{eq} = \frac{18}{11}\Omega$

Using Ohm's law, $= IR_{eq} = 1 \times \frac{18}{11} = \frac{18}{11}$ V.

$\therefore$ Current through shunt

$= \frac{V}{R_S} = \frac{18/11}{2} = \frac{9}{11} \simeq 0.8$amp

92. **(a)** : To convert a galvanometer into ammeter, one needs to connect a low resistance in parallel so that maximum current passes through the shunt wire and ammeter remains protected.

Chapter: 19 MAGNETISM AND MATTER

1. A 250-turn rectangular coil of length 2.1 cm and width 1.25 cm carries a current of $85 \mu A$ and subjected to a magnetic field of strength 0.85 T. Work done for rotating the coil by 180° against the torque is

(2017)

(a) $4.55 \mu J$ (b) $2.3 \mu J$
(c) $1.15 \mu J$ (d) $9.1 \mu J$

2. A bar magnet is hung by a thin cotton thread in a uniform horizontal magnetic field and is in equilibrium state. The energy required to rotate it by 60° is W. Now the torque required to keep the magnet in this new position is

(NEET-II 2016)

(a) $\frac{W}{\sqrt{3}}$ (b) $\sqrt{3} W$
(c) $\frac{\sqrt{3} W}{2}$ (d) $\frac{2 W}{\sqrt{3}}$

3. Following figures show the arrangement of bar magnets in different configurations. Each magnet has magnetic dipole moment $\vec{m}$. Which configuration has highest net magnetic dipole moment? **(2014)**

(1) 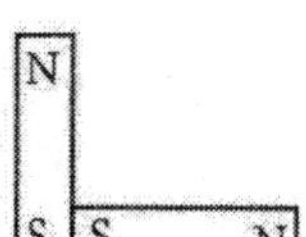

(2) 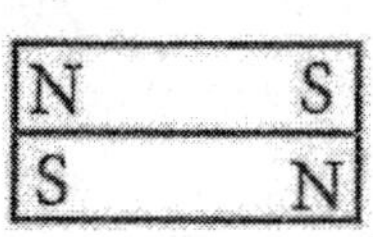

(3) 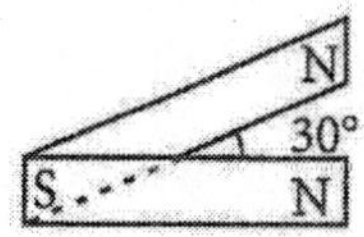

(4) 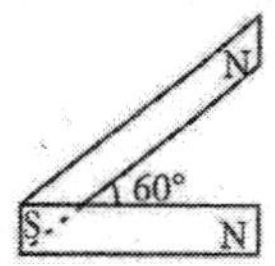

(a) (1) (b) (2)
(c) (3) (d) (4)

4. A bar magnet of length ' P and magnetic dipole moment ' M ' is bent in the form of an arc as shown in figure. The new magnetic dipole moment will be **(2013)**

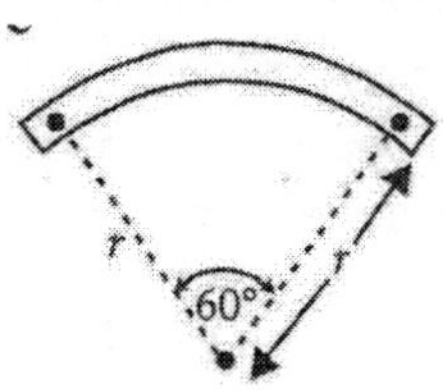

(a) $\frac{2}{\pi} M$ (b) $\frac{M}{2}$
(c) M (d) $\frac{3}{\pi} M$

5. A bar magnet of magnetic moment M is placed at right angles to a magnetic induction B. If a force F is experienced by each pole of the magnet, the length of the magnet will be

(Karnataka NEET 2013)

(a) $M B / F$ (b) $B F / M$
(c) $M F / B$ (d) $F / M B$

6. A magnetic needle suspended parallel to a magnetic field requires $\sqrt{3}$ J of work to

turn it through 60°. The torque needed to maintain the needle in this position will be

(Mains 2012)

(a) $2\sqrt{3}$ J (b) 3J

(c) $\sqrt{3}$ J (d) $\frac{3}{2}$ J

7. A short bar magnet of magnetic moment $0.4\ \mathrm{J\,T^{-1}}$ is placed in a uniform magnetic field of 0.16 T. The magnet is in stable equilibrium when the potential energy is

(Mains 2011)

(a) 0.064 J (b) −0.064J

(c) zero (d) -0.082 J

8. A vibration magnetometer placed in magnetic meridian has a small bar magnet. The magnet executes oscillations with a time period of 2sec in earth's horizontal magnetic field of 24 microtesla. When a horizontal field of 18 microtesla is produced opposite to the earth's field by placing a current carrying wire, the new time period of magnet will be **(2010)**

(a) 1 s (b) 2 s

(c) 3 s (d) 4 s

9. Two identical bar magnets are fixed with their centres at a distance d apart. A stationary charge Q is placed at P in between the gap of the two magnets at a distance D from the centre O as shown in the figure

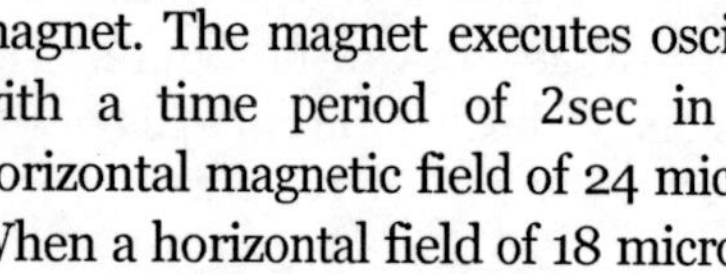

The force on the charge Q is

(a) zero

(b) directed along OP

(c) directed along PO

(d) directed perpendicular to the plane of paper

10. A closely wound solenoid of 2000 turns and area of cross-section $1.5 \times 10^{-4}\ \mathrm{m^2}$ carries a current of 2.0 A. It is suspended through its centre and perpendicular to its length, allowing it to turn in a horizontal plane in a uniform magnetic field 5×10^{-2} tesla making an angle of 30° with the axis of the solenoid. The torque on the solenoid will be

(Mains 2010)

(a) 3×10^{-3} N m

(b) 1.5×10^{-3} N m

(c) 1.5×10^{-2} N m

(d) 3×10^{-2} N m

11. A bar magnet having a magnetic moment of $2 \times 10^{4}\ \mathrm{J\,T^{-1}}$ is free to rotate in a horizontal plane. A horizontal magnetic field $B = 6 \times 10^{-4}$ T exists in the space. The work done in taking the magnet slowly from a direction parallel to the field to a direction 60° from the field is **(2009)**

(a) 12 J (b) 6 J

(c) 2 J (d) 0.6 J

12. A bar magnet is oscillating in the Earth's magnetic field with a period T. What happens to its period and motion if its mass is quadrupled? **(2003, 1994)**

(a) Motion remains simple harmonic with time period = $T/2$

(b) Motion remains S.H.M with time period = $2T$

(c) Motion remains S.H.M with time period $= 4T$

(d) Motion remains S.H.M and period remains nearly constant

13. Two bar magnets having same geometry with magnetic moments M and $2M$, are firstly placed in such a way that their similar poles are in same side then its time period of oscillation is T_1. Now the polarity of one of the magnet is reversed then time period of oscillation is T_2, then **(2002)**

(a) $T_1 < T_2$ (b) $T_1 = T_2$

(c) $T_1 > T_2$ (d) $T_2 = \infty$

14. A bar magnet of magnetic moment $\vec{M}$, is placed in a magnetic field of induction $\vec{B}$. The torque exerted on it is **(1999)**

(a) $\vec{M} \times \vec{B}$ (b) $-\vec{M} \cdot \vec{B}$

(c) $\vec{M} \cdot \vec{B}$ (d) $-\vec{B} \times \vec{M}$

15. A bar magnet of magnetic moment M is cut into two parts of equal length. The magnetic moment of each part will be

(1997)

(a) M (b) $2M$

(c) zero (d) 0.5M

16. The work done in turning a magnet of magnetic moment M by an angle of $90°$ from the meridian, is n times the corresponding work done to turn it through an angle of $60°$. The value of n is given by **(1995)**

(a) ½ (b) ¼

(c) 2 (d) 1

17. At a point A on the earth's surface the angle of dip, $\delta = +25°$. At a point B on the earth's surface the angle of dip, $\delta = -25°$. We can interpret that **(2019)**

(a) A and B are both located in the southern hemisphere.

(b) A and B are both located in the northern hemisphere.

(c) A is located in the southern hemisphere and B is located in the northern hemisphere.

(d) A is located in the northern hemisphere and B is located in the southern hemisphere.

18. If θ_1 and θ_2 be the apparent angles of dip observed in two vertical planes at right angles to each other, then the true angle of dip θ is given by **(2017)**

(a) $\tan^2\theta = \tan^2\theta_1 + \tan^2\theta_2$

(b) $\cot^2\theta = \cot^2\theta_1 - \cot^2\theta_2$

(c) $\tan^2\theta = \tan^2\theta_1 - \tan^2\theta_2$

(d) $\cot^2\theta = \cot^2\theta_1 + \cot^2\theta_2$

19. A compass needle which is allowed to move in a horizontal plane is taken to a geomagnetic pole. It **(2012)**

(a) will become rigid showing no movement

(b) will stay in any position

(c) will stay in north-south direction only

(d) will stay in east-west direction only

20. Tangent galvanometer is used to measure

(2001)

(a) potential difference

(b) current

(c) resistance

(d) charge.

21. An iron rod of susceptibility 599 is subjected to a magnetising field of $1200\ \mathrm{A\ m^{-1}}$. The permeability of the material of the rod is ($\mu_0 = 4\pi \times 10^{-7}\ \mathrm{T\ m\ A^{-1}}$) **(2020)**

(a) $2.4\pi \times 10^{-4}\ \mathrm{T\ m\ A^{-1}}$

(b) $8.0 \times 10^{-5}\ \mathrm{T\ m\ A^{-1}}$

(c) $2.4\pi \times 10^{-5}\ \mathrm{T\ m\ A^{-1}}$

(d) $2.4\pi \times 10^{-7}\ \mathrm{T\ m\ A^{-1}}$

22. A thin diamagnetic rod is placed vertically between the poles of an electromagnet. When the current in the electromagnet is switched on, then the diamagnetic rod is pushed up, out of the horizontal magnetic field. Hence the rod gains gravitational potential energy. The work required to do this comes from **(2018)**

(a) the current source

(b) the magnetic field

(c) the lattice structure of the material of the rod

(d) the induced electric field due to the changing magnetic field

23. The magnetic susceptibility is negative for **(NEET-I 2016)**

(a) ferromagnetic material only

(b) paramagnetic and ferromagnetic materials

(c) diamagnetic material only

(d) paramagnetic material only

24. There are four light-weight-rod samples A, B, C, D separately suspended by threads. A bar magnet is slowly brought near each sample and the following observations are noted **(2011)**

(i) A is feebly repelled

(ii) B is feebly attracted

(iii) C is strongly attracted

(iv) D remains unaffected

Which one of the following is true?

(a) B is of a paramagnetic material

(b) C is of a diamagnetic material

(c) D is of a ferromagnetic material

(d) A is of a non-magnetic material

25. The magnetic moment of a diamagnetic atom is **(Mains 2010)**

(a) much greater than one

(b) 1

(c) between zero and one

(d) equal to zero

26. If a diamagnetic substance is brought near the north or the south pole of a bar magnet, it is **(2009-1999)**

(a) repelled by the north pole and attracted by the south pole

(b) attracted by the north pole and repelled by the south pole

(c) attracted by both the poles

(d) repelled by both the poles

27. Curie temperature above which **(2008,2006)**

(a) paramagnetic material becomes ferromagnetic material

(b) ferromagnetic material becomes diamagnetic material

(c) ferromagnetic material becomes paramagnetic material

(d) paramagnetic material becomes diamagnetic material

28. Nickel shows ferromagnetic property at room temperature. If the temperature is increased beyond Curie temperature, then it will show **(2007)**

(a) anti ferromagnetism

(b) no magnetic property

(c) diamagnetism

(d) paramagnetism.

29. If the magnetic dipole moment of an atom of diamagnetic material, paramagnetic material and ferromagnetic material are denoted by μ_d, μ_p and μ_f respectively, then **(2005)**

(a) $\mu_d = 0$ and $\mu_p \neq 0$

(b) $\mu_d \neq 0$ and $\mu_p = 0$

(c) $\mu_p = 0$ and $\mu_f \neq 0$

(d) $\mu_d \neq 0$ and $\mu_f \neq 0$

30. A diamagnetic material in a magnetic field moves **(2003)**

(a) from stronger to the weaker parts of the field

(b) from weaker to the stronger parts of the field

(c) perpendicular to the field

(d) in none of the above directions

31. According to Curie's law, the magnetic susceptibility of a substance at an absolute temperature T is proportional to **(2003)**

(a) $1/T$ (b) T

(c) $1/T^2$ (d) T^2

32. Among which the magnetic susceptibility does not depend on the temperature? **(2001)**

(a) Diamagnetism

(b) Paramagnetism

(c) Ferromagnetism

(d) Ferrite.

33. For protecting a sensitive equipment from the external magnetic field, it should be **(1998)**

(a) surrounded with fine copper sheet

(b) placed inside an iron can

(c) wrapped with insulation around it when passing current through it

(d) placed inside an aluminium can

34. Electromagnets are made of soft iron because soft iron has **(2010)**

(a) low retentivity and high coercive force

(b) high retentivity and high coercive force

(c) low retentivity and low coercive force

(d) high retentivity and low coercive force

ANSWER KEY

1.	(d)	2.	(b)	3.	(c)	4.	(d)	5.	(a)	6.	(b)	7.	(b)
8.	(d)	9.	(a)	10.	(c)	11.	(b)	12.	(b)	13.	(a)	14.	(a,d)
15.	(d)	16.	(c)	17.	(d)	18.	(d)	19.	(b)	20.	(b)	21.	(a)
22.	(a)	23.	(c)	24.	(a)	25.	(d)	26.	(d)	27.	(c)	28.	(d)
29.	(a)	30.	(a)	31.	(a)	32.	(a)	33.	(b)	34.	(c)		

Hints & Explanations

1. (d): Work done in a coil

$W = mB(\cos\theta_1 - \cos\theta_2)$ ......(i)

When it is rotated by angle 180° then

$W = 2mB = 2(NIA)B$

Given: $N = 250, I = 85\mu\text{A} = 85 \times 10^{-6}$ A

$A = 1.25 \times 2.1 \times 10^{-4}\ \text{m}^2$
$\approx 2.6 \times 10^{-4}\ \text{m}^2$

$B = 0.85$ T

Putting these values in eqn. (i), we get

$W = 2 \times 250 \times 85 \times 10^{-6} \times 2.6 \times 10^{-4} \times 0.85$

$\approx 9.1 \times 10^{-6}\ \text{J} = 9.1\mu\text{J}$

2. **(b)**
At equilibrium, potential energy of dipole
$U_i = -MB_H$

Final potential energy of dipole,

$$U_f = -MB_H\cos 60° = -\frac{MB_H}{2}$$

$$W = U_f - U_i = -\frac{MB_H}{2} - (-MB_H) = \frac{MB_H}{2} \quad ....(ii)$$

$$\tau = MB_H\sin 60° = 2W \times \frac{\sqrt{3}}{2}$$

[Using eqn. (i)]

$= \sqrt{3}W$

3. **(c)** : The direction of magnetic dipole moment is from south to north pole of the magnet.

In configuration (1),

$$m_{\text{net}} = \sqrt{m^2 + m^2 + 2mm\cos 90°} = \sqrt{m^2 + m^2} = m\sqrt{2}$$

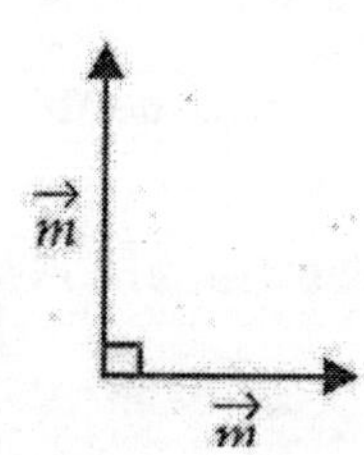

In configuration (2),

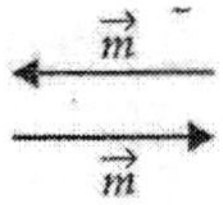

$m_{net} = m - m = 0$

In configuration (3),

$$m_{net} = \sqrt{m^2 + m^2 + 2mm\cos 30°}$$

$$= \sqrt{2m^2 + 2m^2\left(\frac{\sqrt{3}}{2}\right)} = m\sqrt{2+\sqrt{3}}$$

In configuration (4),

$$m_{net} = \sqrt{m^2 + m^2 + 2mm\cos 60°}$$

$$= \sqrt{2m^2 + 2m^2\left(\frac{1}{2}\right)} = m\sqrt{3}$$

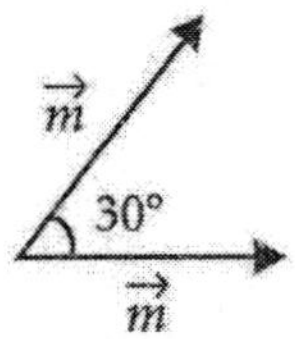

4. **(d) :** Let m be strength of each pole of bar magnet of length l. Then

$$M = m \times l$$

When the bar magnet is bent in the form of an arc as shown in figure. Then

$l = \frac{\pi}{3} \times r = \frac{\pi r}{3}$ or $r = \frac{3l}{\pi}$

New magnetic dipole moment

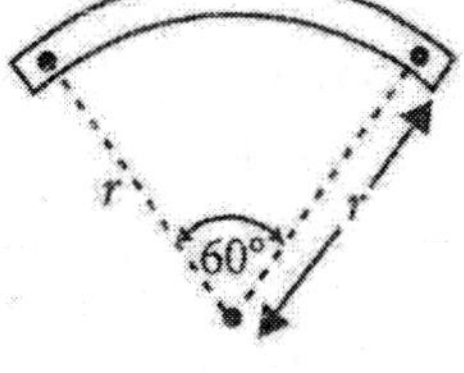

$$M' = m \times 2r\sin 30°$$

$= m \times 2 \times \frac{3l}{\pi} \times \frac{1}{2} = \frac{3ml}{\pi} = \frac{3M}{\pi}$ (Using (i))

5. **(a)**

6. **(b):** Work done in changing the orientation of a magnetic needle of magnetic moment M in a magnetic field B from position θ_1 to θ_2 is given by

$W = MB(\cos\theta_1 - \cos\theta_2)$

Here, $\theta_1 = 0°, \theta_2 = 60°$

$= MB\left(1 - \frac{1}{2}\right) = \frac{MB}{2}$ .....(i)

The torque on the needle is $\vec{\tau} = \vec{M} \times \vec{B}$

In magnitude,

$\tau = MB\sin\theta = MB\sin 60° = \frac{\sqrt{3}}{2}MB$ ...(ii)

Dividing (ii) by (i), we get

$$\frac{\tau}{W^T} = \sqrt{3} \text{ or } \tau = \sqrt{3}W = \sqrt{3} \times \sqrt{3}\text{ J} = 3\text{ J}$$

7. **(b)** : Here, Magnetic moment, $M = 0.4\text{ J T}^{-1}$

Magnetic field, $B = 0.16$ T

When a bar magnet of magnetic moment is placed in a uniform magnetic field, its potential energy is

$$U = -\vec{M} \cdot \vec{B} = -MB\cos\theta$$

For stable equilibrium, $\theta = 0°$

$$\therefore U = -MB = -(0.4\text{JT}^{-1})(0.16\text{ T})$$
$$= -0.064\text{ J}$$

8. **(d) :** The time period T of oscillation of a magnet is given by

$$T = 2\pi\sqrt{\frac{I}{MB}}$$

where,

I = Moment of inertia of the magnet about the axis of rotation

M = Magnetic moment of the magnet

B = Uniform magnetic field

As I and M remain the same

$\therefore T \propto \frac{1}{\sqrt{B}}$ or $\frac{T_2}{T_1} = \sqrt{\frac{B_1}{B_2}}$

According to given problem,

$B_1 = 24\mu T, B_2 = 24\mu T - 18\mu T = 6\mu T, T_1 = 2$ s

$$\therefore T_2 = (2 \text{ s})\sqrt{\frac{(24\mu T)}{(6\mu T)}} = 4 \text{ s}$$

9. **(a) :** Magnetic field due to bar magnets exerts force on moving charges only. Since the charge is at rest, no force acts on it.

10. **(c) :** Magnetic moment of the loop

$$M = NIA = 2000 \times 2 \times 1.5 \times 10^{-4} - 0.6 \text{ J/T}$$

Torque $\tau = MB\sin 30°$

$$= 0.6 \times 5 \times 10^{-2} \times \frac{1}{2} = 1.5 \times 10^{-2}\text{Nm}$$

11. **(b):** Here, $M = 2 \times 10^4 \text{JT}^{-1}$

$B = 6 \times 10^{-4}$ T, $\theta_1 = 0°, \theta_2 = 60°$

$$W = MB(\cos\theta_1 - \cos\theta_2) = MB(1 - \cos 60°)$$

$$W = 2 \times 10^4 \times 6 \times 10^{-4}\left(1 - \frac{1}{2}\right) = 6J$$

12. **(b) :** Initial mass of the magnet $(m_1) = m$ and final mass of the magnet $(m_2) = 4m$.

The time period, $T = 2\pi\sqrt{\frac{I}{MB}} = 2\pi\sqrt{\frac{mk^2}{MB}} \propto \sqrt{m}$

Therefore $\frac{T_1}{T_2} = \frac{\sqrt{m_1}}{\sqrt{m_2}} = \frac{\sqrt{m}}{\sqrt{4m}} = \frac{1}{2}$

or $T_2 = 2T_1 = 2T$

13. **(a):**

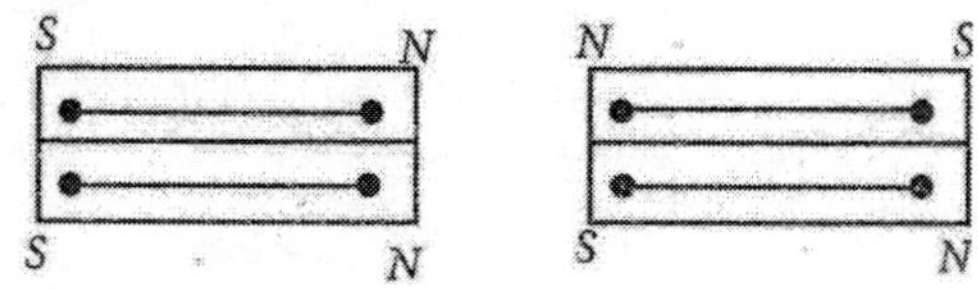

(i) $M = M_1 + M_2$

(ii) $M = M_1 - M_2$ $I = I_1 + I_2$ $I = I_1 + I_2$

(i) Similar poles are placed at the same side (sum position)

(ii) Opposite poles are placed at the same side (difference position) I_1 and I_2 are the moments of inertia of the magnets and M_1 and M_2 are the moments of the magnets.

Here $M_1 = M$ and $M_2 = 2M, I_1 = I_2 = I$ (say), for same geometry.

For sum position

$$T_1 = 2\pi\sqrt{\frac{I_1 + I_2}{(M_1 + M_2)H}} = 2\pi\sqrt{\frac{2I}{(M + 2M)H}}$$

For difference position.

$$T_2 = 2\pi\sqrt{\frac{I_1 + I_2}{(M_2 - M_1)H}} = 2\pi\sqrt{\frac{2I}{(2M - M)H}}$$

$\therefore \frac{T_1}{T_2} = \sqrt{\frac{M}{3M}} = \frac{1}{\sqrt{3}} < 1$ or $T_1 < T_2$

14. **(a, d):** Option (a) and (d) has equal magnitude.

15. **(d) :** Magnetic moment = pole strength × length

$\therefore M' = M/2 = 0.5M$

16. **(c) :** Angle of magnet (θ) = 90° and 60°.

Work done in turning the magnet through 90°

$W_1 = MB(\cos 0° - \cos 90°) = MB(1 - 0) = MB.$

Similarly,

$$W_2 = MB(\cos 0° - \cos 60°) = MB\left(1 - \frac{1}{2}\right) = \frac{MB}{2}$$

Therefore, $W_1 = 2W_2$ or $n = 2$

17. **(d) :** At a point A, the angle of dip is positive and the earth's magnetic north pole is in northern hemisphere. So, point A is located in the northern hemisphere and B is located in the southern hemisphere.

18. **(d):** Let B_H and B_V be the horizontal and vertical components of earth's magnetic field $\vec{B}$. Since θ is the angle of dip

$\therefore \tan\theta = \frac{B_V}{B_H}$ or $\cot\theta = \frac{B_H}{B_V}$

Suppose planes 1 and 2 are two mutually perpendicular planes and respectively make angles θ and $90° - \theta$ with the magnetic meridian. The vertical components of earth's magnetic field remain same in the two planes but the effective horizontal components in the planes will be $B_1 = B_H \cos\theta$ and $B_2 = B_H \sin\theta$

The angles of dip θ_1 and θ_2 in the two planes are given by

$$\tan\theta_1 = \frac{B_V}{B_1}$$

$$\tan\theta_1 = \frac{B_V}{B_H \cos\theta}$$

or $\cot\theta_1 = \frac{B_H \cos\theta}{B_V}$

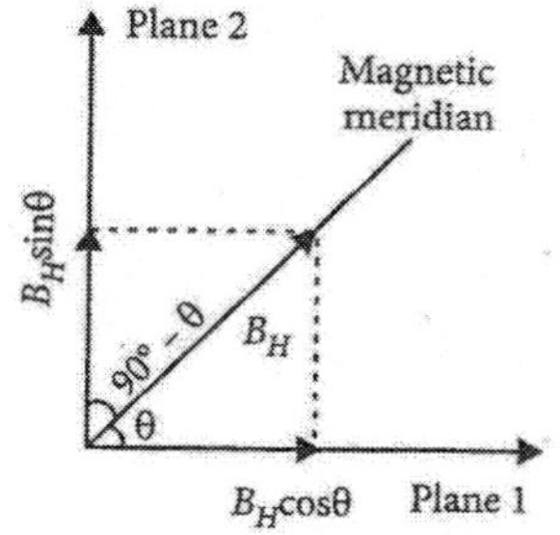

Similarly, $\cot\theta_2 = \frac{B_H \sin\theta}{B_V}$

From eqns. (ii) and (iii)

$$\cot^2\theta_1 + \cot^2\theta_2 = \frac{B_H^2}{B_V^2}(\cos^2\theta + \sin^2\theta) = \frac{B_H^2}{B_V^2}$$

$\therefore \cot^2\theta_1 + \cot^2\theta_2 = \cot^2\theta$ [from eqn. (i)]

19. **(b) :** A compass needle which is allowed to move in a horizontal plane is taken to a geomagnetic pole. It will stay in any position as the horizontal component of earth's magnetic field becomes zero at the geomagnetic pole.

20. **(b) :** $I = K\tan\theta$

21. **(a) :** Given, $X_m = 599$

Relative permeability of the material, $\mu_r = 1 + X_m$

or $\mu_r = 1 + 599 = 600$

$\therefore \mu = \mu_r\mu_0 = 600 \times (4\pi \times 10^{-7})$

$= 24\pi \times 10^{-5}$ T m A^{-1}

22. (a) : Energy of current source will be converted into gravitational potential energy of the rod.

23. (c) : Magnetic susceptibility is negative for diamagnetic material only.

24. (a) : Diamagnetic will be feebly repelled.

Paramagnetic will be feebly attracted.

Ferromagnetic will be strongly attracted.

Therefore, A is of diamagnetic material. B is of paramagnetic material. C is of ferromagnetic material. D is of non-magnetic material.

25. (d): The magnetic moment of a diamagnetic atom is equal to zero.

26. (d) : A diamagnet is always repelled by a magnetic field. Therefore it is repelled by both the north pole as well as the south pole.

27. (c) : Above Curie temperature, there is a change from ferromagnetic to paramagnetic behaviour.

28. (d)

29. (a) : Materials with no unpaired, or isolated electrons are considered diamagnetic. Diamagnetic substances do not have magnetic dipole moments and have negative susceptibilities. However, materials having unpaired electrons whose spins do not cancel each other are called paramagnetic. These substances have positive magnetic moments and susceptibilities.

$$\mu_d = 0, \mu_p \neq 0$$

30. (a)

31. (a): According to Curie's law $\chi \propto \frac{1}{T}$

32. (a)

33. (b)

34. (c) : Electromagnets are made of soft iron because soft iron has low retentivity and low coercive force or low coercivity. Soft iron is a soft magnetic material.

Chapter: 20 ELECTROMAGNETIC INDUCTION

Magnetic Flux

1. The net magnetic flux through any closed surface is : **(2023)**

(a) Positive (b) Infinity
(c) Negative (d) Zero

2. A square loop of side 1 m and resistance 1Ω is placed in a magnetic field of 0.5 T. If the plane of loop is perpendicular to the direction of magnetic field, the magnetic flux through the loop is **(2022)**

(a) 2 weber (b) 0.5 weber
(c) 1 weber (d) zero weber

3. A circular disc of radius 0.2 meter is placed in a uniform magnetic field of induction $\frac{1}{\pi}\left(\frac{\text{Wb}}{\text{m}^2}\right)$ in such a way that its axis makes an angle of 60° with $\vec{B}$. The magnetic flux linked with the disc is **(2008)**

(a) 0.08 Wb (b) 0.01 Wb
(c) 0.02 Wb (d) 0.06 Wb

Faraday's Law of Induction

4. A big circular coil of 1000 turns and average radius 10 m is rotating about its horizontal diameter at 2rads^{-1}. If the vertical component of earth's magnetic field at that place is 2×10^{-5} T and electrical resistance of the coil is 12.56Ω, then the maximum induced current in the coil will be **(2022)**

(a) 0.25 A (b) 1.5 A
(c) 1 A (d) 2 A

5. A 800 turn coil of effective area $0.05\ \text{m}^2$ is kept perpendicular to a magnetic field 5×10^{-5} T. When the plane of the coil is rotated by 90° around any of its coplanar axis in 0.1 s, the emf induced in the coil will be **(2019)**

(a) 0.02 V (b) 2 V
(c) 0.2 V (d) 2×10^{-3} V

6. A uniform magnetic field is restricted within a region of radius r. The magnetic field changes with time at a rate $\frac{d\vec{B}}{dt}$. Loop 1 of radius $R > r$ encloses the region r and loop 2 of radius R is outside the region of magnetic field as shown in the figure. Then the e.m.f. generated is **(NEET-II 2016)**

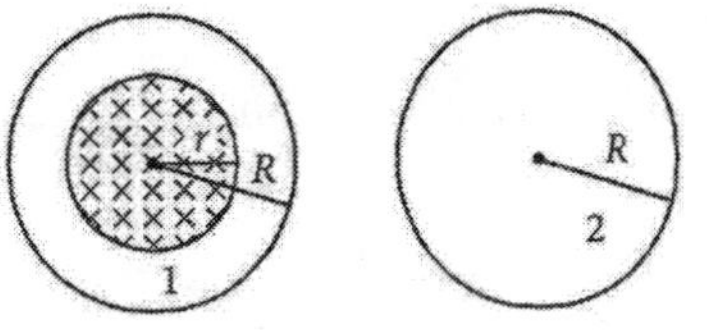

(a) zero in loop 1 and zero in loop 2

(b) $-\frac{d\vec{B}}{dt}\pi r^2$ in loop 1 and $-\frac{d\vec{B}}{dt}\pi r^2$ in loop 2

(c) $-\frac{d\vec{B}}{dt}\pi R^2$ in loop 1 and zero in loop 2

(d) $-\frac{d\vec{B}}{dt}\pi r^2$ in loop 1 and zero in loop 2

7. A coil of resistance 400Ω is placed in a magnetic field. If the magnetic flux ϕ(Wb)

linked with the coil varies with time t(sec) as $\phi = 50t^2 + 4$. The current in the coil at $t = 2$sec is **(2012)**

(a) 0.5 A (b) 0.1 A

(c) 2 A (d) 1 A

8. A conducting circular loop is placed in a uniform magnetic field, $B = 0.025$ T with its plane perpendicular to the loop. The radius of the loop is made to shrink at a constant rate of 1 mm s^{-1}. The induced emf when the radius is 2 cm, is **(2010)**

(a) $2\pi\mu V$ (b) $\pi\mu V$

(c) $\frac{\pi}{2}\mu V$ (d) $2\mu V$

9. A rectangular, a square, a circular and an elliptical loop, all in the $(x-y)$ plane, are moving out of a uniform magnetic field with a constant velocity, $\vec{V} = v\hat{i}$. The magnetic field is directed along the negative z axis direction. The induced emf, during the passage of these loops, out of the field region, will not remain constant for **(2009)**

(a) the circular and the elliptical loops

(b) only the elliptical loop

(c) any of the four loops

(d) the rectangular, circular and elliptical loops

10. A conducting circular loop is placed in a uniform magnetic field 0.04 T with its plane perpendicular to the magnetic field. The radius of the loop starts shrinking at 2 mm/s. The induced emf in the loop when the radius is 2 cm is **(2009)**

(a) $4.8\pi\mu V$ (b) $0.8\pi\mu V$

(c) $1.6\pi\mu V$ (d) $3.4\pi\mu V$

11. As a result of change in the magnetic flux linked to the closed loop as shown in the figure, an e.m.f. V volt is induced in the loop. The work done (joule) in taking a charge Q coulomb once along the loop is **(2005)**

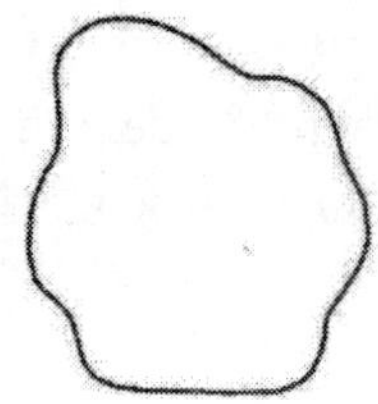

(a) QV (b) $2QV$

(c) $QV/2$ (d) zero.

12. A rectangular coil of 20 turns and area of cross-section 25sq. cm has a resistance of 100Ω. If a magnetic field which is perpendicular to the plane of coil changes at a rate of 1000 tesla per second, the current in the coil is **(1992)**

(a) 1 A (b) 50 A

(c) 0.5 A (d) 5 A

13. A magnetic field of 2×10^{-2} T acts at right angles to a coil of area 100 cm^2, with 50 turns. The average e.m.f. induced in the coil is 0.1 V, when it is removed from the field in $t$sec. The value of t is

(a) 10 s (b) 0.1 s

(c) 0.01 s (d) 1 s(1991)

Lenz's Law and Conservation of Energy

14. An electron moves on a straight line path XY as shown. The abcd is a coil adjacent to the path of electron. What will be the direction of current, if any, induced in the coil? **(2015)**

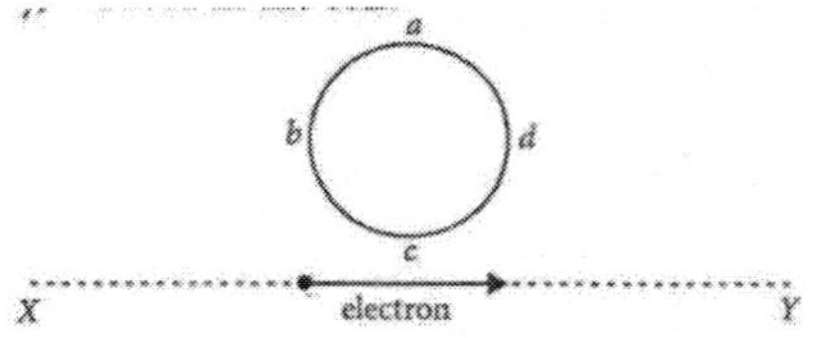

(a) The current will reverse its direction as the electron goes past the coil

(b) No current induced

(c) $abcd$ (d) $adcb$

15. A metal ring is held horizontally and bar magnet is dropped through the ring with its length along the axis of the ring. The acceleration of the falling magnet is **(1996)**

(a) more than g (b) equal to g

(c) less than g (d) either(a) or (c)

16. Faraday's laws are consequence of conservation of **(1991)**

(a) energy

(b) energy and magnetic field

(c) charge

(d) magnetic field

Motional Electromotive Force

17. A cycle wheel of radius 0.5 m is rotated with constant angular velocity of 10rad/s in a region of magnetic field of 0.1 T which is perpendicular to the plane of the wheel. The EMF generated between its centre and the rim is **(Odisha NEET 2019)**

(a) 0.25 V (b) 0.125 V

(c) 0.5 V (d) zero

18. A conducting square frame of side ' a ' and a long straight wire carrying current I are located in the same plane as shown in the figure. The frame moves to

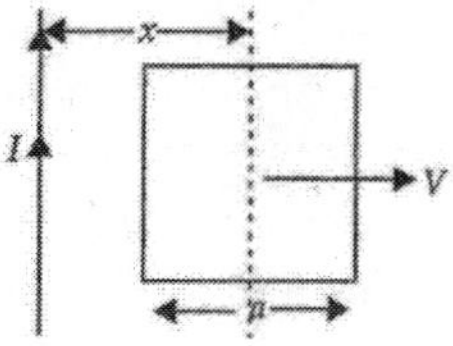

the right with a constant velocity ' V. The emf induced in the frame will be proportional to **(2015 Cancelled)**

(a) $\frac{1}{(2x+a)^2}$ (b) $\frac{1}{(2x-a)(2x+a)}$

(c) $\frac{1}{x^2}$ (d) $\frac{1}{(2x-a)^2}$.

19. A thin semicircular conducting x ××× ring (PQR) of radius r is falling with its plane vertical in a horizontal magnetic field B, as

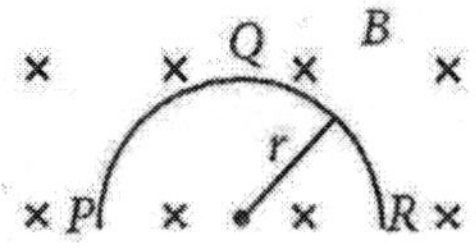

shown in the figure. The potential difference developed across the ring when its speed is v, is **(2014)**

(a) zero

(b) $\frac{Bv\pi r^2}{2}$ and P is at higher potential

(c) πrBv and R is at higher potential

(d) $2rBv$ and R is at higher potential

20. A straight line conductor of length 0.4 m is moved with a speed of $7\,m/s$ perpendicular to a magnetic field of intensity $0.9\,Wb/m^2$. The induced e.m.f. across the conductor is **(1995)**

(a) 5.04 V (b) 25.2 V

(c) 1.26 V (d) 2.52 V

Energy Consideration : A Quantitative Study

21. A long solenoid of diameter 0.1 m has 2×10^4 turns per meter. At the centre of the solenoid, a coil of 100 turns and radius 0.01 m is placed with its axis coinciding with the solenoid axis. The current in the solenoid reduces at a constant rate to 0 A from 4 A in 0.05 s. If the resistance of the coil is $10\pi^2\Omega$, the total charge flowing through the coil during this time is **(2017)**

(a) $16\mu C$ (b) $32\mu C$

(c) $16\pi\mu C$ (d) $32\pi\mu C$

22. In a coil of resistance 10Ω, the induced current developed by changing magnetic flux through it, is shown in figure as a function of time. The magnitude of change in flux through the coil in weber is

(Mains 2012)

(a) 8 (b) 2

(c) 6 (d) 4

23. The magnetic flux through a circuit of resistance R changes by an amount $\Delta\phi$ in a time Δt. Then the total quantity of electric charge Q that passes any point in the circuit during the time Δt is represented by

(2004)

(a) $Q = \frac{1}{R} \cdot \frac{\Delta\phi}{\Delta t}$ (b) $Q = \frac{\Delta\phi}{R}$

(c) $Q = \frac{\Delta\phi}{\Delta t}$ (d) $Q = R \cdot \frac{\Delta\phi}{\Delta t}$

24. The total charge, induced in a conducting loop when it is moved in magnetic field depends on **(1992)**

(a) the rate of change of magnetic flux

(b) initial magnetic flux only

(c) the total change in magnetic flux

(d) final magnetic flux only.

Eddy Currents

25. In which of the following devices, the eddy current effect is not used? **(2019)**

(a) electric heater

(b) induction furnace

(c) magnetic braking in train

(d) electromagnet

26. Eddy currents are produced when **(1988)**

(a) a metal is kept in varying magnetic field

(b) a metal is kept in steady magnetic field

(c) a circular coil is placed in a magnetic field

(d) current is passed through a circular coil

Inductance

27. The magnetic energy stored in an inductor of inductance 4 μH carrying a current of 2 A is **(2023)**

(a) 4 mJ (b) 8 mJ

(c) 8 μJ (d) 4 μJ

28. Two conducting circular loops of radii R_1 and R_2 are placed in the same plane with their centres coinciding. If $R_1 >> R_2$, the mutual inductance M between them will be directly proportional to **(2021)**

(a) $\frac{R_2^2}{R_1}$ (b) $\frac{R_1}{R_2}$

(c) $\frac{R_2}{R_1}$ (d) $\frac{R_1^2}{R_2}$

29. The magnetic potential energy stored in a certain inductor is 25 mJ, when the current in the inductor is 60 mA. This inductor is of inductance **(2018)**

(a) 0.138H (b) 138.88H

(c) 1.389H (d) 13.89H

30. A current of 2.5 A flows through a coil of inductance 5H. The magnetic flux linked with the coil is **(Karnataka NEET 2013)**

(a) 0.5 Wb (b) 12.5 Wb

(c) zero (d) 2 Wb

31. The current (I) in the inductance is varying with time according to the plot shown in figure.

Which one of the following is the correct variation of voltage with time in the coil?

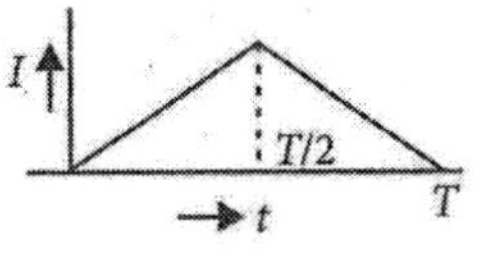

(2012)

(a) 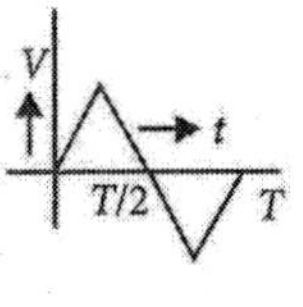

(b) 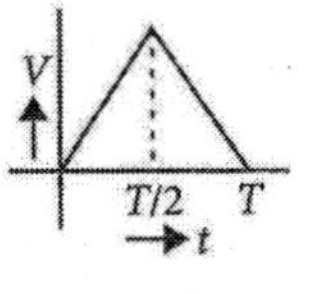

(c) 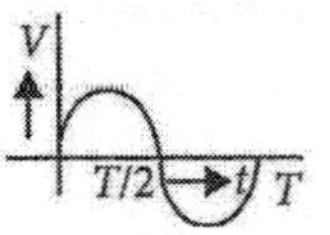

(d) 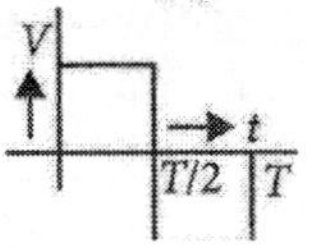

32. The current i in a coil varies with time as shown in the figure. The variation of induced emf with time would be **(2011)**

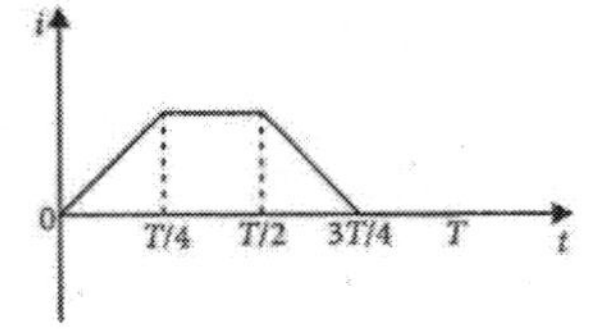

(a) 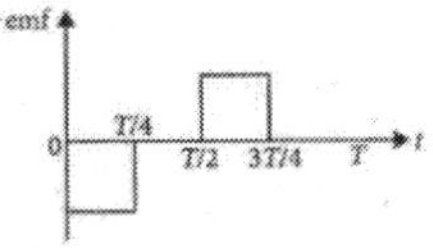

(b) 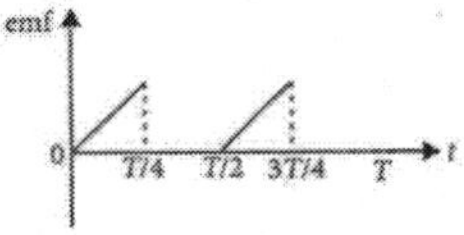

(c) 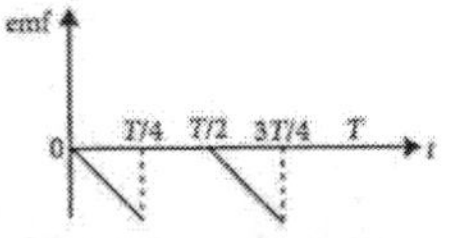

(d) 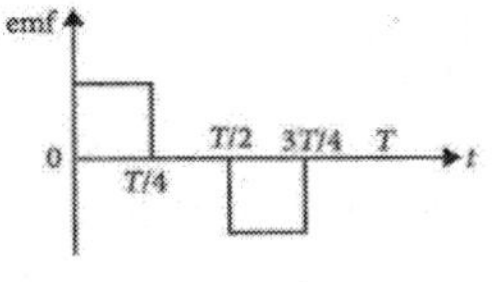

33. A long solenoid has 500 turns. When a current of 2 ampere is passed through it, the resulting magnetic flux linked with each turn of the solenoid is 4×10^{-3} Wb. The self-inductance of the solenoid is

(2008)

(a) 1.0 henry (b) 4.0 henry

(c) 2.5 henry (d) 2.0 henry

34. Two coils of self inductance 2mH and 8mH are placed so close together that the effective flux in one coil is completely linked with the other. The mutual inductance between these coils is **(2006)**

(a) 16mH (b) 10Mh

(c) 6mH (d) 4mH

35. For a coil having $L = 2\text{mH}$, current flow through it is $I = t^2e^{-t}$ then, the time at which emf becomes zero **(2001)**

(a) 2sec (b) 1sec

(c) 4sec (d) 3sec

36. Two coils have a mutual inductance 0.005H. The current changes in the first coil according to equation $I = I_0 \sin \omega t$, where $I_0 = 10$ A and $\omega = 100\pi \text{rad/sec}$. The maximum value of e.m.f. in the second coil is **(1998)**

(a) π (b) 5π

(c) 2π (d) 4π

37. If N is the number of turns in a coil, the value of self inductance varies as **(1993)**

(a) N^0 (b) N

(c) N^2 (d) N^{-2}

38. What is the self-inductance of a coil which produces 5 V when the current changes from 3 ampere to 2 ampere in one millisecond? **(1993)**

(a) 5000 henry (b) 5 milli-henry

(c) 50 henry (d) 5 henry

39. If the number of turns per unit length of a coil of solenoid is doubled, the self-inductance of the solenoid will **(1991)**

(a) remain unchanged

(b) be halved

(c) be doubled

(d) become four times

40. A 100 millihenry coil carries a current of 1A. Energy stored in its magnetic field is **(1991)**

(a) 0.5 J (b) 1 J

(c) 0.05 (d) 0.1 J

41. The current in self inductance $L = 40\text{mH}$ is to be increased uniformly from 1amp to 11amp in 4 milliseconds. The e.m.f. induced in inductor during process is **(1990)**

(a) 100 volt (b) 0.4 volt

(c) 4.0 volt (d) 440 volt

42. An inductor may store energy in **(1990)**

(a) its electric field

(b) its coils

(c) its magnetic field

(d) both in electric and magnetic fields

AC Generator

43. A wire loop is rotated in a magnetic field. The frequency of change of direction of the induced e.m.f. is **(2013)**

(a) four times per revolution

(b) six times per revolution

(c) once per revolution

(d) twice per revolution

44. In a region of magnetic induction $B = 10^{-2}$ tesla, a circular coil of radius 30 cm

and resistance π^2ohm is rotated about an axis which is perpendicular to the direction of B and which forms a diameter of the coil. If the coil rotates at 200rpm the amplitude of the alternating current induced in the coil is **(1988)**

(a) $4\pi^2$ mA (b) 30 mA

(c) 6 mA (d) 200 mA

ANSWER KEY

1.	(d)	2.	(b)	3.	(c)	4.	(c)	5.	(a)	6.	(d)	7.	(a)
8.	(b)	9.	(a)	10.	(d)	11.	(a)	12.	(c)	13.	(b)	14.	(a)
15.	(c)	16.	(a)	17.	(b)	18.	(b)	19.	(d)	20.	(d)	21.	(b)
22.	(b)	23.	(b)	24.	(c)	25.	(a)	26.	(a)	27.	(c)	28.	(a)
29.	(d)	30.	(b)	31.	(d)	32.	(a)	33.	(a)	34.	(d)	35.	(a)
36.	(b)	37.	(c)	38.	(b)	39.	(d)	40.	(c)	41.	(a)	42.	(c)
43.	(d)	44.	(c)										

Hints & Explanations

1. (d)

2. (b) : Given,

Side length of square, $l = 1$ m

Resistance, $R = 1\Omega$

Magnetic field, $B = 0.5$ T

The angle between the area vector and magnetic field is zero as the plane of coil is perpendicular to the magnetic field.

Magnetic flux, $\phi = BA\cos\theta$

$\phi = 0.5 \times 1 \times 1 \times \cos 0° = 0.5$ Wb

3. (c) : $B = \frac{1}{\pi}\left(\frac{\text{Wb}}{\text{m}^2}\right)$

Area of the disc normal to B is $\pi R^2 \cos 60°$.

Flux $= B \times$ Area normal

$\therefore$ Flux $= \frac{1}{2} \times 0.04 = 0.02$ Wb

4. (c): Given, number of turns $(N) = 1000$

Radius $(r) = 10$ m

Angular velocity $(\omega) = 2\text{rads}^{-1}$

Magnetic field $(B) = 2 \times 10^{-5}$ T

Electrical resistance $(R) = 12.56\Omega$

Maximum induced emf $= N\omega AB$

Here area of the circular coil $A = \pi r^2$

$$\varepsilon = N\omega\pi r^2 B = 1000 \times 2 \times 3.14 \times (10)^2 \times 2 \times 10^{-5}$$

$\varepsilon = 12.56$ V

The maximum induced current is, $i_{\max} = \frac{\varepsilon}{R}$

$$\Rightarrow i_{\max} = \frac{12.56}{12.56} = 1 \text{ A}$$

5. (a): Here $N = 800, A = 0.05\ m^2, \Delta t = 0.1\ s$

$B = 5 \times 10^{-5}\ T$

Induced emf, $\varepsilon = -\frac{\Delta\phi}{\Delta t} = -\frac{(\phi_f - \phi_i)}{\Delta t}$

$$\phi_i = N(\vec{B}\cdot\vec{A}) = 800 \times 5 \times 10^{-5} \times 0.05 \times \cos 0° = 2 \times 10^{-3}\ T\ m^2$$

$$\phi_f = 0 \Rightarrow \therefore \varepsilon = \frac{-(0 - 2 \times 10^{-3})}{0.1} = 2 \times 10^{-2}\ V = 0.02\ V$$

6. (d) : Emf generated in loop 1,

$$\varepsilon_1 = -\frac{d\phi}{dt} = -\frac{d}{dt}(\vec{B}\cdot\vec{A}) = -\frac{d}{dt}(BA) = -A \times \frac{dB}{dt}$$

$\varepsilon_1 = -\left(\pi r^2 \frac{dB}{dt}\right)$ ($\because A = \pi r^2$ because $\frac{dB}{dt}$ is restricted upto radius r.)

Emf generated in loop 2, $\varepsilon_2 = -\frac{d}{dt}(BA) = -\frac{d}{dt}(0 \times A) = 0$

7. (a): Here, $\phi = 50t^2 + 4$ Wb, $R = 400\Omega$

Induced emf, $\varepsilon = -\frac{d\phi}{dt} = -\frac{d}{dt}(50t^2 + 4) = -100t$ V

At $t = 2$ s, $\varepsilon = -200$ V; $|\varepsilon| = 200$ V

Induced current in the coil at $t = 2$ s is

$$I = \frac{|\varepsilon|}{R} = \frac{200\ V}{400\Omega} = \frac{1}{2}\ A = 0.5\ A$$

8. (b) : Here, Magnetic field, $B = 0.025$ T

Radius of the loop, $r = 2$ cm $= 2 \times 10^{-2}$ m

Constant rate at which radius of the loop shrinks,

$$\frac{dr}{dt} = 1 \times 10^{-3}\ m\ s^{-1}$$

Magnetic flux linked with the loop is

$$\phi = BA\cos\theta = B(\pi r^2)\cos 0° = B\pi r^2$$

The magnitude of the induced emf is

$$|\varepsilon| = \frac{d\phi}{dt} = \frac{d}{dt}(B\pi r^2) = B\pi 2r\frac{dr}{dt}$$

$$= 0.025 \times \pi \times 2 \times 2 \times 10^{-2} \times 1 \times 10^{-3} = \pi \times 10^{-6}\ V = \pi\mu V$$

9. (a): Once a rectangular loop or a square loop is being drawn out of the field, the rate of cutting the lines of field will be a constant for a square and rectangle, but not for circular or elliptical areas.

10. (d): Rate of decrease in the radius of the loop is 2 mm/s. Final radius $= 2$ cm $= 0.02$ m

Initial radius $= 2.2$ cm $= 0.022$ m, $B = 0.04$ T

$$\varepsilon = -\frac{d\phi}{dt} = -B\frac{dA}{dt}$$

$$\varepsilon = -\pi(0.022^2 - 0.02^2) \times 0.04 = -\pi \times 3.36 \times 10^{-6}\ V$$

$$|\varepsilon| = \pi \times 3.36 \times 10^{-6}\ V = 3.4\pi\mu V$$

11. (a): Work done due to a charge $W = QV$

12. (c) : $i = \frac{\varepsilon}{R} = \frac{\frac{NAdB}{dt}}{R} = \frac{20\times(25\times10^{-4})\times1000}{100} = 0.5$ A

13. (b) : $\varepsilon = \frac{-(\phi_2-\phi_1)}{t} = \frac{-(0-NBA)}{t} = \frac{NBA}{t}$

$$t = \frac{NBA}{\varepsilon} = \frac{50 \times 2 \times 10^{-2} \times 10^{-2}}{0.1} = 0.1\ s$$

14. (a):

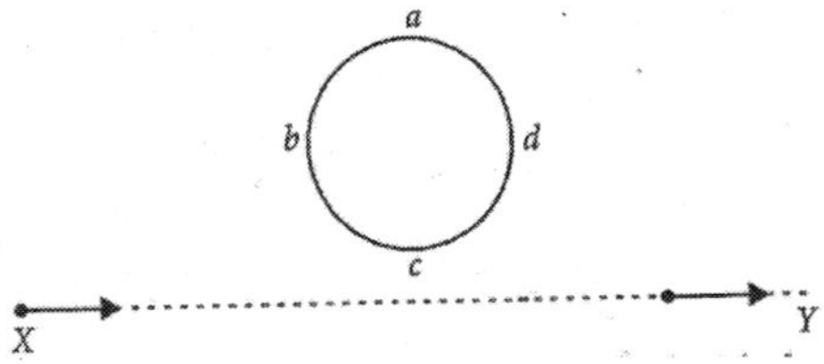

When the electron moves from X to Y, the flux linked with the coil $abcd$ (which is into the page) will first increase and then decrease as the electron passes by. So the induced current in the coil will be first anticlockwise and will reverse its direction (i.e., will become clockwise) as the electron goes past the coil.

15. (c): When the magnet is dropped through the ring, an induced current is developed into the ring in the direction opposing the motion of magnet (Lenz's law). Therefore this induced current decreases the acceleration of bar magnet.

16. (a): According to Faraday's law, it is the conservation of energy.

17. (b) : Here, $B = 0.1$ T, $r = 0.5$ m, $\omega = 10$rad/s

So, the emf generated between its centre and rim is,

$$\varepsilon = \frac{1}{2}B\omega r^2 = \frac{1}{2} \times 0.1 \times 10 \times (0.5)^2$$
$$= 0.125 \text{ V}$$

18. (b): Here, $PQ = RS = PR = QS = a$

Emf induced in the frame, $\varepsilon = B_1(PQ)V - B_2(RS)V$

$$= \frac{\mu_0 I}{2\pi(x - a/2)}aV - \frac{\mu_0 I}{2\pi(x + a/2)}aV$$

$$= \frac{\mu_0 I}{2\pi}\left[\frac{2}{(2x-a)} - \frac{2}{(2x+a)}\right]aV$$

$$= \frac{\mu_0 I}{2\pi} \times 2\left[\frac{2a}{(2x-a)(2x+a)}\right]aV$$

$$\therefore \varepsilon \propto \frac{1}{(2x-a)(2x+a)}$$

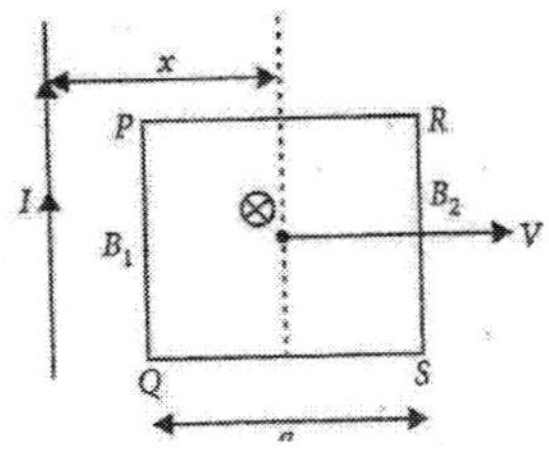

19. (d): Motional emf induced in the semicircular ring PQR is equivalent to the motional emf induced in the imaginary conductor PR.

i.e., $\varepsilon_{PQR} = \varepsilon_{PR} = Bvl = Bv(2r)$

$(l = PR = 2r)$

Therefore, potential difference developed across the ring is $2rBv$ with R at higher potential.

20. (d): Length of conductor $(l) = 0.4$ m,

Speed $(v) = 7$ m/s and magnetic field $(B) = 0.9$ Wb/m^2

Induced e.m.f. $(\varepsilon) = Blv = 0.9 \times 0.4 \times 7 = 2.52$ V.

21. (b) : Given $n = 2 \times 10^4, I = 4$ A

Initially $I = 0$ A $\therefore B_i = 0$ or $\phi_i = 0$

Finally, the magnetic field at the centre of the solenoid is given as

$$B_f = \mu_0 nI = 4\pi \times 10^{-7} \times 2 \times 10^4 \times 4$$
$$= 32\pi \times 10^{-3} \text{ T}$$

Final magnetic flux through the coil is given as

$$\phi_f = NBA = 100 \times 32\pi \times 10^{-3} \times \pi \times (0.01)^2$$

$$\phi_f = 32\pi^2 \times 10^{-5}\ \text{T m}^2$$

Induced charge, $q = \frac{|\Delta\phi|}{R} = \frac{|\phi_f - \phi_i|}{R} = \frac{32\pi^2 \times 10^{-5}}{10\pi^2}$

$$= 32 \times 10^{-6}\text{C} = 32\mu\text{C}$$

22. (b) : $q =$ Area under i - t graph $= \frac{1}{2} \times 4 \times 0.1 = 0.2\text{C}$

As $\quad q = \frac{\Delta\phi}{R} \therefore \Delta\phi = qR = (0.2\text{C})(10\Omega) = 2$ weber

23. (b): Induced emf is given by $V = \frac{\Delta\phi}{\Delta t}$

current $(i) = \frac{Q}{\Delta t} \Rightarrow \frac{\Delta\phi}{\Delta t} \times \frac{1}{R} = \frac{Q}{\Delta t}$

[where Q is total charge in time Δt]

$$\Rightarrow Q = \frac{\Delta\phi}{R}$$

24. (c) :

$$q = \int i dt = \frac{1}{R}\int \varepsilon dt = \left(\frac{-d\phi}{dt}\right)\frac{1}{R}\int dt = \frac{1}{R}\int d\phi$$

Hence total charge induced in the conducting loop depend upon the total change in magnetic flux.

As the emf or iR depends on rate of change of ϕ, charge induced depends on change of flux.

25. (a): Electric heater works on the principle of Joule's heating effect.

26. (a) : Eddy currents are produced when a metal is kept in a varying magnetic field.

27. (c): Energy $= \frac{1}{2}Li^2$

$$= \frac{1}{2}4 \times 10^{-6} \times 2^2$$

$$= 8 \times 10^{-6} J$$

energy $= 8\mu J$

28. (a): Let a current I_1 flows through the outer circular coil of radius R_1.

The magnitude field at the centre of the coil is $B_1 = \frac{\mu_0 I_1}{2R_1}$

As the inner coil of radius R_2 placed coaxially therefore, B_1 may be taken constant over its cross sectional area.

Hence flux associated with inner coil is

$$\phi_2 = B_1 \pi R_2^2 = \frac{\mu_0 I_1}{2R_1}\pi R_2^2 \Rightarrow$$

As $M = \frac{\phi_2}{I_1} = \frac{\mu_0 \pi R_2^2}{2R_1} \therefore M \propto \frac{R_2^2}{R_1}$

29. (d): Magnetic potential energy stored in an inductor is given by

$$U = \frac{1}{2}LI^2 \Rightarrow 25 \times 10^{-3} = \frac{1}{2} \times L \times (60 \times 10^{-3})^2$$

$$L = \frac{25 \times 2 \times 10^{6} \times 10^{-3}}{3600} = \frac{500}{36} = 13.89\text{H}$$

30. (b) : Here, $I = 2.5$ A, $L = 5$H

Magnetic flux linked with the coil is

$$\phi_B = LI = (5\text{H})(2.5\text{ A}) = 12.5\text{ Wb}$$

31. (d) : $|V| = \left|-L\frac{dI}{dt}\right| \Rightarrow |V| \propto$ slope of I - t graph

32. (a): Induced emf, $e = -L\frac{di}{dt}$

For $0 \leq t \leq \frac{T}{4}$,

i - t graph is a straight line with positive constant slope.

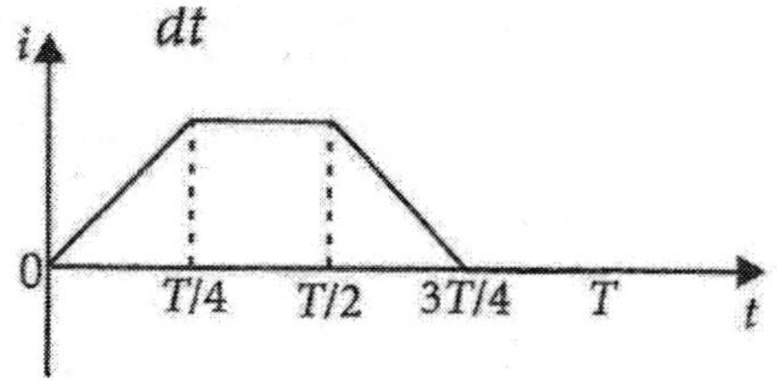

$\therefore \frac{di}{dt}$ = constant ⇒ $e = -$ ve and constant

For $\frac{T}{4} \leq t \leq \frac{T}{2}$

i is constant $\therefore \frac{di}{dt} = 0 \Rightarrow e = 0$

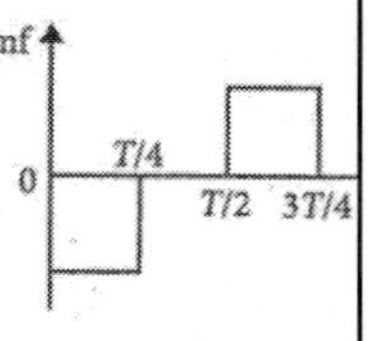

For $\frac{T}{2} \leq t \leq \frac{3T}{4}$

$i - t$ graph is a straight line with negative constant slope.

$\therefore \frac{di}{dt}$ = constant ⇒ $e = +$ ve and constant

For $\frac{3T}{4} \leq t \leq T$

i is zero $\therefore \frac{di}{dt} = 0 \Rightarrow e = 0$

From this analysis, the variation of induced emf with time is as shown in the figure.

33. (a) : Net flux $N\phi = Li$

Flux per turn $= 4 \times 10^{-3}$ Wb, $i = 2$ A

$$L = \frac{N\phi}{i} = \frac{4 \times 10^{-3} \times 500}{2} = 1 \text{ henry}$$

34. (d): Mutual inductance between coils is

$$M = K\sqrt{L_1 L_2} = 1\sqrt{2 \times 10^{-3} \times 8 \times 10^{-3}}$$

($\because$ K = 1)

$= 4 \times 10^{-3} = 4$mH

35. (a) : $I = t^2 e^{-t}$

$|\varepsilon| = L\frac{dI}{dt}$ here emf is zero when $\frac{dI}{dt} = 0$

$$\frac{dI}{dt} = 2te^{-t} - t^2e^{-t} = 0; 2te^{-t} = t^2e^{-t}$$

i.e., $te^{-t}(t-2) = 0 \Rightarrow t \neq \infty$ and $t \neq 0$ $\therefore$ $t = 2$sec

36. (b) : As, $|\varepsilon| = M\frac{dI}{dt} = M\frac{d}{dt}(I_0 \sin \omega t) = MI_0\omega\cos\omega t$

$\therefore \varepsilon_{max} = 0.005 \times 10 \times 100\pi \times 1 = 5\pi$

37. (c) : $L = \frac{N\phi}{i}; \phi = BA; B = \mu_0 ni = \frac{\mu_0 Ni}{l}$

$$L = \frac{\mu_0 N^2}{l}A = \mu_0 n^2 Al$$

where n is the number of turns per unit length $L \propto N^2$

38. (b) : $\varepsilon = -L\frac{di}{dt} \Rightarrow L = \frac{-\varepsilon}{\frac{di}{dt}} = \frac{-5 \times 10^{-3}}{(2-3)}$H = 5mH

39. (d) : Self inductance of a solenoid = $\mu_0 n^2 Al$

where n is the number of turns per length.

So self induction $\propto n^2$

So inductance becomes 4 times when n is doubled.

40. (c) : $E = \frac{1}{2}Li^2 = \frac{1}{2}(100 \times 10^{-3}) \times 1^2 = 0.05$ J

41. (a) : $|\varepsilon| = L\frac{di}{dt}$

Given that, $L = 40 \times 10^{-3}$H, $di = 11\text{ A} - 1\text{ A} = 10\text{ A}$

and $dt = 4 \times 10^{-3}$ s

$$\therefore |\varepsilon| = 40 \times 10^{-3} \times \left(\frac{10}{4 \times 10^{-3}}\right) = 100\text{ V}$$

42. (c)

43. (d)

44. (c): $I_0 = \frac{E_0}{R} = N\frac{BA\omega}{R}$

Given, $N = 1, B = 10^{-2}$ T, $A = \pi(0.3)^2$ m^2, $R = \pi^2\Omega$

$f = (200/60)$ and $\omega = 2\pi(200/60)$

Substituting these values and solving, we get

$I_0 = 6 \times 10^{-3}\text{ A} = 6\text{ mA}$

Chapter: 21 ALTERNATING CURRENT

AC Voltage Applied to a Resistor

1. The peak voltage of the ac source is equal to **(2022)**

   (a) the value of voltage supplied to the circuit

   (b) the rms value of the source

   (c) $\sqrt{2}$ times the rms value of the ac source

   (d) $1/\sqrt{2}$ times the rms value of the ac source

2. The r.m.s. value of potential difference V shown in the figure is **(Mains 2011)**

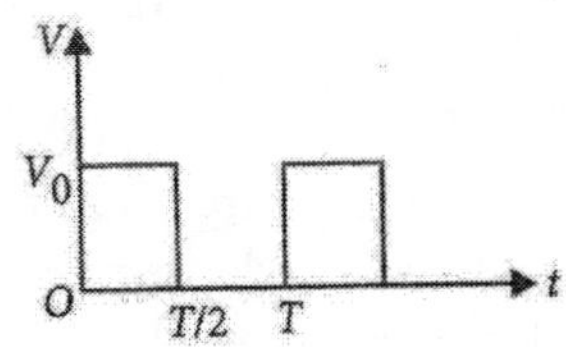

   (a) $\frac{V_0}{\sqrt{3}}$ (b) V_0

   (c) $\frac{V_0}{\sqrt{2}}$ (d) $\frac{V_0}{2}$

3. In an A.C. circuit, I_{rms} and I_0 are related as **(Mains 2011)**

   (a) $I_{rms} = \pi I_0$ (b) $I_{rms} = \sqrt{2} I_0$

   (c) $I_{rms} = I_0/\pi$ (d) $I_{rms} = I_0/\sqrt{2}$

4. Two cables of copper are of equal lengths. One of them has a single wire of area of cross-section A, while other has 10 wires of cross-sectional area $A/10$ each. Give their suitability for transporting A.C. and D.C. **(1994)**

   (a) only multiple strands for A.C., either for D.C.

   (b) only multiple strands for A.C., only single strand for D.C.

   (c) only single strand for D.C., either for A.C.

   (d) only single strand for A.C., either for D.C.

AC Voltage Applied to an Inductor

5. A coil of self-inductance L is connected in series with a bulb B and an AC source. Brightness of the bulb decreases when **(2013)**

   (a) a capacitance of reactance $X_C = X_L$ is included in the same circuit.

   (b) an iron rod is inserted in the coil.

   (c) frequency of the AC source is decreased.

   (d) number of turns in the coil is reduced.

6. The current I in an A.C. circuit with inductance coil varies with time according to the graph given below.

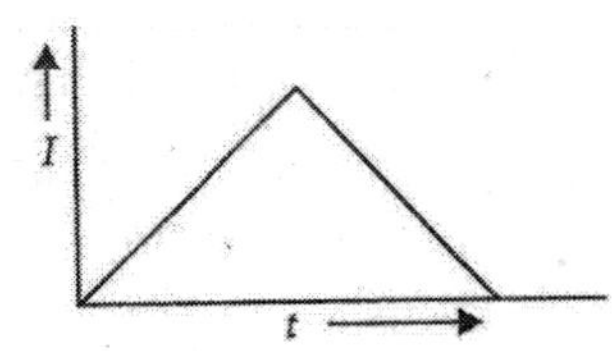

Which one of the following graphs gives the variation of voltage with time? **(1994)**

(a) 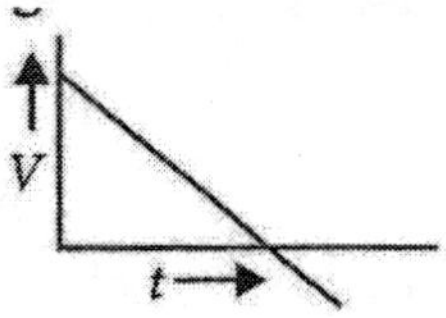

(b) 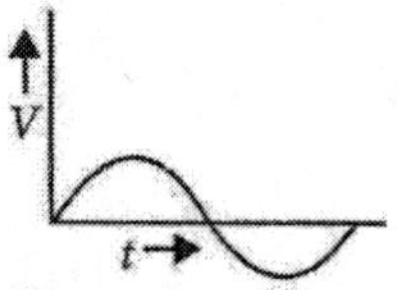

(c) 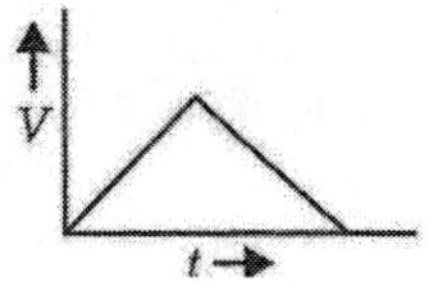

(d) 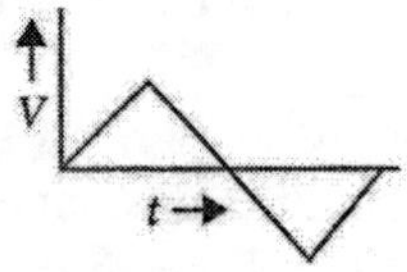

AC Voltage Applied to a Capacitor

7. An ac source is connected to a capacitor C. Due to decrease in its operating frequency **(2023)**

(a) Displacement current increases

(b) Displacement current decreases

(c) Capacitive reactance remains constant

(d) Capacitive reactance decreases

8. A $40\mu F$ capacitor is connected to a $200\ V, 50\ Hz$ ac supply. The r.m.s value of the current in the circuit is, nearly **(2020)**

(a) 1.7 A (b) 2.05 A

(c) 2.5 A (d) 25.1 A

9. A small signal voltage $V(t) = V_0 \sin \omega t$ is applied across an ideal capacitor C **(NEET-I 2016)**

(a) Current $I(t)$ is in phase with voltage $V(t)$.

(b) Current $I(t)$ leads voltage $V(t)$ by $180°$.

(c) Current $I(t)$, lags voltage $V(t)$ by $90°$.

(d) Over a full cycle the capacitor C does not consume any energy from the voltage source.

10. In an ac circuit an alternating voltage $200\sqrt{2}\sin 100t$ volts is connected to a capacitor of capacity $1\mu F$. The r.m.s. value of the current in the circuit is **(2011)**

(a) 10 mA (b) 100 mA

(c) 200 mA (d) 20 mA

11. A capacitor of capacity C has reactance X. If capacitance and frequency become double hen reactance will be **(2001)**

(a) $4X$ (b) $X/2$

(c) $X/4$ (d) $2X$

AC Voltage Applied to a Series LCR Circuit

12. In a series LCR circuit, the inductance L is 10 mH, capacitance C is 1 μF and resistance R is 100Ω. The frequency at which resonance occurs is **(2023)**

(a) 15.9 kHz (b) 1.59 rad/s

(c) 1.59 kHz (d) 15.9 rad/s

13. The net impedance of circuit (as shown in figure) will be **(2023)**

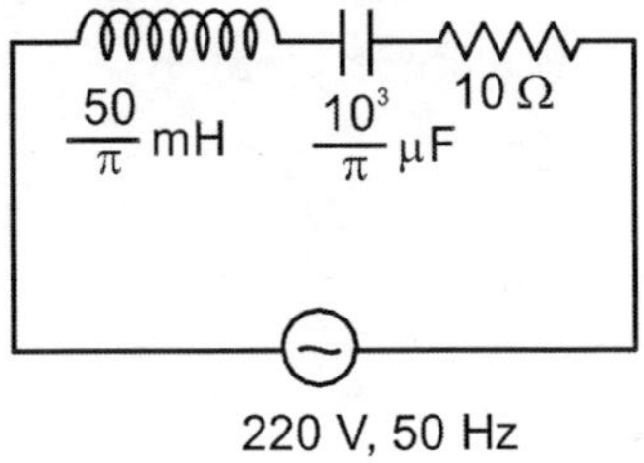

(a) 15 Ω (b) $5\sqrt{5}$ Ω

(c) 25 Ω (d) $10\sqrt{2}$ Ω

14. A series LCR circuit with inductance 10H, capacitance $10\mu\text{F}$, resistance 50Ω is connected to an ac source of voltage, $V = 200\sin(100t)$ volt. If the resonant frequency of the LCR circuit is v_0 and the frequency of the ac source is v, then **(2022)**

(a) $v_0 = v = 50$ Hz

(b) $v_0 = v = \frac{50}{\pi}$ Hz

(c) $v_0 = \frac{50}{\pi}$ Hz, $v = 50$ Hz

(d) $v = 100$ Hz, $v_0 = \frac{100}{\pi}$ Hz

15. A series LCR circuit containing 5.0H inductor $80\mu\text{F}$ capacitor and 40Ω resistor is connected to 230 V variable frequency ac source. The angular frequencies of the source at which power transferred to the circuit half the power at the resonant angular frequency are likely to be **(2021)**

(a) 42rad/s and 58rad/s

(b) 25rad/s and 75rad/s

(c) 50rad/s and 25rad/s

(d) 46rad/s and 54rad/s

16. An inductor of inductance L, a capacitor of capacitance C and a resistor of resistance 'R' are connected in series to an ac source of potential difference 'V' volts as shown in figure.

Potential difference across L, C and R is 40 V, 10 V and 40 V, respectively. The amplitude of current flowing through LCR series circuit is $10\sqrt{2}$ A. The impedance of the circuit is **(2021)**

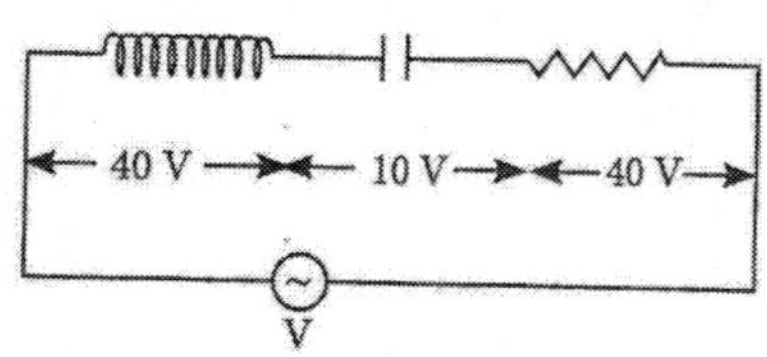

(a) 5Ω (b) $4\sqrt{2}\Omega$

(c) $5/\sqrt{2}\Omega$ (d) 4Ω

17. A series LCR circuit is connected to an ac voltage source. When L is removed from the circuit, the phase difference between current and voltage is $\pi/3$. If instead C is removed from the circuit, the phase difference is again $\pi/3$ between current and voltage. The power factor of the circuit is **(2020)**

(a) zero (b) 0.5

(c) 1.0 (d) -1.0

18. A circuit when connected to an AC source of 12 V gives a current of 0.2 A. The same circuit when connected to a DC source of 12 V, gives a current of 0.4 A. The circuit is

(Odisha NEET 2019)

(a) series LR (b) series RC

(c) series LC (d) series LCR

19. Which of the following combinations should be selected for better tuning of an $L-C-R$ circuit used for communication? **(NEET-II 2016)**

(a) $R = 20\Omega, L = 1.5\text{H}, C = 35\mu\text{F}$

(b) $R = 25\Omega, L = 2.5\text{H}, C = 45\mu\text{F}$

(c) $R = 15\Omega, L = 3.5\text{H}, C = 30\mu\text{F}$

(d) $R = 25\Omega, L = 1.5\text{H}, C = 45\mu\text{F}$

20. A series $R-C$ circuit is connected to an alternating voltage source. Consider two situations :

(i) When capacitor is air filled.

(ii) When capacitor is mica filled.

Current through resistor is i and voltage across capacitor is V then **(2015)**

(a) $i_a > i_b$ (b) $V_a = V_b$

(c) $V_a < V_b$ (d) $V_a > V_b$

21. An ac voltage is applied to a resistance R and an inductor L in series. If R and the inductive reactance are both equal to 3Ω, the phase difference between the applied voltage and the current in the circuit is **(2011)**

(a) $\pi/6$ (b) $\pi/4$

(c) $\pi/2$ (d) zero

22. A coil has resistance 30ohm and inductive reactance 20ohm at 50 Hz frequency. If an ac source, of 200 volt, 100 Hz, is connected across the coil, the current in the coil will be **(Mains 2011)**

(a) 2.0 A (b) 4.0 A

(c) 8.0 A (d) $\frac{20}{\sqrt{13}}$ A

23. In the given circuit the reading of voltmeter V_1 and V_2 are 300 volts each. The reading of the voltmeter V_3 and ammeter A are respectively **(2010)**

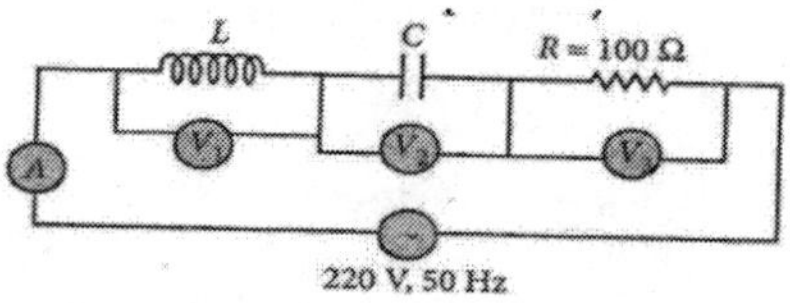

(a) 150 V, 2.2 A (b) 220 V, 2.2 A

(c) 220 V, 2.0 A (d) 100 V, 2.0 A

24. What is the value of inductance L for which the current is maximum in a series LCR circuit with $C = 10\mu\text{F}$ and $\omega = 1000\ \text{s}^{-1}$? **(2007)**

(a) 1mH

(b) cannot be calculated unless R is known

(c) 10mH (d) 100mH

25. In a circuit L, C and R are connected in series with an alternating voltage source of frequency f. The current leads the voltage by 45°. The value of C is **(2005)**

(a) $\frac{1}{\pi f(2\pi fL-R)}$ (b) $\frac{1}{2\pi f(2\pi fL-R)}$

(c) $\frac{1}{\pi f(2\pi fL+R)}$ (d) $\frac{1}{2\pi f(2\pi fL+R)}$

26. The value of quality factor is **(2000)**

(a) $\frac{\omega L}{R}$ (b) $\frac{1}{\omega RC}$

(c) $\sqrt{LC}$ (d) L/R

27. An series $L-C-R$ circuit is connected to a source of A.C. current. At resonance, the phase difference between the applied voltage and the current in the circuit, is **(1994)**

(a) π (b) zero

(c) $\pi/4$ (d) $\pi/2$

Power in AC Circuit: The Power Factor

28. An inductor 20mH, a capacitor $100\mu F$ and a resistor 50Ω are connected in series across a source of emf, $V = 10\sin 314t$. The power loss in the circuit is **(2018)**

(a) 0.79 W (b) 0.43 W

(c) 2.74 W (d) 1.13 W

29. The potential differences across the resistance, capacitance and inductance are 80 V, 40 V and 100 V respectively in an $L-C-R$ circuit. The power factor of this circuit is **(NEET-II 2016)**

(a) 0.4 (b) 0.5

(c) 0.8 (d) 1.0

30. An inductor 20mH, a capacitor $50\mu F$ and a resistor 40Ω are connected in series across a source of emf $V = 10\sin 340t$. The power loss in A.C. circuit is

(NEET-I 2016)

(a) 0.76 W (b) 0.89 W

(c) 0.51 W (d) 0.67 W

31. In an electrical circuit R, L, C and ac voltage source are all connected in series. When L is removed from the circuit, the phase difference between the voltage and the current in the circuit is $\pi/3$. If instead, C is removed from the circuit, the phase difference is again $\pi/3$. The power factor of the circuit is **(2012)**

(a) $\frac{1}{2}$ (b) $\frac{1}{\sqrt{2}}$

(c) 1 (d) $\frac{\sqrt{3}}{2}$

32. The instantaneous values of alternating current and voltages in a circuit are given as

$i = \frac{1}{\sqrt{2}}\sin(100\pi t)$ ampere

$e = \frac{1}{\sqrt{2}}\sin\left(100\pi t + \frac{\pi}{3}\right)$ volt

The average power in watts consumed in the circuit is **(Mains 2012)**

(a) $\frac{1}{4}$ (b) $\frac{\sqrt{3}}{4}$

(c) $\frac{1}{2}$ (d) $\frac{1}{8}$

33. Power dissipated in an LCR series circuit connected to an A.C. source of emf ε is

(2009)

(a) $\frac{\varepsilon^2\sqrt{R^2+\left(L\omega-\frac{1}{C\omega}\right)^2}}{R}$

(b) $\frac{\varepsilon^2\left[R^2+\left(L\omega-\frac{1}{C\omega}\right)^2\right]}{R}$

(c) $\frac{\varepsilon^2 R}{\sqrt{R^2+\left(L\omega-\frac{1}{C\omega}\right)^2}}$

(d) $\frac{\varepsilon^2 R}{\left[R^2+\left(L\omega-\frac{1}{C\omega}\right)^2\right]}$

34. In an a.c. circuit the e.m.f. (ε) and the current (i) at any instant are given respectively by

$e = E_0\sin\omega t, i = I_0\sin(\omega t - \phi)$

The average power in the circuit over one cycle of a.c. is **(2008)**

(a) $\frac{E_0 I_0}{2}\cos\phi$ (b) $E_0 I_0$

(c) $\frac{E_0 I_0}{2}$ (d) $\frac{E_0 I_0}{2}\sin\phi$

35. A coil of inductive reactance 31Ω has a resistance of 8Ω. It is placed in series with a condenser of capacitative reactance 25Ω. The combination is connected to an a.c. source of 110 V. The power factor of the circuit is **(2006)**

(a) 0.33 (b) 0.56

(c) 0.64 (d) 0.80

36. For a series LCR circuit, the power loss at resonance is **(2002)**

(a) $\frac{V^2}{\left[\omega L-\frac{1}{\omega C}\right]}$ (b) $I^2 L\omega$

(c) $I^2 R$ (d) $\frac{V^2}{C\omega}$

37. In an a.c. circuit with phase voltage V and current I, the power dissipated is **(1997)**

(a) V.I

(b) depends on phase angle between V and I

(c) $\frac{1}{2}\times V\cdot I$

(d) $\frac{1}{\sqrt{2}}\times V.I$

38. In an A.C. circuit, the current flowing is $I=5\sin(100t-\pi/2)$ ampere and the potential difference is $V=200\sin(100t)$ volts. The power consumption is equal to **(1995)**

(a) 20 W (b) 0 W

(c) 1000 W (d) 40 W

LC Oscillations

39. A condenser of capacity C is charged to a potential difference of V_1. The plates of the condenser are then connected to an ideal inductor of inductance L. The current through the inductor when the potential difference across the condenser reduces to V_2 is **(Mains 2010)**

(a) $\left(\frac{C(V_1-V_2)^2}{L}\right)^{\frac{1}{2}}$ (b) $\frac{C(V_1^2-V_2^2)}{L}$

(c) $\frac{C(V_1^2+V_2^2)}{L}$ (d) $\left(\frac{C(V_1^2-V_2^2)}{L}\right)^{\frac{1}{2}}$

40. A transistor-oscillator using a resonant circuit with an inductor L (of negligible resistance) and a capacitor C in series produces oscillations of frequency f. If L is doubled and C is changed to $4C$, the frequency will be **(2006)**

(a) $f/2$ (b) $f/4$

(c) $8f$ (d) $f/2\sqrt{2}$

Transformers

41. A 12 V, 60 W lamp is connected to the secondary of a step down transformer, whose primary is connected to ac mains of 220 V. Assuming the transformer to be ideal, what is the current in the primary winding? **(2023)**

(a) 2.7 A (b) 3.7 A

(c) 0.37 A (d) 0.27 A

42. A step down transformer connected to an ac mains supply of 220 V is made to operate at 11 V, 44 W lamp. Ignoring power losses in the transformer, what is the current in the primary circuit? **(2021)**

(a) 4 A (b) 0.2 A
(c) 0.4 A (d) 2 A

43. A transformer having efficiency of 90% is working on 200 V and 3 kW power supply. If the current in the secondary coil is 6 A, the voltage across the secondary coil and the current in the primary coil respectively are **(2014)**

(a) 300 V, 15 A (b) 450 V, 15 A
(c) 450 V, 13.5 A (d) 600 V, 15 A

44. The primary of a transformer when connected to a dc battery of 10 volt draws a current of 1 mA. The number of turns of the primary and secondary windings are 50 and 100 respectively. The voltage in the secondary and the current drawn by the circuit in the secondary are respectively

(Karnataka NEET 2013)

(a) 20 V and 2.0 mA
(b) 10 V and 0.5 mA
(c) Zero volt and therefore no current
(d) 20 V and 0.5 mA

45. A 220 volt input is supplied to a transformer. The output circuit draws a current of 2.0 ampere at 440 volts. If the efficiency of the transformer is 80%, the current drawn by the primary windings of the transformer is **(2010)**

(a) 3.6 ampere (b) 2.8 ampere
(c) 2.5 ampere (d) 5.0 ampere

46. The primary and secondary coils of a transformer have 50 and 1500 turns respectively. If the magnetic flux ϕ linked with the primary coil is given by $\phi = \phi_0 + 4t$, where ϕ is in webers, t is time in seconds and ϕ_0 is a constant, the output voltage across the secondary coil is **(2007)**

(a) 120 volts (b) 220 volts
(c) 30 volts (d) 90 volts

47. A transformer is used to light a 100 W and 110 V lamp from a 220 V mains. If the main current is 0.5amp, the efficiency of the transformer is approximately **(2007)**

(a) 50% (b) 90%
(c) 10% (d) 30%

48. The core of a transformer is laminated because **(2006)**

(a) ratio of voltage in primary and secondary may be increased
(b) energy losses due to eddy currents may be minimised
(c) the weight of the transformer may be reduced
(d) rusting of the core may be prevented.

49. A step-up transformer operates on a 230 V line and supplies a load of 2 ampere. The ratio of the primary and secondary windings is 1:25. The current in the primary is **(1998)**

(a) 15 A (b) 50 A
(c) 25 A (d). 12.5 A

50. The primary winding of a transformer has 500 turns whereas its secondary has 5000 turns. The primary is connected to an A.C. supply of 20 V, 50 Hz. The secondary will have an output of **(1997)**

(a) 2 V, 50 Hz (b) 2 V, 5 Hz

(c) 200 V, 50 Hz (d) 200 V, 500 Hz.

RC/RL Circuits with DC Source

51. Figure shows a circuit that contains three identical resistors with resistance $R = 9.0\Omega$ each, two identical inductors with inductance $L = 2.0$mH each, and an ideal battery with emf $\varepsilon = 18$ V. The current i through the battery just after the switch closed is **(2017)**

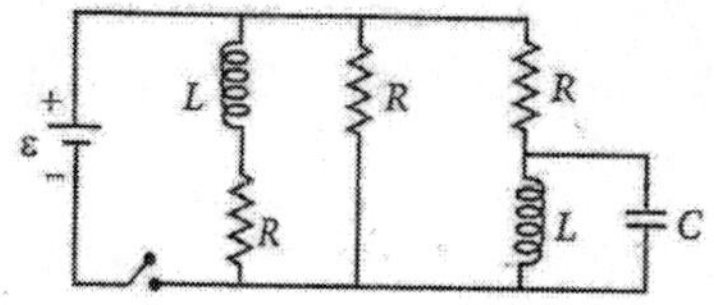

(a) 0.2 A (b) 2 A

(c) 0 ampere (d) 2 mA

52. A coil of 40 henry inductance is connected in series with a resistance of 8ohm and the combination is joined to the terminals of a 2 volt battery. The time constant of the circuit is **(2004)**

(a) 5 seconds (b) 1/5 seconds

(c) 40 seconds (d) 20 seconds

53. In the circuit given in figure, 1 and 2 are ammeters. Just after key K is pressed to complete the circuit, the reading will be

(1999)

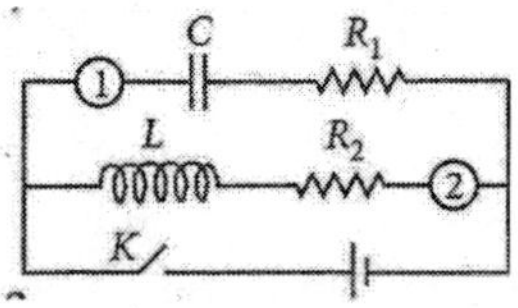

(a) zero in 1, maximum in 2

(b) maximum in both 1 and 2

(c) zero in both 1 and 2

(d) maximum in 1, zero in 2.

54. When the key K is pressed at time $t = 0$, then which of the following statement about the current I in the resistor AB of the given circuit is true?

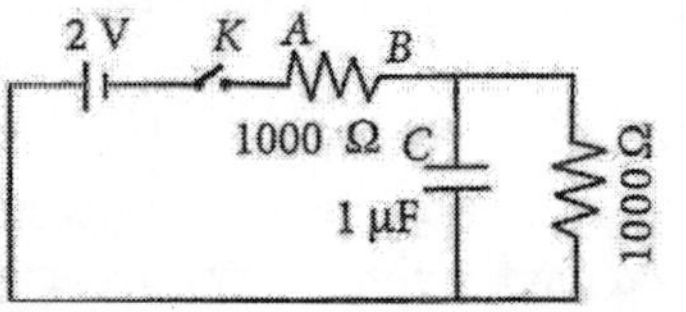

(a) I oscillates between 1 mA and 2 mA

(b) At $t = 0, I = 2$ mA and with time it goes to 1 mA

(c) $I = 1$ mA at all t

(d) $I = 2$ mA at all t.

55. The time constant of C - R circuit is

(1992)

(a) $1/CR$ (b) C/R

(c) CR (d) R/C

ANSWER KEY

1.	(c)	2.	(c)	3.	(d)	4.	(a)	5.	(b)	6.	(a)	7.	(b)
8.	(c)	9.	(d)	10.	(d)	11.	(c)	12.	(3)	13.	(2)	14.	(b)
15.	(d)	16.	(a)	17.	(c)	18.	(a)	19.	(c)	20.	(d)	21.	(b)
22.	(b)	23.	(b)	24.	(d)	25.	(d)	26.	(a,b)	27.	(b)	28.	(a)
29.	(c)	30.	(c)	31.	(c)	32.	(d)	33.	(d)	34.	(a)	35.	(d)
36.	(c)	37.	(b)	38.	(b)	39.	(d)	40.	(d)	41.	(4)	42.	(b)
43.	(b)	44.	(c)	45.	(d)	46.	(a)	47.	(b)	48.	(b)	49.	(b)
50.	(c)	51.	(*)	52.	(a)	53.	(d)	54.	(b)	55.	(c)		

Hints & Explanations

1. **(c)** : The relation between the peak value and the rms value is:

$$V_{rms} = \frac{V_0}{\sqrt{2}}$$

so, $V_0 = \sqrt{2}V_{rms}$

2. **(c) :**

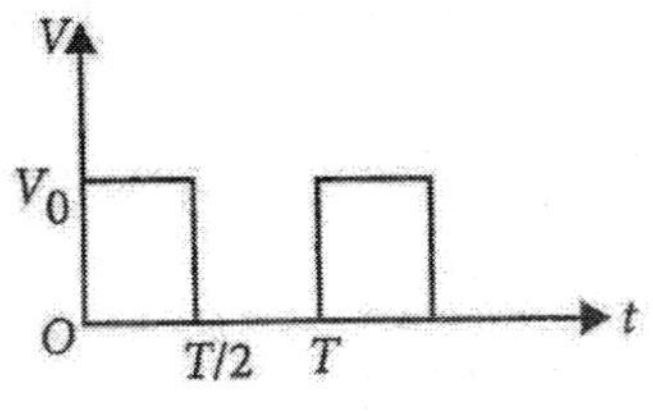

$V = V_0$ for $0 \le t \le \frac{T}{2} \Rightarrow V = 0$ for $\frac{T}{2} \le t \le T$

$$V_{\text{rms}} = \left[\frac{\int_0^T V^2 dt}{\int_0^T dt}\right]^{1/2}$$

$$= \left[\frac{\int_0^{T/2} V_0^2 dt + \int_{T/2}^{T} (0) dt}{\int_0^T dt}\right]^{1/2}$$

$$= \left[\frac{V_0^2}{T}[t]_0^{T/2}\right]^{1/2} = \left[\frac{V_0^2}{T}\left(\frac{T}{2}\right)\right]^{1/2} = \left[\frac{V_0^2}{2}\right]^{1/2}$$

$$\therefore V_{\text{rms}} = \frac{V_0}{\sqrt{2}}$$

3. **(d)** : $I_{\text{rms}} = \frac{I_0}{\sqrt{2}}$

4. **(a)** : The major portion of the A.C. flows on the surface of the wire. So where a thick wire is required, a number of thin wires are joined together to give an equivalent effect of a thick wire. Therefore multiple strands are suitable for transporting A.C. Similarly multiple strands can also be used for D.C.

5. **(b)** : The situation is as shown in the figure.

As the iron rod is inserted, the magnetic field inside the coil magnetizes the iron, increasing the magnetic field inside it.

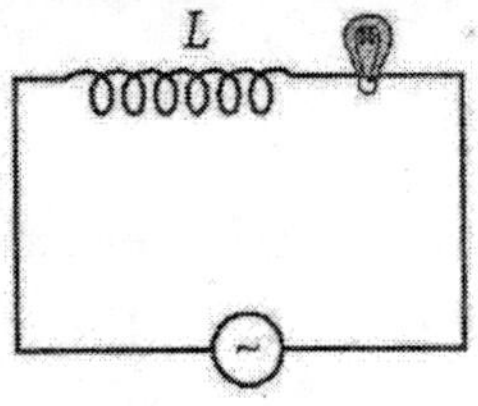

Hence,the inductance of the coil increases. Consequently, the inductive reactance of the coil increases. As a result, a larger fraction of the applied AC voltage appears across the inductor, leaving less voltage across the bulb. Therefore, the brightness of the light bulb decreases.

6. **(a)** : In an A.C. circuit with inductance coil, the voltage V leads the current I by a phase difference of 90° or the current I lags behind the voltage V by a phase difference of 90°. Thus the voltage goes on decreasing with the increase in time as shown in the graph (a).

7. **(b)** : $i_C = i_D = \frac{V_O}{X_C} \sin \omega t$

$i_C = i_D = (V_O \omega C) \sin \omega t$

On decreasing frequency $i_C \downarrow$

8. **(c)** : Here, $C = 40\mu F = 40 \times 10^{-6}$ F

$V_{rms} = 200$ V; $v = 50$ Hz

The value of the current,

$I_{rms} = \frac{\varepsilon_{rms}}{\frac{1}{\omega C}} = \varepsilon_{rms} \omega C$

or $I_{rms} = 200(2\pi \times 50) \times (40 \times 10^{-6}) = 2.51$ A ($\because \omega = 2\pi v$)

9. **(d)** : When an ideal capacitor is connected with an ac voltage source, current leads voltage by 90°. Since, energy stored in capacitor during charging is spent in maintaining charge on the capacitor during discharging. Hence over a full cycle the capacitor does not consume any energy from the voltage source.

10. **(d):** The given equation of alternating voltage is

$$e = 200\sqrt{2} \sin 100t$$

The standard equation of alternating voltage is

$$e = e_0 \sin \omega t$$

Comparing (i) and (ii), we get

$$e_0 = 200\sqrt{2}\text{ V}, \omega = 100\text{rads}^{-1}$$

The capacitive reactance is

$$X_C = \frac{1}{\omega C} = \frac{1}{100 \times 1 \times 10^{-6}} \Omega$$

The r.m.s. value of the current in the circuit is

$$i_{\text{r.m.s.}} = \frac{v_{\text{r.m.s.}}}{X_C} = \frac{e_0/\sqrt{2}}{1/\omega C} = \frac{(200\sqrt{2}/\sqrt{2})}{(1/100 \times 10^{-6})}$$

$$= 200 \times 100 \times 10^{-6}\text{ A} = 2 \times 10^{-2}\text{ A}$$
$$= 20\text{ mA}$$

11. **(c)** I : $X = \frac{1}{C\omega}$ and $X' = \frac{1}{4C\omega}$ $\therefore X' = \frac{X}{4}$

12. **(c)** : $L = 10 \times 10^{-3} H$

$C = 1 \times 10^{-6} F$

$R = 100\Omega$

At resonance $X_L = X_C$

$$\omega L = \frac{1}{\omega C}$$

$$f = \frac{1}{2\pi\sqrt{LC}} = \frac{1}{2\pi\sqrt{10\times10^{-3}\times10^{-6}}}$$
$$=1.59 KHz$$

13. **(b) :** $X_L = \frac{50}{L}\times10^{-3}\times2\pi\times50 = 5\Omega$

$$X_C = \frac{1}{2\pi\times50\times\frac{10^3}{\pi}\times10^{-6}} = 10\Omega$$

$$Z = \sqrt{R^2+(X_L-X_C)^2}$$

$$= \sqrt{(10)^2+(5)^2}$$

$$= 5\sqrt{5}\Omega$$

14. **(b)**: Here, $L = 10\text{H}; C = 10\mu\text{F}; R = 50\Omega;$

$V = 200\sin(100t)\text{V}$

We know that $\omega = 2\pi v \Rightarrow v = \frac{\omega}{2\pi}$

From eq. (i), $v = \frac{100}{2\pi} = \frac{50}{\pi} (\because \omega = 100\text{rad/s})$

$\therefore$ Frequency $v = \frac{50}{\pi}\text{Hz}$

At resonance, $v_r = v_0 = \frac{1}{2\pi\sqrt{LC}}$

$$= \frac{1}{2\pi\sqrt{10\times10\times10^{-6}}} = \frac{1}{2\pi\sqrt{10^{-4}}}$$

$$\therefore v_0 = \frac{1}{2\pi\times10^{-2}} = \frac{100}{2\pi} = \frac{50}{\pi}\text{Hz}$$

15. **(d)** : $\omega_r = \frac{1}{\sqrt{LC}} = \frac{1}{\sqrt{5\times80\times10^{-6}}} = 50\text{rad/s}$

Power transferred = half of power at resonance

So, frequencies at which power transferred is half

$$= \omega_r \pm \Delta\omega \Rightarrow \Delta\omega = \frac{R}{2L} = \frac{40}{2\times5} = 4\text{rad/s}$$

So, range is $\omega_r \pm \Delta\omega = 50 \pm 4 = 54\text{rad/s}$ and 46rad/s

16. **(a)**: Given, $V_L = 40\text{ V}$

$V_C = 10\text{ V}, V_R = 40\text{ V}$

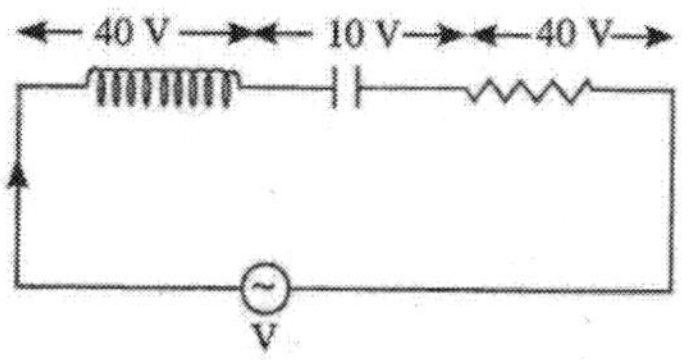

$$V_{\text{rms}} = \sqrt{V_R^2+(V_L-V_C)^2} \Rightarrow V_{\text{rms}}$$
$$= \sqrt{40^2+(40-10)^2}$$
$$= 50\text{ V}$$

$$I_0 = 10\sqrt{2}\text{ A} \Rightarrow I_{\text{rms}} = \frac{I_0}{\sqrt{2}} = 10\text{ A}$$

Impedance, $Z = \frac{V_{\text{rms}}}{I_{\text{rms}}} = \frac{50}{10} = 5\Omega.$

17. **(c):** When L is removed

$$\tan\phi = \frac{|X_C|}{R} \Rightarrow \tan\frac{\pi}{3} = \frac{X_C}{R}$$

When C is removed,

$$\tan\phi = \frac{|X_L|}{R} \Rightarrow \tan\frac{\pi}{3} = \frac{X_L}{R}$$

From (i) and (ii), $X_C = X_L$

Since, $X_L = X_C$, the circuit is in resonance.

$Z = R$

Power factor, $\cos\phi = \frac{Z}{R} = \frac{R}{R} = 1$

18. **(a):** When circuit is connected to an AC source of 12 V gives a current of 0.2 A.

$\therefore$ Impedance, $Z = \frac{12}{0.2} = 60\Omega$

When the same circuit is connected to a DC source of 12 V, gives a current of 0.4 A.

$\therefore$ Resistance, $R = \frac{12}{0.4} = 30\Omega$

As, power factor, $\cos\phi = \frac{R}{Z} = \frac{30}{60} = \frac{1}{2} = \cos 60°$

$\Rightarrow \phi = 60°$, i.e., current lags behind the emf.

So, we can conclude that the circuit is a series LR.

19. **(c) :** Quality factor of an $L-C-R$ circuit is given by,

$$Q = \frac{1}{R}\sqrt{\frac{L}{C}}$$

$$Q_1 = \frac{1}{20}\sqrt{\frac{1.5}{35\times10^{-6}}} = 50\times\sqrt{\frac{3}{70}} = 10.35$$

$$Q_2 = \frac{1}{25}\times\sqrt{\frac{2.5}{45\times10^{-6}}} = 40\times\sqrt{\frac{5}{90}} = 9.43$$

$$Q_3 = \frac{1}{15}\sqrt{\frac{3.5}{30\times10^{-6}}} = \frac{100}{15}\sqrt{\frac{35}{3}} = 22.77$$

$$Q_4 = \frac{1}{25}\times\sqrt{\frac{1.5}{45\times10^{-6}}} = \frac{40}{\sqrt{30}} = 7.30$$

Clearly Q_3 is maximum of Q_1, Q_2, Q_3, and Q_4.

Hence, option (c) should be selected for better tuning of an $L-C-R$ circuit.

20. **(d):** Current through resistor,

i = Current in the circuit

$$= \frac{V_0}{\sqrt{R^2+X_C^2}} = \frac{V_0}{\sqrt{R^2+(1/\omega C)^2}}$$

Voltage across capacitor, $V = iX_C$

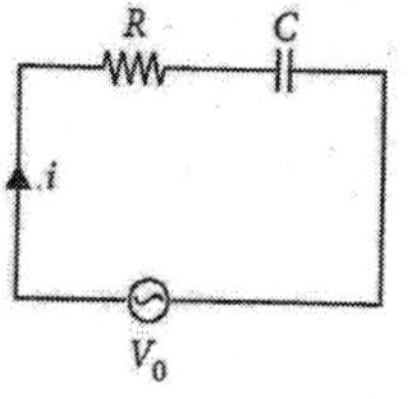

$$= \frac{V_0}{\sqrt{R^2+(1/\omega C)^2}}\times\frac{1}{\omega C} = \frac{V_0}{\sqrt{R^2\omega^2C^2+1}}$$

As $C_a < C_b$ $\therefore$ $i_a < i_b$ and $V_a > V_b$

21. **(b):** Here, $R = 3\Omega, X_L = 3\Omega$

The phase difference between the applied voltage and the current in the circuit is

$\tan\phi = \frac{X_L}{R} = \frac{3\Omega}{3\Omega} = 1$ or $\phi = \tan^{-1}(1) = \frac{\pi}{4}$

22. **(b) :** Here, Resistance, $R = 30\Omega$

Inductive reactance, $X_L = 20\Omega$ at 50 Hz

$\because X_L = 2\pi\upsilon L$

$$X_L' = \frac{\upsilon'}{\upsilon}\times X_L = \left(\frac{100}{50}\right)\times 20\Omega = 40\Omega$$

Impedance, $Z = \sqrt{R^2+(X_L')^2} = \sqrt{(30)^2+(40)^2} = 50\Omega$

Current in the coil, $I = \frac{V}{Z} = \frac{200\text{ V}}{50\Omega} = 4$ A

23. (b)

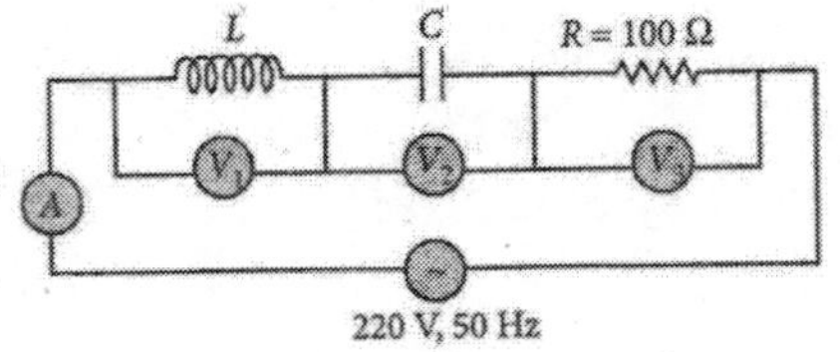

As $V_L = V_C = 300$ V, therefore the given series LCR circuit is in resonance.

$\therefore V_R = V = 220\text{ V}, Z = R = 100\Omega$

Current, $I = \frac{V}{Z} = \frac{220\text{ V}}{100\Omega} = 2.2$ A

Hence, the reading of the voltmeter V_3 is 220 V and the reading of ammeter A is 2.2 A.

24. (d): In series LCR, current is maximum at resonance.

$\therefore$ Resonant frequency, $\omega = \frac{1}{\sqrt{LC}}$

$\therefore \omega^2 = \frac{1}{LC}$ or, $L = \frac{1}{\omega^2 C}$

Given $\omega = 1000\text{ s}^{-1}$ and $C = 10\mu\text{F}$

$\therefore L = \frac{1}{1000\times1000\times10\times10^{-6}} = 0.1\text{H} = 100\text{mH}.$

25. (d) : $\tan\phi = \frac{X_C - X_L}{R}$ or $\tan\left(\frac{\pi}{4}\right) = \frac{\frac{1}{\omega C} - \omega L}{R}$

$R = \frac{1}{\omega C} - \omega L$ or $(R + 2\pi fL) = \frac{1}{2\pi fC}$ or $C = \frac{1}{2\pi f(R+2\pi fL)}$

26. (, *b*) : Quality factor, $Q = \frac{\omega L}{R}$

Since $\omega^2 = \frac{1}{LC}$ $\therefore$ Quality factor, $Q = \frac{1}{\omega RC}$

27. (b) : For resonance condition, the impedance will be minimum and the current will be maximum. This is only possible when $X_L = X_C$.

Therefore $\tan\phi = \frac{X_L + X_C}{R} = 0$ or $\phi = 0$.

28. (a) : Impedance Z in an ac circuit is

$Z = \sqrt{R^2 + (X_C - X_L)^2}$; where $X_C =$ capacitive reactance and $X_L =$ inductive reactance.

Also $X_C = \frac{1}{\omega C}$ and $X_L = \omega L$

$\therefore Z =$

$$\sqrt{(50)^2 + \left(\frac{1}{314\times100\times10^{-6}} - 314\times20\times10^{-3}\right)^2}$$

or $Z = 56\Omega$

The power loss in the circuit is $P_{av} = \left(\frac{V_{rms}}{Z}\right)^2 R$

$$\therefore P_{av} = \left(\frac{10}{(\sqrt{2})56}\right)^2 \times 50 = 0.79\text{ W}$$

29. (c): Here, $V_R = 80\text{ V}, V_C = 40\text{ V}, V_L = 100$ V

Power factor, $\cos\phi = \frac{R}{Z} = \frac{V_R}{V} = \frac{V_R}{\sqrt{V_R^2 + (V_L - V_C)^2}}$

$$= \frac{80}{\sqrt{(80)^2 + (100-40)^2}} = \frac{80}{100} = 0.8$$

30. (c) : Here, $L = 20\text{mH} = 20\times10^{-3}\text{H}$,

$C = 50\mu\text{F} = 50\times10^{-6}\text{ F}, R = 40\Omega$,

$V = 10\sin 340t = V_0 \sin\omega t$

$\omega = 340\text{rads}^{-1}, V_0 = 10$ V

$X_L = \omega L = 340\times20\times10^{-3} = 6.8\Omega$

$$X_C = \frac{1}{\omega C} = \frac{1}{340\times50\times10^{-6}} = \frac{10^4}{34\times5} = 58.82\Omega$$

$Z = \sqrt{R^2 + (X_C - X_L)^2}$
$= \sqrt{(40)^2 + (58.82 - 6.8)^2}$

$= \sqrt{(40)^2 + (52.02)^2} = 65.62\Omega$

The peak current in the circuit is

$$I_0 = \frac{V_0}{Z} = \frac{10}{65.62}\text{ A}, \cos\phi = \frac{R}{Z} = \left(\frac{40}{65.62}\right)$$

Power loss in A.C. circuit, $= V_{\text{rms}} I_{\text{rms}} \cos\phi = \frac{1}{2} V_0 I_0 \cos\phi$

$$= \frac{1}{2} \times 10 \times \frac{10}{65.62} \times \frac{40}{65.62} = 0.46\text{ W}$$

31. **(c)** : When L is removed, the phase difference between the voltage and current is

$$\tan\phi_1 = \frac{X_C}{R}$$

$\tan\frac{\pi}{3} = \frac{X_C}{R}$ or $X_C = R\tan 60°$ or $X_C = \sqrt{3}R$

When C is removed, the phase difference between the voltage and current is

$\tan\phi_2 = \frac{X_L}{R}$ or $\tan\frac{\pi}{3} = \frac{X_L}{R}$ or $X_L = R\tan 60° = \sqrt{3}R$

As $X_L = X_C$, the series LCR circuit is in resonance.

Impedance of the circuit,

$$Z = \sqrt{R^2 + (X_L - X_C)^2} = R$$

Power factor, $\cos\phi = \frac{R}{Z} = \frac{R}{R} = 1$

32. **(d)** : Given : $i = \frac{1}{\sqrt{2}}\sin(100\pi t)$ ampere

Compare it with $i = i_0\sin(\omega t)$, we get

$$i_0 = \frac{1}{\sqrt{2}}\text{ A}$$

Given : $e = \frac{1}{\sqrt{2}}\sin\left(100\pi t + \frac{\pi}{3}\right)$ volt

Compare it with $e = e_0\sin(\omega t + \phi)$, we get

$$e_0 = \frac{1}{\sqrt{2}}\text{ V}, \phi = \frac{\pi}{3}$$

$$\therefore\ i_{\text{rms}} = \frac{i_0}{\sqrt{2}} = \frac{1}{2}\text{ A and } e_{\text{rms}} = \frac{e_0}{\sqrt{2}} = \frac{1}{2}\text{ V}$$

Average power consumed in the circuit,

$P = i_{\text{rms}}\, e_{\text{rms}} \cos\phi$

$$= \left(\frac{1}{2}\right)\left(\frac{1}{2}\right)\cos\frac{\pi}{3} = \left(\frac{1}{2}\right)\left(\frac{1}{2}\right)\left(\frac{1}{2}\right) = \frac{1}{8}\text{ W}$$

33. **(d):** Average power, $P = E_{\text{r.m.s}} I_{\text{r.m.s}} \cos\phi$

$$Z = \sqrt{R^2 + (X_L - X_C)^2}, \cos\phi = \frac{R}{Z}$$

But $I_{\text{r.m.s}} = \frac{E_{\text{r.m.s}}}{Z}$ $\therefore\ P = E^2_{\text{r.m.s}} \cdot \frac{R}{Z^2}$

$$\therefore P = E^2_{\text{r.m.s}} \frac{R}{\{R^2 + (X_L - X_C)^2\}}$$

$$= \frac{\varepsilon^2 R}{\left[R^2 + \left(L\omega - \frac{1}{C\omega}\right)^2\right]}$$

34. **(a):** Average power $= \frac{E_0 I_0}{2}\cos\phi$

35. **(d)** : $X_L = 31\Omega, X_C = 25\Omega, R = 8\Omega$

Impedance of series LCR is

$Z = \sqrt{(R^2) + (X_L - X_C)^2}$
$= \sqrt{(8)^2 + (31 - 25)^2} = \sqrt{64 + 36} = 10\Omega.$

Power factor, $\cos\phi = \frac{R}{Z} = \frac{8}{10} = 0.8$

36. **(c):** The impedance Z of a series LCR circuit is given by, $Z = \sqrt{R^2 + (X_L - X_C)^2}$

where $X_L = \omega L$ and $X_C = \frac{1}{\omega C}$, ω is angular frequency.

At resonance, $X_L = X_C$, hence $Z = R$.

$\therefore\ V_R = V$ (supply voltage)

$\therefore$ r.m.s. current, $I = \frac{V_R}{R} = \frac{V}{R}$

$\therefore$ Power loss $= I^2R = V^2/R$

37. **(b):** The dissipation of power in an a.c. circuit is $(P) = V \times I \times \cos\theta$. Therefore current flowing in the circuit depends upon the phase angle between voltage (V) and current (I) of the a.c. circuit.

38. **(b):** Current $(I) = 5\sin(100t - \pi/2)$ and voltage $(V) = 200\ \sin(100t)$. Comparing the given equation, with the standard equation, we find that phase between current and voltage is $\phi = \frac{\pi}{2} = 90°$

Power consumption $P = I_{\text{rms}}V_{\text{rms}}\cos\phi = I_{\text{rms}}V_{\text{rms}}\cos 90° = 0$

39. **(d):** In case of oscillatory discharge of a capacitor through an inductor, charge at instant t is given by

$$q = q_0\cos\omega t;\ \text{where, } \omega = \frac{1}{\sqrt{LC}}$$

$$\therefore \cos\omega t = \frac{q}{q_0} = \frac{CV_2}{CV_1} = \frac{V_2}{V_1}\ (\because q = CV)$$

Current through the inductor

$$I = \frac{dq}{dt} = \frac{d}{dt}(q_0\cos\omega t) = -q_0\omega\sin\omega t$$

$$|I| = CV_1\frac{1}{\sqrt{LC}}[1 - \cos^2\omega t]^{1/2}$$

$$= V_1\sqrt{\frac{C}{L}}\left[1 - \left(\frac{V_2}{V_1}\right)^2\right]^{1/2} = \left[\frac{C(V_1^2 - V_2^2)}{L}\right]^{1/2}$$

40. **(d) :** Frequency of LC oscillation $= \frac{1}{2\pi\sqrt{LC}}$

or, $\frac{f_1}{f_2} = \left(\frac{L_2C_2}{L_1C_1}\right)^{1/2} = \left(\frac{2L\times 4C}{L\times C}\right)^{1/2} = (8)^{1/2}$

$\therefore \frac{f_1}{f_2} = 2\sqrt{2} \Rightarrow f_2 = \frac{f_1}{2\sqrt{2}}$ or, $f_2 = \frac{f}{2\sqrt{2}}$

41. **(d)** :

$V_SI_S = V_PI_P$ (ideal Transformer)

$\Rightarrow P_{\text{out}} = P_{\text{in}}$

$\Rightarrow 60 = 220 \times I_P$

$$I_P = \frac{60}{220} = 0.27A$$

42. **(b)** : Here $P = 44$ W, $V_p = 220$ V, $V_s = 11$ V

Power, $P = V_sI_s$

$44 = I_s \Rightarrow I_s = 4$ A

Now, $V_pI_p = V_sI_s$

$$220 \times I_p = 11 \times 4 \Rightarrow I_P = \frac{11\times 4}{220} = \frac{4}{20} = 0.2\text{ A}$$

43. **(b) :** Here, Efficiency of the transformer, $\eta = 90\%$

Input power, $P_{\text{in}} = 3\text{ kW} = 3\times 10^3\text{ W} = 3000\text{ W}$

Voltage across the primary coil, $V_p = 200$ V

Current in the secondary coil, $I_s = 6$ A

As $P_{\text{in}} = I_pV_p$

$\therefore$ Current in the primary coil,

$$I_p = \frac{P_{\text{in}}}{V_p} = \frac{3000\text{ W}}{200\text{ V}} = 15\text{ A}$$

Efficiency of the transformer,

$\eta = \frac{P_{out}}{P_{in}} = \frac{V_S I_S}{V_P I_P} \therefore \frac{90}{100} = \frac{6V_S}{3000}$ or $V_s = \frac{90\times3000}{100\times6} = 450\text{ V}$

44. (c): Transformer cannot work on dc.

$\therefore V_s = 0$ and $I_s = 0$

45. (d): Here, Input voltage, $V_p = 220\text{ V}$

Output voltage, $V_s = 440\text{ V}$

Input current, $I_p = ?$

Output current, $I_s = 2\text{ A}$

Efficiency of the transformer, $\eta = 80\%$

Efficiency of the transformer,

$$\eta = \frac{\text{Output power}}{\text{Input power}}$$

$$\eta = \frac{V_s I_s}{V_p I_p} \text{ or } I_p = \frac{V_s I_s}{\eta V_p} = \frac{(440\text{ V})(2\text{ A})}{\left(\frac{80}{100}\right)(220\text{ V})}$$

$$= \frac{(440\text{ V})(2\text{ A})(100)}{(80)(220\text{ V})} = 5\text{ A}$$

46. (a) : No. of turns across primary $N_p = 50$

Number of turns across secondary

$N_s = 1500$

Magnetic flux linked with primary,

$\phi = \phi_0 + 4t$

$\therefore$ Voltage across the primary,

$$V_p = \frac{d\phi}{dt} = \frac{d}{dt}(\phi_0 + 4t) = 4\text{ volt}$$

$$\frac{V_S}{V_P} = \frac{N_S}{N_P} \text{ or } V_s = \left(\frac{1500}{50}\right) \times 4 = 120\text{ V}$$

47. (b) : Given : Output power $P = 100\text{ W}$

Voltage across primary $V_p = 220\text{ V}$

Current in the primary $I_p = 0.5\text{ A}$

Efficiency of a transformer, $\eta = \frac{\text{output power}}{\text{input power}} \times 100$

$$= \frac{P}{V_P I_P} \times 100 = \frac{100}{220\times0.5} \times 100 = 90\%.$$

48. (b) : The core of a transformer is laminated to minimise the energy losses due to eddy currents.

49. (b) : $\frac{E_P}{E_S} = \frac{I_S}{I_P} = \frac{N_P}{N_S} = \frac{1}{25}$;

Here, $I_S = 2\text{ A}$

$$I_P = 25 I_S = 50\text{ A}$$

50. (c) : Turns on primary winding = 500; Turns on secondary winding = 5000; Primary winding voltage $(E_p) = 20\text{ V}$ and frequency = 50 Hz.

$\frac{N_S}{N_P} = \frac{E_S}{E_P}$ or $\frac{5000}{500} = \frac{E_S}{20}$ or $E_s = \frac{5000\times20}{500} = 200\text{ V}$ and frequency remains the same. Therefore secondary winding will have an output of 200 V, 50 Hz.

51. (*) : At time, $t = 0$ i.e., when switch is closed, inductor in the circuit provides very high resistance (open circuit) while capacitor starts charging with maximum current (low resistance).

Equivalent circuit of the given circuit

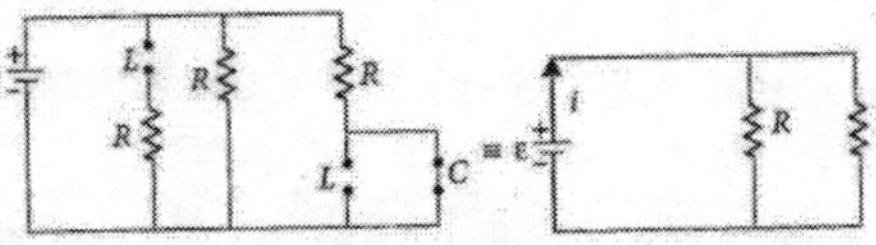

Current drawn from battery,

$$i = \frac{\varepsilon}{(R/2)} = \frac{2\varepsilon}{R} = \frac{2\times18}{9} = 4\text{ A}$$

* None of the given options is correct.

52. (a) : Time constant of LR circuit is $\tau = L/R$.

$$\therefore \tau = \frac{40}{8} = 5 \text{ s}$$

53. (d) : At $t = 0$

(i) capacitor offers negligible resistance.

(ii) inductor offers large resistance to current flow.

54. (b) : Initially, the current will pass through the capacitor (and not through the resistance which is parallel to the capacitor). So effective resistance in the circuit is R_{AB}. Therefore the current in the resistor is 2 mA. After some time, the capacitor will become fully charged and will bc in its steady state. Now no current will pass through the capacitor and the effective resistance of the circuit that is, $(1000 + 1000) = 2000\Omega$.

Therefore final current in the resistor

$$= \frac{V}{R} = \frac{2}{2000} = 1 \times 10^{-3} \text{ A} = 1 \text{ mA}$$

55. (c) : The time constant for $R - C$. circuit, $\tau = CR$

Growth of charge in a circuit containing capacitance and resistance is given by the formula, $q = q_0\left(1 - e^{-t/CR}\right)$

CR is known as time constant in this formula.

Chapter: 22 ELECTROMAGNETIC WAVES

Displacement Current

1. A capacitor of capacitance ' C ', is connected across an ac source of voltage V, given by $V = V_0 \sin \omega t$

The displacement current between the plates of the capacitor, would then be given by **(2021)**

(a) $I_d = V_0 \omega C \sin \omega t$

(b) $I_d = V_0 \omega C \cos \omega t$

(c) $I_d = \frac{V_0}{\omega C} \cos \omega t$

(d) $I_d = \frac{V_0}{\omega C} \sin \omega t$

2. A parallel plate capacitor of capacitance $20 \mu F$ is being charged by a voltage source whose potential is changing at the rate of $3 V/s$. The conduction current through the connecting wires, and the displacement current through the plates of the capacitor, would be, respectively **(2019)**

(a) zero, zero (b) zero, $60 \mu A$

(c) $60 \mu A, 60 \mu A$ (d) $60 \mu A$, zero

3. A 100Ω resistance and a capacitor of 100Ω reactance are connected in series across a 220 V source. When the capacitor is 50% charged, the peak value of the displacement current is **(NEET-II 2016)**

(a) 2.2 A (b) 11 A

(c) 4.4 A (d) $11\sqrt{2}$ A

Electromagnetic Waves

4. In a plane electromagnetic wave travelling in free space, the electric field component oscillates sinusoidally at a frequency of 2.0×10^{10} Hz and amplitude 48 V m^{-1}. Then the amplitude of oscillating magnetic field is (Speed of light in free space = 3×108 m s^{-1}) **(2023)**

(a) 1.6×10^{-8} T (b) $1.6 \times 10–7$ T

(c) 1.6×10^{-6} T (d) 1.6×10^{-9} T

5. When light propagates through a material medium of relative permittivity ε_r and relative permeability μ_r the velocity of light, v is given by (c-velocity of light in vacuum) **(2022)**

(a) $v = c$ (b) $v = \sqrt{\frac{\mu_r}{\varepsilon_r}}$

(c) $v = \sqrt{\frac{\varepsilon_r}{\mu_r}}$ (d) $v = \frac{c}{\sqrt{\varepsilon_r \mu_r}}$

6. For a plane electromagnetic wave propagating in x-direction, which one of the following combination gives the correct possible directions for electric field (E) and magnetic field (B) respectively?

(2021)

(a) $-\hat{j} + \hat{k}, -\hat{j} + \hat{k}$ (b) $\hat{j} + \hat{k}, \hat{j} + \hat{k}$

(c) $-\hat{j} + \hat{k}, -\hat{j} - \hat{k}$ (d) $\hat{j} + \hat{k}, -\hat{j} - \hat{k}$

7. Light with an average flux of $20 W/cm^2$ falls on a non-reflecting surface at normal incidence having surface area $20 cm^2$. The energy received by the surface during time span of 1 minute is **(2020)**

(a) 10×10^3 J (b) 12×10^3 J

(c) 24×10^3 J (d) 48×10^3 J

8. The ratio of contributions made by the electric field and magnetic field components to the intensity of an electromagnetic wave is ($c =$ speed of electromagnetic waves) **(2020)**

(a) $c:1$ (b) $1:1$

(c) $1:c$ (d) $1:c^2$

9. For a transparent medium relative permeability and permittivity, μ_r and ε_r are 1.0 and 1.44 respectively. The velocity of light in this medium would be

(Odisha NEET 2019)

(a) 2.5×10^8 m/s (b) 3×10^8 m/s

(c) 2.08×10^8 m/s (d) 4.32×10^8 m/s

10. An em wave is propagating in a medium with a velocity $\vec{v} = v\hat{i}$. The instantaneous oscillating electric field of this em wave is along $+y$ axis. Then the direction of oscillating magnetic field of the em wave will be along **(2018)**

(a) $-z$ direction (b) $+z$ direction

(c) $-y$ direction (d) $-x$ direction

11. In an electromagnetic wave in free space the root mean square value of the electric field is $E_{rms} = 6$ V m^{-1}. The peak value of the magnetic field is **(2017)**

(a) 2.83×10^{-8} T (b) 0.70×10^{-8} T

(c) 4.23×10^{-8} T (d) 1.41×10^{-8} T

12. Out of the following options which one can be used to produce a propagating electromagnetic wave? **(NEET-I 2016)**

(a) A chargeless particle

(b) An accelerating charge

(c) A charge moving at constant velocity

(d) A stationary charge

13. Light with an energy flux of 25×10^4 W m^{-2} falls on a perfectly reflecting surface at normal incidence. If the surface area is 15 cm^2, the average force exerted on the surface is **(2014)**

(a) 1.25×10^{-6} N (b) 2.50×10^{-6} N

(c) 1.20×10^{-6} N (d) 3.0×10^{-6} N

14. An electromagnetic wave of frequency $v =$ 3.0MHz passes from vacuum into a dielectric medium with relative permittivity $\varepsilon = 4.0$. Then

(Karnataka NEET 2013)

(a) Wavelength is doubled and frequency becomes half.

(b) Wavelength is halved and frequency remains unchanged.

(c) Wavelength and frequency both remain unchanged.

(d) Wavelength is doubled and frequency unchanged

15. The electric field associated with an em wave in vacuum is given by

$[E = \hat{i}40\cos(kz - 6 \times 10^8 t)]$; where E, z and t are in volt /m, meter and seconds respectively. The value of wave vector k is

(2012)

(a) 2 m^{-1} (b) 0.5 m^{-1}

(c) 6 m^{-1} (d) 3 m^{-1}

16. The ratio of amplitude of magnetic field to the amplitude of electric field for an electromagnetic wave propagating in vacuum is equal to **(Mains 2012)**

(a) the speed of light in vacuum

(b) reciprocal of speed of light in vacuum

(c) the ratio of magnetic permeability to the electric susceptibility of vacuum

(d) unity.

17. The electric and the magnetic field, associated with an e.m. wave, propagating along the $+z$-axis, can be represented by **(2011)**

(a) $[\vec{E} = E_0\hat{\imath}, \vec{B} = B_0\hat{\jmath}]$

(b) $[\vec{E} = E_0\hat{k}, \vec{B} = B_0\hat{\imath}]$

(c) $[\vec{E} = E_0\hat{\jmath}, \vec{B} = B_0\hat{\imath}]$

(d) $[\vec{E} = E_0\hat{\jmath}, \vec{B} = B_0\hat{k}]$

18. Which of the following statement is false for the properties of electromagnetic waves? **(2010)**

(a) Both electric and magnetic field vectors attain the maxima and minima at the same place and same time.

(b) The energy in electromagnetic wave is divided equally between electric and magnetic vectors.

(c) Both electric and magnetic field vectors are parallel to each other and perpendicular to the direction of propagation of wave.

(d) These waves do not require any material medium for propagation

19. The electric field of an electromagnetic wave in free space is given by $\vec{E} = 10\cos(10^7 t + kx)\hat{\jmath}$ V/m, where t and x are in seconds and metres respectively. It can be inferred that

(1) the wavelength λ is 188.4 m.

(2) the wave number k is 0.33rad/m.

(3) the wave amplitude is 10 V/m.

(4) the wave is propagating along $+x$ direction.

Which one of the following pairs of statements is correct? **(Mains 2010)**

(a) (3) and (4) (b) (1) and (2)

(c) (2) and (3) (d) (1) and (3)

20. The electric field part of an electromagnetic wave in a medium is represented by $E_x = 0$;

$E_y = 2.5\frac{\text{N}}{\text{C}}\cos\left[\left(2\pi \times 10^6 \frac{\text{rad}}{\text{m}}\right)t - \left(\pi \times 10^{-2}\frac{\text{rad}}{\text{s}}\right)x\right]$;

$E_z = 0$. The wave is **(2009)**

(a) moving along x direction with frequency 10^6 Hz and wavelength 100 m

(b) moving along x direction with frequency 10^6 Hz and wavelength 200 m

(c) moving along $-x$ direction with frequency 10^6 Hz and wavelength 200 m

(d) moving along y direction with frequency $2\pi \times 10^6$ Hz and wavelength 200 m.

21. The velocity of electromagnetic radiation in a medium of permittivity ε_0 and permeability μ_0 is given by **(2008)**

(a) $\frac{1}{\sqrt{\mu_0 \varepsilon_0}}$ (b) $\sqrt{\frac{\mu_0}{\varepsilon_0}}$

(c) $\sqrt{\frac{\varepsilon_0}{\mu_0}}$ (d) $\sqrt{\mu_0 \varepsilon_0}$

22. The electric and magnetic field of an electromagnetic wave are **(2007-1994)**

(a) in opposite phase and perpendicular to each other

(b) in opposite phase and parallel to each other

(c) in phase and perpendicular to each other

(d) in phase and parallel to each other.

23. The velocity of electromagnetic wave is parallel to **(2002)**

(a) $\vec{B} \times \vec{E}$ (b) $\vec{E} \times \vec{B}$

(c) $\vec{E}$ (d) $\vec{B}$

24. Wavelength of light of frequency 100 Hz is **(1999)**

(a) 4×10^6 m (b) 3×10^6 m

(c) 2×10^6 m (d) 5×10^{-5} m

25. If ε_0 and μ_0 are the electric permittivity and magnetic permeability in a free space, ε and μ are the corresponding quantities in medium, the index of refraction of the medium is **(1997)**

(a) $\sqrt{\frac{\varepsilon_0 \mu_0}{\varepsilon \mu}}$ (b) $\sqrt{\frac{\varepsilon \mu}{\varepsilon_0 \mu_0}}$

(c) $\sqrt{\frac{\varepsilon_0 \mu}{\varepsilon \mu_0}}$ (d) $\sqrt{\frac{\varepsilon}{\varepsilon_0}}$

26. The frequency of electromagnetic wave, which best suited to observe a particle of radius 3×10^{-4} cm is of the order of **(1991)**

(a) 10^{15} (b) 10^{14}

(c) 10^{13} (d) 10^{12}

Electromagnetic Spectrum

27. Match List-I with List-II **(2022)**

List-I (Electromagnetic waves)	**List-II** (Wavelength)
(A) AM radio waves	(i) 10^{-10} m
(B) Microwaves	(ii) 10^2 m
(C) Infrared radiations	(iii) 10^{-2} m
(D) X-rays	(iv) 10^{-4} m

Choose the correct answer from the options given below.

(a) (A)-(iv), (B)-(iii), (C)-(ii), (D)-(i)

(b) (A)-(iii), (B)-(ii), (C)-(i), (D)-(iv)

(c) (A)-(iii), (B)-(iv), (C)-(ii), (D)-(i)

(d) (A)-(ii), (B)-(iii), (C)-(iv), (D)-(i)

28. The energy of the em waves is of the order of 15keV. To which part of the spectrum does it belong? **(2015)**

(a) Ultraviolet rays (b) γ-rays

(c) X-rays (d) Infra-red rays

29. The condition under which a microwave oven heats up a food item containing water molecules most efficiently is **(2013)**

(a) microwaves are heat waves, so always produce heating

(b) infra-red waves produce heating in a microwave oven

(c) the frequency of the microwaves must match the resonant frequency of the water molecules

(d) the frequency of the microwaves has no relation with natural frequency of water molecules.

30. The decreasing order of wavelength of infrared, microwave, ultraviolet and gamma rays is **(2011)**

(a) microwave, infrared, ultraviolet, gamma rays

(b) gamma rays, ultraviolet, infrared, microwaves

(c) microwaves, gamma rays, infrared, ultraviolet

(d) infrared, microwave, ultraviolet, gamma rays

31. If λ_v, λ_x and λ_m represent the wavelengths of visible light, X-rays and microwaves respectively, then **(2005)**

(a) $\lambda_m > \lambda_x > \lambda_v$ (b) $\lambda_m > \lambda_v > \lambda_x$

(c) $\lambda_v > \lambda_x > \lambda_m$ (d) $\lambda_v > \lambda_m > \lambda_x$

32. We consider the radiation emitted by the human body. Which one of the following statements is true? **(2003)**

(a) The radiation emitted is in the infrared region.

(b) The radiation is emitted only during the day.

(c) The radiation is emitted during the summers and absorbed during the winters.

(d) The radiation emitted lies in the ultraviolet region and hence is not visible.

33. Which of the following rays are not electromagnetic waves? **(2003)**

(a) X-rays (b) γ-rays

(c) β-rays (d) heat rays

34. What is the cause of Green house effect? **(2002)**

(a) Infra-red rays

(b) Ultra violet rays

(c) X-rays

(d) Radio waves

35. Biological importance of ozone layer is **(2001)**

(a) it stops ultraviolet rays

(b) ozone layer reduces green house effect

(c) ozone layer reflects radio waves

(d) ozone layer controls O_2/H_2 ratio in atmosphere.

36. The frequency order for γ-rays (B), X-rays (A), UV rays (C) is **(2000)**

(a) $B > A > C$ (b) $A > B > C$

(c) $C > B > A$ (d) $A > C > B$.

37. Ozone layer blocks the radiations of wavelength **(1999)**

(a) more than 3×10^{-7} m

(b) equal to 3×10^{-7} m

(c) iess than 3×10^{-7} m

(d) all of these

38. Which of the following electromagnetic radiations have the smaller wavelength? **(1994)**

(a) X-rays (b) γ-rays

(c) UV waves (d) microwaves

39. A signal emitted by an antenna from a certain point can be received at another point of the surface in the form of **(1993)**

(a) sky wave (b) ground wave

(c) sea wave (d) both (a) and (b)

40. The structure of solids is investigated by using **(1992)**

(a) cosmic rays

(b) X-rays

(c) γ-rays

(d) infra-red radiations

41. Which of the following electromagnetic radiations have the longest wavelength? **(1989)**

(a) X-rays (b) γ-rays

(c) Microwaves (d) Radiowaves

ANSWER KEY

1.	(b)	2.	(c)	3.	(a)	4.	(b)	5.	(d)	6.	(c)	7.	(c)
8.	(b)	9.	(a)	10.	(b)	11.	(a)	12.	(b)	13.	(b)	14.	(b)
15.	(a)	16.	(b)	17.	(a)	18.	(c)	19.	(d)	20.	(b)	21.	(a)
22.	(c)	23.	(b)	24.	(b)	25.	(b)	26.	(b)	27.	(d)	28.	(c)
29.	(c)	30.	(a)	31.	(b)	32.	(a)	33.	(c)	34.	(a)	35.	(a)
36.	(a)	37.	(d)	38.	(b)	39.	(d)	40.	(b)	41.	(d)		

Hints & Explanations

1. **(b) :** The instantaneous voltage,

$$V = V_0 \sin \omega t$$

Displacement current is given by

$$i_d = \frac{CdV}{dt}$$

$$i_d = \frac{Cd}{dt}(V_0 \sin \omega t) \Rightarrow i_d = CV_0 \omega \cos \omega t$$

2. **(c):** Here, $C = 20\mu\text{F}$

The rate of change of potential $= 3\ \text{V/s}$

The charge on the capacitor, $Q = CV$

$$\therefore \frac{dQ}{dt} = I_D = C\frac{dV}{dt} = 20\mu\text{F} \times \frac{3\ \text{V}}{\text{s}} = 60\mu\text{A}$$

Displacement current is equal to the conduction current.

3. **(a):** Here, $R = 100\Omega, X_c = 100\Omega$

Net impedance, $Z = \sqrt{R^2 + X_C^2} = 100\sqrt{2}\Omega$

Peak value of displacement current

= Maximum conduction current in the circuit $= \frac{\varepsilon_0}{Z} = \frac{220\sqrt{2}}{100\sqrt{2}} = 2.2\ \text{A}$

4. **(b) :** $C = \dfrac{E_0}{B_0}$

$$B_0 = \frac{E_0}{C}$$

$$= \frac{48}{3 \times 10^8}$$

$$= 1.6 \times 10^{-7} T$$

5. **(d):** The velocity of light in vacuum in given by

$$c = \frac{1}{\sqrt{\mu_0 \varepsilon_0}}$$

For any medium, velocity is

$$v = \frac{1}{\sqrt{\mu_0 \mu_r \varepsilon_0 \varepsilon_r}} = \frac{1}{\sqrt{\mu_0 \varepsilon_0}\sqrt{\mu_r \varepsilon_r}}$$

using equation (i)

$$v = \frac{c}{\sqrt{\mu_r \varepsilon_r}}$$

6. **(c) :** As $\vec{E}$ and $\vec{B}$ are perpendicular to each other, their dot product must be zero.

$$\vec{E} \cdot \vec{B} = 0$$

Also, the wave is propagating along x-axis i.e. cross product of $\vec{E} \times \vec{B}$ is along $\hat{\imath}$.

Out of given options, only $(-\hat{\jmath} + \hat{k}), (-\hat{\jmath} - \hat{k})$ follow the above conditions.

7. **(c) :** Energy received in 1 minute = Intensity × Area × Time $E = (20\ \text{W/cm}^2) \times (20\ \text{cm}^2) \times (1 \times 60\ \text{s}) = 24 \times 10^3\ \text{J}$

8. **(b) :** Energy of electromagnetic wave is equally distributed in the form of electric and magnetic field energy, so ratio $\frac{U_E}{U_B} = \frac{1}{1}$.

9. **(a) :** Given : relative permittivity, $\varepsilon_r = 1.44$ and relative permeability, $\mu_r = 1$

Now, as we know that, $\varepsilon_r = \frac{\varepsilon}{\varepsilon_0} \Rightarrow \varepsilon = \varepsilon_r \varepsilon_0$

and $\mu_r = \frac{\mu}{\mu_0} \Rightarrow \mu = \mu_r \mu_0$

where, ε and μ are the permittivity and permeability of the medium.

$\therefore$ Velocity of light in the medium will be

$$v = \frac{1}{\sqrt{\mu\varepsilon}} = \frac{1}{\sqrt{\mu_r \mu_0 \varepsilon_r \varepsilon_0}} = \frac{c}{\sqrt{\mu_r \varepsilon_r}}$$

$$= \frac{3 \times 10^8}{\sqrt{1 \times 1.44}}$$

$= 2.5 \times 10^8$ m/s

10. **(b) :** Velocity of em wave in a medium is given by $\vec{v} = \vec{E} \times \vec{B}$

$\therefore \hat{v\imath} = (\hat{E\jmath}) \times (\vec{B})$ [$\because \vec{E} = \hat{E\jmath}$ (Given)]

As $\hat{\imath} = \hat{\jmath} \times \hat{k}$, so $\vec{B} = B\hat{k}$

Direction of oscillating magnetic field of the em wave will be along $+z$ direction.

11. **(a):** Given: $E_{\text{rms}} = 6 \text{ V m}^{-1}$

$\frac{E_{\text{rms}}}{B_{\text{rms}}} = c$ or $B_{\text{rms}} = \frac{E_{\text{rms}}}{c} \Rightarrow B_{\text{rms}} = \frac{6}{3\times10^8} = 2 \times 10^{-8}$ T

Since, $B_{\text{rms}} = \frac{B_0}{\sqrt{2}}$

where B_0 is the peak value of magnetic field.

$$\therefore B_0 = B_{\text{rms}}\sqrt{2} = 2 \times 10^{-8} \times \sqrt{2} \text{ T}$$
$$B_0 \approx 2.83 \times 10^{-8} \text{ T}$$

12. **(b) :** An accelerating charge is used to produce oscillating electric and magnetic fields, hence the electromagnetic wave.

13. **(b):** Here, Energy flux, $I = 25 \times 10^4 \text{ W m}^{-2}$

Area, $A = 15 \text{ cm}^2 = 15 \times 10^{-4} \text{ m}^2$

Speed of light, $c = 3 \times 10^8 \text{ m s}^{-1}$

For a perfectly reflecting surface, the average force exerted on the surface is

$$F = \frac{2IA}{c}$$
$$= \frac{2 \times 25 \times 10^4 \text{Wm}^{-2} \times 15 \times 10^{-4} \text{ m}^2}{3 \times 10^8 \text{ m s}^{-1}}$$
$$= 250 \times 10^{-8} \text{ N} = 2.50 \times 10^{-6} \text{ N}$$

14. **(b):** Frequency of electromagnetic wave does not change with change in medium but wavelength and velocity of wave changes with change in medium.

Velocity of electromagnetic wave in vacuum

$$c = \frac{1}{\sqrt{\mu_0 \varepsilon_0}} = v\lambda_{\text{vacuum}}$$

Velocity of electromagnetic wave in the medium

$$v_{\text{medium}} = \frac{1}{\sqrt{\mu_0 \mu_r \varepsilon_0 \varepsilon_r}} = \frac{c}{\sqrt{\mu_r \varepsilon_r}}$$

where μ_r and ε_r be relative permeability and relative permittivity of the medium.

For dielectric medium, $\mu_r = 1$

$$\therefore v_{\text{medium}} = \frac{c}{\sqrt{\varepsilon_r}}$$

Here, $\varepsilon_r = 4.0$

$$\therefore v_{\text{medium}} = \frac{c}{\sqrt{4}} = \frac{c}{2}$$

Wavelength of the wave in medium

$$\lambda_{\text{medium}} = \frac{v_{\text{medium}}}{v} = \frac{c}{2v} = \frac{\lambda_{\text{vacuum}}}{2}$$

(Using (i) and (ii))

15. (a): Compare the given equation with

$$E = E_0\cos(kz - \omega t)$$

we get, $\omega = 6 \times 10^8\ s^{-1}$

Wave vector, $k = \frac{\omega}{c} = \frac{6\times10^8\ s^{-1}}{3\times10^8\ m\ s^{-1}} = 2\ m^{-1}$

16. (b) : The amplitude of magnetic field and electric field for an electromagnetic wave propagating in vacuum are related as

$$E_0 = B_0 c$$

where c is the speed of light in vacuum.

$$\therefore \frac{B_0}{E_0} = \frac{1}{c}$$

17. (a): The electromagnetic wave is propagating along the $+z$ axis.

Since the electric and magnetic fields are perpendicular to each other and also perpendicular to the direction of propagation of wave.

Also, $\vec{E} \times \vec{B}$ gives the direction of wave propagation.

$\therefore\ \vec{E} = E_0\hat{\imath}, B = B_0\hat{\jmath}\ (\because \hat{\imath} \times \hat{\jmath} = \hat{k})$

18. (c): In an electromagnetic wave both electric and magnetic vectors are perpendicular to each other as well as perpendicular to the direction of propagation of wave.

19. (d) : As given

$$E = 10\cos(10^7 t + kx)$$

Comparing it with standard equation of e.m. wave,

$$E = E_0\cos(\omega t + kx)$$

Amplitude $E_0 = 10\ V/m$ and $\omega = 10^7 rad/s$

$$\because c = v\lambda = \frac{\omega\lambda}{2\pi}$$

or $\lambda = \frac{2\pi c}{\omega} = \frac{2\pi\times3\times10^8}{10^7} = 188.4\ m$

Also, $c = \frac{\omega}{k}$ or $k = \frac{\omega}{c} = \frac{10^7}{3\times10^8} = 0.033\ m^{-1}$

The wave is propagating along $-x$ direction.

20. (b) : $E_y = 2.5\frac{N}{C}\left[\left(2\pi \times 10^6 \frac{rad}{m}\right)t - \left(\pi \times 10^{-2}\frac{rad}{s}\right)x\right]$ $E_z = 0$ and $E_x = 0$

The wave is moving in the positive direction of x.

This is the form $E_y = E_0(\omega t - kx)$

$\omega = 2\pi \times 10^6$ or $2\pi v = 2\pi \times 10^6 \Rightarrow v = 10^6$ Hz

$$\frac{2\pi}{\lambda} = k \Rightarrow \frac{2\pi}{\lambda} = \pi \times 10^{-2} \Rightarrow \lambda = 2 \times 10^2$$
$$= 200\ m$$

21. (a): The velocity of electromagnetic radiation in vacuum is

$\frac{1}{\sqrt{\mu_0\varepsilon_0}}$, where μ_0 and ε_0 are the permeability and permittivity of vacuum.

22. (c): In electromagnetic wave, electric and magnetic field are in phase and perpendicular to each other and also perpendicular to the direction of the propagation of the wave.

23. (b) : According to Maxwell, the electromagnetic waves are those waves in which there are sinusoidal variation of electric and magnetic field vectors at right angles to each other as well as at right angles to the direction of wave propagation.

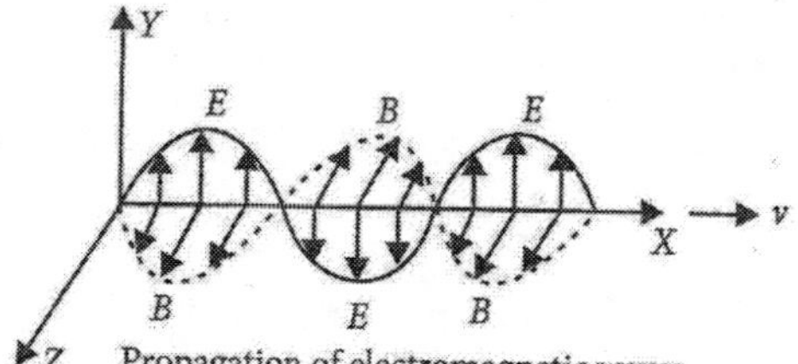

Propagation of electromagnetic waves

If the electric field ($\vec{E}$) and magnetic field ($\vec{B}$) are vibrating along Y and Z direction, propagation of electromagnetic wave will be along the X-axis. Therefore, the velocity of electromagnetic wave is parallel to $\vec{E} \times \vec{B}$.

24. **(b) :** $\lambda = \frac{3\times10^8}{100 \text{ Hz}} = 3 \times 10^6$ m

25. **(b) :** $c = \frac{1}{\sqrt{\mu_0 \varepsilon_0}}$ (free space)

$v = \frac{1}{\sqrt{\mu\varepsilon}}$ (medium) $\therefore \mu = \frac{c}{v} = \sqrt{\frac{\mu\varepsilon}{\mu_0\varepsilon_0}}$

26. **(b) :** The wavelength of radiation used should be less than the size of the particle

Size of particle = $\lambda = \frac{c}{v}$

$3 \times 10^{-4} = \frac{3\times10^{10}}{v}$ or $v = 10^{14}$ hertz

However, when frequency is higher than this, wavelength is still smaller. Resolution becomes better.

27. **(d) :** The wavelength of AM radio waves is 10^2 m. The wavelength of microwaves ranges between 10^{-3} m to 10^{-1} m. Infrared radiations wavelength lines between 4×10^{-7} m to 7×10^{-3} m. X-rays wavelength ranges from 10^{-8} m to 10^{-12} m.

28. **(c) :** As $\lambda = \frac{hc}{E}$

where the symbols have their usual meanings.

Here, $E = 15\text{keV} = 15 \times 10^3\text{eV}$ and $hc = 1240\text{eVnm}$

$$\therefore \lambda = \frac{1240\text{eVnm}}{15 \times 10^3\text{eV}} = 0.083 \text{ nm}$$

As the wavelength range of X-rays is from 1 nm to 10^{-3} nm, so this wavelength belongs to X-rays.

29. **(c):** In microwave oven, the frequency of the microwaves must match the resonant frequency of water molecules so that energy from the waves is transferred efficiently to the kinetic energy of the molecules.

30. **(a):** The decreasing order of wavelength of the given electromagnetic waves is as follows:

$$\lambda_{\text{Microwave}} > \lambda_{\text{Infrared}} > \lambda_{\text{Ultraviolet}} > \lambda_{\text{Gamma rays}}$$

31. **(b) :** $\lambda_m > \lambda_v > \lambda_x$.

In spectrum X-rays has minimum wavelength and microwave has maximum wavelength.

32. **(a):** Every body at all time, at all temperatures emit radiation (except at $T = 0$), which fall in the infrared region.

33. **(c)**

34. **(a):** As the electromagnetic radiations from Sun pass through the atmosphere, some of them are absorbed by it while other reach the surface of earth. The range of wavelength which reaches earth lies in infrared region. This part of the radiation from the sun has shorter wavelength and can penetrate through the layer of gases like CO_2 and reach earth surface. But the radiation from the earth being of longer wavelength can escape through this layer. As a result the earth surface gets warm. This is known as green house effect.

35. **(a) :** The ozone layer absorbs the harmful ultraviolet rays coming from sun.

36. **(a)**

37. **(d):** The range is from 380 nm to even 200 nm to 120 nm.

38. **(b)**

39. **(d)**

40. **(b) :** X-rays are used for the investigation of structure of solids.

41. **(d) :** Radiations

Wavelength [Range in m]

X-rays

1×10^{-11} to 3×10^{-8}

γ-rays

6×10^{-14} to 1×10^{-11}

Microwaves

10^{-3} to 0.3

Radiowaves

10 to 10^4

Chapter: 23 RAY OPTICS AND OPTICAL INSTRUMENTS

Reflection of Light by Sphere Mirrors

1. An object is placed at a distance of 40 cm from a concave mirror of focal length 15 cm. If the object is displaced through a distance of 20 cm towards the mirror, the displacement of the image will be **(2018)**

(a) 30 cm away from the mirror

(b) 36 cm away from the mirror

(c) 30 cm towards the mirror

(d) 36 cm towards the mirror.

2. A beam of light from a source L is incident normally on a plane mirror fixed at a certain distance x from the source. The beam is reflected back as a spot on a scale placed just above the source L. When the mirror is rotated through a small angle θ, the spot of the light is found to move through a distance y on the scale. The angle θ is given by **(2017)**

(a) $\frac{y}{x}$ (b) $\frac{x}{2y}$

(c) $\frac{x}{y}$ (d) $\frac{y}{2x}$

3. Match the corresponding entries of Column 1 with Column 2. [Where m is the magnification produced by the mirror]

(NEET-I 2016)

Column 1	Column 1
(A) $m = -2$	(p) Convex mirror
(B) $m = -\frac{1}{2}$	(q) Concave mirror
(C) $m = +2$	(r) Real image
(D) $m = +\frac{1}{2}$	(s) Virtual image

(a) A → p and s; B → q and r; C → q and s; D → q and r

(b) A → r and s; B → q and s; C → q and r; D → p and s

(c) A → q and r; B → q and r; C → q and s; D → p and s

(d) A → p and r; B → p and s; C → p and q; D → r and s

4. Two plane mirrors are inclined at 70°. A ray incident on one mirror at angle, θ after reflection falls on second mirror and is reflected from there parallel to first mirror. The value of θ is

(Karnataka NEET 2013)

(a) 45° (b) 30°

(c) 55° (d) 50°

5. A rod of length 10 cm lies along the principal axis of a concave mirror of focal length 10 cm in such a way that its end closer to the pole is 20 cm away from the mirror. The length of the image is

(Mains 2012)

(a) 10 cm (b) 15 cm

(c) 2.5 cm (d) 5 cm.

6. A tall man of height 6 feet, want to see his full image. Then required minimum length of the mirror will be **(2000)**

(a) 12 feet (b) 3 feet

(c) 6 feet (d) any length

Refraction

7. A light ray falls on a glass surface of refractive index $\sqrt{3}$, at an angle 60°. The angle between the refracted and reflected rays would be **(2022)**

(a) 30° (b) 60°

(c) 90° (d) 120°

8. An air bubble in a glass slab with refractive index 1.5 (near normal incidence) is 5 cm deep when viewed from one surface and 3 cm deep when viewed from the opposite face. The thickness (in cm) of the slab is

(NEET-II 2016)

(a) 8 (b) 10

(c) 12 (d) 16

9. A microscope is focussed on a mark on a piece of paper and then a slab of glass of thickness 3 cm and refractive index 1.5 is placed over the mark. How should the microscope be moved to get the mark in focus again? **(2006)**

(a) 2 cm upward (b) 1 cm upward

(c) 4.5 cm downward (d) 1 cm downward

10. A beam of light composed of red and green ray is incident obliquely at a point on the face of rectangular glass slab. When coming out on the opposite parallel face, the red and green ray emerge from

(2004)

(a) two points propagating in two different non parallel directions

(b) two points propagating in two different parallel directions

(c) one point propagating in two different directions

(d) one point propagating in the same directions.

11. A ray of light travelling in air have wavelength λ, frequency n, velocity v and intensity I. If this ray enters into water then these parameters are λ', n', v' and I' respectively. Which relation is correct from following? **(2001)**

(a) $\lambda = \lambda'$ (b) $n = n'$

(c) $v = v'$ (d) $I = I'$

12. A bubble in glass slab ($\mu = 1.5$) when viewed from one side appears at 5 cm and 2 cm from other side, then thickness of slab is **(2000)**

(a) 3.75 cm (b) 3 cm

(c) 10.5 cm (d) 2.5 cm

Total Internal Reflection

13. Light travels a distance x in time t_1 in air and 10x in time t_2 in another denser medium. What is the critical angle for this medium? **(2023)**

(a) $\sin^{-1}\left(\frac{10t_2}{t_1}\right)$ (b) $\sin^{-1}\left(\frac{t_1}{10t_2}\right)$

(c) $\sin^{-1}\left(\frac{10t_1}{t_2}\right)$ (d) $\sin^{-1}\left(\frac{t_2}{t_1}\right)$

14. Two transparent media A and B are separated by a plane boundary. The speed of light in those media are 1.5×10^8 m/s and 2.0×10^8 m/s respectively. The critical angle for a ray of light for these two media is **(2022)**

(a) $\sin^{-1}(0.500)$ (b) $\sin^{-1}(0.750)$

(c) $\tan^{-1}(0.500)$ (d) $\tan^{-1}(0.750)$

15. In total internal reflection when the angle of incidence is equal to the critical angle for the pair of media in contact, what will be angle of refraction? **(2019)**

(a) 90° (b) 180° (c) 0°

(d) equal to angle of incidence

16. Which of the following is not due to total internal reflection? **(2011)**

(a) Working of optical fibre

(b) Difference between apparent and real depth of a pond

(c) Mirage on hot summer days

(d) Brilliance of diamond

17. A ray of light travelling in a transparent medium of refractive index μ, falls on a surface separating the medium from air at an angle of incidence of 45°. For which of the following value of μ the ray can undergo total internal reflection? **(2010)**

(a) $\mu = 1.33$ (b) $\mu = 1.40$

(c) $\mu = 1.50$ (d) $\mu = 1.25$

18. The speed of light in media M_1 and M_2 are 1.5×10^8 m/s and 2.0×10^8 m/s respectively. A ray of light enters from medium M_1 to M_2 at an incidence angle i. If the ray suffers total internal reflection, the value of i is **(Mains 2010)**

(a) equal to $\sin^{-1}\left(\frac{2}{3}\right)$

(b) equal to or less than $\sin^{-1}\left(\frac{3}{5}\right)$

(c) equal to or greater than $\sin^{-1}\left(\frac{3}{4}\right)$

(d) less than $\sin^{-1}\left(\frac{2}{3}\right)$

19. A small coin is resting on the bottom of a beaker filled with liquid. A ray of light 4 cm from the coin travels upto the surface of the liquid and moves along its surface. **(2007)**

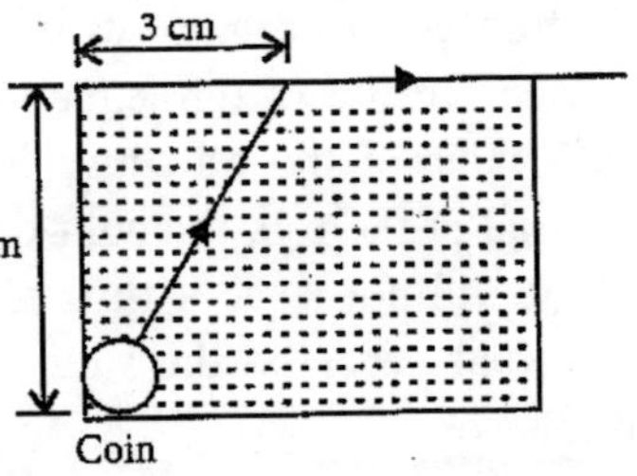

How fast is the light travelling in the liquid?

(a) 2.4×10^8 m/s (b) 3.0×10^8 m/s

(c) 1.2×10^8 m/s (d) 1.8×10^8 m/s.

20. For the given incident ray as shown in figure, the condition of total internal reflection of this ray the required refractive index of prism will be **(2002)**

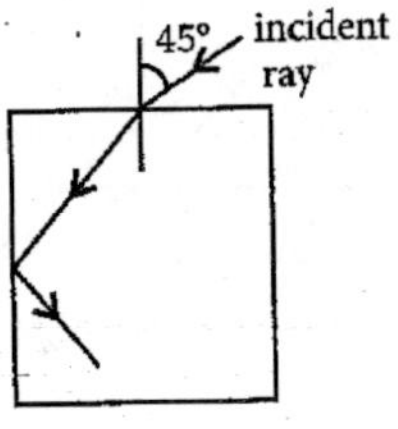

(a) $\frac{\sqrt{3}+1}{2}$ (b) $\frac{\sqrt{2}+1}{2}$

(c) $\sqrt{\frac{3}{2}}$ (d) $\sqrt{\frac{7}{6}}$

21. Optical fibre are based on **(2001)**

(a) total internal reflection

(b) less scattering (c) refraction

(d) less absorption coefficient.

22. A disc is placed on a surface of pond which has refractive index 5/3. A source of light is placed 4 m below the surface of liquid. The minimum radius of disc needed so that light is not coming out is, **(2001)**

(a) ∞ (b) 3 m

(c) 6 m (d) 4 m

23. Light enters at an angle of incidence in a transparent rod of refractive index n. For what value of the refractive index of the material of the rod, the light once entered into it will not leave it through its lateral face whatsoever be the value of angle of incidence? **(1998)**

(a) $n = 1.1$ (b) $n = 1$

(c) $n > \sqrt{2}$ (d) $n = 1.3$

24. A ray of light from a denser medium strikes a rare medium as shown in figure. The reflected and refracted rays make an angle of 90° with each other. The angles of Rarer reflection and refraction are r and r'. The critical angle would be **(1996)**

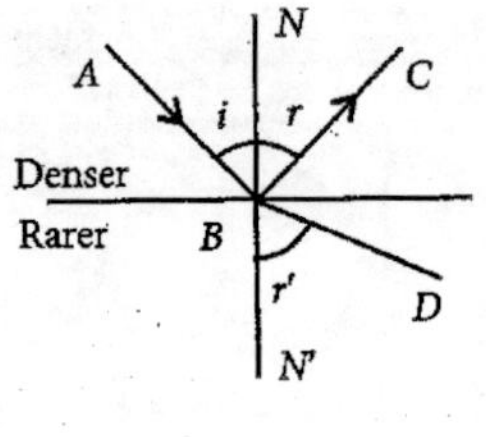

(a) $\sin^{-1}(\tan r)$ (b) $\sin^{-1}(\sin r)$

(c) $\cos^{-1}(\tan r)$ (d) $\tan^{-1}(\sin r)$

25. A small source of light is 4 m below the surface of water of refractive index 5/3. In order to cut off all the light, coming out of water surface, minimum diameter of the disc placed on the surface of water is **(1994)**

(a) 6 m (b) ∞

(c) 3 m (d) 4 m

Diameter of disc = $2r = 6$ m

Refraction at Spherical Surfaces and by Lenses

26. Two thin lenses are of same focal lengths (f), but one is convex and the other one is concave. When they are placed in contact with each other, the equivalent focal length of the combination will be **(2023)**

(a) $\frac{f}{4}$ (b) $\frac{f}{2}$

(c) Infinite (d) Zero

27. In the figure shown here, what is the equivalent focal length of the combination of lenses (Assume that all layers are thin)? **(2023)**

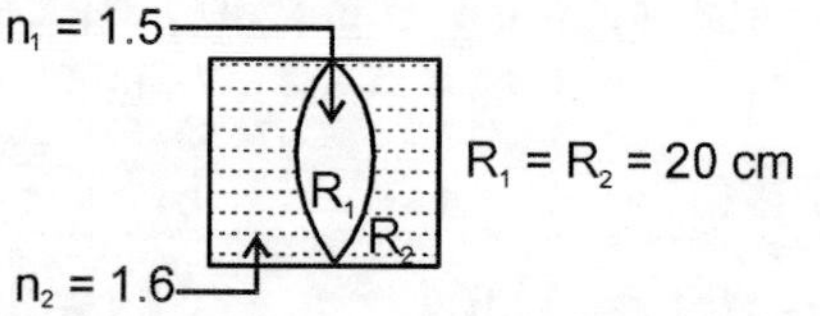

(a) −40 cm (b) −100 cm

(c) −50 cm (d) 40 cm

28. A biconvex lens has radii of curvature, 20 cm each. If the refractive index of the material of the lens is 1.5 , the power of the lens is **(2022)**

(a) +2D (b) +20D

(c) +5D (d) infinity

29. A point object is placed at a distance of 60 cm from a convex lens of focal length 30 cm. If a plane mirror were put perpendicular to the principal axis of the lens and at a distance of 40 cm from it, the final image would be formed at a distance of **(2021)**

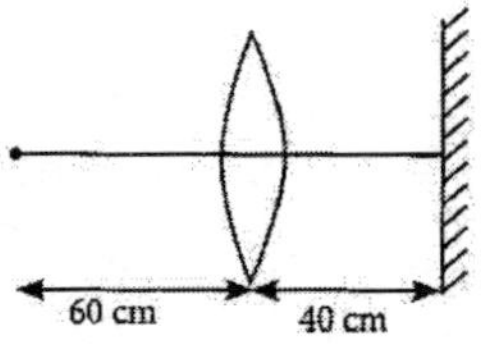

(a) 20 cm from the plane mirror, it would be a virtual image.

(b) 20 cm from the lens, it would be a real image.

(c) 30 cm from the lens, it would be a real image.

(d) 30 cm from the plane mirror, it would be a virtual image.

30. A convex lens ' A ' of focal length 20 cm and a concave lens ' B ' of focal length 5 cm are kept along the same axis with a distance ' d ' between them. If a parallel beam of light falling on ' A ' leaves ' B ' as a parallel beam, then the distance ' d ' in cm will be **(2021)**

(a) 30 (b) 25

(c) 15 (d) 50

31. Two similar thin equi-convex lenses, of focal length f each, are kept coaxially in contact with each other such that the focal length of the combination is F_1. When the space between the two lenses is filled with glycerin (which has the same refractive index (= 1.5) as that of glass) then the equivalent focal length is F_2. The ratio $F_1 : F_2$ will be **(2019)**

(a) 3: 4 (b) 2: 1

(c) 1: 2 (d) 2: 3

32. An equiconvex lens has power P. It is cut into two symmetrical halves by a plane containing the principal axis. The power of one part will be **(Odisha NEET 2019)**

(a) 0 (b) $\frac{P}{2}$

(c) $\frac{P}{4}$ (d) P

33. Two identical glass $(\mu_g = 3/2)$ equiconvex lenses of focal length f each are kept in contact. The space between the two lenses is filled with water $(\mu_w = 4/3)$. The focal length of the combination is

(NEET-II 2016)

(a) $f/3$ (b) f

(c) $4f/3$ (d) 3f/4

34. A plano convex lens fits exactly into a plano concave lens. Their plane surfaces are parallel to each other. If lenses are made of different materials of refractive indices μ_1 and μ_2 and R is the radius of curvature of the curved surface of the lenses, then the focal length of the combination is **(2013)**

(a) $\frac{R}{(\mu_1 - \mu_2)}$ (b) $\frac{2R}{(\mu_2 - \mu_1)}$

(c) $\frac{R}{2(\mu_1+\mu_2)}$ (d) $\frac{R}{2(\mu_1-\mu_2)}$

35. When a biconvex lens of glass having refractive index 1.47 is dipped in a liquid, it acts as a plane sheet of glass. This implies that the liquid must have refractive index **(2012)**

(a) equal to that of glass
(b) less than one
(c) greater than that of glass
(d) less than that of glass.

36. A concave mirror of focal length f_1 is placed at a distance of d from a convex lens of focal length f_2. A beam of light coming from infinity and falling on this convex lens - concave mirror combination returns to infinity. The distance d must equal **(2012)**

(a) $f_1 + f_2$ (b) $-f_1 + f_2$
(c) $2f_1 + f_2$ (d) $-2f_1 + f_2$

37. A biconvex lens has a radius of curvature of magnitude 20 cm. Which one of the following options describe best the image formed of an object of height 2 cm placed 30 cm from the lens? **(2011)**

(a) Virtual, upright, height = 1 cm
(b) Virtual, upright, height = 0.5 cm
(c) Real, inverted, height = 4 cm
(d) Real, inverted, height = 1 cm

38. A converging beam of rays is incident on a diverging lens. Having passed through the lens the rays intersect at a point 15 cm from the lens on the opposite side. If the lens is removed, the point where the rays meet will move 5 cm closer to the lens. The focal length of the lens is **(Mains 2011)**

(a) 5 cm (b) −10 cm
(c) 20 cm (d) −30 cm

39. A lens having focal length f and aperture of diameter d forms an image of intensity I. Aperture of diameter $\frac{d}{2}$ in central region of lens is covered by a black paper. Focal length of lens and intensity of image now will be respectively **(2010)**

(a) f and $\frac{I}{4}$ (b) $\frac{3f}{4}$ and $\frac{I}{2}$
(c) f and $\frac{3I}{4}$ (d) $\frac{f}{2}$ and $\frac{I}{2}$.

40. Two thin lenses of focal lengths f_1 and f_2 are in contact and coaxial. The power of the combination is **(2008)**

(a) $\frac{f_1+f_2}{2}$ (b) $\frac{f_1+f_2}{f_1 f_2}$
(c) $\sqrt{\frac{f_1}{f_2}}$ (d) $\sqrt{\frac{f_2}{f_1}}$

41. A boy is trying to start a fire by focusing sunlight on a piece of paper using an equiconvex lens of focal length 10 cm. The diameter of the sun is 1.39×10^9 m and its mean distance from the earth is 1.5×10^{11} m. What is the diameter of the sun's image on the paper? **(2008)**

(a) 6.5×10^{-5} m (b) 12.4×10^{-4} m
(c) 9.2×10^{-4} m (d) 6.5×10^{-4} m

42. A convex lens and a concave lens, each having same focal length of 25 cm, are put in contact to form a combination of lenses. The power in diopters of the combination is **(2006)**

(a) zero (b) 25
(c) 50 (d) infinite.

43. An equiconvex lens is cut into two halves along (i) XOX' and (ii) YOY' as shown in the figure. Let f, f', f' be the focal lengths of the complete lens, of each half in case (i), and of each half in case (ii), respectively.

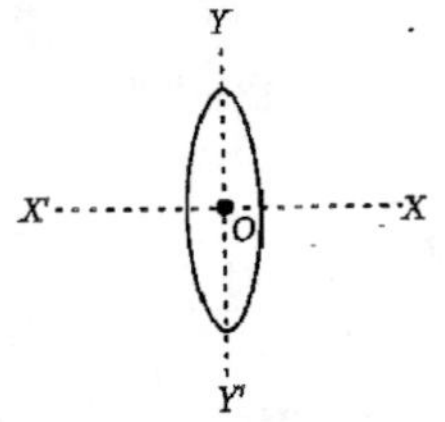

Choose the correct statement from the following. **(2003)**

(a) $f' = f, f'' = 2f$

(b) $f' = 2f, f'' = f$

(c) $f' = f, f'' = f$

(d) $f' = 2f, f'' = 2f$

44. A convex lens is dipped in a liquid whose refractive index is equal to the refractive index of the lens. Then its focal length will **(2003)**

(a) become zero

(b) become infinite

(c) become small, but non-zero

(d) remain unchanged.

45. A bulb is located on a wall. Its image is to be obtained on a parallel wall with the help of convex lens. The lens is placed at a distance d ahead of second wall, then required focal length will be **(2002)**

(a) only $\frac{d}{4}$ (b) only $\frac{d}{2}$

(c) more than $\frac{d}{4}$ but less than $\frac{d}{2}$

(d) less than $\frac{d}{4}$

46. For a plano convex lens ($\mu = 1.5$) has radius of curvature 10 cm. It is silvered on its plane surface. Find focal length after silvering. **(2000)**

(a) 10 cm (b) 20 cm

(c) 15 cm (d) 25 cm

47. A plano convex lens is made of refractive index 1.6. The radius of curvature of the curved surface is 60 cm. The focal length of the lens is **(1999)**

(a) 200 cm (b) 100 cm

(c) 50 cm (d) 400 cm

48. A luminous object is placed at a distance of 30 cm from the convex lens of focal length 20 cm. On the other side of the lens, at what distance from the lens a convex mirror of radius of curvature 10 cm be placed in order to have an upright image of the object coincident with it ? **(1998)**

(a) 50 cm (b) 30 cm

(c) 12 cm (d) 60 cm

49. The focal length of converging lens is measured for violet, green and red colours. It is respectively f_v, f_g, f_r. We will get **(1997)**

(a) $f_v < f_r$ (b) $f_g > f_r$

(c) $f_v = f_g$ (d) $f_g < f_r$

50. If a convex lens of focal length 80 cm and a concave lens of focal length 50 cm are combined together, what will be their resulting power? **(1996)**

(a) +7.5D (b) −0.75D

(c) +6.5D (d) −6.5D

51. If f_V and f_R are the focal lengths of a convex lens for violet and red light respectively and F_V and F_R are the focal lengths of a concave lens for violet and red light respectively, then we must have **(1996)**

(a) $f_V > f_R$ and $F_V > F_R$

(b) $f_V < f_R$ and $F_V > F_R$

(c) $f_V > f_R$ and $F_V < F_R$

(d) $f_V < f_R$ and $F_V < F_R$

52. A lens is placed between a source of light and a wall. It forms images of area A_1 and A_2 on the wall, for its two different positions. The area of the source of light is **(1995)**

(a) $\frac{A_1-A_2}{2}$ (b) $\frac{1}{A_1}+\frac{1}{A_2}$

(c) $\sqrt{A_1A_2}$ (d) $\frac{A_1+A_2}{2}$

53. Focal length of a convex lens of refractive index 1.5 is 2 cm. Focal length of lens when immersed in a liquid of refractive index of 1.25 will be **(1988)**

(a) 10 cm (b) 2.5 cm

(c) 5 cm (d) 7.5 cm

Refraction through a Prism

54. Find the value of the angle of emergence from the prism. Refractive index of the glass is $\sqrt{3}$. **(2021)**

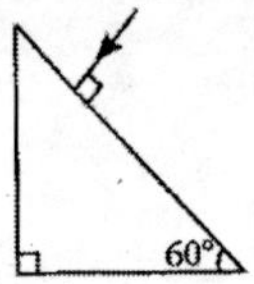

(a) 90° (b) 60°

(c) 30° (d) 45°

55. A ray is incident at an angle of incidence i on one surface of a small angle prism (with angle of prism) and emerges normally from the opposite surface. If the refractive index of the material of the prism is μ, then the angle of incidence is nearly equal to **(2020)**

(a) $A/2\mu$ (b) $2A/\mu$

(c) μA (d) $\mu A/2$

56. The refractive index of the material of a prism is $\sqrt{2}$ and the angle of the prism is 30°. One of the two refracting surfaces of the prism is made a mirror inwards, by silver coating. A beam of monochromatic light entering the prism from the other face will retrace its path (after reflection from the silvered surface) if its angle of incidence on the prism is **(2018, 2004, 1992)**

(a) 60° (b) 45°

(c) 30° (d) zero

57. The angle of incidence for a ray of light at a refracting surface of a prism is 45°. The angle of prism is 60°. If the ray suffers minimum deviation through the prism, the angle of minimum deviation and refractive index of the material of the prism respectively, are **(NEET-I 2016)**

(a) $45°; \sqrt{2}$ (b) $30°; \frac{1}{\sqrt{2}}$

(c) $45°; \frac{1}{\sqrt{2}}$ (d) $30°; \sqrt{2}$

58. A beam of light consisting of red, green and blue colours is incident on a right angled prism. The refractive index of the material of the prism for the above red, green and blue wavelengths are 1.39, 1.44 and 1.47 respectively.

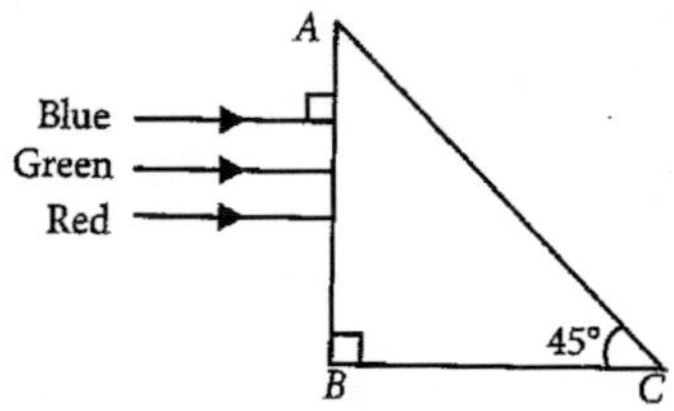

The prism will **(2015)**

(a) not separate the three colours at all

(b) separate the red colour part from the green and blue colours

(c) separate the blue colour part from the red and green colours

(d) separate all the three colours from one another

59. The refracting angle of a prism is A, and refractive index of the material of the prism is $\cot(A/2)$. The angle of minimum deviation is **(2015 Cancelled)**

(a) $90° - A$ (b) $180° + 2A$

(c) $180° - 3A$ (d) $180° - 2A$

60. The angle of a prism is A. One of its refracting surfaces is silvered. Light rays falling at an angle of incidence 2 A on the first surface returns back through the same path after suffering reflection at the silvered surface. The refractive index μ, of the prism is **(2014)**

(a) $2\sin A$ (b) $2\cos A$

(c) $\frac{1}{2}\cos A$ (d) $\tan A$

61. For the angle of minimum deviation of a prism to be equal to its refracting angle, the prism must be made of a material whose refractive index **(Mains 2012)**

(a) lies between $\sqrt{2}$ and 1

(b) lies between 2 and $\sqrt{2}$

(c) is less than 1

(d) is greater than 2

62. A ray of light is incident on a 60° prism at the minimum deviation position. The angle of refraction at the first face (i.e., incident face) of the prism is

(Mains 2010)

(a) zero (b) 30°

(c) 45° (d) 60°

63. If the refractive index of a material of equilateral prism is $\sqrt{3}$, then angle of minimum deviation of the prism is

(1999)

(a) 60° (b) 45°

(c) 30° (d) 75°

Some Natural Phenomena due to Sunlight

64. Pick the wrong answer in the context with rainbow. **(2019)**

(a) Rainbow is a combined effect of dispersion, refraction and reflection of sunlight.

(b) When the light rays undergo two internal reflections in a water drop, a secondary rainbow is formed.

(c) The order of colours is reversed in the secondary rainbow.

(d) An observer can see a rainbow when his front is towards the sun.

65. Which colour of the light has the longest wavelength? **(2019)**

(a) violet (b) red

(c) blue (d) green

66. A thin prism having refracting angle 10° is made of glass of refractive index 1.42. This prism is combined with another thin prism of glass of refractive index 1.7. This combination produces dispersion without deviation. The refracting angle of second prism should be **(2017)**

(a) 6° (b) 8°

(c) 10° (d) 4°

67. The reddish appearance of the sun at sunrise and sunset is due to

(Karnataka NEET 2013)

(a) the scattering of light

(b) the polarisation of light

(c) the colour of the sun

(d) the colour of the sky.

68. A thin prism of angle 15° made of glass of refractive index $\mu_1 = 1.5$ is combined with another prism of glass of refractive index $\mu_2 = 1.75$. The combination of the prisms produces dispersion without deviation. The angle of the second prism should be

(Mains 2011)

(a) 5° (b) 7°

(c) 10° (d) 12°

69. Rainbow is formed due to **(2000)**

(a) scattering and refraction

(b) internal reflection and dispersion

(c) reflection only

(d) diffraction and dispersion.

70. The blue colour of the sky is due to the phenomenon of **(1994)**

(a) scattering (b) dispersion

(c) reflection (d) refraction.

Optical Instruments

71. A lens of large focal length and large aperture is best suited as an objective of an astronomical telescope since **(2021)**

(a) a large aperture contributes to the quality and visibility of the images.

(b) a large area of the objective ensures better light gathering power.

(c) a large aperture provides a better resolution

(d) all of the above.

72. A person can see clearly objects only when they lie between 50 cm and 400 cm from his eyes. In order to increase the maximum distance of distinct vision to infinity, the type and power of the correcting lens, the person has to use, will be **(NEET-II 2016)**

(a) convex, +2.25 dioptre

(b) concave, -0.25 dioptre

(c) concave, -0.2 dioptre

(d) convex, +0.15 dioptre.

73. A astronomical telescope has objective and eyepiece of focal lengths 40 cm and 4 cm respectively. To view an object 200 cm away from the objective, the lenses must be separated by a distance **(NEET-I 2016)**

(a) 50.0 cm (b) 54.0 cm

(c) 37.3 cm (d) 46.0 cm.

74. In an astronomical telescope in normal adjustment a straight black line of length L is drawn on inside part of objective lens. The eye-piece forms a real image of this line. The length of this image is I. The magnification of the telescope is **(2015)**

(a) $\frac{L+I}{L-I}$ (b) $\frac{L}{I}$

(c) $\frac{L}{I}+1$ (d) $\frac{L}{I}-1$

75. If the focal length of objective lens is increased then magnifying power of **(2014)**

(a) microscope will increase but that of telescope decrease

(b) microscope and telescope both will increase

(c) microscope and telescope both will decrease

(d) microscope will decrease but that of telescope will increase

76. For a normal eye, the cornea of eye provides a converging power of 40D and the least converging power of the eye lens behind the cornea is 20D. Using this information, the distance between the retina and the cornea-eye lens can be estimated to be **(2013)**

(a) 1.67 cm (b) 1.5 cm

(c) 5 cm (d) 2.5 cm

77. The magnifying power of a telescope is 9. When it is adjusted for parallel rays the distance between the objective and eyepiece is 20 cm. The focal length of lenses are **(2012)**

(a) 10 cm, 10 cm (b) 15 cm, 5 cm

(c) 18 cm, 2 cm (d) 11 cm, 9 cm.

78. An astronomical telescope of tenfold angular magnification has a length of 44 cm. The focal length of the objective is **(1997)**

(a) 44 cm (b) 440 cm

(c) 4 cm (d) 40 cm

79. Exposure time of camera lens at $f/2.8$ setting is $1/200$ second. The correct time of exposure at $f/5.6$ is **(1995)**

(a) 0.20 second (b) 0.40 second

(c) 0.02 second (d) 0.04 second.

80. Four lenses of focal length ± 15 cm and ± 150 cm are available for making a telescope. To produce the largest magnification, the focal length of the eyepiece should be **(1994)**

(a) +15 cm (b) +150 cm

(c) −150 cm (d) −15 cm

ANSWER KEY

1.	(b)	2.	(d)	3.	(c)	4.	(d)	5.	(d)	6.	(b)	7.	(c)
8.	(c)	9.	(b)	10.	(b)	11.	(b)	12.	(c)	13.	(c)	14.	(b)
15.	(a)	16.	(b)	17.	(c)	18.	(c)	19.	(d)	20.	(c)	21.	(a)
22.	(b)	23.	(c)	24.	(a)	25.	(a)	26.	(c)	27.	(b)	28.	(c)
29.	(a)	30.	(c)	31.	(c)	32.	(d)	33.	(d)	34.	(a)	35.	(a)
36.	(c)	37.	(c)	38.	(d)	39.	(c)	40.	(b)	41.	(c)	42.	(a)
43.	(a)	44.	(b)	45.	(b)	46.	(a)	47.	(b)	48.	(a)	49.	(a)
50.	(b)	51.	(b)	52.	(c)	53.	(c)	54.	(b)	55.	(c)	56.	(b)
57.	(d)	58.	(b)	59.	(d)	60.	(b)	61.	(b)	62.	(b)	63.	(a)
64.	(d)	65.	(b)	66.	(a)	67.	(a)	68.	(c)	69.	(b)	70.	(a)
71.	(d)	72.	(b)	73.	(b)	74.	(b)	75.	(d)	76.	(a)	77.	(c)
78.	(d)	79.	(c)	80.	(a)								

Hints & Explanations

1. (b) :

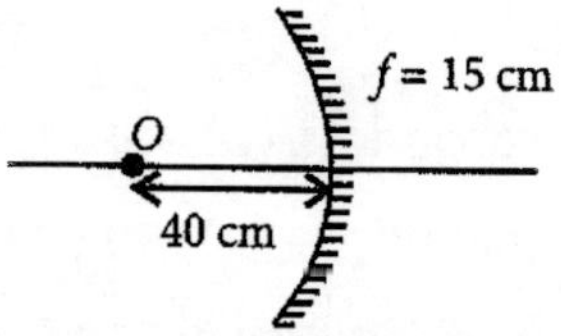

Using mirror formula,

$$\frac{1}{f}=\frac{1}{v_1}+\frac{1}{u_1};-\frac{1}{15}=\frac{1}{v_1}-\frac{1}{40}\Rightarrow\frac{1}{v_1}=\frac{1}{-15}+\frac{1}{40}$$

$v_1 = -24$ cm

When object is displaced by 20 cm towards mirror. Now, $u_2 = -20$ cm

$$\frac{1}{f}=\frac{1}{v_2}+\frac{1}{u_2};\frac{1}{-15}=\frac{1}{v_2}-\frac{1}{20}\Rightarrow\frac{1}{v_2}=\frac{1}{20}-\frac{1}{15};$$

$v_2 = -60$ cm

So, the image will be shift away from mirror by $(60-24)\text{cm} = 36$ cm.

2. (d) : When mirror is rotated by θ angle reflected ray will be rotated by 2θ.

For small angle θ,

$$\tan 2\theta \approx 2\theta = \frac{y}{x}$$

$$\therefore\ \theta = \frac{y}{2x}$$

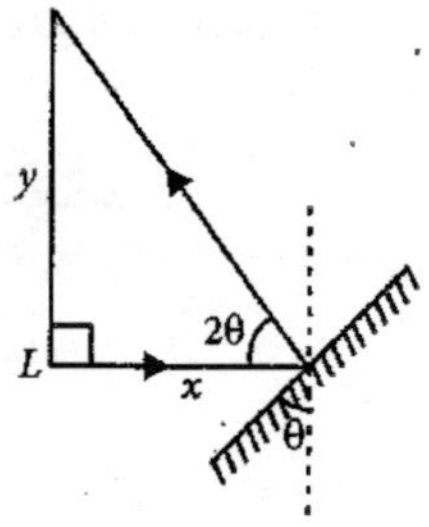

3. (c) : Magnification in the mirror, $m = -\frac{v}{u}$

$$m = -2 \Rightarrow v = 2u$$

As v and u have same signs so the mirror is concave and image formed is real.

$m = -\frac{1}{2} \Rightarrow v = \frac{u}{2} \Rightarrow$ Concave mirror and real image.

$m = +2 \Rightarrow v = -2u$

As v and u have different signs but magnification is 2 so the mirror is concave and image formed is virtual.

$$m = +\frac{1}{2} \Rightarrow v = -\frac{u}{2}$$

As v and u have different signs with magnification $\left(\frac{1}{2}\right)$ so the mirror is convex and image formed is virtual.

4. (d) : Different angles as shown in the figure.

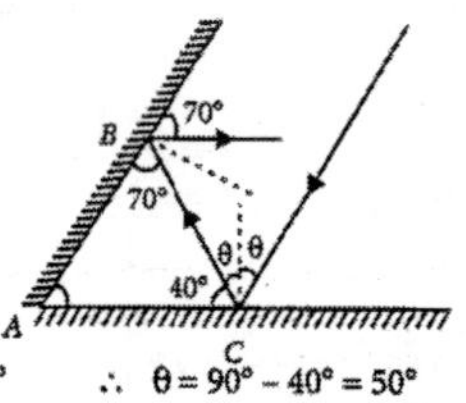

$\theta + 40° = 90°$ $\therefore \theta = 90° - 40° = 50°$

5. (d) :

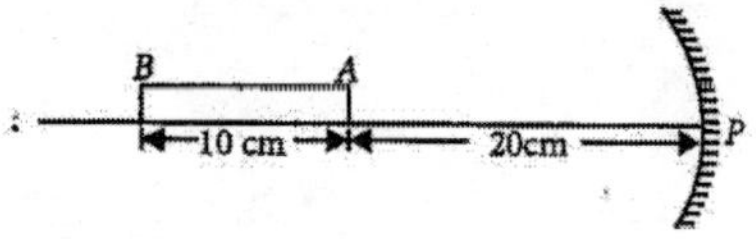

Here, f = -10 cm

For end $A, u_A = -20$ cm

Image position of end A,

$$\frac{1}{v_A} + \frac{1}{u_A} = \frac{1}{f}$$

$\frac{1}{v_A} + \frac{1}{(-20)} = \frac{1}{(-10)}$ or $\frac{1}{v_A} = \frac{1}{-10} + \frac{1}{20} = -\frac{1}{20}$

$v_A = -20$ cm

For end $B, u_B = -30$ cm

Image position of end $B, \frac{1}{v_B} + \frac{1}{u_B} = \frac{1}{f}$

$\frac{1}{v_B} + \frac{1}{(-30)} = \frac{1}{(-10)}$ or $\frac{1}{v_B} = \frac{1}{-10} + \frac{1}{30} =$

$-\frac{2}{30} v_B = -15$ cm

Length of the image

$= |v_A| - |v_B| = 20$ cm $- 15$ cm $= 5$ cm

6. (b) : The minimum mirror length should be half of the height of man.

7. (c) : The refractive index of glass, $\mu = \sqrt{3}$

Angle of incidence $= 60°$

Let 'r' be the angle of refraction.

Now, applying Snell's law

$1 \times \sin 60° = \mu \times \sin r$

$\Rightarrow \frac{\sqrt{3}}{2} = \sqrt{3} \times \sin r \Rightarrow \sin r = \frac{1}{2}$

$\Rightarrow r = 30°$

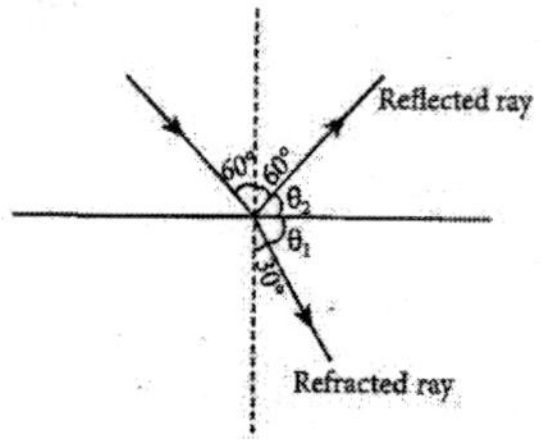

Let $\theta_1 + \theta_2$, be the angle between reflected ray and refracted ray. Hence, from figure we can say that

$$\theta_1 + \theta_2 = 60° + 30° = 90°$$

8. (c) : Here $\mu = 1.5$

l = length of the slab

x = position of air bubble

from one side

As per question, total

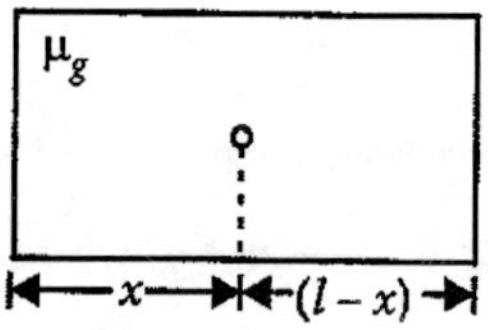

apparent length of slab = 5 + 3

or $\frac{x}{\mu} + \frac{(l-x)}{\mu} = 8$ or

$\frac{l}{\mu} = 8 \therefore l = 8\mu = 8 \times 1.5 = 12$ cm

9. (b) : Apparent depth $= \frac{\text{real depth}}{\mu} = \frac{3}{1.5} =$ 2 cm

As image appears to be raised by 1 cm, therefore, microscope must be moved upwards by 1 cm.

10. (b) : The velocities of different colours is different in a given medium. Red and green are refracted at different angle of refraction.

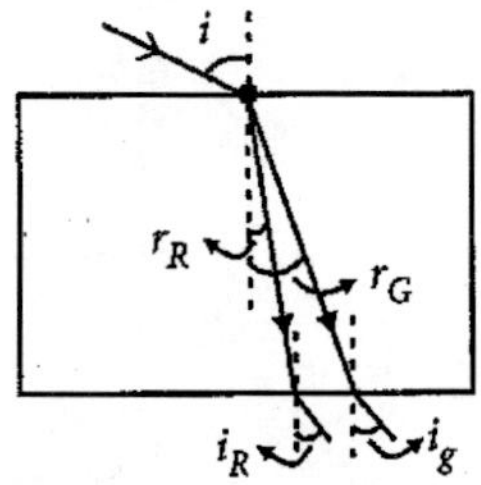

$$\frac{\sin i}{\sin r_R} = \mu$$

$$\frac{\sin i}{\sin r_G} = \mu$$

$$\frac{\sin r_p}{\sin i_p} = \mu$$

From equations (i), (ii) and (iii), we get

$$i = i_R = i_G$$

Thus two point propagation in two different parallel direction.

11. (b) : Frequency remains same.

12. (c) : Total apparent depth,

$$y = y_1 + y_2 = 5 + 2 = 7 \text{ cm.}$$

If x is real depth = thickness of slab, then as

$$\mu = \frac{\text{real depth}}{\text{apparent depth}} = \frac{x}{y}$$

or, $x = \mu y = 1.5 \times 7 = 10.5$ cm.

13. (c) : Speed of light is air $V_1 = \frac{x}{t_1}$ speed of light is a medium $V_2 = \frac{10x}{t_2}$

$$\sin\theta_c = \frac{V_2}{V_1} = \frac{10x}{t_2}\frac{t_1}{x}$$

$$\theta_c = \sin^{-1}\left(\frac{10t_1}{t_2}\right)$$

14. (b) : For medium A, speed of light $v_A = 1.5 \times 10^8$ m/s.

For medium B, speed of light

$v_B = 2.0 \times 10^8$ m/s

For medium A, $n_A = \frac{c}{v_A} = \frac{3\times10^8}{1.5\times10^8} = 2$

For medium B, $n_B = \frac{c}{v_B} = \frac{3\times10^8}{2\times10^8} = 1.5$

The critical angle for a ray of light is,

$$\sin C = \frac{n_B}{n_A}$$

$$C = \sin^{-1}\left(\frac{1.5}{2}\right)$$

$$C = \sin^{-1}(0.750)$$

15. (a) : When the angle of refraction is equal to 90°, the angle of incidence is called the critical angle.

16. (b) : Difference between apparent and real depth of a pond is due to refraction. Other three are due to total internal reflection.

17. (c) : For total internal reflection, $\sin i > \sin C$

where, i = angle of incidence, C = critical angle But, $\sin C = \frac{1}{\mu}$ $\therefore$ $\sin i > \frac{1}{\mu}$ or $\mu > \frac{1}{\sin i}$

$\mu > \frac{1}{\sin 45^\circ}$ ($i = 45^\circ$ (Given))

$\mu > \sqrt{2}$

Hence, option (c) is correct.

18. (c) : Refractive index for medium M_1 is

$$\mu_1 = \frac{c}{v_1} = \frac{3\times10^8}{1.5\times10^8} = 2$$

Refractive index for medium M_2 is

$$\mu_2 = \frac{c}{v_2} = \frac{3\times10^8}{2.0\times10^8} = \frac{3}{2}$$

For total internal reflection, $\sin i \geq \sin C$ where i = angle of incidence, C = critical angle

But $\sin C = \frac{\mu_2}{\mu_1}$ $\therefore \sin i \geq \frac{\mu_2}{\mu_1} \geq \frac{3/2}{2} \Rightarrow i \geq \sin^{-1}\left(\frac{3}{4}\right)$

19. (d) :

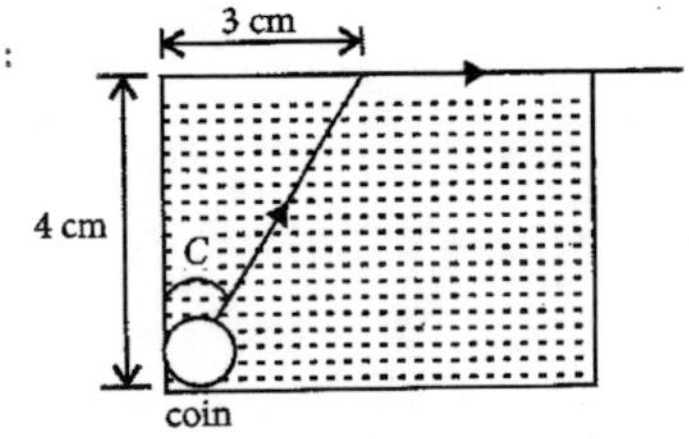

From figure, $\sin C = \frac{3}{\sqrt{(4)^2+(3)^2}} = \frac{3}{5}$

where C is the critical angle.

Also, $\sin C = {}^l\mu_a \Rightarrow \sin C = \frac{1}{{}^a\mu_l}$ [since ${}^l\mu_a = \frac{1}{{}^a\mu_l}$]

Also ${}^a\mu_l = \frac{\text{velocity of light in air } (c)}{\text{velocity of light in liquid } (v)}$

$\therefore \sin C = \frac{v}{c} = \frac{v}{3\times10^8}$

or, $v = 3\times10^8 \times \frac{3}{5} = 1.8\times10^8$ m s^{-1}.

20. (c) : Applying Snell's law of refraction at A, we get

$\mu = \frac{\sin i}{\sin r} = \frac{\sin 45^\circ}{\sin r}$

$\therefore \sin r = 1/\sqrt{2}\mu$

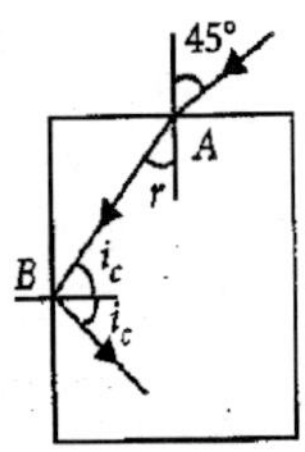

$\therefore\ r = \sin^{-1}\left(\frac{1}{\sqrt{2}\mu}\right)$

Applying the condition of total internal reflection at B, we get

$$i_c = \sin^{-1}(1/\mu)$$

where i_c is the critical angle.

Now, $r + i_c = 90° = \pi/2$

$\therefore\ \sin^{-1}\frac{1}{\sqrt{2}\mu} = \frac{\pi}{2} - \sin^{-1}\frac{1}{\mu}$

or, $\sin^{-1}\frac{1}{\sqrt{2}\mu} = \cos^{-1}\frac{1}{\mu}$

$\therefore\ \frac{1}{\sqrt{2}\mu} = \frac{\sqrt{\mu^2-1}}{\mu}$ or $\frac{1}{2} = \mu^2 - 1\ \therefore\ \mu = \sqrt{3/2}$

21. (a)

22. (b) : θ is the critical angle.

$\therefore\ \theta = \sin^{-1}(1/\mu) = \sin^{-1}(3/5)$

or, $\sin\theta = 3/5$

$\therefore\ \tan\theta = 3/4 = r/4$

or, $r = 3$ m.

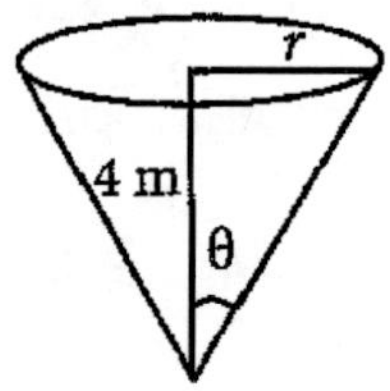

23. (c) : $n > \frac{\sin r}{\sin i}$

i.e., $n > \frac{\sin 90°}{\sin 45°} \Rightarrow n > \sqrt{2}$

24. (a) : According to Snell's law,

$$\mu = \frac{\sin i}{\sin r'} = \frac{\sin i}{\sin(90° - r)} = \frac{\sin i}{\cos r}$$

From law of reflection,

$i = r\ \therefore\ \mu = \frac{\sin r}{\cos r} = \tan r$

Critical angle $= \sin^{-1}(\mu) = \sin^{-1}(\tan r)$.

25. (a) : In order to cut off all the light coming out of water surface, angle C should be equal to critical angle.

i.e. $\sin C = \frac{1}{\mu} = \frac{1}{5/3} = \frac{3}{5}$

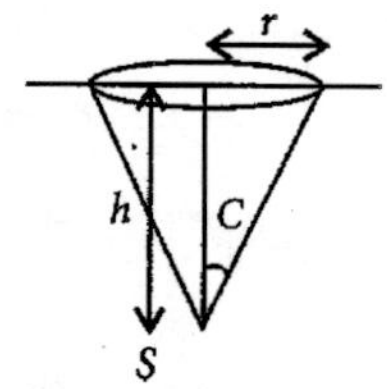

$\therefore\ \tan C = 3/4.$

Now, $\tan C = \frac{r}{h}$;

$r = h\tan C = 4 \times \frac{3}{4} = 3$ m

Diameter of disc $= 2r = 6$ m

26. (3) : $\frac{1}{f_{eq}} = \frac{1}{f_1} + \frac{1}{f_2}$

$$\frac{1}{f_{eq}} = \frac{1}{f} - \frac{1}{f}$$

$$f_{eq} = \infty$$

27. (b) :

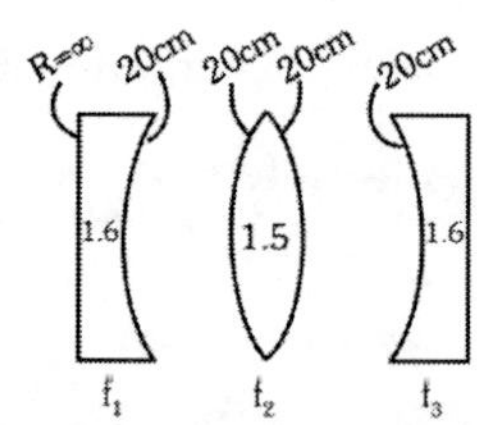

Use $\frac{1}{f} = [\mu - 1]\left[\frac{1}{R_1} - \frac{1}{R_2}\right]$

$$\frac{1}{f_1} = [1.6 - 1]\left[\frac{1}{\infty} - \frac{1}{20}\right] = \frac{-3}{100}$$

$$\frac{1}{f_2} = [1.5 - 1]\left[\frac{1}{20} + \frac{1}{20}\right] = \frac{1}{20}$$

$$\frac{1}{f_3} = \frac{-3}{100}$$

$$\frac{1}{f_{eq}} = \frac{1}{f_1} + \frac{1}{f_2} + \frac{1}{f_3}$$

$$\frac{1}{f_{eq}} = -\frac{3}{100} + \frac{1}{20} - \frac{3}{100} = \frac{-1}{100}$$

28. (c) : Given, refractive index of lens = 1.5

For biconvex lens, $R_1 = +R, R_2 = -R$

$\therefore R_1 = +20$ cm and $R_2 = -20$ cm

According to lens maker's formula,

$$\frac{1}{f} = (\mu - 1)\left(\frac{1}{R_1} - \frac{1}{R_2}\right)$$

$$\therefore \frac{1}{f} = (1.5 - 1)\left(\frac{1}{20} - \frac{1}{(-20)}\right) = 0.5\left(\frac{1}{20} + \frac{1}{20}\right)$$

or $\frac{1}{f} = \frac{1}{20} \Rightarrow f = 20$ cm

Power of lens (in dioptre), $P = \frac{100}{\text{focal length } f \text{ (in cm)}}$

$$\therefore P = \frac{100}{20} = +5\text{D}$$

29. (a) : Distance of object, $u = -60$ cm

Focal length, $f = 30$ cm

Let the image formed by lens is at a distance v.

Using lens equation

$$\frac{1}{v} - \frac{1}{u} = \frac{1}{f} \Rightarrow \frac{1}{v} + \frac{1}{60} = \frac{1}{30} \Rightarrow \frac{1}{v} = \frac{1}{60} \Rightarrow v = 60 \text{ cm}$$

So, image formed behind the mirror at a distance $(60 - 40) = 20$ cm.

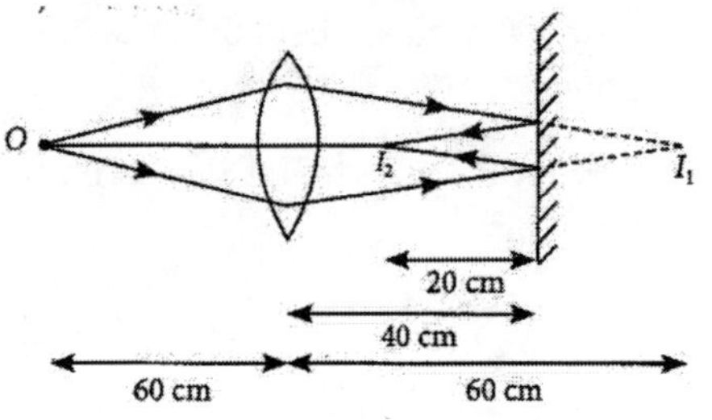

For second refraction from convex lens

$u = -20$ cm, $v = ?, f = 30$ cm

$$\frac{1}{v} - \frac{1}{u} = \frac{1}{f} \Rightarrow \frac{1}{v} + \frac{1}{20} = \frac{1}{30} \Rightarrow \frac{1}{v} = \frac{1}{30} - \frac{1}{20}$$
$$\Rightarrow v = -60 \text{ cm}$$

Thus final image is virtual and at a distance $60 - 40 = 20$ cm from plane mirror.

30. (c) : Given : $f_1 = 20$ cm, $f_2 = -5$ cm

Equivalent focal length, $f = \infty$

(As the rays are parallel)
By using Newton's displacement formula

$$\frac{1}{f} = \frac{1}{f_1} + \frac{1}{f_2} - \frac{d}{f_1 f_2} \Rightarrow \frac{1}{\infty} = \frac{1}{20} - \frac{1}{5} - \frac{d}{20(-5)}$$

$$0 = \frac{5 - 20 + d}{20 \times 5} \Rightarrow d = 15 \text{ cm}$$

31. (c) : According to lens maker's formula

$$\frac{1}{f} = (\mu - 1)\left(\frac{1}{R_1} - \frac{1}{R_2}\right)$$
$$\frac{1}{f} = (\mu - 1)\left(\frac{1}{R} - \frac{1}{-R}\right)$$

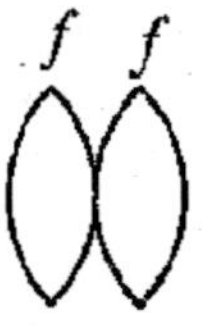

$$= (1.5 - 1)\left(\frac{2}{R}\right) = \frac{1}{R}$$

Two similar equi-convex lenses of focal length f each are held in contact with each other.

The focal length F_1 of the combination is given by

$$\frac{1}{F_1}=\frac{1}{f}+\frac{1}{f}=\frac{2}{f};F_1=\frac{f}{2}=\frac{R}{2}$$

For glycerin in between lenses, there are three lenses, one concave and two convex.

Focal length of the concave lens is given by

$$\frac{1}{f'}=(1.5-1)\left(\frac{-2}{R}\right)=-\frac{1}{R}$$

Now, equivalent focal length of the combination is,

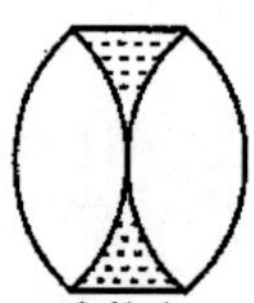

$f\,f'\,f$

$$\frac{1}{F_2}=\frac{1}{f}+\frac{1}{f'}+\frac{1}{f};\frac{1}{F_2}=\frac{1}{R}-\frac{1}{R}+\frac{1}{R}=\frac{1}{R}$$

$F_2=R$

Dividing equation (i) by (ii), we get $\frac{F_1}{F_2}=\frac{1}{2}$

32. (d) : When an equiconvex lens is cut into two symmetrical halves along the principal axis, then there will be no change in focal length of the lens.

$\therefore$ Power of lens, $P=\frac{1}{f}$

So, the power of each part will be P.

33. (d) : Here, $\mu_g=\frac{3}{2}, \mu_w=\frac{4}{3}$

Focal length (f) of glass convex lens is given by

$$\frac{1}{f}=(\mu_g-1)\left(\frac{2}{R}\right)$$

or $\frac{1}{f}=\left(\frac{3}{2}-1\right)\frac{2}{R}=\frac{1}{R}$ or $f=R$

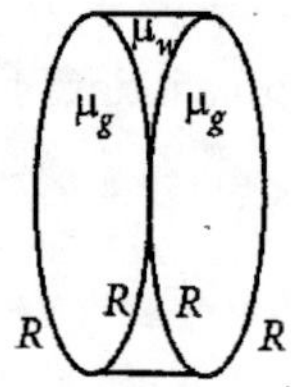

Focal length (f') of water filled concave lens is given by

$$\frac{1}{f'}=(\mu_w-1)\left(-\frac{2}{R}\right) \text{ or } \frac{1}{f'}=\left(\frac{4}{3}-1\right)\left(-\frac{2}{R}\right)$$

$$=-\frac{2}{3R}=-\frac{2}{3f} \text{ [Using eqn. (i)]}$$

Equivalent focal length (f_{eq}) of lens system

$$\frac{1}{f_{eq}}=\frac{1}{f}-\frac{2}{3f}+\frac{1}{f}=\frac{3-2+3}{3f}=\frac{4}{3f}$$

$$\therefore f_{eq}=\frac{3f}{4}$$

34. (a) : The combination of two lenses 1 and 2 is as shown in figure.

$$\therefore\frac{1}{f}=\frac{1}{f_1}+\frac{1}{f_2}$$

According to lens maker's formula

$$\frac{1}{f_1}=(\mu_1-1)\left(\frac{1}{\infty}-\frac{1}{-R}\right)=\frac{(\mu_1-1)}{R}$$

$$\frac{1}{f_2} = (\mu_2 - 1)\left(\frac{1}{-R} - \frac{1}{\infty}\right)$$

$$= (\mu_2 - 1)\left(-\frac{1}{R}\right) = -\frac{(\mu_2 - 1)}{R}$$

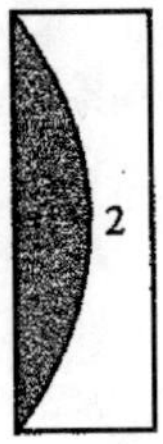

$$\therefore \frac{1}{f} = \frac{(\mu_1 - 1)}{R} - \frac{(\mu_2 - 1)}{R} \Rightarrow \frac{1}{f} = \frac{(\mu_1 - \mu_2)}{R}; f = \frac{R}{(\mu_1 - \mu_2)}$$

35. (a) : According to lens maker's formula

$$\frac{1}{f} = \left(\frac{\mu_g}{\mu_L} - 1\right)\left(\frac{1}{R_1} - \frac{1}{R_2}\right)$$

where μ_g is the refractive index of the material of the lens and μ_L is the refractive index of the liquid in which lens is dipped. As the biconvex lens dipped in a liquid acts as a plane sheet of glass, therefore

$f = \infty \Rightarrow \frac{1}{f} = 0 \therefore \frac{\mu_g}{\mu_L} - 1 = 0$ or $\mu_g = \mu_L$

36. (c) :

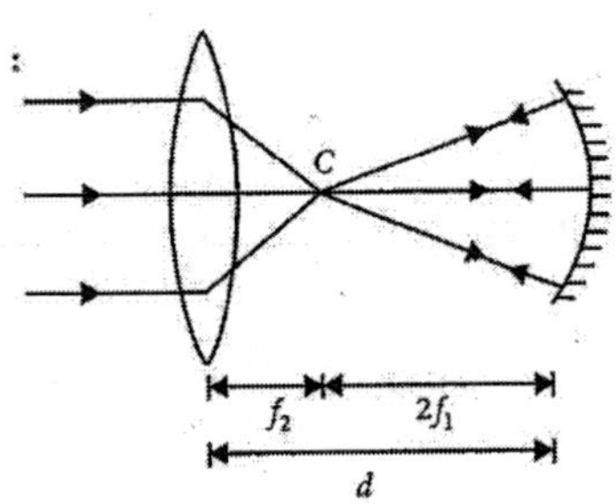

$$\therefore d = 2f_1 + f_2$$

37. (c) :

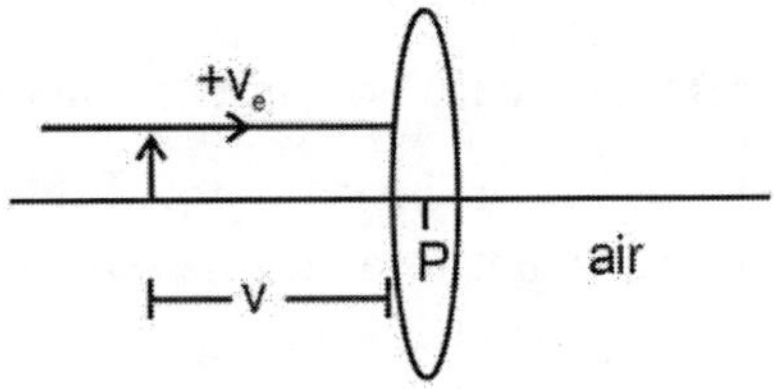

sfqn convention +ve direction along incident ray distance of object from lens v = −30 cm

R_1 = +2 cm

R_2 = −20 cm

$$\frac{1}{f} = \left(\frac{u_2}{u_1} - 1\right)\left(\frac{1}{R_1} - \frac{1}{R_2}\right)$$

$$\frac{1}{f} = (1.5 - 1)\left(\frac{1}{20} - \frac{1}{(-20)}\right)$$

$$\frac{1}{f} = (1.5 - 1) \times \frac{2}{20}$$

f = +20 cm

We know $m = \frac{f}{f+v} = \frac{20}{20-30} = -2$

$$m = \frac{\text{height of image}(h_i)}{\text{Height of object}(h_0)}$$

$$\frac{h_i}{+2} = -2$$

h_i = −4cm [Real and inverted]

hence option (c) is correct

38. (d) : Here, $v = +15$ cm, $u = +(15 - 5) = +10$ cm

According to lens formula

$$\frac{1}{v}-\frac{1}{u}=\frac{1}{f}\Rightarrow\frac{1}{15}-\frac{1}{10}=\frac{1}{f}\Rightarrow f=-30\text{ cm}$$

39. (c) : Focal length of the lens remains same.

Intensity of image formed by lens is proportional to area exposed to incident light from object.

i.e., Intensity ∝ area or $\frac{I_2}{I_1}=\frac{A_2}{A_1}$

Initial area, $A_1=\pi\left(\frac{d}{2}\right)^2=\frac{\pi d^2}{4}$

After blocking, exposed area,

$$A_2=\frac{\pi d^2}{4}-\frac{\pi(d/2)^2}{4}=\frac{\pi d^2}{4}-\frac{\pi d^2}{16}=\frac{3\pi d^2}{16}$$

$$\therefore\ \frac{I_2}{I_1}=\frac{A_2}{A_1}=\frac{\frac{3\pi d^2}{16}}{\frac{\pi d^2}{4}}=\frac{3}{4}\text{ or}$$

$$I_2=\frac{3}{4}I_1=\frac{3}{4}I\ (\because I_1=I)$$

Hence, focal length of a lens $= f$, intensity of the image $=\frac{3I}{4}$

40. (b) :

$\frac{1}{f}=\frac{1}{f_1}+\frac{1}{f_2}$; ∴ Power $P=\frac{f_1+f_2}{f_1f_2}$

41. (c) :

$$\frac{\text{size of image}}{\text{size of object}}=\left|\frac{v}{u}\right|$$

⇒ size of the image $=\frac{1.39\times10^9\times10^{-1}}{1.5\times10^{11}}$

$=0.92\times10^{-3}$ m

size of the image $=9.2\times10^{-4}$ m

42. (a) : Focal length of convex lens $f_1=$ 25 cm

Focal length of concave lens $f_2=-25$ cm

Power of combination in dioptres,

$$P=P_1+P_2=\frac{100}{f_1}+\frac{100}{f_2}=\frac{100}{25}-\frac{100}{25}=0.$$

43. (a) : Since the lens is equiconvex, the radius of curvature of each half is same, say R. We know from Lens maker's formula

$$\frac{1}{f}=(\mu-1)\left(\frac{1}{R_1}-\frac{1}{R_2}\right)$$

(considering the lens to be placed in air).

Here $R_1=R, R_2=-R$ by convention

$$\therefore\frac{1}{f}=(\mu-1)\frac{2}{R}\Rightarrow(\mu-1)\frac{1}{R}=\frac{1}{2f}$$

If we cut the lens along XOX' then the two halves of the lens will be having the same radii of curvature and so, focal length $f'=f$

But when we cut it along YOY' then, we will have $R_1=R$ but $R_2=\infty$

$$\therefore\frac{1}{f''}=(\mu-1)\left(\frac{1}{R}-\frac{1}{\infty}\right)=(\mu-1)\frac{1}{R}$$

$$=\frac{1}{2f}\Rightarrow f''=2f$$

44. (b) : When refractive index of lens is equal to the refractive index of liquid, the lens behave like a plane surface with focal length infinity.

45. (b) : A real image is to be formed on the 2nd wall of the bulb placed on the first wall by the convex lens. The lens is placed at a distance of d from the 2nd wall.

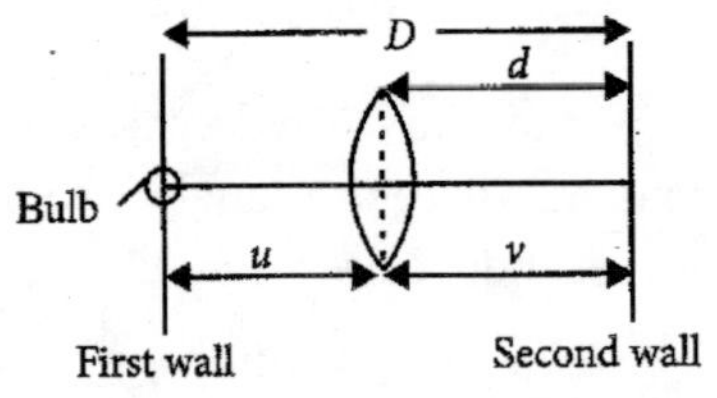

Now, we know that to form a real image of an object on a screen by a convex lens, the distance between the source and the screen (D) should be equal to $4f$, where f is the focal length of the lens.

In that case, $u = v = D/2 = d$.

$$\therefore f = D/4 = d/2$$

46. (a) : $\frac{1}{f} = (\mu - 1)\left[\frac{1}{R_1} - \frac{1}{R_2}\right]$

$$= (1.5 - 1)\left[\frac{1}{\infty} - \frac{1}{(-10)}\right] = 0.5\left[\frac{1}{10}\right] \Rightarrow f$$
$$= 20 \text{ cm}$$

When plane surface is silvered,

$$F = \frac{f}{2} = \frac{20}{2} = 10 \text{ cm}$$

47. (b) : $R_1 = +\infty, R_2 = -60$ cm

$$\frac{1}{f} = (\mu - 1)\left(\frac{1}{R_1} - \frac{1}{R_2}\right)$$
$$= (1.6 - 1)\left(\frac{1}{\infty} - \frac{1}{-60}\right)$$

or $f = 100$ cm

48. (a) : For lens, $\frac{1}{v} - \frac{1}{u} = \frac{1}{f}$

$$u = -30, f = 20, v = 60 \text{ cm}$$

To have an upright image of the object, coincide with it, image should tend to form at centre of curvature of convex mirror Therefore, the distance of convex mirror from the lens $= 60 - 10 = 50$ cm.

49. (a) :

$$\frac{1}{f} = (\mu - 1)\left(\frac{1}{R_1} - \frac{1}{R_2}\right)$$

Since the refractive index of violet colour (μ_v) is greater than the refractive index of red colour (μ_r), therefore focal length of violet colour is less than the focal length of red colour or in other words, $f_v < f_r$.

50. (b) : Focal length $f_1 = 80$ cm and $f_2 = -50$ cm (Minus sign due to concave lens)

Power of the combination (P)

$$= P_1 + P_2 = \frac{100}{f_1} + \frac{100}{f_2} = \frac{100}{80} - \frac{100}{50}$$
$$= -0.75\text{D}$$

51. (b) : For a convex lens, $f_R > f_V$ or $f_V < f_R$. For a concave lens, focal length is negative.

$\therefore |F_V| < |F_R|$ or $F_V > F_R$ as the smaller negative value is bigger.

52. (c) : By displacement method, size of object

$(O) = \sqrt{I_1 \times I_2}$.

Therefore area of source of light

$(A) = \sqrt{A_1 A_2}$.

53. (c) :

$$\frac{f_a}{f_e} = \frac{\left(\frac{\mu_g}{\mu_l} - 1\right)}{(\mu_g - 1)} = \frac{\left(\frac{1.5}{1.25} - 1\right)}{1.5 - 1} = \frac{1/5}{1/2} = \frac{2}{5}$$

$$f_e = \frac{5}{2} f_a = \frac{5}{2} \times 2 = 5 \text{ cm}$$

54. (b) : Let $\angle e$ is angle of emergence and $\angle i$ is angle of incidence.

Form Snell's law at point P

$$\frac{\sin i}{\sin r} = \frac{\mu_a}{\mu_g}$$
$$\angle i = 30^\circ$$

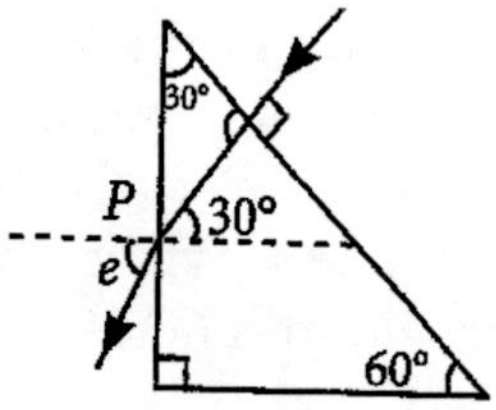

So, $\frac{\sin 30^\circ}{\sin e} = \frac{\mu_a}{\mu_g} \Rightarrow \sin e = \frac{\sqrt{3}}{1} \times \frac{1}{2}$ or $e = 60^\circ$

55. (c) : Light ray emerges normally from another surface so angle of emergence $(e) = 0$

$r_2 = 0 \Rightarrow r_1 + r_2 = A \Rightarrow r_1 = A$

Using Snell's law on first surface,

$1 \times \sin i = \mu \sin r_1 \; \sin i = \mu \sin A$

For small angles, $\sin A \approx A$

Hence, $i = \mu A$

56. (b) : For retracing the path shown in figure, light ray should be incident normally on the silvered face. Applying Snell's law at point M,

$$\frac{\sin i}{\sin 30^\circ} = \frac{\sqrt{2}}{1} \Rightarrow \sin i = \sqrt{2} \times \frac{1}{2}$$

$\sin i = \frac{1}{\sqrt{2}}$ i.e., $i = 45^\circ$.

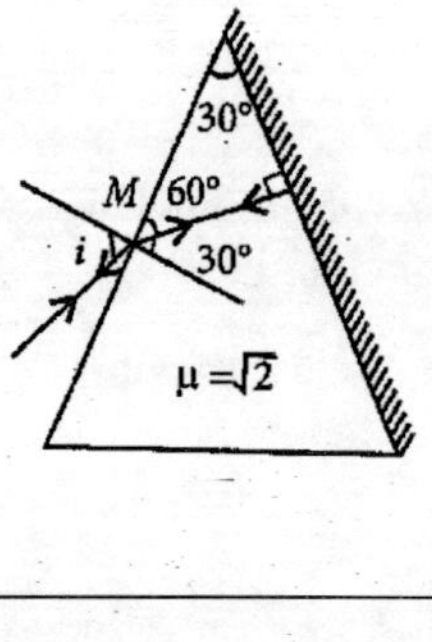

57. (d) : Given, $i = 45^\circ, A = 60^\circ$

Since the ray undergoes minimum deviation, therefore, angle of emergence from second face, $e = i = 45^\circ$

$\therefore \delta_m = i + e - A = 45^\circ + 45^\circ - 60^\circ = 30^\circ$

$$\mu = \frac{\sin\left(\frac{A+\delta_m}{2}\right)}{\sin\left(\frac{A}{2}\right)} = \frac{\sin\left(\frac{60^\circ + 30^\circ}{2}\right)}{\sin\left(\frac{60^\circ}{2}\right)}$$
$$= \frac{\sin 45^\circ}{\sin 30^\circ} = \frac{1}{\sqrt{2}} \times \frac{2}{1} = \sqrt{2}$$

58. (b) : As beam of light is incident normally on the face AB of the right angled prism ABC, so no deviation occurs at face AB and it passes straight and strikes the face AC at an angle of incidence, $i = 45^\circ$.

For total reflection to take place at face AC,

$$i > i_c \text{ or } \sin i > \sin i_c$$

where i_c is the critical angle.

But as here $i = 45^\circ$ and $\sin i_c = \frac{i}{\mu}$

$\therefore \; \sin 45^\circ > \frac{1}{\mu}$ or $\frac{1}{\sqrt{2}} > \frac{1}{\mu}$ or $\mu > \sqrt{2} = 1.414$

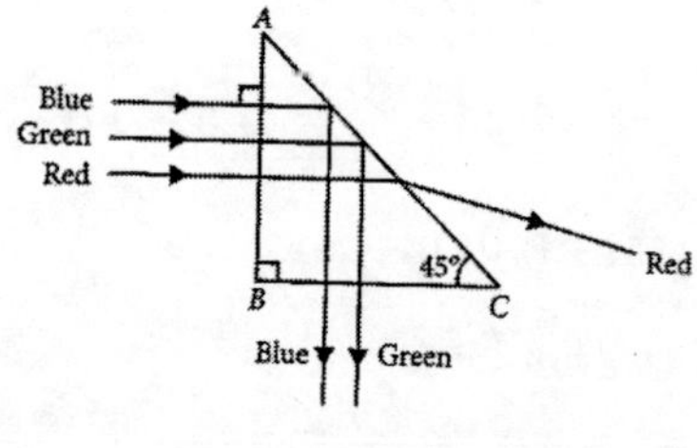

As $\mu_{red} (= 1.39) < \mu (= 1.414)$ while $\mu_{green} (= 1.44)$ and $\mu_{blue} (= 1.47) > \mu (= 1.414)$, so only red colour will be transmitted through face AC while green and blue colours will suffer total internal reflection.

So the prism will separate red colour from the green and blue colours as shown in the given figure.

59. (d) : As $\mu = \frac{\sin\left(\frac{A+\delta}{2}\right)}{\sin\left(\frac{A}{2}\right)}$ or $\cot\frac{A}{2} = \frac{\sin\left(\frac{A+\delta}{2}\right)}{\sin\left(\frac{A}{2}\right)}$

$\frac{\cos\left(\frac{A}{2}\right)}{\sin\left(\frac{A}{2}\right)} = \frac{\sin\left(\frac{A+\delta}{2}\right)}{\sin\left(\frac{A}{2}\right)}$ or

$\sin\left(\frac{\pi}{2}-\frac{A}{2}\right) = \sin\left(\frac{A}{2}+\frac{\delta}{2}\right)$;

$\frac{\pi}{2}-\frac{A}{2} = \frac{A}{2}+\frac{\delta}{2}$

$$\therefore \delta = \pi - 2A = 180^\circ - 2A$$

60. (b) : On reflection from the silvered surface, the incident ray will retrace its path, if it falls normally on the surface.

By geometry, $r = A$

Applying Snell's law at surface PQ,

$1\sin i = \mu\sin r$

$$\mu = \frac{\sin i}{\sin r} = \frac{\sin 2A}{\sin A} = 2\cos A$$

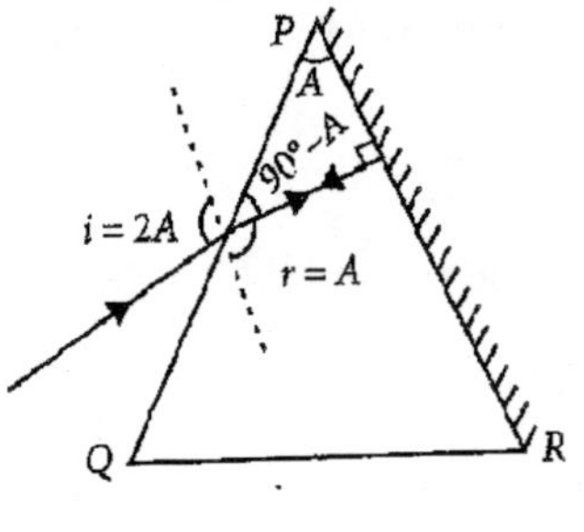

61. (b) : As $\mu = \frac{\sin\left(\frac{A+\delta}{2}\right)}{\sin\left(\frac{A}{2}\right)}$

$$\mu = \frac{\sin\left(\frac{A+A}{2}\right)}{\sin\left(\frac{A}{2}\right)} = \frac{\sin A}{\sin\left(\frac{A}{2}\right)}$$

$$= \frac{2\sin\left(\frac{A}{2}\right)\cos\left(\frac{A}{2}\right)}{\sin\left(\frac{A}{2}\right)}$$

$$= 2\cos\left(\frac{A}{2}\right)$$

As $\delta = i + e - A$

At minimum deviation, $\delta = \delta_m, i = e$

$\therefore \delta_m = 2i - A$ or $2i = \delta_m + A$

$i = \frac{\delta_m+A}{2} = \frac{A+A}{2} = A$ ($\because \delta_m = A$(given))

$i_{\min} = 0^\circ \Rightarrow A_{\min} = 0^\circ$

Then, $\mu_{\max} = 2\cos 0^\circ = 2$

$\because i_{\max} = \frac{\pi}{2} \Rightarrow A_{\max} = \frac{\pi}{2}$

Then, $\mu_{\min} = 2\cos 45^\circ = 2 \times \frac{1}{\sqrt{2}} = \sqrt{2}$

So refractive index lies between 2 and $\sqrt{2}$.

62. (b) : Angle of prism,

$$A = r_1 + r_2$$

For minimum deviation

$$r_1 = r_2 = r \;\therefore A = 2r$$

Given, $A = 60^\circ$

Hence, $r = \frac{A}{2} = \frac{60^\circ}{2} = 30^\circ$

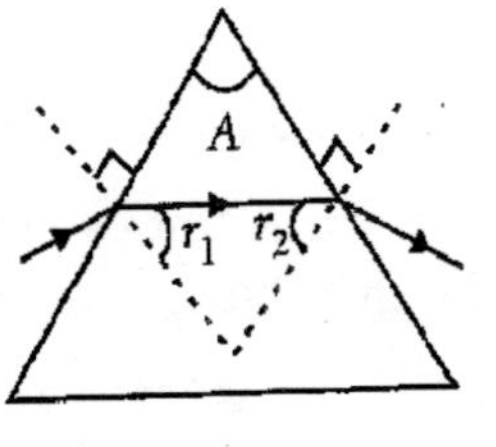

63. (a) : $A = 60°, \mu = \sqrt{3}, \delta_m = ?$

$$\mu = \frac{\sin\left(\frac{A+\delta_m}{2}\right)}{\sin\frac{A}{2}} \quad \therefore \delta_m = 60°$$

64. (d) : An observer can see a rainbow only when his back is towards the sun.

65. (b) : Red light of the visible spectrum is having a maximum wavelength of about 650 nm.

66. (a) : The condition for dispersion without deviation is given as $(\mu - 1)A = (\mu' - 1)A'$

Given $= 1.42, A = 10°, \mu' = 1.7, A' = ?$

$$\therefore (1.42 - 1) \times 10 = (1.7 - 1)A'$$
$$(0.42) \times 10 = 0.7 \times A'$$
$$\text{or } A' = \frac{0.42 \times 10}{0.7} = 6°$$

67. (a) : The reddish appearance of the sun at sunrise and sunset is due to the scattering of light.

68. (c) : For dispersion without deviation

$\delta_1 + \delta_2 = 0$

$$(\mu_1 - 1)A_1 + (\mu_2 - 1)A_2 = 0$$
$$A_2 = -\frac{(\mu_1 - 1)A_1}{(\mu_2 - 1)}$$

Substituting the given values, we get

$$A_2 = -\frac{(1.5 - 1)15°}{(1.75 - 1)} = -10°$$

Negative sign shows that two prisms must be joined in opposition.

69. (b) : The rainbow is an example of the dispersion of sunlight by the water drops in the atmosphere. This is a phenomenon due to a combination of the refraction of sunlight by spherical water droplets and of total internal reflection.

70. (a) : According to Rayleigh, the amount of scattering is inversely proportional to the fourth power of the wavelength.

71. (d) : As the focal length is large so, it enhances the magnifying power of telescope. The large aperture or diameter of lens helps in collecting large amount of light from the object so that the image formed is bright.

The resolving power of telescope is

$$\text{R.P.} = \frac{D}{1.22\lambda}$$

where, D is diameter or aperture of lens and λ is wavelength of light used.

So, all options are correct.

72. (b) : Here, $v = -400 \text{ cm} = -4 \text{ m}, u = \infty, f = ?$

Using lens formula, $\frac{1}{v} - \frac{1}{u} = \frac{1}{f}$

or $\frac{1}{-4} - \frac{1}{\infty} = \frac{1}{f}$ or $f = -4$ m

Lens should be concave.

Power of lens $= \frac{1}{f} = \frac{1}{-4} = -0.25$D

73. (b) : Here $f_o = 40$ cm, $f_e = 4$ cm

Tube length (l) = Distance between lenses

$$= v_0 + f_e$$

For objective lens,

$u_o = -200 \text{ cm}, v_0 = ?$

$$\frac{1}{v_0} - \frac{1}{u_0} = \frac{1}{f_0} \text{ or } \frac{1}{v_0} - \frac{1}{-200} = \frac{1}{40}$$

$$\text{or } \frac{1}{v_0} = \frac{1}{40} - \frac{1}{200} = \frac{4}{200} \therefore v_0 = 50 \text{ cm}$$

$\therefore l = 50 + 4 = 54 \text{ cm}$

74. (b) :

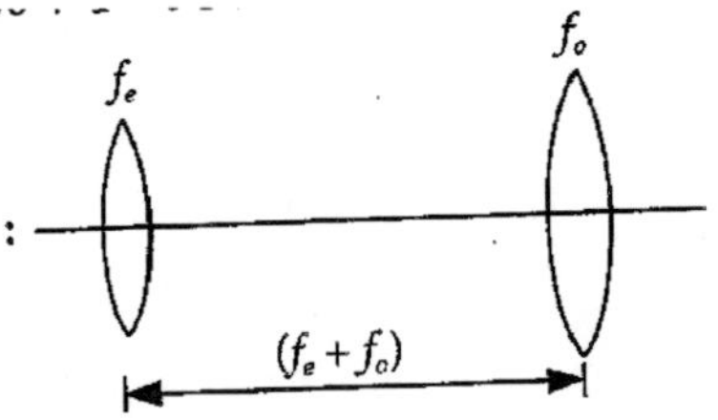

For eye-piece lens,

$$m = \frac{f}{f+u} = \frac{h_1}{h_0} \Rightarrow \frac{f_e}{f_e - (f_o + f_e)} = \frac{I}{L}$$

$\Rightarrow \frac{f_0}{f_e} = -\frac{L}{I} =$ Magnification of the telescope

75. (d) : Magnifying power of a microscope,

$$m = \left(\frac{L}{f_o}\right)\left(\frac{D}{f_e}\right)$$

where f_o and f_e are the focal lengths of the objective and eyepiece respectively and L is the distance between their focal points and D is the least distance of distinct vision.

If f_o increases, then m will decrease.

Magnifying power of a telescope, $m = \frac{f_0}{f_e}$

where f_o and f_e are the focal lengths of the objective and eyepiece respectively.

If f_o increases, then m will increase.

76. (a) : Converging power of cornea,

$P_c = +40\text{D}$

Least converging power of eye lens,

$P_e = +20\text{D}$

Power of the eye-lens, $P = P_c + P_e$

$$= 40\text{D} + 20\text{D} = 60\text{D}$$

Power of the eye lens

$$P = \frac{1}{\text{Focal length of the eye lens } (f)}$$

$$f = \frac{1}{P} = \frac{1}{60\text{D}} = \frac{1}{60} \text{ m} = \frac{100}{60} \text{ cm} = \frac{5}{3} \text{ cm}$$

Distance between the retina and cornea-eye lens = Focal length of the eye lens

$$= \frac{5}{3} \text{ cm} = 1.67 \text{ cm}$$

77. (c) : Magnifying power, $m = \frac{f_0}{f_e} = 9$

where f_o and f_e are the focal lengths of the objective and eyepiece respectively

Also, $f_o + f_e = 20$ cm

On solving (i) and (ii), we get

$$f_o = 18 \text{ cm}, f_e = 2 \text{ cm}$$

78. (d) : Length of astronomical telescope $(f_o + f_e) = 44$ cm and ratio of focal length of the objective lens to that of the eye piece

$\frac{f_0}{f_e} = 10$

From the given ratio, we find that

$f_o = 10 f_e$.

Therefore $10f_e + f_e = 44$ or $f_e = 4$ cm

and focal length of the objective (f_0)

$$= 44 - f_e = 44 - 4 = 40 \text{ cm}$$

79. (c) : Time of exposure $t \propto (f - \text{number})^2$

$$\therefore \frac{t}{\left(\frac{1}{200}\right)} = \left(\frac{5.6}{2.8}\right)^2 = 4 \text{ or } t = 0.02 \text{ s}$$

80. (a) : Magnifying power of telescope,

$M = f_o/f_e$

To produce largest magnifications $f_o > f_e$ and f_o and f_e both should be positive (convex lens).

Therefore $f_e = +15$ cm.

Chapter: 24 WAVE OPTICS

Introduction

1. Which one of the following phenomena is not explained by Huygen's construction of wavefront? **(1988)**

(a) Refraction (b) Reflection
(c) Diffraction (d) Origin of spectra

Refraction and Reflection of Plane Waves using Huygens Principle

2. The frequency of a light wave in a material is 2×10^{14} Hz and wavelength is 5000Å. The refractive index of material will be **(2007)**

(a) 1.50 (b) 3.00
(c) 1.33 (d) 1.40

3. An electromagnetic radiation of frequency n, wavelength λ, travelling with velocity v in air, enters a glass slab of refractive index μ. The frequency, wavelength and velocity of light in the glass slab will be respectively **(1997)**

(a) $n, 2\lambda$ and $\frac{v}{\mu}$ (b) $\frac{2n}{\mu}, \frac{\lambda}{\mu}$ and v
(c) $\frac{n}{\mu}, \frac{\lambda}{\mu}$ and $\frac{v}{\mu}$ (d) $n, \frac{\lambda}{\mu}$ and $\frac{v}{\mu}$

4. The refractive index of water is 1.33 . What will be the speed of light in water? **(1996)**

(a) 4×10^8 m/s (b) 1.33×10^8 m/s
(c) 3×10^8 m/s (d) 2.25×10^8 m/s

5. Light travels through a glass plate of thickness t and having a refractive index μ. If c is the velocity of light in vacuum, the time taken by light to travel this thickness of glass is **(1996)**

(a) $\frac{t}{\mu c}$ (b) $\frac{\mu t}{c}$
(c) $t\mu c$ (d) $\frac{tc}{\mu}$

6. A star, which is emitting radiation at a wavelength of 5000Å, is approaching the earth with a velocity of 1.5×10^4 m/s. The change in wavelength of the radiation as received on the earth is **(1995)**

(a) 25Å (b) 100Å
(c) zero (d) 2.5Å

7. Time taken by sunlight to pass through a window of thickness 4 mm whose refractive index is $\frac{3}{2}$ is **(1993)**

(a) 2×10^{-4} s (b) 2×10^8 s
(c) 2×10^{-11} s (d) 2×10^{11} s

8. A beam of monochromatic light is refracted from vacuum into a medium of refractive index 1.5. The wavelength of refracted light will be **(1992, 1991)**

(a) depend on intensity of refracted light
(b) same
(c) smaller
(d) larger.

9. Green light of wavelength 5460Å is incident on an air-glass interface. If the refractive index of glass is 1.5 , the wavelength of light in glass would be ($c = 3 \times 10^8$ m s^{-1}) **(1991)**

(a) 3640Å (b) 5460Å

(c) 4861Å (d) none of these.

Coherent and Incoherent Addition of Waves

10. The interference pattern is obtained with two coherent light sources of intensity ratio n. In the interference pattern, the ratio $\frac{I_{\max}-I_{\min}}{I_{\max}+I_{\min}}$ will be **(NEET-II 2016)**

(a) $\frac{\sqrt{n}}{n+1}$ (b) $\frac{2\sqrt{n}}{n+1}$

(c) $\frac{\sqrt{n}}{(n+1)^2}$ (d) $\frac{2\sqrt{n}}{(n+1)^2}$

11. Ratio of intensities of two waves are given by 4: 1. Then ratio of the amplitudes of the two waves is **(1991)**

(a) 2: 1 (b) 1: 2

(c) 4: 1 (d) 1: 4

12. Interference is possible in **(1989)**

(a) light waves only

(b) sound waves only

(c) both light and sound waves

(d) neither light nor sound waves.

Interference of Light Waves and Young's Experiment

13. For Young's double slit experiment, two statements are given below : **(2023)**

Statement I : If screen is moved away from the plane of slits, angular separation of the fringes remains constant.

Statement II : If the monochromatic source is replaced by another monochromatic source of larger wavelength, the angular separation of fringes decreases.

In the light of the above statements, choose the correct answer from the options given below:

(a) Both Statement I and Statement II are false

(b) Statement I is true but Statement II is false

(c) Statement I is false but Statement II is true

(d) Both Statement I and Statement II are true

14. In a Young's double slit experiment, a student observes 8 fringes in a certain segment of screen when a monochromatic light of 600 nm wavelength is used. If the wavelength of light is changed to 400 nm, then the number of fringes he would observe in the same region of the screen is **(2022)**

(a) 6 (b) 8

(c) 9 (d) 12

15. In Young's double slit experiment, if the separation between coherent sources is halved and the distance of the screen from the coherent sources is doubled, then the fringe width becomes **(2020)**

(a) double (b) half

(c) four times (d) one-fourth

16. In a double slit experiment, when light of wavelength 400 nm was used, the angular width of the first minima formed on a screen placed 1 m away, was found to be $0.2°$. What will be the angular width of the first minima, if the entire experimental apparatus is immersed in water? ($\mu_{\text{water}} = 4/3$) **(2019)**

(a) $0.1°$ (b) $0.266°$

(c) $0.15°$ (d) $0.05°$

17. In a Young' double slit experiment if there is no initial phase difference between the light from the two slits, a point on the screen corresponding to the fifth minimum has path difference.

(Odisha NEET 2019)

(a) $5\frac{\lambda}{2}$ (b) $10\frac{\lambda}{2}$

(c) $9\frac{\lambda}{2}$ (d) $11\frac{\lambda}{2}$

18. In Young's double slit experiment the separation d between the slits is 2 mm, the wavelength λ of the light used is 5896Å and distance D between the screen and slits is 100 cm. It is found that the angular width of the fringes is $0.20°$. To increase the fringe angular width to $0.21°$ (with same λ and D) the separation between the slits needs to be changed to **(2018)**

(a) 1.8 mm (b) 1.9 mm

(c) 2.1 mm (d) 1.7 mm

19. Young's double slit experiment is first performed in air and then in a medium other than air. It is found that 8th bright fringe in the medium lies where 5th dark fringe lies in air. The refractive index of the medium is nearly **(2017)**

(a) 1.59 (b) 1.69

(c) 1.78 (d) 1.25

20. The intensity at the maximum in a Young's double slit experiment is I_0. Distance between two slits is $d = 5\lambda$, where λ is the wavelength of light used in the experiment. What will be the intensity in front of one of the slits on the screen placed at a distance $D = 10d$?

(NEET-I 2016)

(a) $\frac{3}{4}I_0$ (b) $\frac{I_0}{2}$

(c) I_0 (d) $\frac{I_0}{4}$

21. Two slits in Young's experiment have widths in the ratio $1:25$. The ratio of intensity at the maxima and minima in the interference pattern, $\frac{I_{\max}}{I_{\min}}$ is **(2015)**

(a) $\frac{49}{121}$ (b) $\frac{4}{9}$

(c) $\frac{9}{4}$ (d) $\frac{121}{49}$

22. In the Young's double slit experiment, the intensity of light at a point on the screen where the path difference λ is K, (λ being the wavelength of light used). The intensity at a point where the path difference is $\lambda/4$ will be **(2014)**

(a) K (b) $K/4$

(c) $K/2$ (d) zero

23. In Young's double slit experiment, the slits are 2 mm apart and are illuminated by photons of two wavelengths $\lambda_1 = 12000$Å and $\lambda_2 = 10000$Å. At what minimum distance from the common central bright fringe on the screen 2 m from the slit will a bright fringe from one interference pattern coincide with a bright fringe from the other? **(2013)**

(a) 4 mm (b) 3 mm
(c) 8 mm (d) 6 mm

24. In Young's double slit experiment the distance between the slits and the screen is doubled. The separation between the slits is reduced to half. As a result the fringe width **(Karnataka NEET 2013)**

(a) is halved
(b) becomes four times
(c) remains unchanged
(d) is doubled.

25. Colours appear on a thin soap film and on soap bubbles due to the phenomenon of **(1999)**

(a) interference (b) dispersion
(c) refraction (d) diffraction.

26. In a Fresnel biprism experiment, the two positions of lens give separation between the slits as 16 cm and 9 cm respectively. What is the actual distance of separation? **(1995)**

(a) 13 cm (b) 14 cm
(c) 12.5 cm (d) 12 cm

27. Interference was observed in interference chamber where air was present, now the chamber is evacuated, and if the same light is used, a careful observer will see **(1993)**

(a) no interference
(b) interference with brighter bands
(c) interference with dark bands
(d) interference with larger width.

28. If yellow light emitted by sodium lamp in Young's double slit experiment is replaced by monochromatic blue light of the same intensity **(1992)**

(a) fringe width will decrease
(b) fringe width will increase
(c) fringe width will remain unchanged
(d) fringes will becomes less intense

29. In Young's double slit experiment carried out with light of wavelength $(\lambda) = 5000\text{Å}$, the distance between the slits is 0.2 mm and the screen is at 200 cm from the slits. The central maximum is at $x = 0$. The third maximum (taking the central maximum as zeroth maximum) will be at x equal to **(1992)**

(a) 1.67 cm (b) 1.5 cm
(c) 0.5 cm (d) 5.0 cm

30. In Young's experiment, two coherent sources are placed 0.90 mm apart and fringes are observed one metre away. If it produces second dark fringe at a distance of 1 mm from central fringe, the wavelength of monochromatic light is used would be **(1991)**

(a) 60×10^{-4} cm (b) 10×10^{-4} cm
(c) 10×10^{-5} cm (d) 6×10^{-5} cm

31. In Young's double slit experiment, the fringes width is found to be 0.4 mm. If the whole apparatus is immersed in water of refractive index $\frac{4}{3}$, without disturbing the geometrical arrangement, the new fringe width will be **(1990)**

(a) 0.30 mm (b) 0.40 mm
(c) 0.53 mm (d) 450 micron.

32. The Young's double slit experiment is performed with blue and with green light of wavelengths 4360Å and 5460Å respectively. If x is the distance of 4th maxima from the central one, then

(1990)

(a) x (blue) $= x$ (green)

(b) x (blue) $> x$ (green)

(c) x (blue) $< x$ (green)

(d) $\frac{x\text{ (blue)}}{x\text{ (green)}} = \frac{5460}{4360}$

Diffraction

33. Assume that light of wavelength 600 nm is coming from a star. The limit of resolution of telescope whose objective has a diameter of 2 m is **(2020)**

(a) 3.66×10^{-7}rad (b) 1.83×10^{-7}rad

(c) 7.32×10^{-7}rad (d) 6.00×10^{-7}rad

34. An astronomical refracting telescope will have large angular magnification and high angular resolution, when it has an objective lens of **(2018)**

(a) small focal length and large diameter

(b) large focal length and small diameter

(c) large focal length and large diameter

(d) small focal length and small diameter.

35. The ratio of resolving powers of an optical microscope for two wavelengths $\lambda_1 = 4000$Å and $\lambda_2 = 6000$Å is **(2017)**

(a) 9: 4 (b) 3: 2

(c) 16: 81 (d) 8: 27

36. A linear aperture whose width is 0.02 cm is placed immediately in front of a lens of focal length 60 cm. The aperture is illuminated normally by a parallel beam of wavelength 5×10^{-5} cm. The distance of the first dark band of the diffraction pattern from the centre of the screen is

(NEET-II 2016)

(a) 0.10 cm (b) 0.25 cm

(c) 0.20 cm (d) 0.15 cm

37. In a diffraction pattern due to a single slit of width a, the first minimum is observed at an angle 30° when light of wavelength 5000Å is incident on the slit. The first secondary maximum is observed at an angle of **(NEET-I 2016)**

(a) $\sin^{-1}\left(\frac{1}{2}\right)$ (b) $\sin^{-1}\left(\frac{3}{4}\right)$

(c) $\sin^{-1}\left(\frac{1}{4}\right)$ (d) $\sin^{-1}\left(\frac{2}{3}\right)$

38. In a double slit experiment, the two slits are 1 mm apart and the screen is placed 1 m away. A monochromatic light of wavelength 500 nm is used. What will be the width of each slit for obtaining ten maxima of double slit within the central maxima of single slit pattern?

(2015 Cancelled)

(a) 0.5 mm (b) 0.02 mm

(c) 0.2 mm (d) 0.1 mm

39. At the first minimum adjacent to the central maximum of a single-slit diffraction pattern, the phase difference between the Huygen's wavelet from the edge of the slit and the wavelet from the midpoint of the slit is **(2015)**

(a) π radian (b) $\frac{\pi}{8}$ radian

(c) $\frac{\pi}{4}$ radian (d) $\frac{\pi}{2}$ radian

40. A beam of light of $\lambda = 600$ nm from a distant source falls on a single slit 1 mm wide and the resulting diffraction pattern is observed on a screen 2 m away. The distance between first dark fringes on either side of the central bright fringe is **(2014)**

(a) 1.2 cm (b) 1.2 mm

(c) 2.4 cm (d) 2.4 mm

41. A parallel beam of fast moving electrons is incident normally on a narrow slit. A fluorescent screen is placed at a large distance from the slit. If the speed of the electrons is increased, which of the following statements is correct? **(2013)**

(a) The angular width of the central maximum will decrease.

(b) The angular width of the central maximum will be unaffected.

(c) Diffraction pattern is not observed on the screen in the case of electrons.

(d) The angular width of the central maximum of the diffraction pattern will increase.

42. A parallel beam of light of wavelength λ is incident normally on a narrow slit. A diffraction pattern formed on a screen placed perpendicular to the direction of the incident beam. At the second minimum of the diffraction pattern, the phase difference between the rays coming from the two edges of slit is

(Karnataka NEET 2013)

(a) 2π (b) 3π

(c) 4π (d) $\pi\lambda$

43. The angular resolution of a 10 cm diameter telescope at a wavelength of 5000Å is of the order of **(2005)**

(a) 10^{6}rad (b) 10^{-2}rad

(c) 10^{-4}rad (d) 10^{-6}rad

44. A telescope has an objective lens of 10 cm diameter and is situated at a distance of one kilometre from two objects. The minimum distance between these two objects, which can be resolved by the telescope, when the mean wavelength of light is 5000Å, is of the order of **(2004)**

(a) 0.5 m (b) 5 m

(c) 5 mm (d) 5 cm

45. Diameter of human eye lens is 2 mm. What will be the minimum distance between two points to resolve them, which are situated at a distance of 50 meter from eye? (The wavelength of light is 5000Å.)

(2002)

(a) 2.32 m (b) 4.28 mm

(c) 1.25 cm (d) 12.48 cm

46. Ray optics is valid, when characteristic dimensions are **(1994, 1989)**

(a) much smaller than the wavelength of light

(b) of the same order as the wavelength of light

(c) of the order of one millimetre

(d) much larger than the wavelength of light.

47. A parallel beam of monochromatic light of wavelength 5000Å is incident normally on a single narrow slit of width 0.001 mm. The light is focussed by a convex lens on a screen placed in focal plane.

The first minimum will be formed for the angle of diffraction equal to **(1993)**

(a) 0° (b) 15°

(c) 30° (d) 50°

Polarisation

48. The Brewsters angle i_b for an interface should be **(2020)**

(a) $0° < i_b < 30°$ (b) $30° < i_b < 45°$

(c) $45° < i_b < 90°$ (d) $i_b = 90°$

49. Unpolarised light is incident from air on a plane surface of a material of refractive index μ. At a particular angle of incidence i, it is found that the reflected and refracted rays are perpendicular to each other. Which of the following options is correct for this situation? **(2018)**

(a) Reflected light is polarised with its electric vector parallel to the plane of incidence.

(b) Reflected light is polarised with its electric vector perpendicular to the plane of incidence.

(c) $i = \sin^{-1}\left(\frac{1}{\mu}\right)$

(d) $i = \tan^{-1}\left(\frac{1}{\mu}\right)$

51. Two polaroids P_1 and P_2 are placed with their axis perpendicular to each other. Unpolarised light I_0 is incident on P_1. A third polaroid P_3 is kept in between P_1 and P_2 such that its axis makes an angle 45° with that of P_1. The intensity of transmitted light through P_2 is **(2017)**

(a) $\frac{I_0}{4}$ (b) $\frac{I_0}{8}$

(c) $\frac{I_0}{16}$ (d) $\frac{I_0}{2}$

51. Which of the phenomenon is not common to sound and light waves? **(1988)**

(a) Interference (b) Diffraction

(c) Coherence (d) Polarisation

ANSWER KEY

1.	(d)	2.	(b)	3.	(d)	4.	(d)	5.	(b)	6.	(a)	7.	(c)
8.	(c)	9.	(a)	10.	(b)	11.	(a)	12.	(c)	13.	(b)	14.	(d)
15.	(c)	16.	(c)	17.	(c)	18.	(b)	19.	(c)	20.	(b)	21.	(c)
22.	(c)	23.	(d)	24.	(b)	25.	(a)	26.	(d)	27.	(d)	28.	(a)
29.	(b)	30.	(d)	31.	(a)	32.	(c)	33.	(a)	34.	(c)	35.	(b)
36.	(d)	37.	(b)	38.	(c)	39.	(a)	40.	(d)	41.	(a)	42.	(c)
43.	(c)	44.	(c)	45.	(c)	46.	(d)	47.	(c)	48.	(c)	49.	(b)
50.	(b)	51.	(d)										

Hints & Explanations

1. **(d)**: Huygen's construction of wavefront does not apply to origin of spectra which is explained by quantum theory.

2. **(b)** : $\mu = \frac{\text{velocity of light in vacuum } (c)}{\text{velocity of light in medium (v)}}$

$\therefore\ v = \nu\lambda = 2 \times 10^{14} \times 5000 \times 10^{-10} =$

10^8 m/s $\therefore\ \mu = \frac{c}{v_{med}} = \frac{3\times10^8}{10^8} = 3.54$

3. **(d)**: Frequency $= n$; Wavelength $= \lambda$; Velocity of light in air $= v$ and refractive index of glass slab $= \mu$

Frequency of light remains the same, when it changes the medium. Refractive index is the ratio of wavelengths in vacuum

and in the given medium. Similarly refractive index is also the ratio of velocities in vacuum and in the given medium.

4. **(d)** : Refractive index of water $(\mu_2) =$ 1.33.

$$\frac{v_2}{v_1} = \frac{\mu_1}{\mu_2} = \frac{1}{1.33}$$

Therefore $v_2 = \frac{v_1}{1.33} = \frac{3\times10^8}{1.33} = 2.25 \times$ 10^8 m/s

5. **(b)** : Time $= \frac{\text{distance}}{\text{velocity}} = \frac{t}{v} = \frac{t}{c/\mu} = \frac{\mu t}{c}$

6. **(a)**: Wavelength (λ) = 5000Å and velocity $(v) = 1.5 \times 10^4$ m/s

Wavelength of the approaching star,

$\lambda' == \lambda\frac{c-v}{c}$ or $\frac{\lambda'}{\lambda} = 1 - \frac{v}{c}$ or, $\frac{v}{c} = 1 - \frac{\lambda'}{\lambda} =$ $\frac{\lambda-\lambda'}{\lambda} = \frac{\Delta\lambda}{\lambda}$

Therefore $\Delta\lambda = \lambda \times \frac{v}{c} = 5000Å \times \frac{1.5\times10^6}{3\times10^8} =$ 25Å

(here $\Delta\lambda$ is the change in the wavelength)

$$\text{(c)} : v_g = \frac{c}{\mu} = \frac{3 \times 10^8}{\frac{3}{2}} = 2 \times 10^8 \text{ m/s}$$

$$t = \frac{x}{v_g} = \frac{4 \times 10^{-3}}{2 \times 10^8} = 2 \times 10^{-11} \text{ s}$$

8. **(c)** : λ' of refracted light is smaller, because $\lambda' = \frac{\lambda}{\mu}$

9. **(a)** : $\lambda_g = \frac{\lambda_a}{\mu} = \frac{5460}{1.5} = 3640$Å

10. **(b)**: Here, $\frac{I_1}{I_2} = n$

$$\frac{I_{max}}{I_{min}} = \left(\frac{\sqrt{I_1} + \sqrt{I_2}}{\sqrt{I_1} - \sqrt{I_2}}\right)^2 = \left(\frac{\sqrt{I_1/I_2} + 1}{\sqrt{I_1/I_2} - 1}\right)^2$$

$$= \left(\frac{\sqrt{n} + 1}{\sqrt{n} - 1}\right)^2$$

$$\frac{I_{max} - I_{min}}{I_{max} + I_{min}} = \frac{\frac{I_{max}}{I_{min}} - 1}{\frac{I_{max}}{I_{min}} + 1}$$

$$= \frac{\left(\frac{\sqrt{n} + 1}{\sqrt{n} - 1}\right)^2 - 1}{\left(\frac{\sqrt{n} + 1}{\sqrt{n} - 1}\right)^2 + 1} = \frac{(\sqrt{n} + 1)^2 - (\sqrt{n} - 1)^2}{(\sqrt{n} + 1)^2 + (\sqrt{n} - 1)^2}$$

$$= \frac{4\sqrt{n}}{2(n+1)} = \frac{2\sqrt{n}}{n+1}$$

11. **(a):** $\frac{I_1}{I_2} = \frac{a^2}{b^2} = \frac{4}{1} \therefore \frac{a}{b} = \frac{2}{1}$

12. **(c) :** Interference is a wave phenomenon shown by both the light waves and sound waves.

13. **(b) :** Angular width, $\theta_w = \frac{\lambda}{d}$ θ_w

independent of D but depends on λ

14. **(d):** As we know, wavelength of light is inversely proportional to number of fringes observed.

$\therefore \lambda_1 n_1 = \lambda_2 n_2$

$$n_2 = \frac{\lambda_1 n_1}{\lambda_2} = \frac{600 \times 8}{400} = 12$$

15. **(c)** Fringe width, $\beta = \frac{D\lambda}{d}$

d becomes half $\Rightarrow d' = d/2$ D doubles, so

$\Rightarrow D' = 2D$

New fringe width, $\beta' = \frac{2D\lambda}{\left(\frac{d}{2}\right)} = 4\beta$

16. **(c) :** Angular width for first minima in Young's double slit experiment, $\theta = \frac{\lambda}{a}$

For given value of $a, \theta \propto \lambda$

$$\frac{\theta}{\theta_w} = \frac{\lambda}{\lambda_w} = \frac{\lambda}{\frac{\lambda}{\mu}} = \mu \Rightarrow \theta_w = \frac{\theta}{\mu} = \frac{0.2^\circ}{\frac{4}{3}}$$

$$= 0.15^\circ$$

17. **(c):** Given, there is no initial phase difference.

$\therefore$ Initial phase $= \delta = 0$

Again, phase difference $= \frac{2\pi}{\lambda} \times$ path difference

$$\Rightarrow \delta' = \frac{2\pi}{\lambda} \times \Delta x \Rightarrow \Delta x = \frac{\lambda}{2\pi} \times \delta'$$

Now, for the fifth minima we will consider $n = 4$ as initial phase difference is zero.

$\therefore$ For fifth minimum, $\delta' = (8+1)\pi = 9\pi$

$\therefore$ Path difference, $\Delta x = \frac{\lambda}{2\pi} \times 9\pi = \frac{9\lambda}{2}$

18. **(b) :** Angular width $= \frac{\lambda}{d}$

$0.20^\circ = \frac{\lambda}{2\text{ mm}}$ and $0.21^\circ = \frac{\lambda}{d}$

On dividing we get, $\frac{0.20}{0.21} = \frac{d}{2\text{ mm}}$

$\therefore d = 1.9$ mm

19. **(c) :** Position of 8th bright fringe in medium,

$$x = \frac{8\lambda_m D}{d}$$

Position of 5th dark fringe in air,

$$x' = \frac{\left(5 - \frac{1}{2}\right)\lambda_{air} D}{d} = \frac{4.5\lambda_{air} D}{d}$$

Given $x = x' \Rightarrow \frac{8\lambda_m D}{d} = \frac{4.5\lambda_{air} D}{d}$

$$\mu_m = \frac{\lambda_{air}}{\lambda_m} = \frac{8}{4.5} = 1.78$$

20. **(b):** Here, $d = 5\lambda, D = 10d, y = \frac{d}{2}$

Resultant Intensity at $y = \frac{d}{2}, I_y = ?$

The path difference between two waves at $y = \frac{d}{2}$.

$$\Delta x = d\tan\theta = d\times\frac{y}{D} = \frac{d\times\frac{d}{2}}{10d} = \frac{d}{20} = \frac{5\lambda}{20}$$
$$= \frac{\lambda}{4}$$

Corresponding phase difference, $\phi = \frac{2\pi}{\lambda}\Delta x = \frac{\pi}{2}$

Now, maximum intensity in Young's double slit experiment,

$$I_{\max} = I_1 + I_2 + 2I_1I_2 \text{ or } I_0 = 4I$$

$(\because I_1 = I_2 = I)$

$\therefore \quad I = \frac{I_0}{4}$

Required intensity,

$$I_y = I_1 + I_2 + 2I_1I_2\cos\frac{\pi}{2} = 2I = \frac{I_0}{2}$$

21. **(c) :** As, intensity $I \propto$ width of slit W

Also, intensity $I \propto$ square of amplitude A

$$\therefore \quad \frac{I_1}{I_2} = \frac{W_1}{W_2} = \frac{A_1^2}{A_2^2}$$

But $\frac{W_1}{W_2} = \frac{1}{25}$ (given) $\therefore \frac{A_1^2}{A_2^2} = \frac{1}{25}$ or $\frac{A_1}{A_2} = \sqrt{\frac{1}{25}} = \frac{1}{5}$

$$\therefore \quad \frac{I_{\max}}{I_{\min}} = \frac{(A_1+A_2)^2}{(A_1-A_2)^2} = \frac{\left(\frac{A_1}{A_2}+1\right)^2}{\left(\frac{A_1}{A_2}-1\right)^2}$$

$$= \frac{\left(\frac{1}{5}+1\right)^2}{\left(\frac{1}{5}-1\right)^2} = \frac{\left(\frac{6}{5}\right)^2}{\left(-\frac{4}{5}\right)^2} = \frac{36}{16} = \frac{9}{4}$$

22. **(c):** Intensity at any point on the screen is

$$I = 4I_0\cos^2\frac{\phi}{2}$$

where I_0 is the intensity of either wave and ϕ is the phase difference between two waves.

Phase difference, $\phi = \frac{2\pi}{\lambda}\times$ Path difference

When path difference is λ, then

$$\phi = \frac{2\pi}{\lambda}\times\lambda = 2\pi$$

$$\therefore I = 4I_0\cos^2\left(\frac{2\pi}{2}\right) = 4I_0\cos^2(\pi) = 4I_0 = K$$

When path difference is $\frac{\lambda}{4}$, then

$$\phi = \frac{2\pi}{\lambda}\times\frac{\lambda}{4} = \frac{\pi}{2} \quad \therefore I = 4I_0\cos^2\left(\frac{\pi}{4}\right) = 2I_0 = \frac{K}{2}$$

[Using (i)]

23. **(d) :** Let n_1 bright fringe of λ_1 coincides with n_2 bright fringe of λ_2. Then

$\frac{n_1\lambda_1 D}{d} = \frac{n_2\lambda_2 D}{d}$ or

$$n_1\lambda_1 = n_2\lambda_2 \Rightarrow \frac{n_1}{n_2} = \frac{\lambda_2}{\lambda_1} = \frac{10000}{12000} = \frac{5}{6}$$

Let x be given distance.

$$\therefore x = \frac{n_1\lambda_1 D}{d}$$

Here, $n_1 = 5, D = 2\text{ m}, d = 2\text{ mm} = 2\times 10^{-3}\text{ m}$

$$\lambda_1 = 12000\text{Å} = 12000\times10^{-10}\text{ m}$$
$$= 12\times10^{-7}\text{ m}$$

$$x = \frac{5\times12\times10^{-7}\text{ m}\times 2\text{ m}}{2\times10^{-3}\text{ m}} = 6\times10^{-3}\text{ m}$$
$$= 6\text{ mm}$$

24. **(b) :** Fringe width, $\beta = \frac{\lambda D}{d}$

where D is the distance between slits and screen and d is the distance between the slits.

When D is doubled and d is reduced to half, then fringe width becomes

$$\beta' = \frac{\lambda(2D)}{(d/2)} = \frac{4\lambda D}{d} = 4\beta$$

25. **(a)**

26. **(d) :** Separations between the slits $d_1 =$ 16 cm and $d_2 = 9$ cm Actual distance of separation

$$d = \sqrt{d_1 d_2} = \sqrt{16 \times 9} = 12 \text{ cm}$$

27. **(d):** In vacuum, λ increases very slightly compared to that in air. As $\beta \propto \lambda$, therefore, width of interference fringe increases slightly.

28. **(a) :** As $\beta = \frac{\lambda D}{d}$ and $\lambda_b < \lambda_y$,

$\therefore$ Fringe width β will decrease.

29. **(b) :** $x = (n)\lambda\frac{D}{d} = 3 \times 5000 \times 10^{-10} \times \frac{2}{0.2\times10^{-3}}$

$$= 1.5 \times 10^{-2} \text{ m} = 1.5 \text{ cm}$$

30. **(d) :** For dark fringe, $x = (2n-1)\frac{\lambda D}{2d}$

$$\lambda = \frac{2xd}{(2n-1)D} = \frac{2 \times 10^{-3} \times 0.9 \times 10^{-3}}{(2 \times 2 - 1) \times 1}$$

$$\lambda = 0.6 \times 10^{-6} \text{ m} = 6 \times 10^{-5} \text{ cm}$$

31. **(a):** $\beta' = \frac{\beta}{\mu} = \frac{0.4}{4/3} = 0.3$ mm

32. **(c) :** Distance of nth maxima $x = n\lambda\frac{D}{d} \propto \lambda$

As $\lambda_b < \lambda_g$ $\therefore$ x (blue) < x (green)

33. **(a):** Given $\lambda = 600$ nm $= 600 \times 10^{-9}$ m and $D = 2$ m

$\therefore$ Limit of resolution $= \frac{1.22\lambda}{D} = \frac{1.22\times600\times10^{-9}}{2}$

$$= 366 \times 10^{-9} = 3.66 \times 10^{-7} \text{rad}$$

34. **(c):** For telescope, angular magnification $= \frac{f_0}{f_e}$

Angular resolution $= \frac{D}{1.22\lambda}$ should be large.

So, objective lens should have large focal length (f_0) and large diameter D for large angular magnification and high angular resolution.

35. **(b) :** The resolving power of an optical microscope,

$$\text{RP} = \frac{2\mu\sin\theta}{\lambda}$$

For wavelength $\lambda_1 = 4000$Å, resolving power will be

$$\text{RP}_1 = \frac{2\mu\sin\theta}{4000}$$

For wavelength $\lambda_2 = 6000$Å, resolving power will be

$$\text{RP}_2 = \frac{2\mu\sin\theta}{6000}$$

On dividing eqn. (i) by eqn. (ii)

$$\frac{RP_1}{RP_2} = \frac{6000}{4000} = \frac{3}{2}$$

36. **(d) :** Here, $a = 0.02$ cm $= 2 \times 10^{-4}$ m

$\lambda = 5 \times 10^{-5}$ cm $= 5 \times 10^{-7}$ m $\Rightarrow D$

$= 60$ cm $= 0.6$ m

Position of first minima on the diffraction pattern,

$$y = \frac{D\lambda}{a} = \frac{0.6 \times 5 \times 10^{-7}}{2 \times 10^{-4}} = 15 \times 10^{-4} \text{ m}$$

$= 0.15$ cm

37. **(b) :** For first minimum, the path difference between extreme waves,

$a\sin\theta = \lambda$

Here $\theta = 30° \Rightarrow \sin\theta = \frac{1}{2} \therefore a = 2\lambda$

For first secondary maximum, the path difference between extreme waves

$a\sin\theta' = \frac{3}{2}\lambda$ or $(2\lambda)\sin\theta' = \frac{3}{2}\lambda$. [Using eqn (i)]

or $\sin\theta' = \frac{3}{4} \therefore \theta' = \sin^{-1}\left(\frac{3}{4}\right)$

38. **(c) :** For double slit experiment,

$d = 1$ mm $= 1 \times 10^{-3}$ m, $D = 1$ m, λ

$= 500 \times 10^{-9}$ m

Fringe width $\beta = \frac{D\lambda}{d}$.

Width of central maxima in a single slit

$= \frac{2\lambda D}{a}$

As per question, width of central maxima of single slit pattern = width of 10 maxima of double slit pattern

$\frac{2\lambda D}{a} = 10\left(\frac{\lambda D}{d}\right)$ or $a = \frac{2d}{10} = \frac{2\times10^{-3}}{10} = 0.2 \times$

10^{-3} m $= 0.2$ mm

39. **(a):** The situation is shown in the figure.

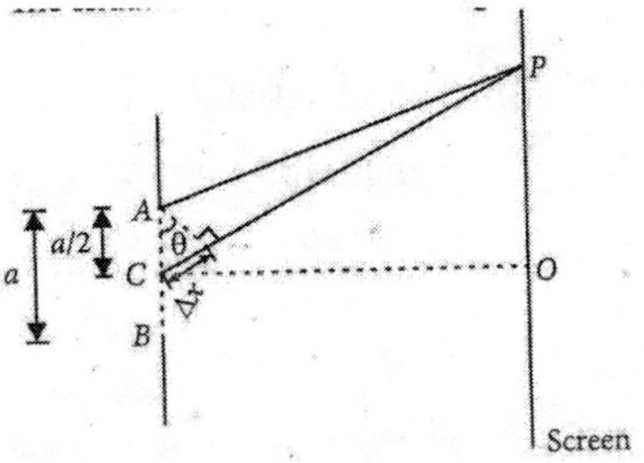

In figure A and B represent the edges of the slit AB of width a and C represents the midpoint of the slit.

For the first minimum at P,

$$a\sin\theta = \lambda$$

where λ is the wavelength of light.

The path difference between the wavelets from A to C is

$$\Delta x = \frac{a}{2}\sin\theta = \frac{1}{2}(a\sin\theta) = \frac{\lambda}{2} \text{ (using(i))}$$

The corresponding phase difference $\Delta\phi$ is

$$\Delta\phi = \frac{2\pi}{\lambda}\Delta x = \frac{2\pi}{\lambda} \times \frac{\lambda}{2} = \pi$$

40. **(d) :** Here, $\lambda = 600$ nm $= 600 \times 10^{-9}$ m

$a = 1$ mm $= 10^{-3}$ m, $D = 2$ m

Distance between the first dark fringes on either side of the central bright fringe is also the width of central maximum.

Width of central maximum $= \frac{2\lambda D}{a}$

$$= \frac{2 \times 600 \times 10^{-9}\ m \times 2\ m}{10^{-3}\ m}$$

$= 24 \times 10^{-4}$ m

$= 2.4 \times 10^{-3}$ m

$= 2.4$ mm

41. **(a)**

42. **(c):** For the second minimum,

Path difference $= 2\lambda$

Therefore, corresponding value of phase difference is

$$\Delta\phi = \frac{2\pi}{\lambda} \times \text{ Path difference } = \frac{2\pi}{\lambda} \times 2\lambda$$

$= 4\pi$

43. **(c) :** R.P. $= 1/\Delta\theta$

The angular resolution, $\Delta\theta = \frac{1.22\lambda}{D}$

$$= \frac{1.22 \times 5000 \times 10^{-8}}{0.1} = 6.1 \times 10^{-4}$$

$\simeq 10^{-4}$rad

44. **(c) :** Resolution of telescope

$$d\theta = 1.22\frac{\lambda}{D} = 1.22 \times \frac{5000 \times 10^{-8}}{10}$$

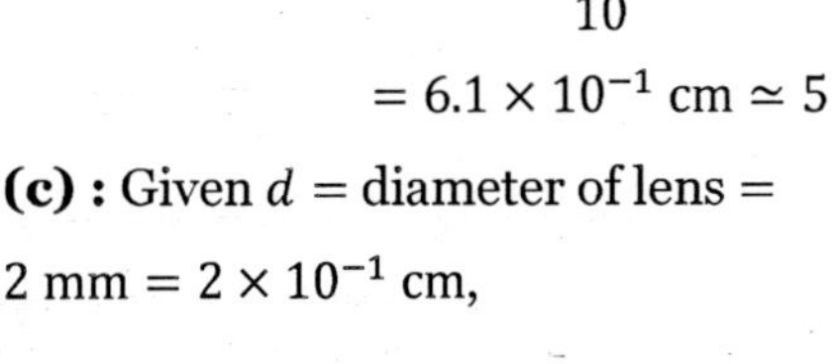

$$x = d\theta \times d = \frac{1.22 \times 5000 \times 10^{-8} \times 10^5}{10}$$

$= 6.1 \times 10^{-1}$ cm $\simeq 5$ mm

45. **(c) :** Given d = diameter of lens =

2 mm $= 2 \times 10^{-1}$ cm,

$\lambda = 5000$Å $= 5000 \times 10^{-8}$ cm

Resolving power of eye lens

$$= \frac{d}{\lambda} = \frac{2 \times 10^{-1}}{5000 \times 10^{-8}} = \frac{1}{d\theta}$$

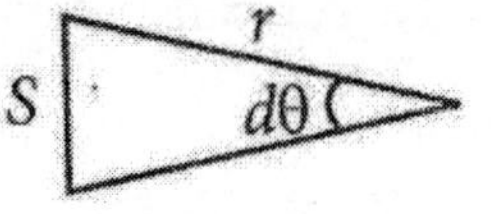

Let S be the minimum distance between two points so that it may be resolved.

$\therefore S = rd\theta$. Here $r = 50$ m $= 5000$ cm

$$\therefore\ S = 5000 \times \frac{5000 \times 10^{-8}}{2 \times 10^{-1}} = 1.25 \text{ cm}$$

46. **(d)**

47. **(c):** For first minimum, $a\sin\theta = n\lambda = 1\lambda$

$$\sin\theta = \frac{\lambda}{a} = \frac{5000 \times 10^{-10}}{0.001 \times 10^{-3}} = 0.5 \text{ or } \theta = 30°$$

48. **(c) :** We know, $\mu = \tan i_b$

As $1 < \mu < \infty\ \therefore\ 1 < \tan i_b < \infty$

$\tan(45°) < \tan i_b < \tan(90°)$ or $45° < i_b < 90°$.

49. **(b) :** When reflected light and refracted light are perpendicular, reflected light is polarised with electric field vector perpendicular to the plane of incidence.

Also, $\tan i = \mu$ (Brewster angle)

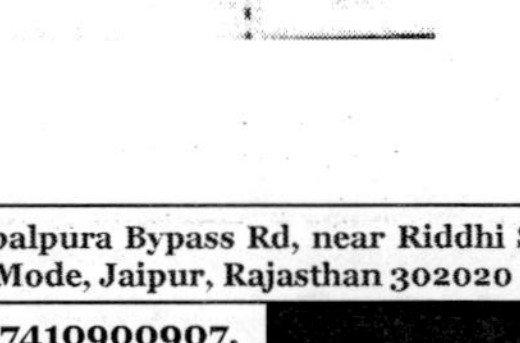

50. **(b) :** The intensity of transmitted light through P_1

$$I_1 = \frac{I_0}{2}$$

The intensity of transmitted light through P_3

$$I_2 = I_1 \cos^2 45° = \frac{I_0}{2}\left(\frac{1}{\sqrt{2}}\right)^2 = \frac{I_0}{2} \cdot \frac{1}{2} = \frac{I_0}{4}$$

Angle between polaroids P_3 and $P_2 = (90° - 45°) = 45°$

∴ Intensity of transmitted light through P_2,

$$I_3 = I_2 \cos^2 45° = \frac{I_0}{4}\left(\frac{1}{\sqrt{2}}\right)^2 = \frac{I_0}{8}$$

51. **(d):** Sound waves can not be polarised as they are longitudinal. Light waves can be polarised as they are transverse.

Chapter: 25 DUAL NATURE OF RADIATON AND MATTER

Introduction

1. A beam of cathode rays is subjected to crossed electric (E) and magnetic fields (B). The fields are adjusted such that the beam is not deflected. The specific charge of the cathode rays is given by **(2010)**

(a) $\frac{B^2}{2VE^2}$ (b) $\frac{2VB^2}{E^2}$

(c) $\frac{2VE^2}{B^2}$ (d) $\frac{E^2}{2VB^2}$

2. In the phenomenon of electric discharge through gases at low pressure, the coloured glow in the tube appears as a result of **(2008)**

(a) collisions between the charged particles emitted from the cathode and the atoms of the gas

(b) collision between different electrons of the atoms of the gas

(c) excitation of electrons in the atoms

(d) collision between the atoms of the gas atoms in the gas.

3. In a discharge tube ionization of enclosed gas is produced due to collisions between **(2006)**

(a) neutral gas atoms/molecules

(b) positive ions and neutral atoms/molecules

(c) negative electrons and neutral atoms/molecules

(d) photons and neutral atoms/molecules.

4. J.J. Thomson's cathode-ray tube experiment demonstrated that **(2003)**

(a) cathode rays are streams of negatively charged ions

(b) all the mass of an atom is essentially in the nucleus

(c) the e/m of electrons is much greater than the e/m of protons

(d) the e/m ratio of the cathode-ray particles changes when a different gas is placed in the discharge tube

5. Which of the following is not the property of cathode rays? **(2002)**

(a) It produces heating effect.

(b) It does not deflect in electric field.

(c) It casts shadow.

(d) It produces fluorescence.

6. Who evaluated the mass of electron indirectly with help of charge? **(2000)**

(a) Thomson (b) Millikan

(c) Rutherford (d) Newton

7. In a discharge tube at 0.02 mm, there is formation of **(1996)**

(a) Crooke's dark space

(b) Faraday's dark space

(c) both space partly

(d) none of these.

Electron Emission

8. In which of the following, emission of electrons does not take place **(1990)**

(a) thermionic emission

(b) X-rays emission

(c) photoelectric emission

(d) secondary emission

9. Thermions are **(1988)**

(a) protons (b) electrons

(c) photons (d) positrons.

Experimental Study of Photoelectric Effect

10. A source of light is placed at a distance of 50 cm from a photo cell and the stopping potential is found to be V_0. If the distance between the light source and photo cell is made 25 cm, the new stopping potential will be : **(Karnataka NEET 2013)**

(a) $V_0/2$ (b) V_0

(c) $4V_0$ (d) $2V_0$

11. Photoelectric emission occurs only when the incident light has more than a certain minimum **(2011)**

(a) power (b) wavelength

(c) intensity (d) frequency

12. In photoelectric emission process from a metal of work function 1.8eV, the kinetic energy of most energetic electrons is 0.5eV. The corresponding stopping potential is

(a) 1.8 V (b) 1.3 V

(c) 0.5 V (d) 2.3 V

13. When monochromatic radiation of intensity I falls on a metal surface, the number of photoelectrons and their maximum kinetic energy are N and T respectively. If the intensity of radiation is $2I$, the number of emitted electrons and their maximum kinetic energy are respectively **(Mains 2010)**

(a) N and 2 T (b) 2 N and T

(c) $2N$ and $2T$ (d) N and T

14. The number of photo electrons emitted for light of a frequency v (higher than the threshold frequency v_0) is proportional to **(2009)**

(a) threshold frequency (v_0)

(b) intensity of light

(c) frequency of light (v)

(d) $v - v_0$

15. The figure shows a plot of photo current versus anode potential for a photo sensitive surface for three different radiations. Which one of the following is a correct statement? **(2009)**

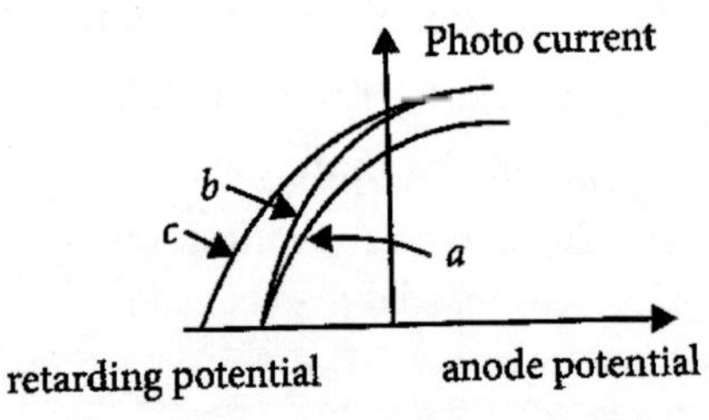

(a) Curves (a) and (b) represent incident radiations of same frequency but of different intensities.

(b) Curves (b) and (c) represent incident radiations of different frequencies and different intensities.

(c) Curves (b) and (c) represent incident radiations of same frequency having same intensity.

(d) Curves (a) and (b) represent incident radiations of different frequencies and different intensities

16. A 5 watt source emits monochromatic light of wavelength 5000. When placed 0.5 m away, it liberates photoelectrons from a photosensitive metallic surface. When the source is moved to a distance of 1.0 m, the number of photoelectrons liberated will be reduced by a factor of **(2007)**

(a) 8 (b) 16

(c) 2 (d) 4

17. A photocell employs photoelectric effect to convert **(2006)**

(a) change in the frequency of light into a change in the electric current

(b) change in the frequency of light into a change in electric voltage

(c) change in the intensity of illumination into a change in photoelectric current

(d) change in the intensity of illumination into a change in the work function of the photocathode.

18. A photoelectric cell is illuminated by a point source of light 1 m away. When the source is shifted to 2 m then **(2003)**

(a) each emitted electron carries one quarter of the initial energy

(b) number of electrons emitted is half the initial number

(c) each emitted electron carries half the initial energy

(d) number of electrons emitted is a quarter of the initial number.

19. When ultraviolet rays incident on metal plate then photoelectric effect does not occur, it occurs by incidence of **(2002)**

(a) infrared rays (b) X-rays

(c) radio wave (d) micro wave.

20. A photo-cell is illuminated by a source of light, which is placed at a distance d from the cell. If the distance become $d/2$, then number of electrons emitted per second will be **(2001)**

(a) remain same (b) four times

(c) two times (d) one-fourth.

21. As the intensity of incident light increases **(1999)**

(a) kinetic energy of emitted photoelectrons increases

(b) photoelectric current decreases

(c) photoelectric current increases

(d) kinetic energy of emitted photoelectrons decreases.

22. Which of the following statement is correct? **(1997)**

(a) The photocurrent increases with intensity of light.

(b) The stopping potential increases with increase of incident light.

(c) The current in photocell increases with increasing frequency.

(d) The photocurrent is proportional to the applied voltage.

23. Number of ejected photoelectrons increases with increase **(1993)**

(a) in intensity of light

(b) in wavelength of light

(c) in frequency of light

(d) never.

24. The cathode of a photoelectric cell is changed such that the work function changes from W_1 to W_2 ($W_2 > W_1$). If the current before and after changes are I_1 and I_2, all other conditions remaining unchanged, then (assuming $h\nu > W_2$) **(1992)**

(a) $I_1 = I_2$ (b) $I_1 < I_2$

(c) $I_1 > I_2$ (d) $I_1 < I_2 < 2I_1$

Photoelectric Effect and Wave Theory of Light

25. Light of frequency 1.5 times the threshold frequency is incident on a photosensitive material. What will be the photoelectric current if the frequency is halved and intensity is doubled? **(2020)**

(a) Doubled (b) Four times

(c) One-fourth (d) Zero

Einstein's Photoelectric Equation Energy Quantum of Radiation

26. The work functions of Caesium (Cs), potassium (K) and Sodium (Na) are 2.14 eV, 2.30 eV and 2.75 eV respectively. If incident electromagnetic radiation has an incident energy of 2.20 eV, which of these photosensitive surfaces may emit photoelectrons ? **(2023)**

(a) Both Na and K (b) K only

(c) Na only (d) Cs only

27. When two monochromatic light of frequency, v and $\frac{v}{2}$ are incident on a photoelectric metal, their stopping potential becomes $\frac{V_s}{2}$ and V_s respectively. The threshold frequency for this metal is **(2022)**

(a) $2v$ (b) $3v$

(c) $\frac{2}{3}v$ (d) $\frac{3}{2}v$

28. The work function of a photosensitive material is 4.0eV. The longest wavelength of light that can cause photon emission from the substance is (approximately) **(Odisha NEET 2019)**

(a) 3100 nm (b) 966 nm

(c) 31 nm (d) 310 nm

29. When the light of frequency $2v_0$ (where v_0 is threshold frequency), is incident on a metal plate, the maximum velocity of electrons emitted is v_1. When the frequency of the incident radiation is increased to $5v_0$, the maximum velocity of electrons emitted from the same plate is v_2. The ratio of v_1 to v_2 is **(2018)**

(a) 1: 2 (b) 1: 4

(c) 4: 1 (d) 2: 1

30. The photoelectric threshold wavelength of silver is 3250×10^{-10} m. The velocity of the electron ejected from a silver surface by ultraviolet light of wavelength 2536×10^{-10} m is [Given $h = 4.14 \times 10^{-15}$eVs and $c = 3 \times 10^8$ m s^{-1}] **(2017)**

(a) $\approx 0.6 \times 10^6$ m s^{-1}

(b) $\approx 61 \times 10^3$ m s^{-1}

(c) $\approx 0.3 \times 10^6$ m s^{-1}

(d) $\approx 6 \times 10^5$ m s^{-1}

31. Photons with energy 5eV are incident on a cathode C in a photoelectric cell. The maximum energy of emitted photoelectrons is 2eV. When photons of energy 6eV are incident on C, no photoelectrons will reach the anode A, if the stopping potential of A relative to C is

(NEET-II 2016)

(a) +3 V (b) +4 V

(c) −1 V (d) −3 V

32. When a metallic surface is illuminated with radiation of wavelength λ, the stopping potential is V. If the same surface is illuminated with radiation of wavelength 2λ, the stopping potential is $\frac{V}{4}$. The threshold wavelength for the metallic surface is **(NEET-I 2016)**

(a) $\frac{5}{2}\lambda$ (b) 3λ

(c) 4λ (d) 5λ

33. A photoelectric surface is illuminated successively by monochromatic light of wavelength λ and $\lambda/2$. If the maximum kinetic energy of the emitted photoelectrons in the second case is 3 times that in the first case, the work function of the surface of the material is (h = Planck's constant, c = speed of light)

(2015)

(a) $\frac{2hc}{\lambda}$ (b) $\frac{hc}{3\lambda}$

(c) $\frac{hc}{2\lambda}$ (d) $\frac{hc}{\lambda}$

34. A certain metallic surface is illuminated with monochromatic light of wavelength, λ. The stopping potential for photoelectric current for this light is $3V_0$. If the same surface is illuminated with light of wavelength 2λ, the stopping potential is V_0. The threshold wavelength for this surface for photoelectric effect is

(2015 Cancelled)

(a) $\frac{\lambda}{4}$ (b) $\frac{\lambda}{6}$

(c) 6λ (d) 4λ

35. When the energy of the incident radiation is increased by 20%, the kinetic energy of the photoelectrons emitted from a metal surface increased from 0.5eV to 0.8eV. The work function of the metal is **(2014)**

(a) 0.65eV (b) 1.0eV

(c) 1.3eV (d) 1.5eV

36. For photoelectric emission from certain metal the cutoff frequency is v. If radiation of frequency $2v$ impinges on the metal plate, the maximum possible velocity of the emitted electron will be (is the electron mass) **(2013)**

(a) $\sqrt{\frac{2hv}{m}}$ (b) $2\sqrt{\frac{hv}{m}}$

(c) $\sqrt{\frac{hv}{(2m)}}$ (d) $\sqrt{\frac{hv}{m}}$

37. Two radiations of photons energies 1eV and 2.5eV, successively illuminate a photosensitive metallic surface of work function 0.5eV. The ratio of the maximum speeds of the emitted electrons is

(Mains 2012, 2011)

(a) 1: 4 (b) 1: 2

(c) 1: 1 (d) 1: 5

38. The threshold frequency for a photosensitive metal is 3.3×10^{14} Hz. If light of frequency 8.2×10^{14} Hz is incident on this metal, the cut-off voltage for the photoelectron emission is nearly

(Mains 2011)

(a) 1 V (b) 2 V

(c) 3 V (d) 5 V

39. The potential difference that must be applied to stop the fastest photoelectrons emitted by a nickel surface, having work function 5.01eV, when ultraviolet light of 200 nm falls on it, must be **(2010)**

(a) 2.4 V (b) −1.2 V

(c) −2.4 V (d) 1.2 V

40. The work function of a surface of a photosensitive material is 6.2eV. The wavelength of the incident radiation for which the stopping potential is 5 V lies in the **(2008)**

(a) Infrared region

(b) X-ray region

(c) Ultraviolet region

(d) Visible region.

41. When photons of energy hv fall on an aluminium plate (of work function E_0), photoelectrons of maximum kinetic energy K are ejected. If the frequency of radiation is doubled, the maximum kinetic energy of the ejected photoelectrons will be **(2006)**

(a) $K + hv$ (b) $K + E_0$

(c) $2K$ (d) K

42. The work functions for metals A, B and C are respectively 1.92eV, 2.0eV and 5eV. According to Einstein's equation the metals which will emit photoelectrons for a radiation of wavelength 4100Å is/are **(2005)**

(a) A only (b) A and B only

(c) all the three metals (d) none.

43. A photosensitive metallic surface has work function, hv_0. If photons of energy $2hv_0$ fall on this surface, the electrons come out with a maximum velocity of 4×10^6 m/s. When the photon energy is increased to $5hv_0$, then maximum velocity of photoelectrons will be **(2005)**

(a) 2×10^7 m/s (b) 2×10^6 m/s

(c) 8×10^6 m/s (d) 8×10^5 m/s

44. According to Einstein's photoelectric equation, the graph between the kinetic energy of photoelectrons ejected and the frequency of incident radiation is

(2004, 1996)

(a) 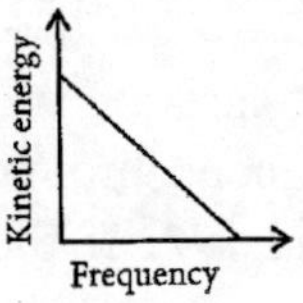

(b) 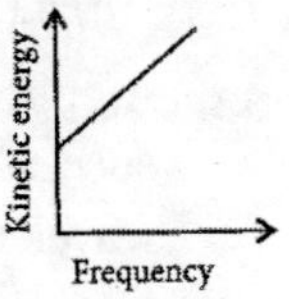

(c) 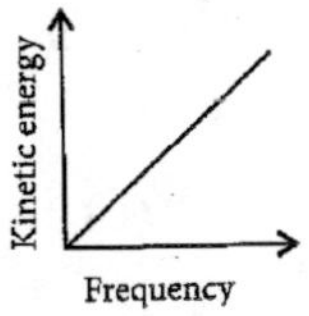

(d) 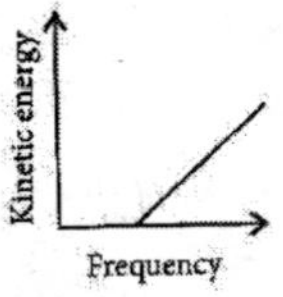

45. The value of Planck's constant is **(2002)**

(a) 6.63×10^{-34} J/sec

(b) 6.63×10^{-34} kg m^2/sec

(c) 6.63×10^{-34} kg m^2

(d) 6.63×10^{-34} Jsec

46. By photoelectric effect, Einstein proved **(2000)**

(a) $E = hv$ (b) K.E. $= \frac{1}{2}mv^2$

(c) $E = mc^2$ (d) $E = \frac{-Rhc^2}{n^2}$

47. The photoelectric work function for a metal surface is 4.125eV. The cut-off wavelength for this surface is **(1999)**

(a) 3000Å (b) 2062.5Å

(c) 4125Å (d) 6000Å

48. In a photo-emissive cell, with exciting wavelength λ, the fastest electron has speed v. If the exciting wavelength is changed to $\frac{3\lambda}{4}$, the speed of the fastest emitted electron will be **(1998)**

(a) less than $v(4/3)^{1/2}$

(b) $v(4/3)^{1/2}$

(c) $v(3/4)^{\frac{1}{2}}$

(d) greater than $v(4/3)^{1/2}$

49. When light of wavelength 300 nm (nanometer) falls on a photoelectric emitter, photoelectrons are liberated. For another emitter, however, light of 600 nm wavelength is sufficient for creating photoemission. What is the ratio of the work functions of the two emitters? **(1993)**

(a) 1: 2 (b) 2: 1

(c) 4: 1 (d) 1: 4

50. Photoelectric work function of a metal is 1eV. Light of wavelength $\lambda = 3000$Å falls on it. The photo electrons come out with a maximum velocity **(1991)**

(a) 10metres/sec

(b) 10^2 metres/ sec

(c) 10^4metres/sec

(d) 10^6metres/sec

51. Ultraviolet radiations of 6.2eV falls on an aluminium surface. Kinetic energy of fastest electron emitted is (work function = 4.2eV) **(1989)**

(a) 3.2×10^{-21} J (b) 3.2×10^{-19} J

(c) 7×10^{-25} J (d) 9×10^{-32} J

52. The threshold frequency for photoelectric effect on sodium corresponds to a wavelength of 5000Å. Its work function is **(1988)**

(a) 4×10^{-19} J (b) 1 J

(c) 2×10^{-19} J (d) 3×10^{-19} J

Particle Nature of Light: The Photon

53. The number of photons per second on an average emitted by the source of monochromatic light of wavelength

600 nm, when it delivers the power of 3.3×10^{-3} watt will be $(h = 6.6 \times 10^{-34} \text{Js})$ **(2021)**

(a) 10^{15} (b) 10^{18}
(c) 10^{17} (d) 10^{16}

54. A 200 W sodium street lamp emits yellow light of wavelength $0.6 \mu m$. Assuming it to be 25% efficient in converting electrical energy to light, the number of photons of yellow light it emits per second is **(2012)**

(a) 1.5×10^{20} (b) 6×10^{18}
(c) 62×10^{20} (d) 3×10^{19}

55. A source S_1 is producing, 10^{15} photons per second of wavelength 5000Å. Another source S_2 is producing 1.02×10^{15} photons per second of wavelength 5100Å. Then, (power of S_2)/(power of S_1) is equal to **(2010)**

(a) 1.00 (b) 1.02
(c) 1.04 (d) 0.98

56. Monochromatic light of wavelength 667 nm is produced by a helium neon laser. The power emitted is 9 mW. The number of photons arriving per second on the average at a target irradiated by this beam is **(2009)**

(a) 3×10^{16} (b) 9×10^{15}
(c) 3×10^{19} (d) 9×10^{17}

57. Monochromatic light of frequency 6.0×10^{14} Hz is produced by a laser. The power emitted is 2×10^{-3} W. The number of photons emitted, on the average, by the source per second is **(2007)**

(a) 5×10^{16} (b) 5×10^{17}
(c) 5×10^{14} (d) 5×10^{15}

58. The momentum of a photon of energy 1MeV in kgm/s will be **(2006)**

(a) 5×10^{-22} (b) 0.33×10^{6}
(c) 7×10^{-24} (d) 10^{-22}

59. If a photon has velocity c and frequency v, then which of the following represents its wavelength? **(1996)**

(a) $\frac{hv}{c^2}$ (b) hv
(c) $\frac{hc}{E}$ (d) $\frac{hv}{c}$

60. The velocity of photons is proportional to (where v = frequency) **(1996)**

(a) $1/\sqrt{v}$ (b) v^2
(c) v (d) None of these

61. Momentum of photon of wavelength λ is **(1993)**

(a) $\frac{hv}{c}$ (b) zero
(c) $\frac{h\lambda}{c^2}$ (d) $\frac{h\lambda}{c}$

62. The wavelength of a 1keV photon is 1.24×10^{-9} m. What is the frequency of 1MeV photon? **(1991)**

(a) 1.24×10^{15} (b) 2.4×10^{20}
(c) 1.24×10^{18} (d) 2.4×10^{23}

63. A radio transmitter operates at a frequency 880kHz and a power of 10 kW. The number of photons emitted per second is **(1990)**

(a) 1.72×10^{31} (b) 1.327×10^{25}
(c) 1.327×10^{37} (d) 1.327×10^{45}

64. The momentum of a photon of an electromagnetic radiation is 3.3×10^{-29} kg m s^{-1}. What is the frequency of the associated waves? [$h = 6.6 \times 10^{-34}$ J s; $c = 3 \times 10^8$ m s^{-1}] **(1990)**

(a) 1.5×10^{13} Hz (b) 7.5×10^{12} Hz

(c) 6×10^3 Hz (d) 3×10^3 Hz

65. The energy of a photon of wavelength λ is **(1998)**

(a) $hc\lambda$ (b) $\frac{hc}{\lambda}$

(c) $\frac{\lambda}{hc}$ (d) $\frac{\lambda h}{c}$

Wave Nature of Matter

66. The graph which shows the variation of the de-Broglie wavelength (λ) of a particle and its associated momentum (p) is **(2022)**

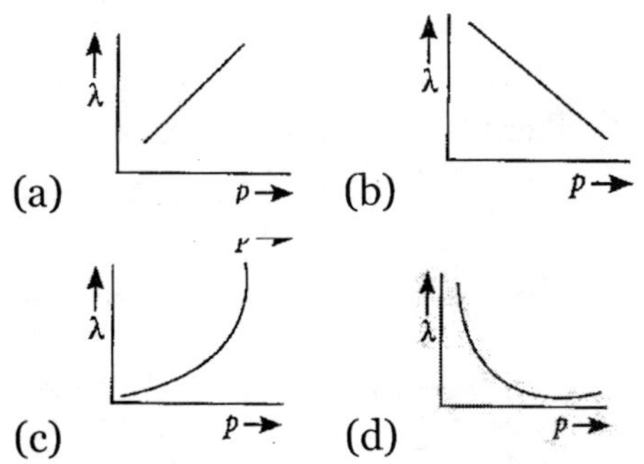

67. An electromagnetic wave of wavelength 'λ' is incident on a photosensitive surface of negligible work function. If 'm' mass is of photoelectron emitted from the surface has de-Broglie wavelength λ_d, then **(2021)**

(a) $\lambda = \left(\frac{2h}{mc}\right)\lambda_d^2$ (b) $\lambda = \left(\frac{2m}{hc}\right)\lambda_d^2$

(c) $\lambda = \left(\frac{2mc}{h}\right)\lambda^2$ (d) $\lambda = \left(\frac{2mc}{h}\right)\lambda_d^2$

68. An electron is accelerated from rest through a potential difference of V volt. If the de Broglie wavelength of the electron is 1.227×10^{-2} nm, the potential difference is **(2020)**

(a) 10 V (b) 10^2 V

(c) 10^3 V (d) 10^4 V

69. An electron is accelerated through a potential difference of 10,000 V. Its de Broglie wavelength is, (nearly) ($m_e = 9 \times 10^{-31}$ kg) **(2019)**

(a) 12.2 nm

(b) 12.2×10^{-13} m

(c) 12.2×10^{-12} m

(d) 12.2×10^{-14} m

70. An electron of mass m with an initial velocity $\vec{v} = v_0\hat{\imath}(v_0 > 0)$ enters an electric field $\vec{E} = -\vec{E}_0\hat{\imath}$ (E_0 = constant > 0) at $t = 0$. If λ_0 is its de-Broglie wavelength initially, then its de- Broglie wavelength at time t is **(2018)**

(a) $\frac{\lambda_0}{\left(1+\frac{eE_0}{mv_0}t\right)}$ (b) $\lambda_0\left(1+\frac{eE_0}{mv_0}t\right)$

(c) $\lambda_0 t$ (d) λ_0

71. The de-Broglie wavelength of a neutron in thermal equilibrium with heavy water at a temperature T (kelvin) and mass m, is **(2017)**

(a) $\frac{h}{\sqrt{3mkT}}$ (b) $\frac{2h}{\sqrt{3mkT}}$

(c) $\frac{2h}{\sqrt{mkT}}$ (d) $\frac{h}{\sqrt{mkT}}$

72. Electrons of mass m with de-Broglie wavelength λ fall on the target in an X-ray tube. The cutoff wavelength (λ_0) of the emitted X-ray is **(NEET-II 2016)**

(a) $\lambda_0 = \frac{2mc\lambda^2}{h}$ (b) $\lambda_0 = \frac{2h}{mc}$

(c) $\lambda_0 = \frac{2m^2c^2\lambda^3}{h^2}$ (d) $\lambda_0 = \lambda$

73. An electron of mass m and a photon have same energy E. The ratio of de-Broglie wavelengths associated with them is

(NEET-I 2016)

(a) $c(2mE)^{\frac{1}{2}}$ (b) $\frac{1}{c}\left(\frac{2m}{E}\right)^{\frac{1}{2}}$

(c) $\frac{1}{c}\left(\frac{E}{2m}\right)^{\frac{1}{2}}$ (d) $\left(\frac{E}{2m}\right)^{\frac{1}{2}}$

(c being velocity of light)

74. Light of wavelength 500 nm is incident on a metal with work function 2.28eV. The de Broglie wavelength of the emitted electron is **(2015)**

(a) $\geq 2.8 \times 10^{-9}$ m

(b) $\leq 2.8 \times 10^{-12}$ m

(c) $< 2.8 \times 10^{-10}$ m

(d) $< 2.8 \times 10^{-9}$ m

75. Which of the following figures represent the variation of particle momentum and the associated de-Broglie wavelength?

(2015 Cancelled)

(a) 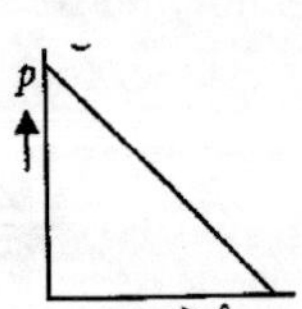

(b) 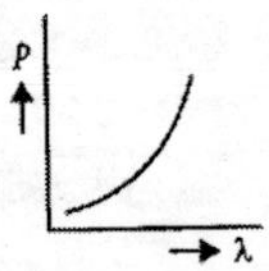

(c) 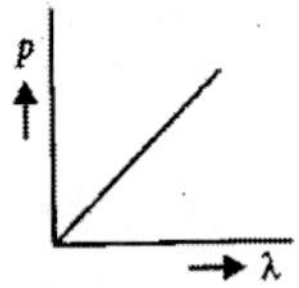

(d) 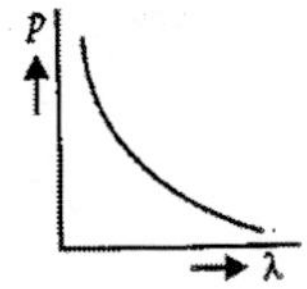

76. If the kinetic energy of the particle is increased to 16 times its previous value, the percentage change in the de Broglie wavelength of the particle is **(2014)**

(a) 25 (b) 75

(c) 60 (d) 50

77. The wavelength λ_e of an electron and λ_p of a photon of same energy E are related by

(2013)

(a) $\lambda_p \propto \sqrt{\lambda_e}$ (b) $\lambda_p \propto \frac{1}{\sqrt{\lambda_e}}$

(c) $\lambda_p \propto \lambda_e^2$ (d) $\lambda_p \propto \lambda_e$.

78. The de-Broglie wavelength of neutrons in thermal equilibrium at temperature T is

(Karnataka NEET 2013)

(a) $\frac{3.08}{\sqrt{T}}$ Å (b) $\frac{0.308}{\sqrt{T}}$ Å

(c) $\frac{0.0308}{\sqrt{T}}$ Å (d) $\frac{30.8}{\sqrt{T}}$ Å

79. An α-particle moves in a circular path of radius 0.83 cm in the presence of a magnetic field of 0.25 Wb/m^2. The de Broglie wavelength associated with the particle will be **(2012)**

(a) 1Å (b) 0.1Å

(c) 10Å (d) 0.01Å

80. If the momentum of an electron is changed by P, then the de Broglie wavelength associated with it changes by

0.5%. The initial momentum of electron will be **(Mains 2012)**

(a) $200P$ (b) $400P$

(c) $P/200$ (d) $100P$

81. Electrons used in an electron microscope are accelerated by a voltage of 25kV. If the voltage is increased to 100kV then the de-Broglie wavelength associated with the electrons would **(2011)**

(a) increase by 2 times

(b) decrease by 2 times

(c) decrease by 4 times

(d) increase by 4 times.

82. A particle of mass 1mg has the same wavelength as an electron moving with a velocity of 3×10^6 m s^{-1}. The velocity of the particle is **(2008)**

(a) 3×10^{-31} ms^{-1}

(b) 2.7×10^{-21} ms^{-1}

(c) 2.7×10^{-18} ms^{-1}

(d) 9×10^{-2} ms^{-1}

(mass of electron $= 9.1 \times 10^{-31}$ kg)

83. If particles are moving with same velocity, then which has maximum de Broglie wavelength? **(2002)**

(a) proton (b) α-particle

(c) neutron (d) β-particle

84. Which one among the following shows particle nature of light? **(2001)**

(a) photoelectric effect

(b) interference

(b) refraction

(d) polarization.

85. When a proton is accelerated through 1 V, then its kinetic energy will be **(1999)**

(a) 1eV (b) 13.6Ev

(c) 1840eV (d) 0.54eV

86. The kinetic energy of an electron, which is accelerated in the potential difference of 100 volts, is **(1997)**

(a) 416.6cal (b) 6.636cal

(c) 1.602×10^{-17} J (d) 1.6×10^4 J

87. An electron beam has a kinetic energy equal to 100eV. Find its wavelength associated with a beam, if mass of electron $= 9.1 \times 10^{-31}$ kg and 1eV $= 1.6 \times 10^{-19}$ J. (Planck's constant $= 6.6 \times 10^{-34}$Js) **(1996)**

(a) 24.6Å (b) 0.12Å

(c) 1.2Å (d) 6.3Å

88. An electron of mass m and charge e is accelerated from rest through a potential difference V in vacuum. Its final velocity will be **(1996)**

(a) $\sqrt{\frac{2eV}{m}}$ (b) $\sqrt{\frac{eV}{m}}$

(c) $\frac{eV}{2m}$ (d) $\frac{eV}{m}$

89. An electron of mass m, when accelerated through a potential difference V, has de Broglie wavelength λ. The de Broglie wavelength associated with a proton of mass M accelerated through the same potential difference, will be **(1995)**

(a) $\lambda \frac{M}{m}$ (b) $\lambda \frac{m}{M}$

(c) $\lambda \sqrt{\frac{M}{m}}$ (d) $\lambda \sqrt{\frac{m}{M}}$

90. If we consider electrons and photons of same wavelength, then they will have same **(1995)**

(a) momentum

(b) angular momentum

(c) energy

(d) velocity.

91. The de Broglie wave corresponding to a particle of mass m and velocity v has a wavelength associated with it **(1989)**

(a) $\frac{h}{mv}$ (b) hmv

(c) $\frac{mh}{v}$ (d) None of these

Davisson and Germer Experiment

92. In the Davisson and Germer experiment, the velocity of electrons emitted from the electron gun can be increased by **(2011)**

(a) increasing the potential difference between the anode and filament

(b) increasing the filament current

(c) decreasing the filament current

(d) decreasing the potential difference between the anode and filament.

ANSWER KEY

1.	(d)	2.	(a)	3.	(c)	4.	(c)	5.	(b)	6.	(a)	7.	(a)
8.	(b)	9.	(b)	10.	(b)	11.	(d)	12.	(c)	13.	(b)	14.	(b)
15.	(a)	16.	(d)	17.	(c)	18.	(d)	19.	(b)	20.	(b)	21.	(c)
22.	(a)	23.	(a)	24.	(a)	25.	(d)	26.	(d)	27.	(d)	28.	(d)
29.	(a)	30.	(a, d)	31.	(d)	32.	(b)	33.	(c)	34.	(d)	35.	(b)
36.	(a)	37.	(b)	38.	(b)	39.	(b)	40.	(c)	41.	(a)	42.	(b)
43.	(c)	44.	(d)	45.	(d)	46.	(a)	47.	(a)	48.	(d)	49.	(b)
50.	(d)	51.	(b)	52.	(a)	53.	(d)	54.	(a)	55.	(a)	56.	(a)
57.	(d)	58.	(a)	59.	(c)	60.	(d)	61.	(a)	62.	(b)	63.	(a)
64.	(a)	65.	(b)	66.	(d)	67.	(d)	68.	(d)	69.	(c)	70.	(a)
71.	(a)	72.	(a)	73.	(c)	74.	(a)	75.	(d)	76.	(b)	77.	(c)
78.	(d)	79.	(d)	80.	(a)	81.	(*)	82.	(c)	83.	(d)	84.	(a)
85.	(a)	86.	(c)	87.	(c)	88.	(a)	89.	(d)	90.	(a)	91.	(a)
92.	(a)												

Hints & Explanations

1. **(d) :** When a beam of cathode rays (or electrons) are subjected to crossed electric (E) and magnetic (B) fields, the beam is not deflected, if

Force on electron due to magnetic field = Force on electron due to electric field

$$Bev = eE \text{ or } v = \frac{E}{B}$$

If V is the potential difference between the anode and the cathode, then

$$\frac{1}{2}mv^2 = eV \text{ or } \frac{e}{m} = \frac{v^2}{2V}$$

Substituting the value of v from equation (i) in equation (ii), we get

$$\frac{e}{m} = \frac{E^2}{2VB^2}$$

Specific charge of the cathode rays

$$\frac{e}{m} = \frac{E^2}{2VB^2}$$

(Where V is the potential difference between cathode and anode)

2. **(a) :** Collisions of the charged particles with the atoms in the gas.

3. **(c) :** ionisation of gas [enclosed] is a result of e^- collision with neutral gas atom/molecule.

4. **(c) :** J.J. Thomson's cathode-ray experiment provide information about charge to the mass ratio of electron s proton.

$$\left(\frac{e}{m}\right)_{electron} > \left[\frac{e}{m}\right]_{proton} \text{ as } \boxed{m_p > m_e}$$

5. **(b) :** Cathode rays are basically negatively charged particles (electrons). If the cathode rays are allowed to pass between two plates kept at a difference of potential, the rays are found to be deflected from the rectilinear path. The direction of deflection shows that the rays carry negative charges.

6. **(a)**

7. **(a)**

8. **(b) :** Thermionic emission : When a metal is heated to a high temperature, the free electron gain kinetic energy and escape from the surface of the metal.

Secondary emission : When an electron strikes the surface of a metallic plate, it emits other electrons from the surface.

Photoelectric emission : Emission of electrons from the metal surface on irradiation with radiation of suitable frequency.

X-rays emission : They are due to transitions in the inner energy levels of the atom.

9. **(b) :** When a metal is heated, electrons are ejected out of it, which are called thermions

10. **(b) :** By changing the position of source of light from photo cell, there will be a change in the intensity of light falling on photo cell.

As stopping potential is independent of the intensity of the incident light, hence stopping potential remains same i.e., V_0.

11. **(d) :** The photoelectic emission occurs only when the incident light has more than a certain minimum frequency. This minimum frequency is called threshold frequency.

12. **(c) :** The stopping potential V_s is related to the maximum kinetic energy of the emitted electrons K_{max} through the relation $K_{max} = eV_s$

$$0.5\text{eV} = eV_s \text{ or } V_s = 0.5 \text{ V}$$

13. **(b) :** The number of photoelectrons ejected is directly proportional to the intensity of incident light. Maximum kinetic energy is independent of intensity of incident light but depends upon the frequency of light. Hence option (b) is correct.

14. **(b) :** The number of photoelectrons decide the photocurrent. Assuming that the number of electrons emitted depends on the number of photons incident, the number of photoelectrons depend on the intensity of light.

15. **(a) :** The energy of the incident photon is hλ.

Hence frequency determine the energy of incident photon. This energy is imparted on the photosensitive surface to cause photo equation. At the point where curve cuts the x-axis, the incident photon energy is equal to the work potential of material.

Hence energy hence frequency, is same for radiation of a & b.

Intensity is the measure of number of photons striking / time. Thus they determine the amount of photocurrent produced. Thus it is same for b & c.

16. **(d) :** For a light source of power P watt, the intensity at a distance d is given by

$I = \frac{P}{4\pi d^2}$

where we assume light to spread out uniformly in all directions i.e., it is a spherical source.

$\therefore\ I \propto \frac{1}{d^2}$ or $\frac{I_1}{I_2} = \frac{d_2^2}{d_1^2}$

or, $\frac{I_1}{I_2} = \left(\frac{1}{0.5}\right)^2$ or, $\frac{I_1}{I_2} = 4$ or, $I_2 = \frac{I_1}{4}$.

In a photoelectric emission, the number of photoelectrons liberated per second from a photosensitive metallic surface is proportional to the intensity of the light. When a intensity of source is reduced by a factor of four, the number of photoelectrons is also reduced by a factor of 4.

17. **(c)** : The photoelectric current is directly proportional to the intensity of illumination. Therefore a change in the intensity of the incident radiation will change the photocurrent.

18. **(d)** : Photoelectric current $I \propto$ intensity of light and intensity $\propto \frac{1}{(\text{distance})^2}$

$$\therefore I \propto \frac{1}{(\text{distance})^2}$$

19. **(b)** : If photo electric effect does not occur by Uv rays then it simply means that wave length of Uvrays is more than threshold wavelength for the metal.

In the given example only the x-rays have lower wavelength than of Uv so it may produce the effect.

so x-ray is current.

20. **(b)** : No of e^- effected/time (Intensity)

$$\text{Intensity} \propto \frac{1}{(\text{distance})^2}$$

$$I_1 \propto \frac{1}{(d)^2} \qquad I_2 \propto \frac{1}{(d/2)^2}$$

$$\frac{I_1}{I_2} = \frac{\frac{d^2}{d^2}}{4} \qquad \frac{I_1}{I_2} = \frac{1}{4} \Rightarrow \boxed{I_2 = 4I_1}$$

21. **(c)** : If the intensity of light of a given frequency is increased, then the number of photons striking the surface per second will increase in the same ratio. This increased number of photons strikes more electrons of metals and hence number of photoelectrons emitted through the surface increase and hence photoelectric current increases.

22. **(a)** : Since the emission of photoelectrons is directly proportional to the intensity of the incident light, therefore photocurrent increases with the intensity of light.

23. **(a)** : Photoelectric current is directly proportional to the intensity of incident light.

24. **(a)** : The work function has no effect on photoelectric current so long as $h\nu > W_0$. The photoelectric current is proportional to the intensity of incident light. Since there is no change in the intensity of light, hence $I_1 = I_2$.

25. **(d)** :Initially, $v = 1.5v_0$

If the frequency is halved,

$$v' = \frac{v}{2} = \frac{1.5v_0}{2} < v_0$$

Hence, no photoelectric emission will take place.

26. **(d)** : Given energy of photon $E = 2.20eV$

Work function of Cs

$\phi_0 = 2.14eV, K\phi_0 = 2.30eV$
, Na $\phi_0 = 2.75eV$

We know that e^- emitts when $hv > \phi_0$

here it is clear that energy of photon is more than the work function of Cs [Caesium] only so Ans. only (Cs)

27. **(d) :** Let the threshold frequency is v_0. By using the equation of photo electric effect, $E = hv_0 + eV_0$

case I : $hv = hv_0 + \frac{eV_s}{2}$

case II : $\frac{hv}{2} = hv_0 + eV_s$

$$\frac{hv}{2} = \frac{-eV_s}{2}$$

$-hv = eV_s$ put in (i)

$hv = hv_0 - \frac{hv}{2}$, so, $v_0 = \frac{3}{2}v$

28. **(d) :** Required wavelength of light,

$$\lambda_0 = \frac{hc}{\phi} = \frac{1240\text{eVnm}}{4\text{eV}} \approx 310 \text{ nm}$$

29. **(a)** : According to the Einstein's photoelectric equation,

$$E = W_0 + \frac{1}{2}mv^2$$

When frequency of incident light is $2v_0$.

$$h(2v_0) = hv_0 + \frac{1}{2}mv_1^2 \Rightarrow hv_0 = \frac{1}{2}mv_1^2$$

When frequency of incident light is $5v_0$

$$h(5v_0) = hv_0 + \frac{1}{2}mv_2^2 \Rightarrow 4hv_0 = \frac{1}{2}mv_2^2$$

Dividing (i) by (ii), $\frac{1}{4} = \frac{v_1^2}{v_2^2}$ or $\frac{v_1}{v_2} = \frac{1}{2}$.

30. **(a, d) :** The maximum kinetic energy is given as

$$K_{\max} = hv - \phi_0 = hv - hv_0 = \frac{hc}{\lambda} - \frac{hc}{\lambda_0}$$

where λ_0 = threshold wavelength

or $\frac{1}{2}mv^2 = \frac{hc}{\lambda} - \frac{hc}{\lambda_0}$

Here, $h = 4.14 \times 10^{-15}$eVs, $c = 3 \times 10^8$ m s^{-1}

$\lambda_o = 3250 \times 10^{-10}$ m $= 3250$Å

$\lambda = 2536 \times 10^{-10}$ m $= 2536$Å,

$m = 9.1 \times 10^{-31}$ kg

$hc = 4.14 \times 10^{-15}\text{eVs} \times 3 \times 10^8 \text{ m s}^{-1}$

$= 12420$eVÅ

$$\therefore \frac{1}{2}mv^2 = 12420\left[\frac{1}{2536} - \frac{1}{3250}\right]\text{eV}$$

$= 1.076$eV

$$v^2 = \frac{2.152\text{eV}}{m} = \frac{2.152 \times 1.6 \times 10^{-19}}{9.1 \times 10^{-31}}$$

$\therefore v \approx 6 \times 10^5 \text{ m s}^{-1} = 0.6 \times 10^6 \text{ m s}^{-1}$

Note: Options (a) and (d) are same. So both are correct.

31. **(d)** : According to Einstein's photoelectric equation maximum kinetic energy of photoelectrons,

$$KE_{\max} = E_v - \phi$$

or $2 = 5 - \phi \therefore \phi = 3$eV

When $E_\gamma = 6\text{eV}$ then, $KE_{\max} = 6 - 3 = 3\text{eV}$

or $e\left(V_{\text{cathode}} - V_{\text{anode}}\right) = 3\text{eV}$

or $V_{\text{cathode}} - V_{\text{anode}} = 3\text{ V} = -V_{\text{stopping}}$

$$\therefore V_{\text{stopping}} = -3\text{ V}$$

32. **(b)** : According to Einstein's photoelectric equation,

$$eV_s = \frac{hc}{\lambda} - \frac{hc}{\lambda_0}$$

$\therefore$ As per question, $eV = \frac{hc}{\lambda} - \frac{hc}{\lambda_0}$

$$\frac{eV}{4} = \frac{hc}{2\lambda} - \frac{hc}{\lambda_0}$$

From equations (i) and (ii), we get

$$\frac{hc}{2\lambda} - \frac{hc}{4\lambda} = \frac{hc}{\lambda_0} - \frac{hc}{4\lambda_0}, \Rightarrow \frac{hc}{4\lambda} = \frac{3hc}{4\lambda_0} \text{ or } \lambda_0 = 3\lambda$$

33. **(c)** : Let ϕ_0 be the work function of the surface of the material.

According to Einstein's photoelectric equation, the maximum kinetic energy of the emitted photoelectrons in the first case is

$$K_{\max_1} = \frac{hc}{\lambda} - \phi_0$$

and that in the second case is

$$K_{\max_2} = \frac{hc}{\frac{\lambda}{2}} - \phi_0 = \frac{2hc}{\lambda} - \phi_0$$

But $K_{\max_2} = 3K_{\max_1}$ (given)

$$\therefore \frac{2hc}{\lambda} - \phi_0 = 3\left(\frac{hc}{\lambda} - \phi_0\right); \frac{2hc}{\lambda} - \phi_0$$

$$= \frac{3hc}{\lambda} - 3\phi_0$$

34. **(d)** :

$$3\phi_0 - \phi_0 = \frac{3hc}{\lambda} - \frac{2hc}{\lambda} \text{ or } 2\phi_0 = \frac{hc}{\lambda} \text{ or } \phi_0$$

$$= \frac{hc}{2\lambda}$$

35. **(b)** : According to Einstein's photoelectric equation, the kinetic energy of emitted photoelectrons is

$$K = hv - \phi_0$$

where hv is the energy of incident radiation and ϕ_0 is work function of the metal.

As per question,

$$0.5\text{eV} = hv - \phi_0$$
$$0.8\text{eV} = 1.2hv - \phi_0$$

On solving eqns. (i) and (ii), we get

$$\phi_0 = 1.0\text{eV}$$

36. **(a)** : Work function, $\phi = hv$

According to Einstein's photoelectric equation

$$\frac{1}{2}mv_{\max}^2 = h(2v) - hv \text{ or } \frac{1}{2}mv_{\max}^2 = hv$$

$$v_{\max}^2 = \frac{2hv}{m} \Rightarrow v_{\max} = \sqrt{\frac{2hv}{m}}$$

37. **(b)** : According to Einstein's photoelectric equation

$$\frac{1}{2}mv_{\max}^2 = hv - \phi_0$$

where $\frac{1}{2}mv_{max}^2$ is the maximum kinetic energy of the emitted electrons, $h\nu$ is the incident energy and ϕ_0 is the work function of the metal.

$\therefore \frac{1}{2}mv_{max_1}^2 = 1eV - 0.5eV = 0.5eV$ and

$\frac{1}{2}mv_{max_2}^2 = 2.5eV - 0.5eV = 2eV$

Divide (i) and (ii), we get

$$\frac{v_{max_1}^2}{v_{max_2}^2} = \frac{0.5}{2} \text{ or } \frac{v_{max_1}}{v_{max_2}} = \sqrt{\frac{0.5}{2}} = \frac{1}{2}$$

38. **(b)** : According to Einstein's photoelectric equation $eV_0 = h\nu - h\nu_0$

where, ν = Incident frequency

ν_0 = Threshold frequency

V_0 = Cut-off or stopping potential

or $V_0 = \frac{h}{e}(\nu - \nu_0)$

Substituting the given values, we get

$$V_0 = \frac{6.63 \times 10^{-34}(8.2 \times 10^{14} - 3.3 \times 10^{14})}{1.6 \times 10^{-19}}$$

$$\approx 2\text{ V}$$

39. **(b)** : Here, Incident wavelength,

$\lambda = 200$ nm

Work function, $\phi_0 = 5.01eV$

According to Einstein's photoelectric equation

$$eV_s = h\nu - \phi_0 \text{ or } eV_s = \frac{hc}{\lambda} - \phi_0$$

where V_s is the stopping potential

$$eV_s = \frac{(1240eVnm)}{(200\text{ nm})} - 5.01eV$$

$$= 6.2eV - 5.01eV$$

$$= 1.2eV$$

Stopping potential, $V_s = 1.2$ V

The potential difference that must be applied to stop photoelectrons

$= -V_s = -1.2$ V

40. **(c)** : $\phi_0 = 6.2eV$

$K_{max} = 5eV \therefore h\nu = 11.2eV$

$$\therefore \lambda = \frac{hc}{E} = \frac{12400eVÅ}{11.2eV} = 1107Å$$

This wavelength is in the ultraviolet region.

41. **(a)** : Let K and K' be the maximum kinetic energy of photoelectrons for incident light of frequency ν and 2ν respectively.

According to Einstein's photoelectric equation,

$K = h\nu - E_0$

$$K' = h(2\nu) - E_0 = 2h\nu - E_0$$

$$= h\nu + h\nu$$

$$- E_0 \text{ [using (i)]}$$

$$K' = h\nu + K$$

42. **(b)** :

43. **(c)** : K.E. $= h\nu - W$ i.e., $\frac{1}{2}mv_{max}^2 = h\nu - W$

$$\Rightarrow \frac{1}{2}m \times (4 \times 10^6)^2 = 2h\nu_0 - h\nu_0$$

or, $\frac{1}{2}m \times (4 \times 10^6)^2 = h\nu_0$

Another case, $2h\nu_0 \to 5h\nu_0$

$\frac{1}{2}mv_{\max}^2 = 4h\nu_0 \Rightarrow \frac{1}{2}mv_{\max}^2$

$= 4 \times \frac{1}{2} \times m \times (4 \times 10^6)^2$

$\Rightarrow v_{\max}^2 = 64 \times 10^{12} \Rightarrow v_{\max} = 8 \times 10^6$ m/s

44. **(d) :** The maximum kinetic energy of photoelectron ejected is given by

K.E. $= h\nu - W = h\nu - h\nu_0$

where work function depends on the type of material.

If the frequency of incident radiation is greater than ν_0 only then the ejection of Frequency

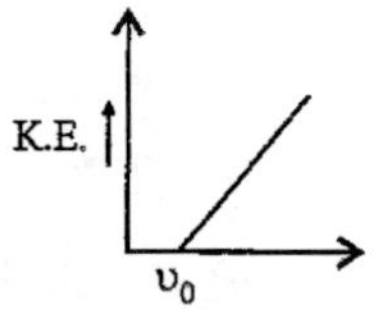

photoelectrons start. After that as frequency increases kinetic energy also increases.

45. **(d) :** The value of Planck's constant is 6.63×10^{-34} J s.

46. **(a) :** Einstein P.E. proues

E = h ν [for metals]

were ν if greater ν_0 of metal e^- ejection can be possible.

47. **(a) :** $\phi = h\nu_0 = \frac{hc}{\lambda_0}$

$$\Rightarrow \lambda_0 = \frac{hc}{\phi} = \frac{1242\text{eVnm}}{4.125\text{eV}} \approx 3000\text{Å}$$

48. **(d) :** According to Einstein's photoelectric equation,

$$\frac{1}{2}mv^2 = \frac{hc}{\lambda} - W_0 \text{ or, } \frac{hc}{\lambda} = \frac{1}{2}mv^2 + W_0$$

$$\frac{1}{2}mv_1^2 = \frac{hc}{3\lambda/4} - W_0 = \frac{4}{3}\left(\frac{1}{2}mv^2 + W_0\right) - W_0$$

$$v_1^2 = \frac{4}{3}v^2 + \frac{2}{3}W_0$$

So, v_1 is greater than $v(4/3)^{1/2}$.

49. **(b) :**

$W_0 = \frac{hc}{\lambda_0}$ or $W_0 \propto \frac{1}{\lambda_0}$

$$\Rightarrow \frac{W_1}{W_2} = \frac{\lambda_2}{\lambda_1} = \frac{600}{300} = \frac{2}{1}$$

50. **(d) :** $h\nu = W + \frac{1}{2}mv^2$ or $\frac{hc}{\lambda} = W + \frac{1}{2}mv^2$

Here $\lambda = 3000\text{Å} = 3000 \times 10^{-10}$ m

and $W = 1\text{eV} = 1.6 \times 10^{-19}$ joule

$$\frac{(6.6 \times 10^{-34})(3 \times 10^8)}{3000 \times 10^{-10}} = (1.6 \times 10^{-19}) + \frac{1}{2} \times (9.1 \times 10^{-31})v^2$$

Solving we get $v \cong 10^6$ m/s

51. **(b) :** Kinetic energy of fastest electron

$= E - W_0 = 6.2 - 4.2 = 2.0$eV

$= 2 \times 1.6 \times 10^{-19}$ J $= 3.2 \times 10^{-19}$ J

52. **(a) :** $W_0 = \frac{hc}{\lambda_0}$

$$= \frac{6.63 \times 10^{-34} \times 3 \times 10^{8}}{5000 \times 10^{-10}} = 4 \times 10^{-19}\ \text{J}$$

53. **(d) :** Given, Power $= 3.3 \times 10^{-3}$ Watt

Wavelength, $\lambda = 600\ \text{nm} = 600 \times 10^{-9}\ \text{m}$

Number of photons emitted per second is

$$n_1 = \frac{P\lambda}{hc} = \frac{3.3 \times 10^{-3} \times 600 \times 10^{-9}}{6.6 \times 10^{-34} \times 3 \times 10^{8}} \Rightarrow n = 10^{16}$$

54. **(a) :** Energy of a photon

$$= \frac{(6.6 \times 10^{-34}\ \text{J s})(3 \times 10^{8}\ \text{m s}^{-1})}{0.6 \times 10^{-6}\ \text{m}} = 33 \times 10^{-20}\ \text{J}$$

Number of photons emitted per second is

$$N = \frac{\frac{25}{100}P}{E} = \frac{\frac{25}{100} \times 200\ \text{W}}{33 \times 10^{-20}\ \text{J}} = 1.5 \times 10^{20}$$

55. **(a) :** For a source S_1,

Wavelength, $\lambda_1 = 5000\text{Å}$

Number of photons emitted per second, $N_1 = 10^{15}$

Energy of each photon, $E_1 = \frac{hc}{\lambda_1}$

Power of source $S_1, P_1 = E_1 N_1 = \frac{N_1 hc}{\lambda_1}$

For a source S_2,

Wavelength, $\lambda_2 = 5100\text{Å}$

Number of photons emitted per second, $N_2 = 1.02 \times 10^{15}$

Energy of each photon, $E_2 = \frac{hc}{\lambda_2}$

Power of source $S_2, P_2 = N_2 E_2 = \frac{N_2 hc}{\lambda_2}$

$$\therefore \frac{\text{Power of } S_2}{\text{Power of } S_1} = \frac{P_2}{P_1} = \frac{\frac{N_2 hc}{\lambda_2}}{\frac{N_1 hc}{\lambda_1}} = \frac{N_2 \lambda_1}{N_1 \lambda_2}$$

$$= \frac{(1.02 \times 10^{15}\ \text{photons}/\text{s}) \times (5000\text{Å})}{(10^{15}\ \text{photons}/\text{s}) \times (5100\text{Å})}$$

$$= \frac{51}{51} = 1$$

56. **(a) :** $\lambda = 6670\text{Å}$

E of a photon $= \frac{12400\text{eVÅ}}{6670\text{Å}} = \frac{12400}{6670} \times 1.6 \times 10^{-19}\ \text{J}.$

Energy emitted per second,

power $P = 9 \times 10^{-3}\ \text{J}$

$\therefore$ Number of photons incident $= \frac{\text{Power}}{\text{Energy}} = \frac{P}{E}$

$$= \frac{9 \times 10^{-3} \times 6670}{12400 \times 1.6 \times 10^{-19}} = 3 \times 10^{16}$$

57. **(d) :** Power $P = 2 \times 10^{-3}\ \text{W}$

Energy of one photon $E = h\nu = 6.63 \times 10^{-34} \times 6 \times 10^{14}\ \text{J}$

Number of photons emitted per second, $N = P/E$

$$= \frac{2 \times 10^{-3}}{6.63 \times 10^{-34} \times 6 \times 10^{14}} = 0.05 \times 10^{17} = 5 \times 10^{15}.$$

58. **(a) :** Energy of photon $E = 1\text{MeV}$

Momentum of photon $p = E/c$

$$\therefore p = \frac{E}{c} = \frac{1 \times 10^{6} \times 1.6 \times 10^{-19}\ \text{J}}{3 \times 10^{8}\ \text{m s}^{-1}} = 0.53 \times 10^{-21}$$

$$\approx 5 \times 10^{-22}\ \text{kg m/s}$$

59. **(c) :** Energy of the photon $E = \frac{hc}{\lambda}$ or $\lambda = \frac{hc}{E}$, where λ is the wavelength.

60. **(d) :** The velocity of a photon in vacuum is a constant. $c = v\lambda$. But $c =$ constant and one cannot say that it is proportional to v or λ but only $c = v\lambda$. In media, for a particular medium, v remain the same, velocity changes. Therefore λ changes. The question is wrong.

61. **(a) :** Momentum of the photon $= \frac{hv}{c}$

62. **(b) :**

Here, $\frac{hc}{\lambda} = 10^3\text{eV}$ and $hv = 10^6\text{eV}$

Hence, $v = \frac{10^3 c}{\lambda} = \frac{10^3 \times 3 \times 10^8}{1.24 \times 10^{-9}} = 2.4 \times 10^{20}$ Hz

63. **(a) :** No. of photons emitted per sec,

$$n = \frac{\text{Power}}{\text{Energy of photon}}$$

$$= \frac{P}{hv} = \frac{10000}{6.6 \times 10^{-34} \times 880 \times 10^3} = 1.72 \times 10^{31}$$

64. **(a) :** Momentum of the photon $= \frac{hv}{c}$

$$\Rightarrow \frac{c}{v} = \frac{h}{p} = \lambda$$

$$v = \frac{c}{\lambda} = \frac{cp}{h} = 3 \times 10^8 \times \frac{3.3 \times 10^{-29}}{6.6 \times 10^{-34}}$$

$$= 1.5 \times 10^{13} \text{ Hz}$$

65. **(b):** Energy of a photon $E = hv = \frac{hc}{\lambda}$

66. **(d) :** de-broglie wavelength, $\lambda = \frac{h}{p}$ or $\lambda \propto \frac{1}{p}$

Shape of graph is rectangular hyperbola.

Hence, curve (d) is correct option.

67. **(d) :** As work function is negligible, therefore Kinetic energy of emitted electron = Energy of incident photon

i.e., $\frac{1}{2}mv^2 = hv$

$$\Rightarrow \frac{p^2}{2m} = \frac{hc}{\lambda}, \Rightarrow p = \sqrt{\frac{2mhc}{\lambda}}$$

de-broglie wavelength of emitted electrons is

$$\lambda_d = \frac{h}{p} = \frac{h}{\sqrt{\frac{2mhc}{\lambda}}}$$

$$\Rightarrow \lambda_d = \sqrt{\frac{h\lambda}{2mc}}$$

$$\Rightarrow \lambda = \left(\frac{2mc}{h}\right)\lambda_d^2$$

68. **(d) :** Given : de-Broglie wavelength of electron $\lambda = 1.227 \times 10^{-2}$ nm $=$ 0.1227Å

$$\because \lambda = \frac{h}{\sqrt{2meV}} = \frac{12.27}{\sqrt{V}} \text{Å}$$

We have, $\sqrt{V} = \frac{12.27}{0.1227} = 100 \Rightarrow V = 10^4$ V.

69. **(c) :** de Broglie wavelength of electron,

$$\lambda_e = \frac{12.27\text{Å}}{\sqrt{V(\text{ in V})}}$$

Here, $V = 10000$ V

$$\therefore \lambda_e = \frac{12.27}{\sqrt{10000}} \times 10^{-10} \text{ m}$$

$$= 12.27 \times 10^{-12} \text{ m}$$

70. **(a)** : Here, $\vec{E} = -E_0\hat{\imath}$; initial velocity $\vec{v} = v_0\hat{\imath}$

Force acting on electron due to electric field

$$\vec{F} = (-e)(-E_0\hat{\imath}) = eE_0\hat{\imath}$$

Acceleration produced in the electron,

$$\vec{a} = \frac{\vec{F}}{m} = \frac{eE_0}{m}\hat{\imath}$$

Now, velocity of electron after time t,

$$\vec{v}_t = \vec{v} + \vec{a}t = \left(v_0 + \frac{eE_0t}{m}\right)\hat{\imath} \text{ or } |\vec{v}_t| = v_0 + \frac{eE_0t}{m}$$

Now, $\lambda_t = \frac{h}{mv_t} = \frac{h}{m\left(v_0+\frac{eE_0t}{m}\right)} = \frac{h}{mv_0\left(1+\frac{eE_0t}{mv_0}\right)}$

$$= \frac{\lambda_0}{\left(1+\frac{eE_0t}{mv_0}\right)} \qquad \left(\because \lambda_0 = \frac{h}{mv_0}\right)$$

71. **(a)** : Kinetic energy of a neutron in thermal equilibrium with heavy water at a temperature T is given as

$$K = \frac{3}{2}kT$$

Also momentum (p) is, $p = \sqrt{2mK}$

From eqn. (i)

$$p = \sqrt{2m \cdot \frac{3}{2}kT} = \sqrt{3mkT}$$

Required de-Broglie wavelength is given as

$$\lambda = \frac{h}{p} = \frac{h}{\sqrt{3mkT}}$$

72. **(a)** : Kinetic energy of electrons

$$K = \frac{p^2}{2m} = \frac{(h/\lambda)^2}{2m} = \frac{h^2}{2m\lambda^2}$$

So, maximum energy of photon (X-ray) $= K$

$$\frac{hc}{\lambda_0} = \frac{h^2}{2m\lambda^2} \quad \therefore \lambda_0 = \frac{2mc\lambda^2}{h}$$

73. **(c)** : For electron of energy E,

de-Broglie wavelength, $\lambda_e = \frac{h}{p} = \frac{h}{\sqrt{2mE}}$

For photon of energy, $E = h\nu = \frac{hc}{\lambda_p} \Rightarrow$

$$\lambda_p = \frac{hc}{E}$$

$$\therefore \frac{\lambda_e}{\lambda_p} = \frac{h}{\sqrt{2mE}} \times \frac{E}{hc} = \frac{1}{c}\left(\frac{E}{2m}\right)^{1/2}$$

74. **(a)** : According to Einstein's photoelectric equation, the maximum kinetic energy of the emitted electron is

$$K_{\text{max}} = \frac{hc}{\lambda} - \phi_0$$

where λ is the wavelength of incident light and ϕ_0 is the work function.

Here, $\lambda = 500$ nm, $hc = 1240$eVnm and $\phi_0 = 2.28$eV

$$\therefore K_{\text{max}} = \frac{1240\text{eVnm}}{500\text{ nm}} - 2.28\text{eV}$$

$$= 2.48\text{eV} - 2.28\text{eV} = 0.2\text{eV}$$

The de Broglie wavelength of the emitted electron is

$$\lambda_{\min} = \frac{h}{\sqrt{2mK_{\max}}}$$

where h is the Planck's constant and m is the mass of the electron.

As $h = 6.6 \times 10^{-34}$ J s, $m = 9 \times 10^{-31}$ kg and $K_{\max} = 0.2\text{eV} = 0.2 \times 1.6 \times 10^{-19}$ J

$\therefore \lambda_{\min}$

$$= \frac{6.6 \times 10^{-34}\text{ J s}}{\sqrt{2(9 \times 10^{-31}\text{ kg})(0.2 \times 1.6 \times 10^{-19}\text{ J})}}$$

$$= \frac{6.6}{2.4} \times 10^{-9}\text{ m} \approx 2.8 \times 10^{-9}\text{ m So, } \lambda \geq 2.8 \times 10^{-9}\text{ m}$$

75. **(d)** : de-Broglie wavelength, $\lambda = \frac{h}{p}$

or $\lambda p =$ constant

This represents a rectangular hyperbola.

76. **(b)** : de Broglie wavelength,

$$\lambda = \frac{h}{\sqrt{2mK}}$$

where m is the mass and K is the kinetic energy of the particle. When kinetic energy of the particle is increased to 16 times, then its de Broglie wavelength becomes,

$$\lambda' = \frac{h}{\sqrt{2m(16K)}} = \frac{1}{4}\frac{h}{\sqrt{2mK}}$$

$$= \frac{\lambda}{4}\text{(Using(i))}$$

% change in the de Broglie wavelength

$$= \frac{\lambda - \lambda'}{\lambda} \times 100 = \left(1 - \frac{\lambda'}{\lambda}\right) \times 100$$

$$= \left(1 - \frac{1}{4}\right) \times 100 = 75\%$$

77. **(c)** : Wavelength of an electron of energy E is

$$\lambda_e = \frac{h}{\sqrt{2m_eE}}$$

Wavelength of a photon of same energy E is

$$\lambda_p = \frac{hc}{E} \text{ or } E = \frac{hc}{\lambda_p}$$

Squaring both sides of eq. (i), we get

$$\lambda_e^2 = \frac{h^2}{2m_eE} \text{ or } E = \frac{h^2}{2m_e\lambda_e^2}$$

Equating (ii) and (iii), we get

$$\frac{hc}{\lambda_p} = \frac{h^2}{2m_e\lambda_e^2} \text{ or } \lambda_p = \frac{2m_ec}{h}\lambda_e^2$$

$$\lambda_p \propto \lambda_e^2$$

78. **(d)** : de Broglie wavelength of neutrons in thermal equilibrium at temperature T is

$$\lambda = \frac{h}{\sqrt{2mk_BT}},$$

where m is the mass of the neutron

Here, $m = 1.67 \times 10^{-27}$ kg, $k_B = 1.38 \times 10^{-23}$ J K^{-1}

$h = 6.63 \times 10^{-34}$ J s

$\therefore \lambda$

$$= \frac{6.63 \times 10^{-34}}{\sqrt{2 \times 1.67 \times 10^{-27} \times 1.38 \times 10^{-23} \times T}}$$

$$= \frac{3.08 \times 10^{-34} \times 10^{25}}{\sqrt{T}}$$

$$= \frac{30.8 \times 10^{-10}}{\sqrt{T}} \text{ m}$$

$$= \frac{30.8}{\sqrt{T}} \text{Å}$$

79. **(d)** : Radius of the circular path of a charged particle in a magnetic field is given by

$$R = \frac{mv}{Bq} \text{ or } mv = RBq$$

Here, $R = 0.83 \text{ cm} = 0.83 \times 10^{-2}$ m,

$B = 0.25 \text{ Wb m}^{-2}$

$$q = 2e = 2 \times 1.6 \times 10^{-19} \text{C}$$

$$\therefore mv = (0.83 \times 10^{-2})(0.25)(2 \times 1.6 \times 10^{-19})$$

de Broglie wavelength, $\lambda = \frac{h}{mv}$

$$= \frac{6.6 \times 10^{-34}}{0.83 \times 10^{-2} \times 0.25 \times 2 \times 1.6 \times 10^{-19}}$$

$$\times 10^{-12} \text{ m} = 0.01\text{Å}$$

80. **(a)** : de Broglie wavelength associated with an electron is

$$\lambda = \frac{h}{P} \text{ or } P = \frac{h}{\lambda} \therefore \frac{\Delta P}{P} = -\frac{\Delta\lambda}{\lambda}; \frac{P}{P_{\text{initial}}}$$

$$= \frac{0.5}{100}$$

$$P_{\text{initial}} = 200P$$

81. (*) : The de Broglie wavelength λ associated with the electrons is

$$\lambda = \frac{1.227}{\sqrt{V}} \text{ nm}$$

where V is the accelerating potential in volts.

$$\text{or } \lambda \propto \frac{1}{\sqrt{V}}$$

$$\therefore \frac{\lambda_1}{\lambda_2} = \sqrt{\frac{V_2}{V_1}} = \sqrt{\frac{100 \times 10^3}{25 \times 10^3}} = 2 \text{ or } \lambda_2 = \frac{\lambda_1}{2}$$

*None of the given options is correct.

82. **(c)** :

$$\lambda = \frac{h}{10^{-6} \text{ kg} \times v} = \frac{h}{9.1 \times 10^{-31} \text{ kg} \times 3 \times 10^6 \text{ m/s}}$$

$$\therefore v = 2.7 \times 10^{-18} \text{ m/s}$$

83. **(d)** : de Broglie wavelength for a particle is given by $\lambda = \frac{h}{p} = \frac{h}{mv}$, where m, v and p are the mass, velocity and momentum respectively. h is Planck's constant. Now, since all the particles are moving with same velocity, the particle with least mass will have maximum de-Broglie wavelength. Out of the given four particles (proton, neutron, α-particles, i.e., He nucleus and β-particles, i.e., electrons) β-particle has the lowest mass and therefore it has maximum wavelength.

84. **(a)**

85. **(a)** : K.E. $= 1.6 \times 10^{-19} \times 1 \text{ J} = 1\text{eV}$

86. **(c)** : Potential difference $(V) = 100$ volts.

Kinetic energy of an electron (K.E.)

$= eV = (1.6 \times 10^{-19}) \times 100$

$= 1.6 \times 10^{-17}$ J

87. **(c) :** Kinetic energy $(E) = 100\text{eV}$;

Mass of electron $(m) = 9.1 \times 10^{-31}$ kg;

$1\text{eV} = 1.6 \times 10^{-19}$ J and

Planck's constant $(h) = 6.6 \times 10^{-34}$ J s

Energy of an electron

$(E) = 100 \times (1.6 \times 10^{-19})$J

Or $\lambda = \frac{h}{\sqrt{2mE}}$

$$= \frac{6.6 \times 10^{-34}}{\sqrt{2 \times 9.1 \times 10^{-31} \times 100 \times 1.6 \times 10^{-19}}}$$

$= 1.2 \times 10^{-10}$ m $= 1.2$Å

88. **(a) :** The kinetic energy of an electron,

$\frac{1}{2} \times mv^2 = eV$

or final velocity of electron $(v) = \sqrt{\frac{2eV}{m}}$

89. **(d) :** Momentum of electrons, $(p_e) = \sqrt{2meV}$

Momentum for proton $(p_p) = \sqrt{2\text{MeV}}$

Therefore, $\frac{\lambda_p}{\lambda_e} = \frac{h/p_p}{h/p_e} = \frac{p_e}{p_p} = \frac{\sqrt{2meV}}{\sqrt{2MeV}} = \sqrt{\left(\frac{m}{M}\right)}$

Therefore, $\lambda_p = \lambda\sqrt{\left(\frac{m}{M}\right)}$

90. **(a) :** Wavelength $(\lambda) = \frac{h}{mv} = \frac{h}{p}$.

Therefore for same wavelength of electrons and photons, the momentum should

91. **(a) :** de Broglie wavelength, $\lambda = \frac{h}{p} = \frac{h}{mv}$

92. **(a)**

Chapter: 26 ATOMS

Alpha-Particle Scattering and Rutherford's Nuclear Model of Atom

1. When an α-particle of mass m moving with velocity v bombards on a heavy nucleus of charge Ze, its distance of closest approach from the nucleus depends on m as **(NEET-I 2016)**

(a) $\frac{1}{m^2}$ (b) m

(c) $\frac{1}{m}$ (d) $\frac{1}{\sqrt{m}}$

2. An alpha nucleus of energy $\frac{1}{2}mv^2$ bombards a heavy nuclear target of charge Ze. Then the distance of closest approach for the alpha nucleus will be proportional to **(2010)**

(a) $\frac{1}{Ze}$ (b) v^2

(c) $\frac{1}{m}$ (d) $\frac{1}{v^4}$

3. In a Rutherford scattering experiment when a projectile of charge z_1 and mass M_1 approaches a target nucleus of charge z_2 and mass M_2, the distance of closest approach is r_0. The energy of the projectile is **(2009)**

(a) directly proportional to $z_1 z_2$

(b) inversely proportional to z_1

(c) directly proportional to mass M_1

(d) directly proportional to $M_1 \times M_2$

4. An electron is moving round the nucleus of a hydrogen atom in a circular orbit of radius r. The Coulomb force $\vec{F}$ between the two is **(2003)**

(a) $K\frac{e^2}{r^2}\hat{r}$

(b) $-K\frac{e^2}{r^3}\hat{r}$

(c) $K\frac{e^2}{r^3}\vec{r}$

(d) $-K\frac{e^2}{r^3}\vec{r}$ $\left(\text{where } K = \frac{1}{4\pi\varepsilon_0}\right)$

Atomic Spectra

5. In hydrogen spectrum, the shortest wavelength in the Balmer series is λ. The shortest wavelength in the Bracket series is **(2023)**

(a) 4λ (b) 9λ

(c) 16λ (d) 2λ

6. The ratio of wavelengths of the last line of Balmer series and the last line of Lyman series is **(2017)**

(a) 1 (b) 4

(c) 0.5 (d) 2

7. Given the value of Rydberg constant is $10^7\ m^{-1}$, the wave number of the last line of the Balmer series in hydrogen spectrum will be **(NEET-I 2016)**

(a) $0.25 \times 10^7\ m^{-1}$ (b) $2.5 \times 10^7\ m^{-1}$

(c) $0.025 \times 10^4\ m^{-1}$ (d) $0.5 \times 10^7\ m^{-1}$

8. Ratio of longest wavelengths corresponding to Lyman and Balmer series in hydrogen spectrum is **(2013)**

(a) $\frac{7}{29}$ (b) $\frac{9}{31}$

(c) $\frac{5}{27}$ (d) $\frac{5}{23}$

9. The wavelength of the first line of Lyman series for hydrogen atom is equal to that of the second line of Balmer series for a hydrogen like ion. The atomic number Z of hydrogen like ion is **(2011)**

(a) 3 (b) 4

(c) 1 (d) 2

10. Which source is associated with a line emission spectirum? **(1993)**

(a) Electric fire

(b) Neon street sign

(c) Red traffic light

(d) Sun

Bohr Model of the Hydrogen Atom

11. The radius of inner most orbit of hydrogen atom is 5.3×10^{-11} m. What is the radius of third allowed orbit of hydrogen atom?

(2023)

(a) 1.06 Å (b) 1.59 Å

(c) 4.77 Å (d) 0.53 Å

12. Let T_1 and T_2 be the energy of an electron in the first and second excited states of hydrogen atom, respectively. According to the Bohr's model of an atom, the ratio $T_1 : T_2$ is **(2022)**

(a) $1:4$ (b) $4:1$

(c) $4:9$ (d) $9:4$

13. For which one of the following, Bohr model is not valid? **(2020)**

(a) Hydrogen atom

(b) Singly ionised helium atom (He^+)

(c) Deuteron atom

(d) Singly ionised neon atom (Ne^+)

14. The total energy of an electron in an atom in an orbit is -3.4eV. Its kinetic and potential energies are, respectively **(2019)**

(a) 3.4eV, 3.4eV (b) -3.4eV, -3.4Ev

(c) -3.4eV, -6.8eV (d) 3.4eV, -6.8eV

15. The radius of the first permitted Bohr orbit for the electron, in a hydrogen atom equals 0.51Å and its ground state energy equals -13.6eV. If the electron in the hydrogen atom is replaced by muon (μ^-) [charge same as electron and mass $207m_e$], the first Bohr radius and ground state energy will be **(Odisha NEET 2019)**

(a) 0.53×10^{-13} m, -3.6eV

(b) 25.6×10^{-13} m, -2.8eV

(c) 2.56×10^{-13} m, -2.8keV

(d) 2.56×10^{-13} m, -13.6eV

16. The ratio of kinetic energy to the total energy of an electron in a Bohr orbit of the hydrogen atom, is **(2018)**

(a) $1:1$ (b) $1:-1$

(c) $2:-1$ (d) $1:-2$

17. Consider 3rd orbit of He^+(Helium), using non-relativistic approach, the speed of electron in this orbit will be [given $K = 9 \times 10^9$ constant, $Z = 2$ and h (Planck's constant) $= 6.6 \times 10^{-34}$ J s]

(2015 Cancelled)

(a) 0.73×10^6 m/s (b) 3.0×10^8 m/s
(c) 2.92×10^6 m/s (d) 1.46×10^6 m/s

18. An electron in hydrogen atom makes a transition $n_1 \rightarrow n_2$ where n_1 and n_2 are principal quantum numbers of the two states. Assuming Bohr's model to be valid, the time period of the electron in the initial state is eight times that in the final state. The possible values of n_1 and n_2 are

(Karnataka NEET 2013)

(a) $n_1 = 6$ and $n_2 = 2$
(b) $n_1 = 8$ and $n_2 = 1$
(c) $n_1 = 8$ and $n_2 = 2$
(d) $n_1 = 4$ and $n_2 = 2$

19. Monochromatic radiation emitted when electron on hydrogen atom jumps from first excited to the ground state irradiates a photosensitive material. The stopping potential is measured to be 3.57 V. The threshold frequency of the material is

(2012)

(a) 4×10^{15} Hz (b) 5×10^{15} Hz
(c) 1.6×10^{15} Hz (d) 2.5×10^{15} Hz

20. An electron in the hydrogen atom jumps from excited state n to the ground state. The wavelength so emitted illuminates a photosensitive material having work function 2.75eV. If the stopping potential of the photoelectron is 10 V, then the value of n is **(Mains 2011)**

(a) 2 (b) 3
(c) 4 (d) 5

21. Out of the following which one is not a possible energy for a photon to be emitted by hydrogen atom according to Bohr's atomic model? **(Mains 2011)**

(a) 0.65eV (b) 1.9eV
(c) 11.1eV (d) 13.6eV

22. The energy of a hydrogen atom in the ground state is -13.6eV. The energy of a He^+ ion in the first excited state will be

(2010)

(a) -13.6eV (b) -27.2eV
(c) -54.4eV (d) -6.8eV

23. The electron in the hydrogen atom jumps from excited state $(n = 3)$ to its ground state $(n = 1)$ and the photons thus emitted irradiate a photosensitive material. If the work function of the material is 5.1eV, the stopping potential is estimated to be (the energy of the electron in n^{th} state $E_n = \frac{-13.6}{n^2}$ eV) **(Mains 2010)**

(a) 5.1 V (b) 12.1 V
(c) 17.2 V (d) 7 V

24. The ground state energy of hydrogen atom is -13.6eV. When its electron is in the first excited state, its excitation energy is

(2008)

(a) 10.2eV (b) 0
(c) 3.4eV (d) 6.8eV

25. The total energy of electron in the ground state of hydrogen atom is -13.6eV. The kinetic energy of an electron in the first excited state is **(2007)**

(a) 6.8eV (b) 13.6eV
(c) 1.7eV (d) 3.4eV

26. The total energy of an electron in the first excited state of hydrogen atom is about $-3.4eV$. Its kinetic energy in this state is **(2005)**

(a) $3.4eV$ (b) $6.8eV$

(c) $-3.4eV$ (d) $-6.8eV$

27. The Bohr model of atoms **(2004)**

(a) Assumes that the angular momentum of electrons is quantized.

(b) Uses Einstein's photoelectric equation.

(c) Predicts continuous emission spectra for atoms.

(d) Predicts the same emission spectra for all types of atoms.

28. In which of the following systems will the radius of the first orbit $(n = 1)$ be minimum? **(2003)**

(a) doubly ionized lithium

(b) singly ionized helium

(c) deuterium atom

(d) hydrogen atom

29. The energy of hydrogen atom in n^{th} orbit is E_n then the energy in n^{th} orbit of singly ionised helium atom will be **(2001)**

(a) $4E_n$ (b) $E_n/4$

(c) $2E_n$ (d) $E_n/2$

30. The life span of atomic hydrogen is **(2000)**

(a) fraction of one second

(b) one year

(c) one hour (d) one day

31. In the Bohr model of a hydrogen atom, the centripetal force is furnished by the coulomb attraction between the proton and the electron. If a_0 is the radius of the ground state orbit, m is the mass and e is the charge on the electron and ε_0 is the vacuum permittivity, the speed of the electron is **(1998)**

(a) $\frac{e}{\sqrt{4\pi\varepsilon_0 a_0 m}}$ (b) $\frac{e}{\sqrt{\varepsilon_0 a_0 m}}$

(c) 0 (d) $\frac{\sqrt{4\pi\varepsilon_0 a_0 m}}{e}$

32. The energy of the ground electronic state of hydrogen atom is $-13.6eV$. The energy of the first excited state will be **(1997)**

(a) $-27.2eV$ (b) $-52.4eV$

(c) $-3.4eV$ (d) $-6.8eV$

33. When hydrogen atom is in its first excited level, its radius is of the Bohr radius. **(1997)**

(a) twice (b) 4 times

(c) same (d) half

34. According to Bohr's principle, the relation between principal quantum number (n) and radius of orbit (r) is **(1996)**

(a) $r \propto \frac{1}{n}$ (b) $r \propto \frac{1}{n^2}$

(c) $r \propto n$ (d) $r \propto n^2$

35. When a hydrogen atom is raised from the ground state to an excited state, **(1995)**

(a) both K.E. and P.E. increase

(b) both K.E. and P.E. decrease

(c) the P.E. decreases and K.E. increases

(d) the P.E. increases and K.E. decreases.

36. In terms of Bohr radius a_0, the radius of the second Bohr orbit of a hydrogen atom is given by **(1992)**

(a) $4a_0$ (b) $8a_0$

(c) $\sqrt{2}a_0$ (d) $2a_0$

37. The ionization energy of hydrogen atom is 13.6eV. Following Bohr's theory, the energy corresponding to a transition between 3rd and 4th orbit is **(1992)**

(a) 3.40eV (b) 1.51eV

(c) 0.85eV (d) 0.66eV

38. The ground state energy of H-atom is −13.6eV. The energy needed to ionize H-atom from its second excited state **(1991)**

(a) 1.51eV (b) 3.4eV

(c) 13.6eV (d) none of these

39. To explain his theory, Bohr used **(1989)**

(a) conservation of linear momentum

(b) quantisation of angular momentum

(c) conservation of quantum frequency

(d) none of these

40. The ionisation energy of hydrogen atom is 13.6eV, the ionisation energy of a singly ionised helium atom would be **(1988)**

(a) 13.6eV (b) 27.2eV

(c) 6.8eV (d) 54.4eV

The Line Spectra of the Hydrogen Atom

41. If an electron in a hydrogen atom jumps from the 3rd orbit to the 2nd orbit, it emits a photon of wavelength λ. When it jumps from the 4th orbit to the 3rd orbit, the corresponding wavelength of the photon will be **(NEET-II 2016)**

(a) $\frac{16}{25}\lambda$ (b) $\frac{9}{16}\lambda$ (c) $\frac{20}{7}\lambda$ (d) $\frac{20}{13}\lambda$

42. Hydrogen atom in ground state is excited by a monochromatic radiation of $\lambda = 975Å$. Number of spectral lines in the resulting spectrum emitted will be **(2014)**

(a) 3 (b) 2

(c) 6 (d) 10

43. Electron in hydrogen atom first jumps from third excited state to second excited state and then from second excited to the first excited state. The ratio of the wavelengths $\lambda_1 : \lambda_2$ emitted in the two cases is **(2012)**

(a) $\frac{7}{5}$ (b) $\frac{27}{20}$

(c) $\frac{27}{5}$ (d) $\frac{20}{7}$

44. An electron of a stationary hydrogen atom passes from the fifth energy level to the ground level. The velocity that the atom acquired as a result of photon emission will be **(2012)**

(a) $\frac{24hR}{25m}$ (b) $\frac{25hR}{24m}$

(c) $\frac{25m}{24hR}$ (d) $\frac{24m}{25hR}$

(is the mass of the electron, R Rydberg constant and h Planck's constant)

45. The transition from the state $n = 3$ to $n = 1$ in a hydrogen like atom results in ultraviolet radiation. Infrared radiation will be obtained in the transition from

(Mains 2012)

(a) $2 \to 1$ (b) $3 \to 2$

(c) $4 \to 2$ (d) $4 \to 3$

46. The ionization energy of the electron in the hydrogen atom in its ground state is 13.6eV. The atoms are excited to higher energy levels to emit radiations of 6 wavelengths. Maximum wavelength of emitted radiation corresponds to the transition between **(2009)**

(a) $n = 3$ to $n = 1$ states

(b) $n = 2$ to $n = 1$ states

(c) $n = 4$ to $n = 3$ states

(d) $n = 3$ to $n = 2$ states

47. Ionization potential of hydrogen atom is 13.6eV. Hydrogen atoms in the ground state are excited by monochromatic radiation of photon energy 12.1eV. According to Bohr's theory, the spectral lines emitted by hydrogen will be **(2006)**

(a) one (b) two

(c) three (d) four.

48. Energy levels A, B and C of a certain atom corresponding to increasing values of energy i.e., $E_A < E_B < E_C$. If λ_1, λ_2 and λ_3 are wavelengths of radiations corresponding to transitions C to B, B to A and C to A respectively, which of the following relations is correct? **(2005, 1990)**

(a) $\lambda_3 = \lambda_1 + \lambda_2$

(b) $\lambda_3 = \frac{\lambda_1 \lambda_2}{\lambda_1 + \lambda_2}$

(c) $\lambda_1 + \lambda_2 + \lambda_3 = 0$

(d) $\lambda_3^2 = \lambda_1^2 + \lambda_2^2$

49. Maximum frequency of emission is obtained for the transition **(2000)**

(a) $n = 2$ to $n = 1$ (b) $n = 6$ to $n = 2$

(c) $n = 1$ to $n = 2$ (d) $n = 2$ to $n = 6$

50. When an electron does transition from $n = 4$ to $n = 2$, then emitted line spectrum will be **(2000)**

(a) first line of Lyman series

(b) second line of Balmer series

(c) first line of Paschen series

(d) second line of Paschen series.

51. An electron makes a transition from orbit $n = 4$ to the orbit $n = 2$ of a hydrogen atom. What is the wavelength of the emitted radiations? (= Rydberg's constant) **(1995)**

(a) $\frac{16}{4R}$ (b) $\frac{16}{5R}$

(c) $\frac{16}{2R}$ (d) $\frac{16}{3R}$

52. The figure indicates the energy level diagram of an atom and the origin of six spectral lines in emission (e.g., line no. 5 arises from the transition from level B to A).

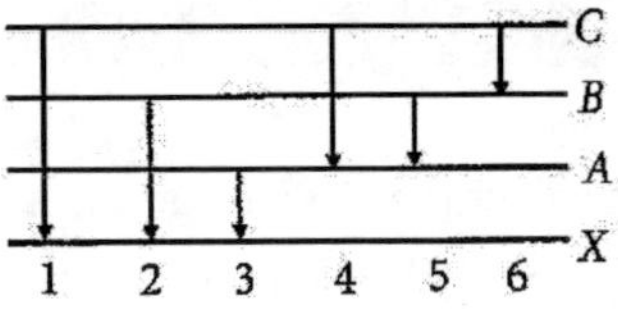

Which of the following spectral lines will occur in the absorption spectrum? **(1995)**

(a) 4,5,6 (b) 1,2,3,4,5,6

(c) 1,2,3 (d) 1,4,6

53. Hydrogen atoms are excited from ground state of the principle quantum number 4 . Then the number of spectral lines observed will be **(1993)**

(a) 3 (b) 6
(c) 5 (d) 2

de Broglie's Explanation of Bohr's Second Postulate of Quantisation

54. Consider an electron in the nth orbit of a hydrogen atom in the Bohr model. The circumference of the orbit can be expressed in terms of de Broglie wavelength λ of that electron as **(1990)**

(a) $(0.529)n\lambda$ (b) $\sqrt{n}\lambda$
(c) $(13.6)\lambda$ (d) $n\lambda$

ANSWER KEY

1.	(c)	2.	(c)	3.	(a)	4.	(d)	5.	(a)	6.	(b)	7.	(a)
8.	(c)	9.	(d)	10.	(b)	11.	(c)	12.	(d)	13.	(d)	14.	(d)
15.	(c)	16.	(b)	17.	(d)	18.	(d)	19.	(c)	20.	(c)	21.	(c)
22.	(a)	23.	(d)	24.	(a)	25.	(d)	26.	(a)	27.	(a)	28.	(a)
29.	(a)	30.	(a)	31.	(a)	32.	(c)	33.	(b)	34.	(d)	35.	(d)
36.	(a)	37.	(d)	38.	(a)	39.	(b)	40.	(d)	41.	(c)	42.	(c)
43.	(d)	44.	(a)	45.	(d)	46.	(c)	47.	(c)	48.	(b)	49.	(a)
50.	(b)	51.	(d)	52.	(c)	53.	(b)	54.	(d)				

Hints & Explanations

1. **(c) :** Distance of closest approach when an α-particle of mass m moving with velocity v is bombarded on a heavy nucleus of charge Ze, is given by

$$r_0 = \frac{Ze^2}{2\pi\varepsilon_0 mv^2} \quad \therefore r_0 \propto \frac{1}{m}$$

2. **(c) :**

3. **(a) :** Energy of the projectile is the potential energy at closest approach, $\frac{1}{4\pi\varepsilon_0}\frac{z_1z_2}{r}$. Therefore energy $\propto z_1z_2$

4. **(d) :** The charge on hydrogen nucleus $q_1 = +e$

charge on electron, $q_2 = -e$

Coulomb force, $F = K\frac{q_1q_2}{r^2} = K\frac{(+e)(-e)}{r^2}$

$$\vec{F} = -\frac{Ke^2}{r^3}\vec{r} = -\frac{Ke^2}{r^2}\hat{r}$$

5. **(a) :** Shortest wavelength in Balmer series when transition of e^- from ∞ to $n = 2$

$$\because \frac{1}{\lambda} = Rz^2\left[\frac{1}{2^2} - \frac{1}{\infty^2}\right]$$

$$\frac{1}{\lambda} = \frac{R}{4}$$

Shortest wavelength is Bracket series when transition of e^- from ∞ to $n = 4$

$$\frac{1}{\lambda'} = R(1)^2\left[\frac{1}{4^2} - \frac{1}{\infty^2}\right] \Rightarrow \frac{1}{\lambda'} = \frac{R}{16}$$

Eq. (1)/Eq. (2)

$$\frac{\lambda'}{\lambda} = \frac{R}{4} \times \frac{16}{R} \Rightarrow \lambda' = 4\lambda$$

6. **(b) :** The wavelength of last line of Balmer series

$$\frac{1}{\lambda_B} = R\left(\frac{1}{2^2} - \frac{1}{\infty^2}\right) = \frac{R}{4}$$

The wavelength of last line of Lyman series

$$\frac{1}{\lambda_L} = R\left(\frac{1}{1^2} - \frac{1}{\infty^2}\right) = R \therefore \frac{\lambda_B}{\lambda_L} = \frac{4}{1} = 4$$

7. **(a) :** Here, $R = 10^7 \text{ m}^{-1}$

The wave number of the last line of the Balmer series in hydrogen spectrum is given by

$$\frac{1}{\lambda} = R\left(\frac{1}{2^2} - \frac{1}{\infty^2}\right) = \frac{R}{4} = \frac{10^7}{4}$$

$$= 0.25 \times 10^7 \text{ m}^{-1}$$

8. **(c) :** The wavelength of different spectral lines of Lyman series is given by

$$\frac{1}{\lambda_L} = R\left[\frac{1}{1^2} - \frac{1}{n^2}\right] \text{ where } n = 2,3,4, \ldots$$

where subscript L refers to Lyman.

For longest wavelength, $n = 2$

$$\therefore \frac{1}{\lambda_{L_{\text{longest}}}} = R\left[\frac{1}{1^2} - \frac{1}{2^2}\right] = \frac{3}{4}R$$

The wavelength of different spectral series of Balmer series is given by

$$\frac{1}{\lambda_B} = R\left[\frac{1}{2^2} - \frac{1}{n^2}\right] \text{ where } n = 3,4,5, \ldots.$$

where subscript B refers to Balmer.

For longest wavelength, $n = 3$

$$\therefore \frac{1}{\lambda_{B_{\text{longest}}}} = R\left[\frac{1}{2^2} - \frac{1}{3^2}\right] = R\left[\frac{1}{4} - \frac{1}{9}\right]$$

$$= \frac{5R}{36}$$

Divide (ii) by (i), we get

$$\frac{\lambda_{L_{\text{longest}}}}{\lambda_{B_{\text{longest}}}} = \frac{5R}{36} \times \frac{4}{3R} = \frac{5}{27}$$

9. **(d) :** The wavelength of the first line of lyman series for hydrogen atom is $\frac{1}{\lambda} = R\left[\frac{1}{1^2} - \frac{1}{2^2}\right]$

The wavelength of the second line of Balmer series for hydrogen like ion is $\frac{1}{\lambda'} = Z^2R\left[\frac{1}{2^2} - \frac{1}{4^2}\right]$

According to question $\lambda = \lambda'$

$$\Rightarrow R\left[\frac{1}{1^2} - \frac{1}{2^2}\right] = Z^2R\left[\frac{1}{2^2} - \frac{1}{4^2}\right]$$

or $\frac{3}{4} = \frac{3Z^2}{16}$ or $Z^2 = 4$ or $Z = 2$

10. **(b) :** Neon street sign is a source of line emission spectrum.

11. **(c) :** Radius of nth orbit in Hydrogen Atom $r_n = 0.53 \times \frac{n^2}{Z} \mathring{A}$

So, radius of third orbit

$$r_3 = 0.53 \times \frac{(3)^2}{(1)} \AA = 4.77 \AA$$

12. **(d) :**

For 1st excited state, $n = 2$

For 2nd excited state, $n = 3$

$$\therefore \frac{T_1}{T_2} = \frac{n_2^2}{n_1^2} = \frac{3^2}{2^2} = \frac{9}{4}$$

13. **(d) :** Bohr's atomic model is valid for single electron species only. A singly ionised neon contains more than one electron. Hence option (d) is correct.

14. **(d) :** Total energy of electron in n^{th} orbit,

$E_n = \frac{-13.6Z^2}{n^2}$ eV.

Kinetic energy of electron in nth orbit,

K. E. $= \frac{13.6Z^2}{n^2}$ eV.

Potential energy of electron in n^{th} orbit,

P.E. $= \frac{-27.2Z^2}{n^2}$ eV

Thus, total energy of electron,

$E_n = -$ K.E. $= \frac{\text{P.E.}}{2}$

$\therefore$ K.E. $= 3.4$eV

P.E. $= 2 \times -3.4 = -6.8$eV

[Given $E_n = -3.4$eV]

15. **(c) :** Given, radius of first Bohr orbit for electron in a hydrogen atom, $r =$ 0.51

and its ground state energy, $E_n =$ -13.6eV

Charge of muon = charge of electron

Mass of muon = 207 × (mass of electron)

Therefore, when electron is replaced by muon then, first Bohr radius, $r_1' =$ $\frac{0.51}{207} = 2.56 \times 10^{-13}$ m and ground state energy, $E_1' = -13.6 \times 207 =$ $-2815.2\text{eV} = -2.815\text{keV}$

16. **(b) :** In a Bohr orbit of the hydrogen atom,

Kinetic energy = −(Total energy)

So, Kinetic energy : Total energy = 1 : -1

17. **(d) :**

Energy of electron in He$^+$ 3rd orbit

$$E_3 = -13.6 \times \frac{Z^2}{n^2}\text{eV} = -13.6 \times \frac{4}{9}\text{eV}$$

$= -13.6 \times \frac{4}{9} \times 1.6 \times 10^{-19}$ J $\simeq -9.7 \times 10^{-19} J$

As per Bohr's model,

Kinetic energy of electron in the 3rd orbit $= -E_3$

$$\therefore 9.7 \times 10^{-19} = \frac{1}{2} m_e v^2 \Rightarrow v$$

$$= \sqrt{\frac{2 \times 9.7 \times 10^{-19}}{9.1 \times 10^{-31}}}$$

$= 1.46 \times 10^6$ m s^{-1}

18. **(d) :** In the nth orgit let r_n = radius and v_n = speed of election

Time period $T_n = \frac{2\pi r_n}{V_n} \propto \frac{r_n}{V_n}$

Now $r_n \propto n^2$, $V_n \propto \frac{1}{n}$

$\frac{r_n}{V_n} \propto n^3 \, Tn \propto n^3$;

$\left(\frac{n_1}{n_2}\right)^3 = \frac{T_1}{T_2} = 8$

$\left(\frac{n_1}{n_2}\right)^3 = 8$; $\frac{n_1}{n_2} = 2$

$n_1 = 2n_2$; $n_1 = 4$

$n_2 = 2$

19. **(c) :** For hydrogen atom, $E_n = -\frac{13.6}{n^2}$ eV

For ground state, $n = 1 \therefore E_1 = -\frac{13.6}{1^2} = -13.6\text{eV}$

For first excited state, $n = 2 \therefore E_2 = -\frac{13.6}{2^2} = -3.4\text{eV}$

The energy of the emitted photon when an electron jumps from first excited state to ground state is

$hv = E_2 - E_1 = -3.4\text{eV} - (-13.6\text{eV})$

$= 10.2\text{eV}$

Maximum kinetic energy,

$K_{max} = eV_s = e \times 3.57 \text{ V} = 3.57\text{eV}$

According to Einstein's photoelectric equation $K_{max} = hv - \phi_0$ where ϕ_0 is the work function and hv is the incident energy $\phi_0 = hv - K_{max} = 10.2\text{eV} - 3.57\text{eV} = 6.63\text{eV}$

Threshold frequency, $v_0 = \frac{\phi_0}{h} = \frac{6.63 \times 1.6 \times 10^{-19}\text{ J}}{6.63 \times 10^{-34}\text{ J s}}$

$= 1.6 \times 10^{15}$ Hz

20. **(c) :** Here, Stopping potential, $V_0 = 10$ V

Work function, $W = 2.75\text{eV}$

According to Einstein's photoelectric equation

$$eV_0 = hv - W \text{ or } hv = eV_0 + W$$
$$= 10\text{eV} + 2.75\text{eV} = 12.75\text{eV}$$

When an electron in the hydrogen atom makes a transition from excited state n to the gound state ($n = 1$), then the frequency (v) of the emitted photon is given by

$$hv = E_n - E_1 \Rightarrow hv = -\frac{13.6}{n^2} - \left(-\frac{13.6}{1^2}\right)$$

$\left[\because \text{ For hydrogen atom, } E_n = -\frac{13.6}{n^2}\text{eV}\right]$

According to given problem

$$-\frac{13.6}{n^2} + 13.6 = 12.75 \text{ (Using(i))}$$

$$\frac{13.6}{n^2} = 0.85 \Rightarrow n^2 = \frac{13.6}{0.85} = 16 \text{ or } n = 4$$

21. **(c) :** The energy of nth orbit of hydrogen atom is given as

$$E_n = -\frac{13.6}{n^2}\text{eV}$$

$$\therefore E_1 = -13.6\text{eV}; E_2 = -\frac{13.6}{2^2} = -3.4\text{eV}$$

$$E_3 = -\frac{13.6}{3^2} = -1.5\text{eV}; E_4 = -\frac{13.6}{4^2}$$
$$= -0.85\text{eV}$$

$$\therefore E_3 - E_2 = -1.5 - (-3.4) = 1.9\text{eV}$$
$$E_4 - E_3 = -0.85 - (-1.5) = 0.65\text{eV}$$

22. **(a) :** The energy of e^- in n^{th} state

$$E_n = \frac{-13.6}{n^2}\text{ev}$$

The energy of He^+ ion in the first excited state

$E_n = -13.6\frac{Z^2}{n^2} = -13.6\times\frac{4}{4} = -13.6 ev$

23. **(d) :** Energy released when electron in the atom jumps from excited state ($n = 3$) to ground state ($n = 1$) is $E = h\nu = E_3 - E_1 = \frac{-13.6}{3^2} - \left(\frac{-13.6}{1^2}\right) = \frac{-13.6}{9} + 13.6 =$ 12.1eV

Therefore, stopping potential

$eV_0 = h\nu - \phi_0 = 12.1 - 5.1 = 7 eV$

$$V_0 = 7 V$$

[$\because$ work function $\phi_0 = 5.1$]

24. **(a) :**

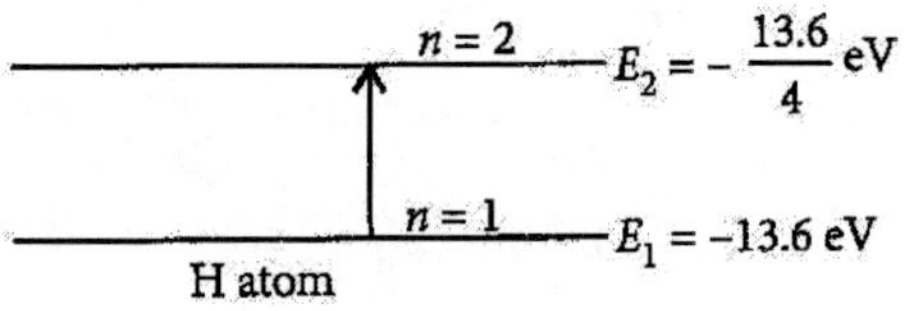

1 st excitation energy

$E_{n2} - E_{n1} = (-3.4 + 13.6) = 10.2 eV$

25. **(d) :** Energy of nth orbit of hydrogen atom is given by $E_n = \frac{-13.6}{n^2} eV$

For ground state,

$n = 1 \therefore E_1 = \frac{-13.6}{1^?} = -13.6 eV$

For first excited state,

$n = 2 \therefore E_2 = \frac{-13.6}{2^2} = -3.4 eV$

Kinetic energy of an electron in the first excited state is $K = -E_2 = 3.4 eV$

26. **(a) :** K.E. $= |\frac{1}{2}$ P.E. $|$

$\therefore$ Total energy $= |\frac{1}{2}$ P.E. $| -$ P.E. $=$

$\frac{-\text{P.E.}}{2} = -3.4 eV.$

$\therefore$ K.E. $= +3.4 eV$

27. **(a)**

28. **(a) :** Radius of first orbit, $r \propto \frac{1}{Z}$, for doubly ionized lithium $Z(= 3)$ will be maximum, hence for doubly ionized lithium, r will be minimum.

29. **(a) :** $E \propto \frac{Z^2}{n^2}$

30. **(a) :**

31. **(a) :** Centripetal force = force of attraction of nucleus on electron $\frac{mv^2}{a_0} = \frac{1}{4\pi\varepsilon_0}\frac{e^2}{a_0^2} \Rightarrow v = \frac{e}{\sqrt{4\pi\varepsilon_0 a_0 m}}$

32. **(c) :** Energy of the ground electronic state of hydrogen atom $E = -13.6 eV$.

We know that energy of the first excited state for second orbit (where = 2)

$$E_n = -\frac{13.6}{(n)^2} = -\frac{13.6}{(2)^2} = -3.4 eV$$

33. **(b) :** When a hydrogen atom is in its excited level, then $n = 2$. Therefore radius of hydrogen atom in its first excited level $(r) = n^2 r_0 = (2)^2 r_0 = 4r_0$.

34. **(d) :** According to Bohr's principle, radius of orbit (r)

$= 4\pi\varepsilon_0 \times \frac{n^2 h^?}{4\pi^2 me^2}; r \propto n^2$

where n = principal quantum number.

35. **(d) :** P.E. of H-atom is given by $= \frac{-KZe^2}{r}$

As atom excited its radius increases. But due to –Ve sign or reverse sign. Its actual P.E. increases and K.E. is given by

$$\text{K.E.} = \frac{KZe^2}{2r}$$

36. **(a) :** As $r \propto n^2$, therefore, radius of 2nd Bohr's orbit $= 4a_0$

37. **(d) :** $E = E_4 - E_3$

$$= -\frac{13.6}{4^2} - \left(-\frac{13.6}{3^2}\right) = -0.85 + 1.51$$

$$= 0.66\text{eV}$$

38. **(a) :** Second excited state corresponds to $n = 3$

Energy needed to ionize, $E = \frac{13.6}{3^2}\text{eV} =$ 1.51eV

39. **(b) :** Bohr used quantisation of angular momentum. For stationary orbits, Angular momentum $mvr = \frac{nh}{2\pi}$ where $n = 1, 2, 3, \ldots$etc.

40. **(d) :** $E \propto Z^2$ and Z for singly ionised helium is 2 (i.e., 2 protons in the nucleus) $\therefore (E)_{\text{He}} = 4 \times 13.6 = 54.4\text{eV}$

41. **(c) :** When electron jumps from higher orbit to lower orbit then, wavelength of emitted photon is given by,

$$\frac{1}{\lambda} = R\left(\frac{1}{n_f^2} - \frac{1}{n_i^2}\right)$$

$$\text{so, } \frac{1}{\lambda} = R\left(\frac{1}{2^2} - \frac{1}{3^2}\right) = \frac{5R}{36} \text{ and}$$

$$\frac{1}{\lambda'} = R\left(\frac{1}{3^2} - \frac{1}{4^2}\right) = \frac{7R}{144}$$

$$\therefore \lambda' = \frac{144}{7} \times \frac{5\lambda}{36} = \frac{20\lambda}{7}$$

42. **(c) :** Energy of the photon, $E = \frac{hc}{\lambda}$

$$E = \frac{6.63\times10^{-34}\times3\times10^{8}}{975\times10^{-10}}\text{ J}$$

$$= \frac{6.63 \times 10^{-34} \times 3 \times 10^{8}}{975 \times 10^{-10} \times 1.6 \times 10^{-19}}\text{eV}$$

$$= 12.75\text{eV}$$

After absorbing a photon of energy 12.75eV, the electron will reach to third excited state of energy -0.85eV, since energy difference corresponding to $n = 1$ and $n = 4$ is 12.75eV.

$\therefore$ Number of spectral lines emitted

$$= \frac{(n)(n-1)}{2} = \frac{(4)(4-1)}{2} = 6$$

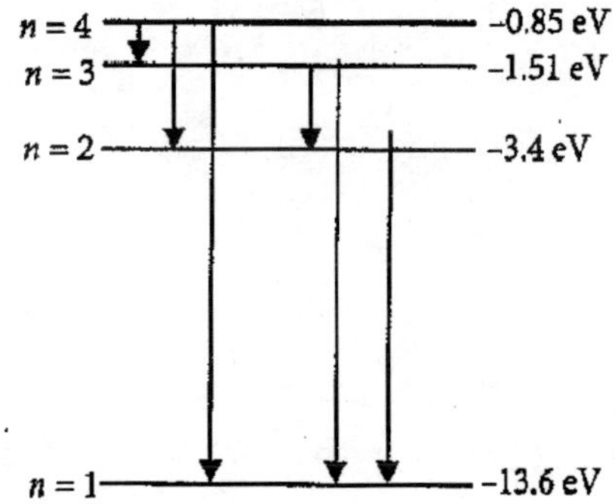

43. **(d) :** As e⁻ is jumping from 3rd exeited state to 2nd excited state

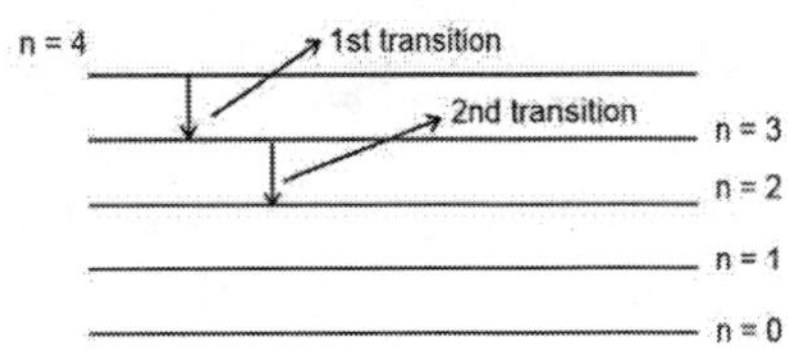

$n_i = 4$ $\qquad$ $n_f = 3$

$$\frac{1}{\lambda} = R_H\left[\frac{1}{n_{f^2}} - \frac{1}{n_{i^2}}\right]$$

$$\frac{1}{\lambda} = R_H\left[\frac{1}{3^2} - \frac{1}{4^2}\right]$$

$$\frac{1}{\lambda}=R_H\left[\frac{16-9}{9\times16}\right]$$

$$\frac{1}{\lambda}=R_H\left[\frac{7}{16\times9}\right] \quad ...(i)$$

then e^- is jumping from 2nd exited state to 1st exited state

$$\frac{1}{\lambda_2}=R_H\left[\frac{1}{2^2}-\frac{1}{9}\right]$$

$$\frac{1}{\lambda_2}=R_H\left[\frac{9-4}{4\times9}\right]$$

$$\frac{1}{\lambda_2}=R_H\left[\frac{5}{4\times9}\right] \quad ...(ii)$$

dividing eqn (ii) by (i)

$$\frac{\frac{1}{\lambda_2}}{\frac{1}{\lambda_1}}=\frac{R_H\left[\frac{5}{4\times9}\right]}{R_H\left[\frac{7}{16\times9}\right]}=\frac{20}{7}$$

44. **(a) :** According to Rydberg formula

$$\frac{1}{\lambda}=R\left[\frac{1}{n_f^2}-\frac{1}{n_i^2}\right]$$

Here, $n_f=1, n_i=5$

$$\therefore \frac{1}{\lambda}=R\left[\frac{1}{1^2}-\frac{1}{5^2}\right]=R\left[\frac{1}{1}-\frac{1}{25}\right]=\frac{24}{25}R$$

According to conservation of linear momentum, we get Momentum of photon = Momentum of atom

$$\frac{h}{\lambda}=mv \text{ or } v=\frac{h}{m\lambda}=\frac{h}{m}\left(\frac{24R}{25}\right)=\frac{24hR}{25m}$$

45. **(d) :** Infrared radiation found in Paschen, Bracket and fund series and is obtained when e^- transition is from a high energy level to min. 3rd energy level.

46. **(c) :**

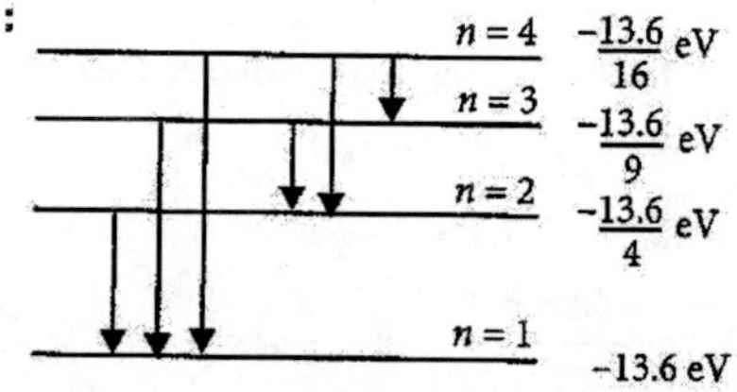

The maximum wavelength emitted here corresponds to the transition $n=4 \rightarrow n=3$ (Pasthen series 1st line)

47. **(c) :** Ionisation potential of hydrogen atom is 13.6eV.

Energy required for exciting the hydrogen atom in the ground state to orbit n is given by

$$E=E_n-E_1$$

i.e., $12.1=-\frac{13.6}{n^2}-\left(\frac{-13.6}{1^2}\right)=-\frac{13.6}{n^2}+13.6$

or, $-1.5=\frac{-13.6}{n^2}$ or, $n^2=\frac{13.6}{1.5}=9$ or, $n=3$

Number of spectral lines emitted

$$=\frac{n(n-1)}{2}=\frac{3\times2}{2}=3$$

48. **(b) :**

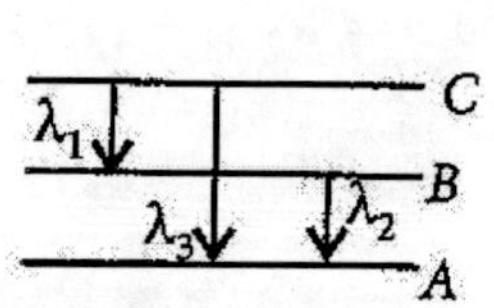

$$(E_C-E_A)=(E_C-E_B)+(E_B-E_A)$$

$$\frac{hc}{\lambda_3}=\frac{hc}{\lambda_1}+\frac{hc}{\lambda_2} \text{ or } \frac{1}{\lambda_3}=\frac{1}{\lambda_1}+\frac{1}{\lambda_2}$$

$$\therefore \frac{1}{\lambda_3}=\frac{\lambda_1+\lambda_2}{\lambda_1\lambda_2} \text{ or } \lambda_3=\frac{\lambda_1\lambda_2}{\lambda_1+\lambda_2}$$

49. (a) :

$v \propto \left[\frac{1}{n_1^2} - \frac{1}{n_2^2}\right]$

50. (b) : Jump to second orbit leads to Balmer series. The jump from 4 th orbit shall give rise to second line of Balmer series.

51. (d) : Transition of hydrogen atom from orbit $n_1 = 4$ to $n_2 = 2$.

Wave number $= \frac{1}{\lambda} = R\left[\frac{1}{n_1^2} - \frac{1}{n_2^2}\right] =$

$R\left[\frac{1}{(2)^2} - \frac{1}{(4)^2}\right]$

$= R\left[\frac{1}{4} - \frac{1}{16}\right] = R\left[\frac{4-1}{16}\right] = \frac{3R}{16} \Rightarrow \lambda$

$= 16/3R$

52. (c) : Absorption spectrum involves only excitation of ground level to higher level. Therefore spectral lines 1, 2, 3 will occur in the absorption spectrum.

53. (b)

54. (d) : The circumference of an orbit in an atom in terms of wavelength of wave associated with electron is given by the relation,

Circumference $= n\lambda$, where $n = 1,2,3,...$

Chapter: 27 NUCLEI

Atomic Masses and Composition of Nucleus

1. Which one of the following pairs of nuclei are isotones? **(2005)**

(a) ${}_{34}Se^{74}$, ${}_{31}Ga^{71}$

(b) ${}_{38}Sr^{84}$, ${}_{38}Sr^{86}$

(c) ${}_{42}Mo^{92}$, ${}_{40}Zr^{92}$

(d) ${}_{20}Ca^{40}$, ${}_{16}S^{32}$

2. A nucleus represented by the symbol ${}_Z^AX$ has **(2004)**

(a) Z neutrons and $A-Z$ protons

(b) Z protons and $A-Z$ neutrons

(c) Z protons and A neutrons

(d) A protons and $Z-A$ neutrons

3. The mass number of a nucleus is **(2003)**

(a) always less than its atomic number

(b) always more than its atomic number

(c) sometimes equal to its atomic number

(d) sometimes less than and sometimes more than its atomic number

4. Atomic weight of Boron is 10.81 and it has two isotopes ${}_5B^{10}$ and ${}_5B^{11}$. Then the ratio of ${}_5B^{10}$: ${}_5B^{11}$ in nature would be **(1998)**

(a) 15: 16 (b) 10: 11

(c) 19: 81 (d) 81: 19

5. The constituents of atomic nuclei are believed to be **(1991)**

(a) neutrons and protons

(b) protons only

(c) electrons and protons

(d) electrons, protons and neutrons

6. In the nucleus of ${}_{11}Na^{23}$, the number of protons, neutrons and electrons are **(1991)**

(a) 11,12,0 (b) 23,12,11

(c) 12,11,0 (d) 23,11,12

7. The nuclei ${}_6C^{13}$ and ${}_7N^{14}$ can be described as **(1990)**

(a) isotones

(b) isobars

(c) isotopes of carbon

(d) isotopes of nitrogen

Size of the Nucleus

8. A nucleus of mass number 189 splits into two nuclei having mass number 125 and 64 . The ratio of radius of two daughter nuclei respectively is **(2022)**

(a) 1: 1 (b) 4: 5

(c) 5: 4 (d) 25: 16

9. If the nuclear radius of ${}^{27}Al$ is 3.6 fermi, the approximate nuclear radius of ${}^{64}Cu$ in fermi is **(2012)**

(a) 2.4 (b) 1.2

(c) 4.8 (d) 3.6

10. Two nuclei have their mass numbers in the ratio of 1: 3. The ratio of their nuclear densities would be **(2008)**

(a) $(3)^{1/3}: 1$ (b) 1: 1

(c) 1: 3 (d) 3: 1

11. If the nucleus $^{27}_{13}Al$ has a nuclear radius of about 3.6fm, then $^{125}_{32}Te$ would have its radius approximately as **(2007)**

(a) 9.6fm (b) 12.0fm

(c) 4.8fm (d) 6.0fm

12. The radius of germanium (Ge) nuclide is measured to be twice the radius of $^{9}_{4}Be$. The number of nucleons in Ge are **(2006)**

(a) 72 (b) 73

(c) 74 (d) 75

13. The volume occupied by an atom is greater than the volume of the nucleus by a factor of about **(2003)**

(a) 10^1 (b) 10^5

(c) 10^{10} (d) 10^{15}

14. A nucleus ruptures into two nuclear parts, which have their velocity ratio equal to 2: 1. What will be the ratio of their nuclear size (nuclear radius)? **(1996)**

(a) $3^{1/2}: 1$ (b) $1: 3^{1/2}$

(c) $2^{1/3}: 1$ (d) $1: 2^{1/3}$

15. The mass number of He is 4 and that of sulphur is 32. The radius of sulphur nucleus is larger than that of helium by the factor of **(1995)**

(a) 4 (b) 2

(c) 8 (d) $\sqrt{8}$

16. The mass density of a nucleus varies with mass number A as **(1992)**

(a) A^2 (b) A

(c) constant (d) $1/A$

17. The ratio of the radii of the nuclei $_{13}Al^{27}$ and $_{52}Te^{125}$ is approximately **(1990)**

(a) 6: 10 (b) 13: 52

(c) 40: 177 (d) 14: 73

Mass-Energy and Nuclear Binding Energy

18. A nucleus with mass number 240 breaks into two fragments each of mass number 120 , the binding energy per nucleon of unfragmented nuclei is 7.6 MeV while that of fragments is 8.5MeV. The total gain in the Binding Energy in the process is **(2021)**

(a) 216MeV (b) 0.9MeV

(c) 9.4MeV (d) 804MeV

19. The energy required to break one bond in DNA is 10^{-20} J. This value in eV is nearly **(2020)**

(a) 6 (b) 0.6

(c) 0.06 (d) 0.006

20. The energy equivalent of 0.5 g of a substance is **(2020)**

(a) 4.5×10^{16} J (b) 4.5×10^{13} J

(c) 1.5×10^{13} J (d) 0.5×10^{13} J

21. How does the Binding Energy per nucleon vary with the increase in the number of nucleons? **(Karnataka NEET 2013)**

(a) Decrease continuously with mass number.

(b) First decreases and then increases with increase in mass number.

(c) First increases and then decreases with increase in mass number.

(d) Increases continuously with mass number.

22. The mass of a ^7_3Li nucleus is 0.042u less than the sum of the masses of all its nucleons. The binding energy per nucleon of ^7_3Li nucleus is nearly **(2010)**

(a) 46MeV (b) 5.6MeV

(c) 3.9MeV (d) 23MeV

23. If $M(A;Z), M_p$ and M_n denote the masses of the nucleus ^A_ZX, proton and neutron respectively in units of $u(1u = 931.5MeV/c^2)$ and BE represents its binding energy in MeV, then

(2008, 2004)

(a) $M(A,Z) = ZM_p + (A - Z)M_n - BE$

(b) $M(A,Z) = ZM_p + (A - Z)M_n + BE/c^2$

(c) $M(A,Z) = ZM_p + (A - Z)M_n - BE/c^2$

(d) $M(A,Z) = ZM_p + (A - Z)M_n + BE$

24. A nucleus ^A_ZX has mass represented by $M(A,Z)$. If M_p and M_n denote the mass of proton and neutron respectively and B.E. the binding energy in MeV, then **(2007)**

(a) B.E. $= [ZM_p + (A - Z)M_n - M(A,Z)]c^2$

(b) B.E. $= [ZM_p + AM_n - M(A,Z)]c^2$

(c) B.E. $= M(A,Z) - ZM_p - (A - Z)M_n$

(d) B.E. $= [M(A,Z) - ZM_p - (A - Z)M_n]c^2$

25. Fission of nuclei is possible because the binding energy per nucleon in them

(2005)

(a) increases with mass number at low mass numbers

(b) decreases with mass number at low mass numbers

(c) increases with mass number at high mass numbers

(d) decreases with mass number at high mass numbers.

26. The mass of proton is 1.0073u and that of neutron is 1.0087u (u = atomic mass unit). The binding energy of ^4_2He is

(Given helium nucleus mass ≈ 4.0015u) **(2003)**

(a) 0.0305 J (b) 0.0305erg

(c) 28.4MeV (d) 0.061u

27. Which of the following are suitable for the fusion process? **(2002)**

(a) Light nuclei

(b) Heavy nuclei

(c) Element lying in the middle of the periodic table

(d) Middle elements, which are lying on binding energy curve.

28. M_n and M_p represent the mass of neutron and proton respectively. An element having mass M has N neutrons and Z protons, then the correct relation will be **(2001)**

(a) $M < \{N \cdot M_n + Z \cdot M_p\}$

(b) $M > \{N \cdot M_n + Z \cdot M_p\}$

(c) $M = \{N \cdot M_n + Z \cdot M_p\}$

(d) $M = N\{M_n + M_p\}$

29. Energy released in nuclear fission is due to **(2001)**

(a) some mass is converted into energy

(b) total binding energy of fragments is more than the binding energy of parental element

(c) total binding energy of fragments is less than the binding energy of parental element

(d) total binding energy of fragments is equal to the binding energy of parental element.

30. The binding energy per nucleon is maximum in case of **(1993)**

(a) $^{4}_{2}He$ (b) $^{56}_{26}Fe$

(c) $^{141}_{56}Ba$ (d) $^{235}_{92}U$

31. The energy equivalent of one atomic mass unit is **(1992)**

(a) 1.6×10^{-19} J (b) 6.02×10^{23} J

(c) 931MeV (d) 9.31MeV

32. The average binding energy of a nucleon inside an atomic nucleus is about **(1989)**

(a) 8MeV (b) 8eV

(c) 8 J (d) 8erg

Nuclear Force

33. If the nuclear force between two protons, two neutrons and between proton and neutron is denoted by F_{pp}, F_{nn} and F_{pn} respectively, then **(1991)**

(a) $F_{pp} \approx F_{nn} \approx F_{pn}$

(b) $F_{pp} \neq F_{nn}$ and $F_{pp} = F_{nn}$

(c) $F_{pp} = F_{nn} = F_{pn}$

(d) $F_{pp} \neq F_{nn} \neq F_{pn}$

34. Which of the following statements is true for nuclear forces? **(1990)**

(a) They obey the inverse square law of distance.

(b) They obey the inverse third power law of distance.

(c) They are short range forces.

(d) They are equal in strength to electromagnetic forces.

Nuclear Energy

35. When a uranium isotope $^{235}_{92}U$ is bombarded with a neutron, it generates $^{89}_{36}Kr$, three neutrons and **(2020)**

(a) $^{144}_{56}Ba$ (b) $^{91}_{40}Zr$

(c) $^{101}_{36}Kr$ (d) $^{103}_{36}Kr$

36. A certain mass of Hydrogen is changed to Helium by the process of fusion. The mass defect in fusion reaction is 0.02866u. The energy liberated per u is (given 1u = 931MeV) **(2013)**

(a) 6.675MeV (b) 13.35MeV

(c) 2.67MeV (d) 26.7MeV

37. The power obtained in a reactor using U^{235} disintegration is 1000 kW. The mass decay of U^{235} per hour is **(2011)**

(a) 10 microgram (b) 20 microgram

(c) 40 microgram (d) 1 microgram

38. Fusion reaction takes place at high temperature because **(2011)**

(a) nuclei break up at high temperature

(b) atoms get ionised at high temperature

(c) kinetic energy is high enough to overcome the coulomb repulsion between nuclei

(d) molecules break up at high temperature

39. The binding energy per nucleon in deuterium and helium nuclei are 1.1 MeV and 7.0 MeV, respectively. When two deuterium nuclei fuse to form a helium nucleus the energy released in the fusion is

(Mains 2010)

(a) 23.6MeV (b) 2.2MeV

(c) 28.0MeV (d) 30.2MeV

40. The binding energy of deuteron is 2.2MeV and that of ^4_2He is 28MeV. If two deuterons are fused to form one ^4_2He then the energy released is **(2006)**

(a) 30.2MeV (b) 25.8MeV

(c) 23.6MeV (d) 19.2MeV

41. In any fission process the ratio $\frac{\text{mass of fission products}}{\text{mass of parent nucleus}}$ is **(2005)**

(a) equal to 1

(b) greater than 1

(c) less than 1

(d) depends on the mass of the parent nucleus.

42. If in a nuclear fusion process the masses of the fusing nuclei be m_1 and m_2 and the mass of the resultant nucleus be m_3, then

(2004)

(a) $m_3 = m_1 + m_2$

(b) $m_3 = |m_1 - m_2|$

(c) $m_3 < (m_1 + m_2)$

(d) $m_3 > (m_1 + m_2)$

43. Solar energy is mainly caused due to

(2003)

(a) burning of hydrogen in the oxygen

(b) fission of uranium present in the Sun

(c) fusion of protons during synthesis of heavier elements

(d) gravitational contraction

44. Nuclear fission is best explained by

(2000)

(a) liquid droplet theory

(b) Yukawa π-meson theory

(c) independent particle model of the nucleus

(d) proton-proton cycle.

45. Which of the following is used as a moderator in nuclear reaction? **(1997)**

(a) Cadmium (b) Plutonium

(c) Uranium (d) Heavy water

46. Energy released in the fission of a single $^{235}_{92}U$ nucleus is 200MeV. The fission rate of $^{235}_{92}U$ filled reactor operating at a power level of 5 W is **(1993)**

(a) $1.56 \times 10^{-10}\ s^{-1}$

(b) $1.56 \times 10^{11}\ s^{-1}$

(c) $1.56 \times 10^{-16}\ s^{-1}$

(d) $1.56 \times 10^{-17}\ s^{-1}$

47. Solar energy is due to **(1992)**

(a) fusion reaction

(b) fission reaction

(c) combustion reaction

(d) chemical reaction

ANSWER KEY

1.	(a)	2.	(b)	3.	(c)	4.	(c)	5.	(a)	6.	(a)	7.	(a)
8.	(c)	9.	(c)	10.	(b)	11.	(d)	12.	(a)	13.	(d)	14.	(d)
15.	(b)	16.	(c)	17.	(a)	18.	(a)	19.	(c)	20.	(b)	21.	(c)
22.	(b)	23.	(c)	24.	(a)	25.	(d)	26.	(c)	27.	(a)	28.	(a)
29.	(a)	30.	(b)	31.	(c)	32.	(a)	33.	(c)	34.	(c)	35.	(a)
36.	(a)	37.	(c)	38.	(c)	39.	(a)	40.	(c)	41.	(c)	42.	(c)
43.	(d)	44.	(a)	45.	(d)	46.	(b)	47.	(a)				

Hints & Explanations

1. **(a) :** Isotones means number of neutron remains same.

2. **(b) :** Z is number of protons and A is the total number of protons and neutrons.

3. **(c) :** Mass number = atomic number + no. of neutrons

For hydrogen, number of neutrons = 0

So, mass number = Atomic number.

Hence mass number is sometimes equal to atomic number.

4. **(c) :** Let ${}_5\text{B}^{10}$ be present as x% so percentage of ${}_5\text{B}^{11} = (100 - x)$

$\therefore$ Average atomic weight

$$= \frac{10x + 11(100 - x)}{100} = 10.81 \Rightarrow x = 19$$

$\therefore$ % of ${}_5\text{B}^{11}$ is $100 - 19 = 81$. Ratio is $19:81$.

5. **(a) :** Nucleus contains only neutrons and protons.

6. **(a) :** $Z = 11$ i.e., number of protons = $11, A = 23$

$\therefore$ Number of neutrons $= A - Z = 12$

Number of electron = 0 (No electron in nucleus)

Therefore 11, 12, 0 is the correct answer.

7. **(a) :** As_6C^{13} and ${}_7\text{N}^{14}$ have same number of neutrons

($13 - 6 = 7$ for C and $14 - 7 = 7$ for N), they are isotones.

8. **(c) :** Nuclear radius, $R = R_0 A^{1/3}$

where R_0 is a constant and A is the mass number.

From eq: (i) $R \propto A^{1/3}$

$$\frac{R_1}{R_2} = \left(\frac{125}{64}\right)^{\frac{1}{3}}, \frac{R_1}{R_2} = \frac{5}{4}$$

9. **(c) :** Nuclear radius, $R = R_0A^{1/3}$
where R_0 is a constant and A is the mass number

$$\therefore \frac{R_{Al}}{R_{Cu}} = \frac{(27)^{1/3}}{(64)^{1/3}} = \frac{3}{4}$$

or $R_{Cu} = \frac{4}{3} \times R_{Al} = \frac{4}{3} \times 3.6\text{fermi} =$ 4.8fermi

10. **(b) :** $A_1 : A_2 = 1 : 3$
Their radii will be in the ratio

$$R_0A_1^{1/3} : R_0A_2^{1/3} = 1 : 3^{1/3}$$

Density $= \frac{A}{\frac{4}{3}\pi R^3}$

$$\therefore \rho_{A_1} : \rho_{A_2} = \frac{1}{\frac{4}{3}\pi R_0^3 \cdot 1^3} : \frac{3}{\frac{4}{3}\pi R_0^3 (3^{1/3})^3}$$

$$= 1 : 1$$

Their nuclear densities will be the same.

11. **(d) :** Nuclear radii $R = (R_0)A^{1/3}$
where A is the mass number.

$$\therefore \frac{R_{Te}}{R_{Al}} = \left(\frac{A_{Te}}{A_{Al}}\right)^{1/3} = \left(\frac{125}{27}\right)^{1/3} = \left(\frac{5}{3}\right)$$

or, $R_{Te} = \frac{5}{3} \times R_{Al} = \frac{5}{3} \times 3.6 = 6\text{fm}$.
(Given $R_{Al} = 3.6\text{fm}$)

12. **(a) :** Nuclear radii $R = R_0(A)^{1/3}$, where $R_0 \approx 1.2\text{fm}$
or $R \propto (A)^{1/3}$

$\therefore \frac{R_{Be}}{R_{Ge}} = \frac{(9)^{1/3}}{(A)^{1/3}}$ or, $\frac{R_{Be}}{2R_{Be}} = \frac{(9)^{1/3}}{(A)^{1/3}}$ ($\because$ given $R_{Ge} = 2R_{Be}$) or, $(A)^{1/3} = 2 \times (9)^{1/3}$
or, $A = 2^3 \times 9 = 8 \times 9 = 72$
$\therefore$ The number of nucleons in Ge is 72

13. **(d) :** $\frac{\text{Volume of atom}}{\text{Volume of nucleus}} = \frac{\frac{4}{3}\pi(10^{-10})^3}{\frac{4}{3}\pi(10^{-15})^3} = 10^{15}$

14. **(d) :** Velocity ratio $(v_1 : v_2) = 2 : 1$
Mass $(m) \propto$ Volume $\propto r^3$.
According to law of conservation of momentum,

$$m_1v_1 = m_2v_2$$

Therefore $\frac{v_1}{v_2} = \frac{m_2}{m_1} = \frac{r_2^3}{r_1^3}$ or $\frac{r_1}{r_2} = \left(\frac{v_2}{v_1}\right)^{1/3} = \left(\frac{1}{2}\right)^{1/3} = \frac{1}{2^{1/3}}$

or $r_1 : r_2 = 1 : 2^{1/3}$

15. **(b) :** Mass number of helium $(A_{He}) =$ 4 and mass number of sulphur $(A_S) =$ 32.
Radius of nucleus, $r = r_0(A)^{1/3}$.
Therefore

$$\frac{r_s}{r_{He}} = \left(\frac{A_s}{A_{He}}\right)^{1/3} = \left(\frac{32}{4}\right)^{1/3} = (8)^{1/3} = 2$$

16. **(c) :** The nuclear radius r varies with mass number A according to the relation

$$r = r_0A^{1/3} \Rightarrow r \propto A^{1/3} \text{ or } A \propto r^3$$

Now density $= \frac{\text{mass}}{\text{volume}}$
Further mass $\propto A$ and volume $\propto r^3$
$\therefore \frac{\text{mass}}{\text{volume}} =$ constant

17. **(a) :** $R \propto (A)^{1/3}$ from $R = R_0A^{1/3}$
$\therefore R_{A1} \propto (27)^{\frac{1}{3}}$ and $R_{Te} \propto (125)^{\frac{1}{5}}$

$$\therefore \frac{R_{Al}}{R_{Te}} = \frac{3}{5} = \frac{6}{10}$$

18. **(a) :** Let the parent nucleus be X which breaks into two fragments Y

$^{240}X \rightarrow 2^{120}Y$

Binding energy X, B.E. $x = 240 \times 7.6 = 1824\text{MeV}$

Binding energy of Y, B.E. $Y = 120 \times 8.5 = 1020\text{MeV}$

Energy released, $E = 2(\text{BE})_Y - (\text{BE})_X$

$$= 2 \times (1020) - 1824 = 216\text{MeV}$$

19. **(c) :** Given : energy, $E = 10^{-20}$ J

Now, $1\text{ J} = \frac{1}{1.6\times10^{-19}}\text{eV}$

$$\therefore\ E = \frac{10^{-20}}{1.6\times10^{-19}}\text{eV} = 0.0625\text{eV}$$

$$\simeq 0.06\text{eV}$$

20. **(b) :**

Given mass $m = 0.5\text{ g} = 0.5\times10^{-3}$ kg

According to Einstein mass-energy equivalence, $E = mc^2 = 0.5\times10^{-3}\times(3\times10^8)^2 = 4.5\times10^{13}$ J

21. **(c) :**

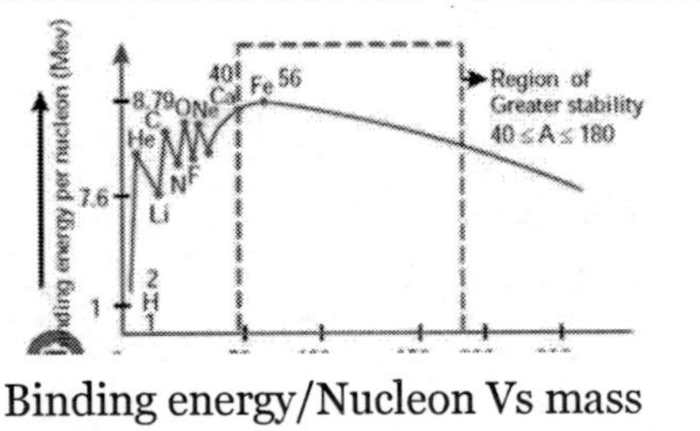

Binding energy/Nucleon Vs mass number curve the binding energy per nucleon first increases and then decreases with increase in mass number.

22. **(b)**

For ^7_3Li nucleus,

Mass defect, $\Delta M = 0.042\text{u}$ $\because 1\text{u} = 931.5\text{MeV/c}^2$

$$\therefore \Delta M = 0.042 \times 931.5\text{MeV/c}^2$$

$$= 39.1\text{MeV/c}^2$$

Binding energy, $E_b = \Delta M c^2$

$$= \left(39.1\frac{\text{MeV}}{c^2}\right)c^2 = 39.1\text{MeV}$$

Binding energy per nucleon,

$$E_{bn} = \frac{E_b}{A} = \frac{39.1\text{MeV}}{7} \approx 5.6\text{MeV}$$

23. **(c) :** $ZM_p + (A-Z)M_n - M(A,Z)$

$$= \text{mass defect } = \frac{B\cdot E}{c^2}$$

$$\Rightarrow M(A,Z) = ZM_p + (A-Z)M_n - \frac{B\cdot E}{c^2}$$

24. **(a) :** In the case of formation of nucleus in the evolution energy equals to the binding energy of the nucleus take place due to disappearance of a fraction of total mass. If the quantity of mass disappearance is Δm then B.E. is

B.E. = ΔmC^2

from the above discussion, it is clear that the mass of nucleus must be less than the sum of the masses of the constituent neutrons & protons. We can write them

$\Delta m = Zm_p + Nm_n - m\,(A, Z)$

where, M (A, Z) is the mass of the atom of mass number 'A' and atomic number 'Z'

Hence B.E. of nucleus is

B.E. $[Zm_p + Nm_n - m\,(A, Z)]C^2$

B.E. $[Zm_p + (A-Z)m_n - m(A, Z)]C^2$

25. **(d) :** For nuclei having $A > 56$ binding energy per nucleon gradually decreases.

26. **(c) :** Mass defect $= 2M_P + 2M_N - M_{He}$

$= 2 \times 1.0073 + 2 \times 1.0087 - 4.0015$

$= 0.0305$

$\Rightarrow$ Binding energy $= (931 \times$ mass defect$)$MeV

$= 931 \times 0.0305\text{MeV} = 28.4\text{MeV}$

27. **(a) :** The nuclei of light elements have a lower binding energy than that for the elements of intermediate mass. They are therefore less stable; consequently the fusion of the light elements results in more stable nucleus.

28. **(a) :** Mass of neutrons = M_n

Mass of proton = M_p

Now we know atomic mass (M) of any stable nucleus always less than the sum of masses of constituent particle therefore $M < [NM_n + ZM_p]$

29. **(a) :**

Energy is released in nuclear fission is due to the total binding energy of fragments is more than B.E. of parental element.

Nuclear fission occurs in heavy nuclei and leads to the formation of lighter nuclei.

30. **(b) :** From binding energy curve, the curve reaches peak for $_{26}Fe^{56}$.

31. **(c) :** 1 a.m.u = 931MeV

32. **(a) :** Average binding energy/nucleon in nuclei is of the order of 8MeV.

33. **(c) :** Nuclear force is the same between any two nucleons.

34. **(c) :** Nuclear forces are short range forces.

35. **(a) :** $_{92}U^{235} + {_0n^1} \longrightarrow {_{36}Kr^{89}} + 3n_0^1 + {_ZX^A}$

$92 + 0 = 36 + Z \Rightarrow Z = 56$

Now, $235 + 1 = 89 + 3 + A \Rightarrow A = 144$

So, $_{56}Ba^{144}$ is generated.

36. **(a) :** As ${}_1^2H + {}_1^2H \longrightarrow {}_2^4He$

Here, $\Delta M = 0.02866$u

$\therefore$ The energy liberated per u is

$= \frac{\Delta M \times 931}{4}$ MeV

$$= \frac{0.02866 \times 931}{4}\text{MeV} = \frac{26.7}{4}\text{MeV}$$

$$= 6.675\text{MeV}$$

37. **(c) :** According to Einstein's mass energy relation

$$E = mc^2 \text{ or } m = \frac{E}{c^2}$$

Mass decay per second

$$= \frac{\Delta m}{\Delta t} = \frac{1}{c^2}\frac{\Delta E}{\Delta t} = \frac{P}{c^2} = \frac{1000 \times 10^3 \text{ W}}{(3 \times 10^8 \text{ m/s})^2}$$

$$= \frac{10^6}{9 \times 10^{16}} \text{ kg/s}$$

Mass decay per hour

$$= \frac{\Delta m}{\Delta t} \times 60 \times 60 = \left(\frac{10^6}{9 \times 10^{16}} \text{ kg/s}\right)(3600 \text{ s})$$

$$= 4 \times 10^{-8} \text{ kg} = 40 \times 10^{-6} \text{ g} = 40\mu g$$

38. **(c) :** Extremely high temperature needed for fusion make kinetic energy large enough to overcome coulomb repulsion between nuclei.

39. **(a) :** ${}_1H^2 + {}_1H^2 \rightarrow {}_2He^4 + \Delta E$

The binding energy per nucleon of a deuteron = 1.1MeV

$\therefore$ Total binding energy = $2 \times 1.1 =$ 2.2MeV

The binding energy per nucleon of a helium nuclei = 7MeV

$\therefore$ Total binding energy = $4 \times 7 =$ 28MeV

Hence, energy released

$$\Delta E = (28 - 2 \times 2.2) = 23.6\text{MeV}$$

40. **(c) :**

41. **(c) :**

42. **(c) :** In nuclear fusion the mass of end product or resultant is always less than the sum of initial product, the rest is liberated in the form of energy, like in Sun energy is liberated due to fusion of two hydrogen atoms.

43. **(d) :**

44. **(a) :**

45. **(d) :** In nuclear fission, the chain reaction is controlled in such way that only one neutron, produced in each fission, causes further fission. Therefore some moderator is used to slow down the neutrons. Heavy water is used for this purpose.

46. **(b) :**

Fission rate

$$= \frac{\text{total power}}{\frac{\text{energy}}{\text{fission}}} = \frac{5}{200 \times 1.6 \times 10^{-13}}$$

$$= 1.56 \times 10^{11}\ \text{s}^{-1}$$

47. **(a) :**

Chapter : 28

SEMICONDUCTOR ELECTRONICS : MATERIALS, DEVICES AND SIMPLE CIRCUITS

Classification of Metals, Conductors and Semiconductors

1. Choose the only false statement from the following. **(2005)**
   (a) In conductors the valence and conduction bands overlap.
   (b) Substances with energy gap of the order of 10eV are insulators.
   (c) The resistivity of a semiconductor increases with increase in temperature.
   (d) The conductivity of a semiconductor increases with increase in temperature.

2. Carbon, silicon and germanium atoms have four valence electrons each. Their valence and conduction bands are separated by energy band gaps represented by $(E_g)_C$, $(E_g)_{Si}$ and $(E_g)_{Ge}$ respectively. Which one of the following relationships is true in their case? **(2005)**
   (a) $(E_g)_C > (E_g)_{Si}$ (b) $(E_g)_C < (E_g)_{Si}$
   (c) $(E_g)_C = (E_g)_{Si}$ (d) $(E_g)_C < (E_g)_{Ge}$

3. In semiconductors at a room temperature **(2004)**
   (a) the valence band is partially empty and the conduction band is partially filled
   (b) the valence band is completely filled and the conduction band is partially filled
   (c) the valence band is completely filled
   (d) the conduction band is completely empty.

Intrinsic Semiconductor

4. C and Si both have same lattice structure; having 4 bonding electrons in each. However, C is insulator whereas Si is intrinsic semiconductor. This is because **(2012)**
   (a) in case of C the valence band is not completely filled at absolute zero temperature
   (b) in case of C the conduction band is partly filled even at absolute zero temperature
   (c) the four bonding electrons in the case of C lie in the second orbit, whereas in the case of Si they lie in the third
   (d) the four bonding electrons in the case of C lie in the third orbit, whereas for Si they lie in the fourth orbit.

5. At absolute zero, Si acts as **(1988)**
   (a) non metal (b) metal

(c) insulator (d) none of these.

Extrinsic Semiconductor

6. The electron concentration in an n-type semiconductor is the same as hole concentration in a p-type semiconductor. An external field (electric) is applied across each of them. Compare the currents in them. **(2021)**

(a) No current will flow in p-type, current will only flow in n-type.

(b) Current in n-type = current in p-type.

(c) Current in p-type > current in n-type.

(d) Current in n-type > current in p-type.

7. For a p-type semiconductor, which of the following statements is true? **(2019)**

(a) Electrons are the majority carriers and pentavalent atoms are the dopants.

(b) Electrons are the majority carriers and trivalent atoms are the dopants.

(c) Holes are the majority carriers and trivalent atoms are the dopants.

(d) Holes are the majority carriers and pentavalent atoms are the dopants.

8. In a n-type semiconductor, which of the following statement is true? **(2013)**

(a) Holes are minority carriers and pentavalent atoms are dopants.

(b) Holes are majority carriers and trivalent atoms are dopants.

(c) Electrons are majority carriers and trivalent atoms are dopants.

(d) Electrons are minority carriers and pentavalent atoms are dopants.

9. If a small amount of antimony is added to germanium crystal **(2011)**

(a) it becomes a p-type semiconductor

(b) the antimony becomes an acceptor atom

(c) there will be more free electrons than holes in the semiconductor

(d) its resistance is increased.

10. Pure Si at 500 K has equal number of electron (n_e) and hole (n_h) concentrations of $1.5 \times 10^{16}\ m^{-3}$. Doping by indium increases n_h to $4.5 \times 10^{22}\ m^{-3}$. The doped semiconductor is of **(Mains 2011)**

(a) p-type having electron concentration

(b) n-type with electron concentration $n_e = 5 \times 10^{9}\ m^{-3}$

(c) p-type with electron concentration $n_e = 5 \times 10^{22}\ m^{-3}$

(d) n-type with electron concentration $n_e = 2.5 \times 10^{23}\ m^{-3}$

11. Which one of the following statement is false? **(2010)**

(a) Pure Si doped with trivalent impurities gives a p-type semiconductor.

(b) Majority carriers in a n-type semiconductor are holes.

(c) Minority carriers in a p-type semiconductor are electrons.

(d) The resistance of intrinsic semiconductor decreases with increase of temperature.

12. In the energy band diagram of a material shown here, the open circles and filled circles denote holes and electrons respectively. The material is **(2007)**

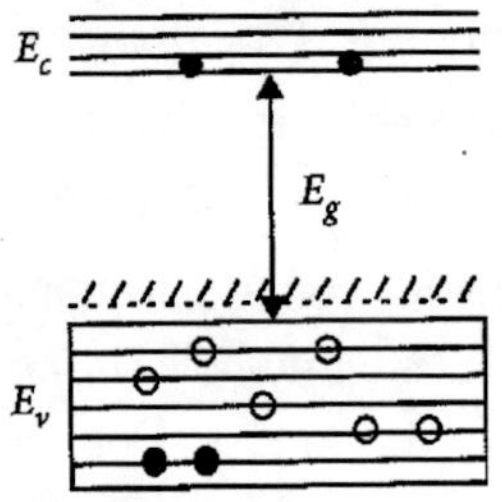

(a) an insulator

(b) a metal

(c) an n-type semiconductor

(d) a p-type semiconductor.

13. In a p type semiconductor, the majority carriers of current are **(1999)**

(a) protons (b) electrons

(c) holes (d) neutrons

14. Which of the following, when added as an impurity into the silicon produces n type semiconductor? **(1999)**

(a) B (b) Al

(c) P (d) Mg

15. To obtain a p-type germanium semiconductor, it must be doped with **(1997)**

(a) indium (b) phosphorus

(c) arsenic (d) antimony.

16. When arsenic is added as an impurity to silicon, the resulting material is **(1996)**

(a) n-type conductor

(b) n-type semiconductor

(c) p-type semiconductor

(d) none of these.

17. When n type semiconductor is heated **(1989)**

(a) number of electrons increases while that of holes decreases

(b) number of holes increases while that of electrons decreases

(c) number of electrons and holes remain same

(d) number of electrons and holes increases equally.

p-n Junction

18. The increase in the width of the depletion region in a $p-n$ junction diode is due to **(2020)**

(a) forward bias only

(b) reverse bias only

(c) both forward bias and reverse bias

(d) increase in forward current

19. The barrier potential of a $p-n$ junction depends on **(2014)**

(1) type of semiconductor material

(2) amount of doping

(3) temperature

Which one of the following is correct?

(a) (1) and (2) only (b) (2) only

(c) (2) and (3) only (d) (1), (2) and (3)

20. In an unbiased $p-n$ junction, holes diffuse from the p-region to n-region because of

(Karnataka NEET 2013)

(a) the attraction of free electrons of n-region

(b) the higher hole concentration in p-region than that in n-region

(c) the higher concentration of electrons in the n-region than that in the p-region

(d) the potential difference across the $p-n$ junction.

21. In a $p-n$ junction **(2002)**

(a) high potential at n side and low potential at p side

(b) high potential at p side and low potential at n side

(c) p and n both are at same potential

(d) undetermined.

22. Depletion layer consists of **(1999)**

(a) mobile ions (b) protons

(c) electrons (d) immobile ions

23. The depletion layer in the $p-n$ junction region is caused by **(1991)**

(a) drift of holes

(b) diffusion of charge carriers

(c) migration of impurity ions

(d) drift of electrons.

Semiconductor Diode

24. Given below are two statements: **(2023)**

Statement I: Photovoltaic devices can convert optical radiation into electricity.

Statement II: Zener diode is designed to operate under reverse bias in breakdown region.

In the light of the above statements, choose the most appropriate answer from the options given below.

(a) Both Statement I and Statement II are incorrect

(b) Statement I is correct but Statement II is incorrect

(c) Statement I is incorrect but Statement II is correct

(d) Both Statement I and Statement II are correct

25. (a) 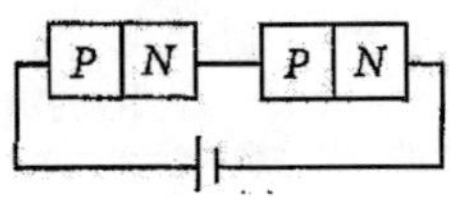

(b) 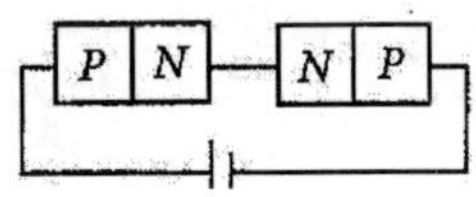

(c) 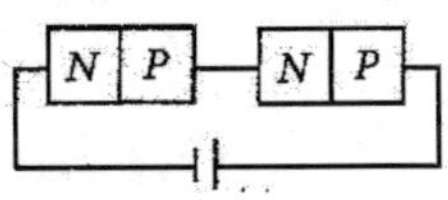

In the given circuits (a), (b) and (c), the potential drop across the two $p-n$ junctions are equal in : **(2022)**

(a) Circuit (a) only

(b) Circuit (b) only

(c) Circuit (c) only

(d) Both circuits (a) and (c)

26. In a $p-n$ junction diode, change in temperature due to heating **(2018)**

(a) affects only reverse resistance

(b) affects only forward resistance

(c) does not affect resistance of $p-n$ junction

(d) affects the overall $V-I$ characteristics of $p-n$ junction.

27. Which one of the following represents forward bias diode? **(NEET 2017, 2006)**

(a) 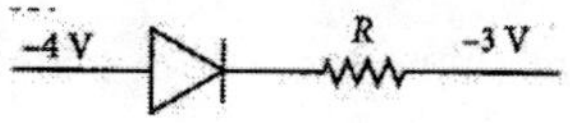

(b) 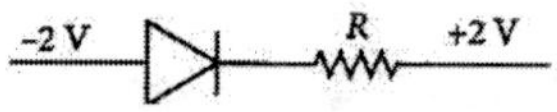

(c) 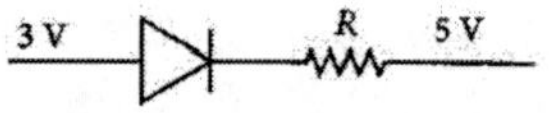

(d) 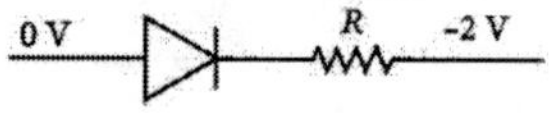

28. The given circuit has two ideal diodes connected as shown in the figure. The current flowing through the resistance R_1 will be **(NEET-II 2016)**

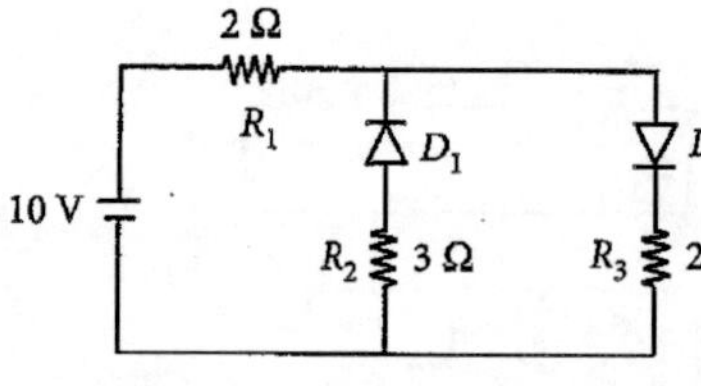

(a) 2.5 A (b) 10.0 A

(c) 1.43 A (d) 3.13 A

29. Consider the junction diode as ideal. The value of current flowing through AB is **(NEET-I 2016)**

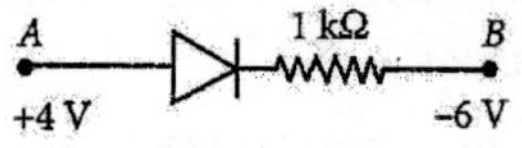

(a) 10^{-1} A (b) 10^{-3} A

(c) 0 A (d) 10^{-2} A

30. In the given figure, a diode D is connected to an external resistance $R = 100\Omega$ and an e.m.f. of 3.5 V. If the barrier potential developed across the diode is 0.5 V, the current in the circuit will be **(2015)**

(a) 20 mA (b) 35 mA

(c) 30 mA (d) 40 mA

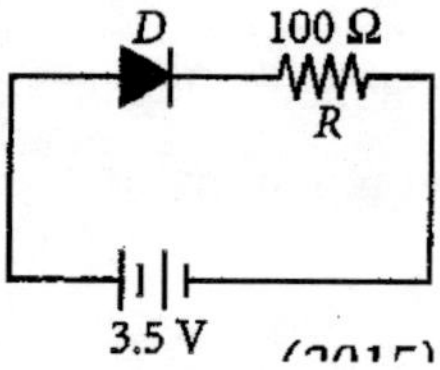

31. If in a $p-n$ junction, a square input signal of 10 V is applied, as shown,

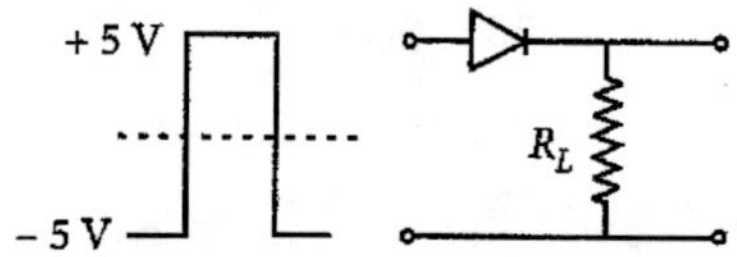

then the output across R_L will be

(2015 Cancelled)

(a) 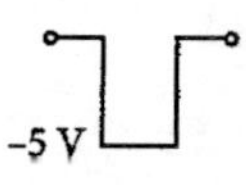

(b) 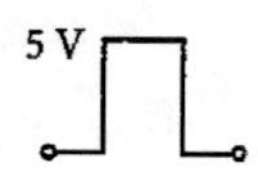

(c) 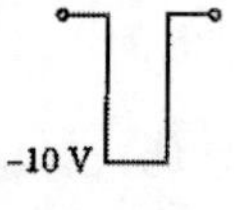

(d) 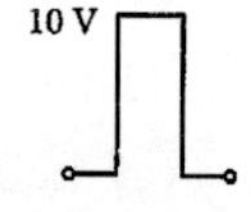

32. Two ideal diodes are connected to a battery as shown in the circuit. The current supplied by the battery is **(2012)**

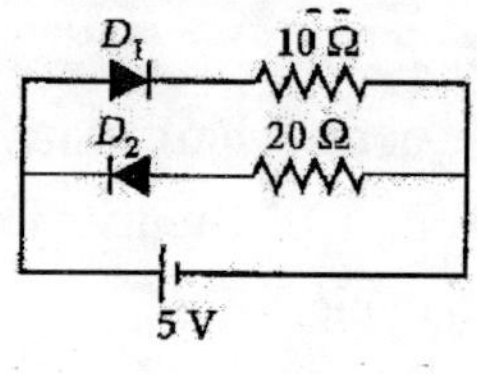

(a) 0.75 A (b) zero
(c) 0.25 A (d) 0.5 A

33. In forward biasing of the $p-n$ junction **(2011, 1988)**

(a) the positive terminal of the battery is connected to p-side and the depletion region becomes thick.
(b) the positive terminal of the battery is connected to n-side and the depletion region becomes thin.
(c) the positive terminal of the battery is connected to n-side and the depletion region becomes thick.
(d) the positive terminal of the battery is connected to p-side and the depletion region becomes thin.

34. In the following figure, the diodes which are forward biased, are **(Mains 2011)**

(A)
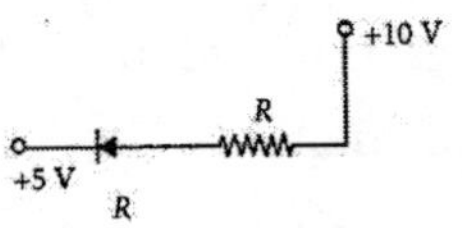

(B)
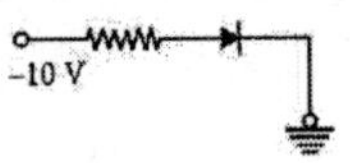

(C)
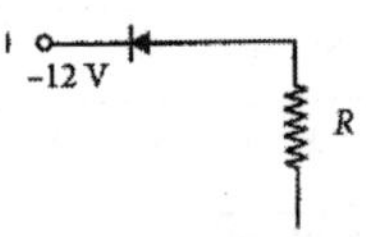

(D)
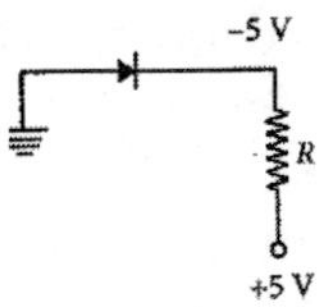

(a) (A), (B) and (D) (b) (C) only
(c) (C) and (A) (d) (B) and (D)

35. Application of a forward bias to a $p-n$ junction **(2005)**

(a) widens the depletion zone
(b) increases the potential difference across the depletion zone
(c) increases the number of donors on the n side
(d) decreases the electric field in the depletion zone.

36. Of the diodes shown in the following diagrams, which one is reverse biased?

(a)
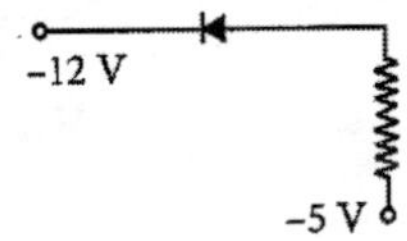

(b)
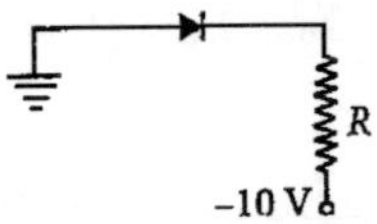

(c)
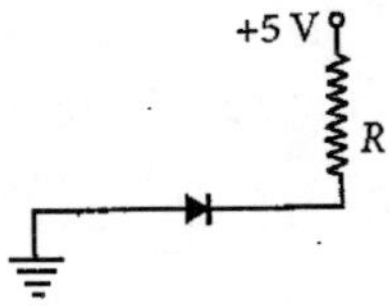

(d)
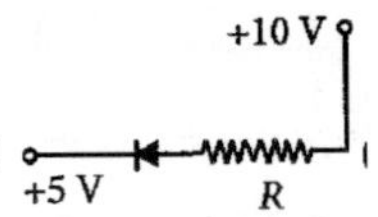

37. Reverse bias applied to a junction diode **(2003)**

(a) lowers the potential barrier
(b) raises the potential barrier
(c) increases the majority carrier current
(d) increases the minority carrier current

38. Barrier potential of a $p-n$ junction diode does not depend on **(2003)**

(a) diode design (b) temperature

(c) forward bias (d) doping density

39. For the given circuit of $p-n$ junction diode which is correct? **(2002)**

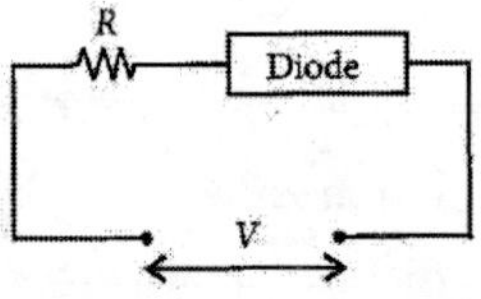

(a) In forward bias the voltage across R is V.

(b) In reverse bias the voltage across R is V.

(c) In forward bias the voltage across R is 2V.

(d) In reverse bias the voltage across R is $2V$.

40. The current in the circuit will be **(2001)**

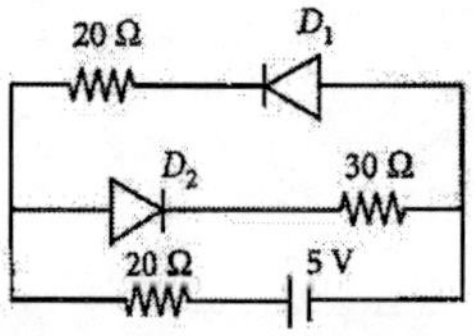

(a) $5/40$ A (b) $5/50$ A

(c) $5/10$ A (d) $5/20$ A

41. From the following diode circuit, which diode is in forward biased condition **(2000)**

(a) 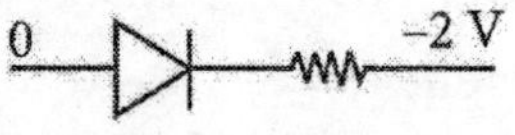

(b) 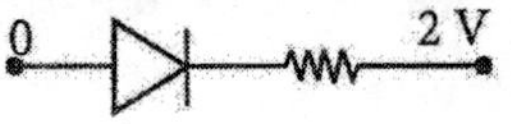

(c) 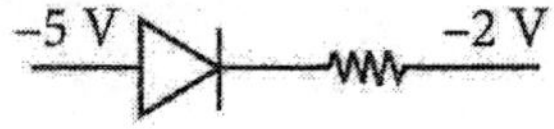

(d) 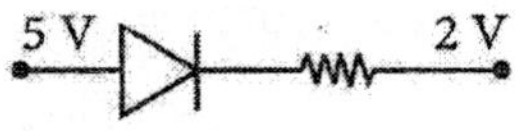

42. In forward bias, the width of potential barrier in a $p-n$ junction diode **(1999)**

(a) remains constant

(b) decreases

(c) increases

(d) first (a) then (b)

43. In a junction diode, the holes are due to **(1999)**

(a) extra electrons

(b) neutrons

(c) protons

(d) missing of electrons

44. The cause of the potential barrier in a $p-n$ junction diode is **(1998)**

(a) depletion of negative charges near the junction

(b) concentration of positive charges near the junction

(c) depletion of positive charges near the junction

(d) concentration of positive and negative charges near the junction.

45. A semiconducting device is connected in a series circuit with a battery and a resistance. A current is found to pass through the circuit. If the polarity of the battery is reversed, the current drops to almost zero. The device may be **(1998)**

(a) a p-type semiconductor

(b) an intrinsic semiconductor

(c) a p - n junction

(d) an n-type semiconductor.

46. The diode used in the circuit shown in the figure has a constant voltage drop at 0.5 V at all currents and a maximum power rating of 100 milli watts. What should be the value of the resistor R, connected in series with diode for obtaining maximum current? **(1997)**

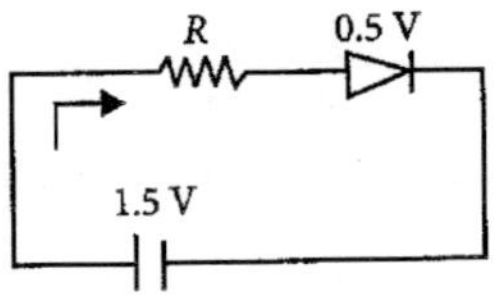

(a) 6.76Ω (b) 20Ω

(c) 5Ω (d) 5.6Ω.

47. In the case of forward biasing of $p-n$ junction, which one of the following figures correctly depicts the direction of flow of carriers? **(1995)**

(a) 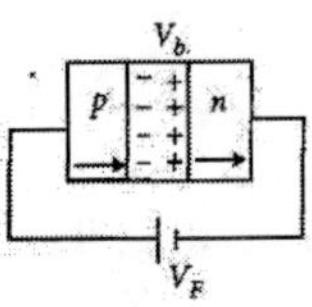

(b) 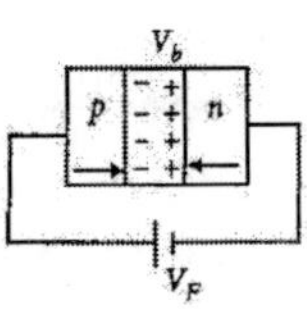

(c) 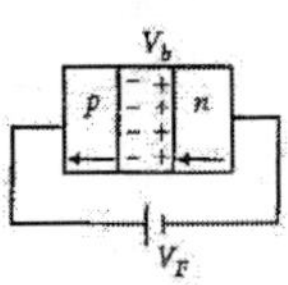

(d) 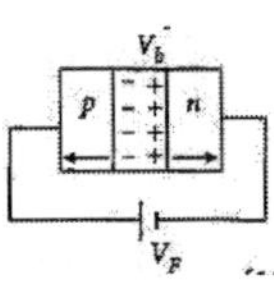

Application of Junction Diode as a Rectifier

48. A full wave rectifier circuit consists of two p-n junction diodes, a centre-tapped transformer, capacitor and a load resistance. Which of these components remove the ac ripple from the rectified output? **(2023)**

(a) p-n junction diodes

(b) Capacitor

(c) Load resistance

(d) A centre-tapped transformer

49. In half wave rectification, if the input frequency is 60 Hz, then the output frequency would be **(2022)**

(a) zero (b) 30 Hz

(c) 60 Hz (d) 120 Hz

50. The peak voltage in the output of a half wave diode rectifier fed with a sinusoidal signal without filter is 10 V. The d.c. component of the output voltage is **(2004)**

(a) $10/\sqrt{2}$ V (b) $10/\pi$V

(c) 10 V (d) $20/\pi$V

51. If a full wave rectifier circuit is operating from 50 Hz mains, the fundamental frequency in the ripple vill be **(2003)**

(a) 25 Hz (b) 50 Hz

(c) 70.7 Hz (d) 100 Hz

52. A p - n junction diode can be used as **(1999)**

(a) condenser (b) regulator

(c) amplifier (d) rectifier

Special Purpose p-n Junction Diodes

53. Consider the following statements (A) and (B) and identify the correct answer. **(2021)**

(A) A zener diode is connected in reverse bias, when used as a voltage regulator.

(B) The potential barrier of $p-n$ junction lies between 0.1 V to 0.3 V.

(a) (A) is incorrect but (B) is correct.
(b) (A) and (B) both are correct.
(c) (A) and (B) both are incorrect.
(d) (A) is correct and (B) is incorrect.

54. An LED is constructed from a $p-n$ junction diode using GaAsP. The energy gap is 1.9eV. The wavelength of the light emitted will be equal to **(Odisha NEET 2019)**

(a) 10.4×10^{-26} m
(b) 654 nm
(c) 654Å
(d) 654×10^{-11} m

55. The given graph represents $V-I$ characteristic for a semiconductor device. Which of the following statement is correct? **(2014)**

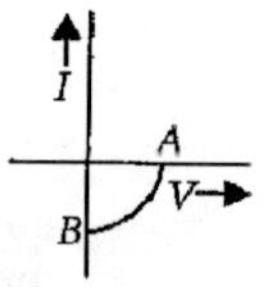

(a) It is V-I characteristic for solar cell where, point A represents open circuit voltage and point B short circuit current.

(b) It is for a solar cell and points A and B represent open circuit voltage and current, respectively.

(c) It is for a photodiode and points A and B represent open circuit voltage and current, respectively.

(d) It is for a LED and points A and B represent open circuit voltage and short circuit current, respectively.

56. A Zener diode, having breakdown voltage equal to 15 V, is used in a voltage regulator circuit shown in figure. The current through the diode is **(Mains 2011)**

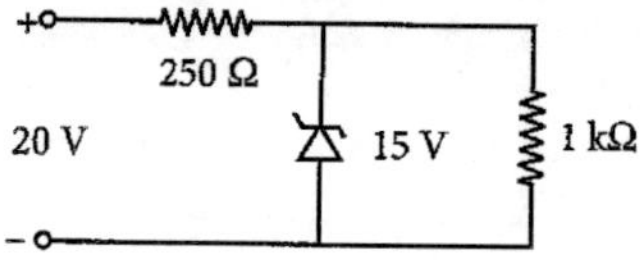

(a) 5 mA (b) 10 Ma
(c) 15 mA (d) 20 mA

57. A $p-n$ photodiode is fabricated from a semiconductor with a band gap of 2.5eV. It can detect a signal of wavelength **(2009)**

(a) 4000 nm (b) 6000 nm
(c) 4000Å (d) 6000Å

58. A $p-n$ photodiode is made of a material with a band gap of 2.0eV. The minimum frequency of the radiation that can be absorbed by the material is nearly **(2008)**

(a) 1×10^{14} Hz (b) 20×10^{14} Hz
(c) 10×10^{14} Hz (d) 5×10^{14} Hz

59. Zener diode is used for **(2005)**

(a) amplification
(b) rectification
(c) stabilization
(d) producing oscillations in an oscillator.

60. In a $p-n$ junction photo cell, the value of the photoelectromotive force produced by monochromatic light is proportional to **(2005)**

(a) the barrier voltage at the $p-n$ junction

(b) the intensity of the light falling on the cell

(c) the frequency of the light falling on the cell

(d) the voltage applied at the $p-n$ junction.

Digital Electronics and Logic Gates

61. For the following logic circuit, the truth table is : **(2023)**

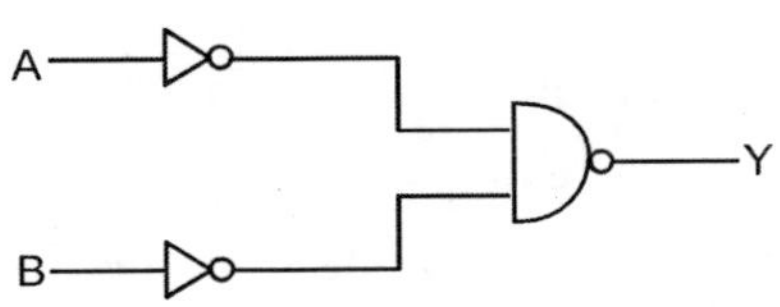

(a)

A	B	C
0	0	0
0	1	1
1	0	1
1	1	1

(b)

A	B	C
0	0	1
0	1	0
1	0	1
1	1	0

(c)

A	B	C
0	0	0
0	1	0
1	0	0
1	1	1

(d)

A	B	C
0	0	1
0	1	1
1	0	1
1	1	0

62.

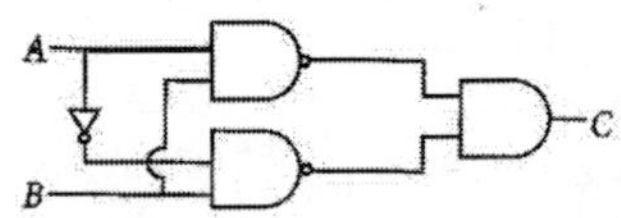

The truth table for the given logic circuit is **(2022)**

(a)

A	B	C
0	0	0
0	1	1
1	0	1
1	1	0

(b)

A	B	C
0	0	1
0	1	0
1	0	0
1	1	1

(c)

A	B	C
0	0	1
0	1	0
1	0	1
1	1	0

(d)

A	B	C
0	0	0
0	1	1
1	0	0
1	1	1

63. For the given circuit, the input digital signals are applied at the terminals A, B and C. What would be the output at the terminal ? **(2021)**

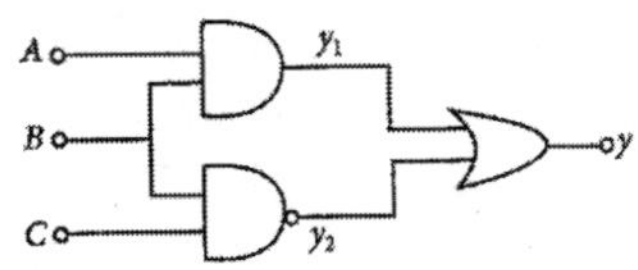

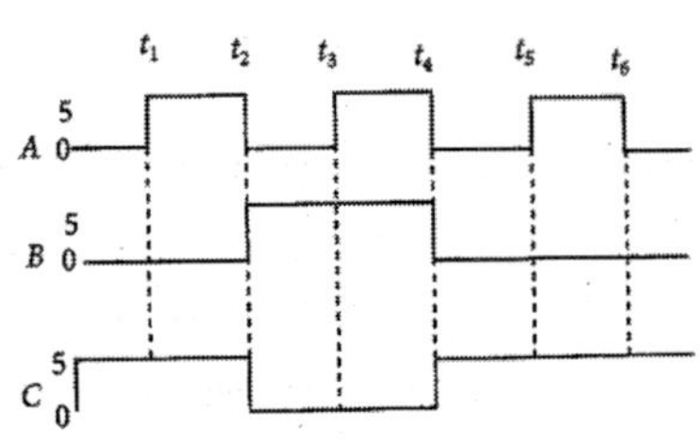

(a) 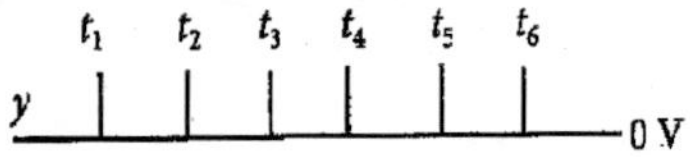

(b) 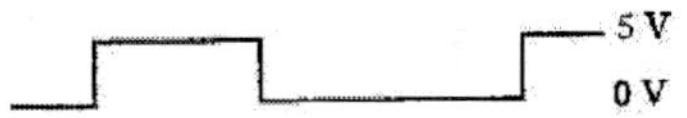

(c) 

(d) 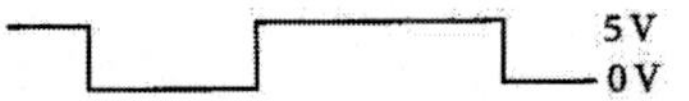

64. For the logic circuit shown, the truth table is

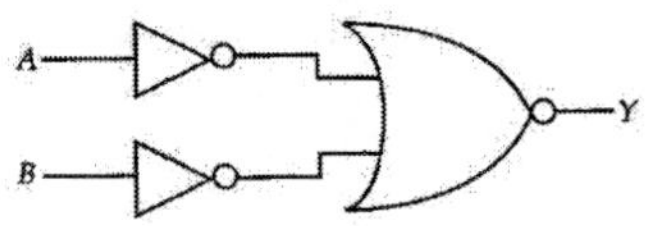

(a)

A	B	C
0	0	0
0	1	0
1	0	0
1	1	1

(b)

A	B	C
0	0	0
0	1	1
1	0	1
1	1	1

(c)

A	B	C
0	0	1
0	1	1
1	0	1
1	1	0

(d)

A	B	C
0	0	1
0	1	0
1	0	0
1	1	0

65.

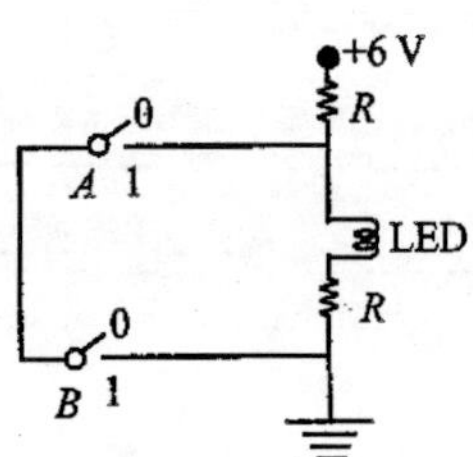

The correct Boolean operation represented by the circuit diagram drawn is **(2019)**

(a) NOR (b) AND

(c) OR (d) NAND

66. In the combination of the following gates the output Y can be written in terms of inputs A and B as **(2018)**

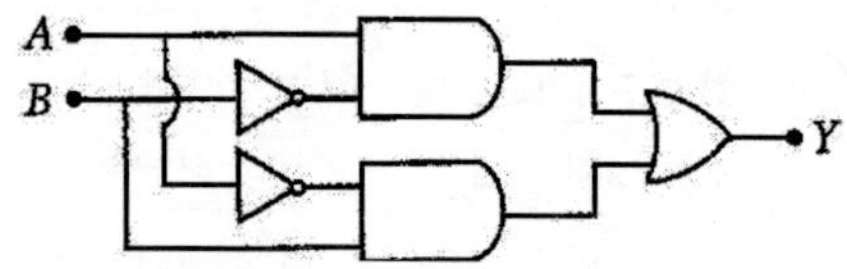

(a) $\overline{A \cdot B}$ (b) $A \cdot \bar{B} + \bar{A} \cdot B$

(c) $\overline{A \cdot B} + A \cdot B$ (d) $\overline{A + B}$

67. The given electrical network is equivalent to **(2017)**

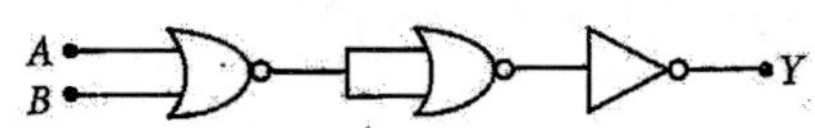

(a) OR gate (b) NOR gate

(c) NOT gate (d) AND gate

68. What is the output Y in the following circuit, when all the three inputs A, B, C are first 0 and then 1 ? **(NEET-II 2016)**

(a) 0,1 (b) 0,0

(c) 1,0 (d) 1,1

69. To get output 1 for the following circuit, the correct choice for the input is

(NEET-I 2016, Mains 2012, 2010)

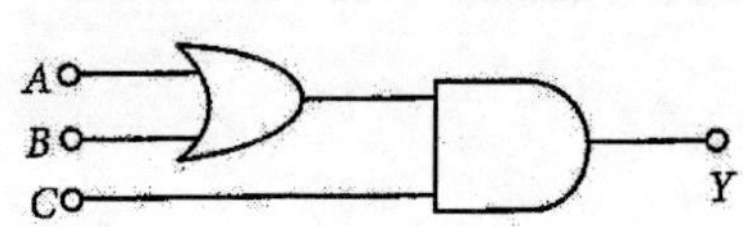

(a) $A = 1, B = 1, C = 0$

(b) $A = 1, B = 0, C = 1$

(c) $A = 0, B = 1, C = 0$

(d) $A = 1, B = 0, C = 0$

70. The output (X) of the logic circuit shown in figure will be **(2013)**

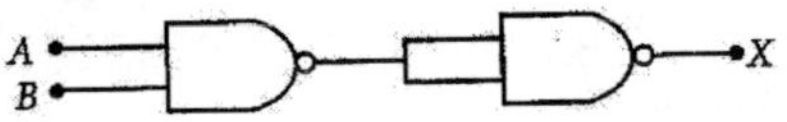

(a) $X = A \cdot B$ (b) $X = \overline{A + B}$

(c) $X = \overline{\bar{A} \cdot B}$ (d) $X = \overline{A \cdot B}$

71. The output from of a NAND gate is divided into two in parallel and fed to another B **(Karnataka NEET 2013)**

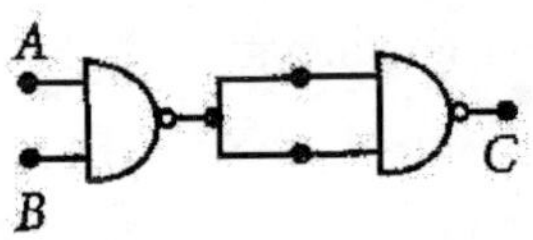

NAND gate. The resulting gate is a

(a) AND gate (b) NOR gate

(c) OR gate (d) NOT gate

72. The figure shows a logic circuit with two inputs A and B and the output C. The voltage wave forms across A, B and C are as given. The logic circuit gate is **(2012)**

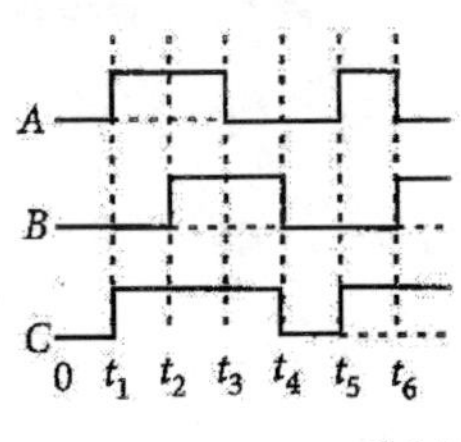

(a) OR gate (b) NOR gate

(c) AND gate (d) NAND gate

73. Symbolic representation of four logic gates are shown as

(i) 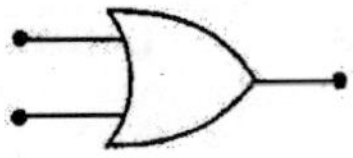

(ii) 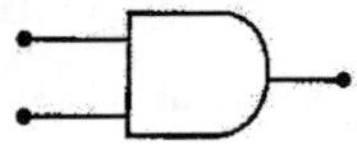

(iii) 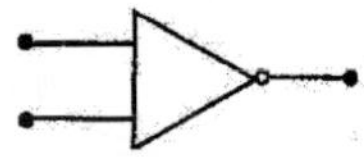

(iv) 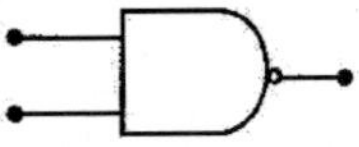

Pick out which ones are for AND, NAND and NOT gates, respectively **(2011)**

(a) (ii), (iii) and (iv)

(b) (iii), (ii) and (i)

(c) (iii), (ii) and (iv)

(d) (ii), (iv) and (iii)

74. The device that can act as a complete electronic circuit is **(2010)**

(a) junction diode

(b) integrated circuit

(c) junction transistor

(d) zener diode.

75. The following figure shows a logic gate circuit with two inputs A and B and the output Y. The voltage waveforms of A, B and Y are as given.

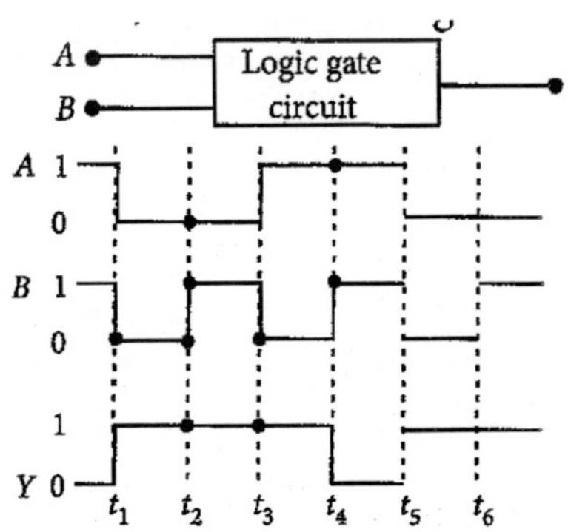

The logic gate is **(Mains 2010)**

(a) NOR gate (c) AND gate

(b) OR gate (d) NAND gate

76. The symbolic representation of four logic gates are given here

(i) 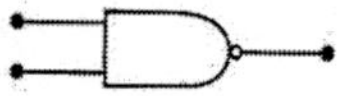

(ii) 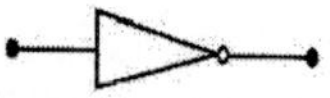

(iii) 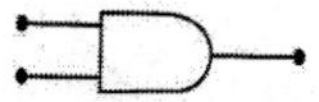

(iv) 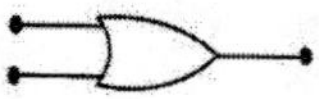

The logic symbols for OR, NOT and NAND gates are respectively **(2009)**

(a) (iv), (i), (iii) (b) (iv), (ii), (i)

(c) (i), (iii), (iv) (d) (iii), (iv), (ii)

77. In the following circuit, the output Y for all possible inputs A and B is expressed by the truth table. **(2007)**

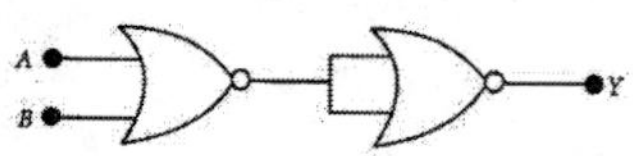

(a)

A	B	Y
0	0	1
0	1	1
1	0	1
1	1	0

(b)

A	B	Y
0	0	1
0	1	0
1	0	0
1	1	0

(c)

A	B	Y
0	0	0
0	1	1
1	0	1
1	1	1

(d)

A	B	Y
0	0	0
0	1	0
1	0	0
1	1	1

78. The following figure shows a logic gate circuit with two inputs A and B and the output C.

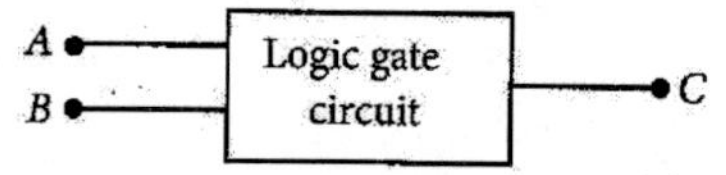

The voltage waveforms of A, B and C are as shown

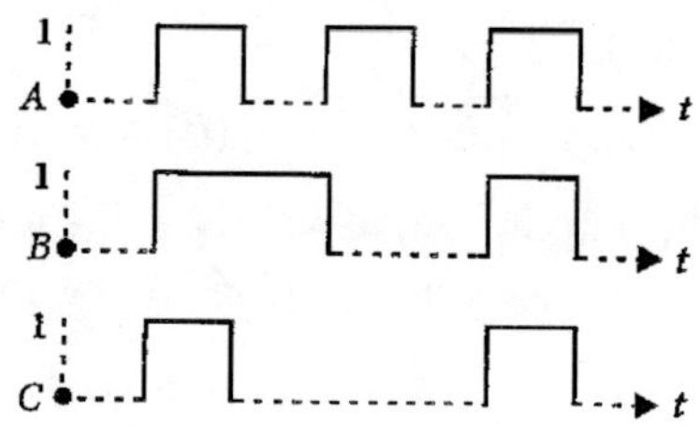

The logic circuit gate is **(2006)**

(a) OR gate (b) AND gate

(c) NAND gate (d) NOR gate.

79. The output of OR gate is 1 **(2004)**

(a) if both inputs are zero

(b) if either or both inputs are 1

(c) only if both inputs are 1

(d) if either input is zero.

80. The given truth table is for which logic gate? **(2002, 2001, 1998, 1994)**

A	B	Y
1	1	0
0	1	1
1	0	1
0	0	1

(a) NAND (b) XOR

(c) NOR (d) OR

81. Which of the following gates will have an output of 1 ? **(1998)**

(a) 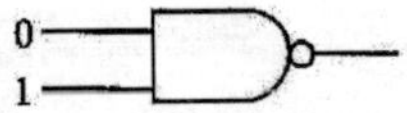

(b) 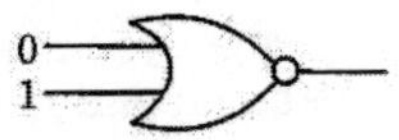

(c) 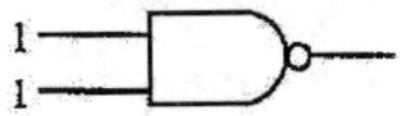

(d) 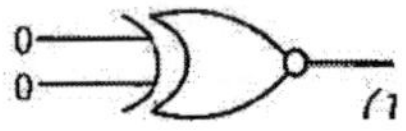

82. The following truth-table belongs to which one of the following four gates?

(1997, 1995)

A	**B**	**Y**
1	1	0
1	0	0
0	1	0
0	0	1

(a) XOR (b) NOR
(c) OR (d) NAND

83. This symbol represents **(1996)**

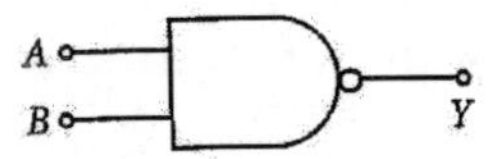

(a) AND gate (b) NOR gate
(c) NAND gate (d) OR gate.

84. The following truth table corresponds to the logical gate **(1991)**

A	B	Y
0	0	0
0	1	1
1	0	1
1	1	1

(a) NAND (b) OR
(c) AND (d) XOR.

ANSWER KEY

1.	(c)	2.	(a)	3.	(a)	4.	(c)	5.	(c)	6.	(d)	7.	(c)
8.	(a)	9.	(c)	10.	(a)	11.	(b)	12.	(d)	13.	(c)	14.	(c)
15.	(a)	16.	(b)	17.	(d)	18.	(b)	19.	(d)	20.	(b)	21.	(a)
22.	(d)	23.	(b)	24.	(d)	25.	(d)	26.	(d)	27.	(d)	28.	(a)
29.	(d)	30.	(c)	31.	(b)	32.	(d)	33.	(d)	34.	(c)	35.	(d)
36.	(c)	37.	(b)	38.	(a)	39.	(a)	40.	(b)	41.	(a)	42.	(b)
43.	(d)	44.	(d)	45.	(c)	46.	(c)	47.	(b)	48.	(b)	49.	(c)
50.	(b)	51.	(d)	52.	(d)	53.	(b)	54.	(b)	55.	(a)	56.	(a)
57.	(c)	58.	(d)	59.	(c)	60.	(b)	61.	(a)	62.	(c)	63.	(c)
64.	(a)	65.	(d)	66.	(b)	67.	(b)	68.	(c)	69.	(b)	70.	(a)
71.	(a)	72.	(a)	73.	(d)	74.	(b)	75.	(d)	76.	(b)	77.	(c)
78.	(b)	79.	(b)	80.	(a)	81.	(a)	82.	(b)	83.	(c)	84.	(b)

Hints & Explanations

1. **(c) :** Resistivity of a semiconductor decreases with increase in the temperature.
2. **(a) :** Band gap of carbon is 5.5eV while that of silicon is 1.1eV. $(E_g)_C > (E_g)_{Si}$
3. **(a) :** In semiconductors at room temperature the electrons get enough energy so that they are able to over come the forbidden gap. Thus at room temperature the valence band is partially empty and conduction band is partially filled. Conduction band in semiconductor is completely empty only at 0 K.
4. **(c) :** Electronic configuration of carbon (^6C) is $1s^2 2s^2 2p^2$. The electronic configuration of silicon $_{14}Si)$ is $1s^2 2s^2 2p^6 3s^2 3p^2$.
   Hence, the four bonding electrons of C and Si respectively lie in second and third orbit.
5. **(c) :** Semiconductors are insulators at room temperature.
6. **(d) :** Mobility of electrons is more as compare to holes and electrons are majority charge carriers in n-type semiconductors. So when we apply electric field, current will be more in n-type semiconductor compare to p-type semiconductor.
7. **(c) :** In p-type semiconductors, holes are the majority carriers and trivalent atoms are the dopants such as B, Al or Ga.
8. **(a) :** In n-type semiconductor, electrons are majority charge carriers and holes are minority charge carriers and pentavalent atoms are dopants:
9. **(c) :** When a small amount of antimony (pentavalent) is added to germanium (tetravalent) crystal, then crystal becomes n-type semiconductor. In n-type semiconductor electrons are the majority charge carriers and the holes are the minority charge carriers.
10. **(a) :** p-type semiconductor is obtained when Si or Ge is doped with a trivalent impurity like aluminium (Al), boron (B), indium (In) etc,
    Here, $n_i = 1.5 \times 10^{16}\ \text{m}^{-3}, n_h = 4.5 \times 10^{22}\ \text{m}^{-3}$
    As $n_e n_h = n_i^2$
    $$n_e = \frac{n_i^2}{n_h} = \frac{(1.5 \times 10^{16}\ \text{m}^{-3})^2}{4.5 \times 10^{22}\ \text{m}^{-3}}$$
    $$= 5 \times 10^9\ \text{m}^{-3}$$
11. **(b) :** In a n-type semiconductors, electrons are majority carriers and holes are minority carriers.
12. **(d) :** p-type semiconductor.
13. **(c) :** p-type semiconductor majority charge carriers are holes.

14. **(c) :** Because P (phosphorus) is pentavalent.

15. **(a) :** In p type germanium semiconductor, it must be doped with a trivalent impurity atom. Since indium is a third group member, therefore germanium must be doped in indium.

16. **(b) :** Arsenic is pentavalent, therefore when added with silicon it leaves one electron as a free electron. In this case the conduction of electricity is due to motion of electrons, so the resulting material is n-type semiconductor.

17. **(d) :** Due to heating, when a free electron is produced then simultaneously a hole is also produced.

18. **(b) :** Width of the depletion layer increases in reverse biasing

19. **(d) :** The barrier potential depends on type of semiconductor (For Si, V_b = 0.7 V and for Ge, V_b = 0.3 V), amount of doping and also on the temperature.

20. **(b) :** The higher hole concentration is in p-region than that in n-region.

21. **(a) :**

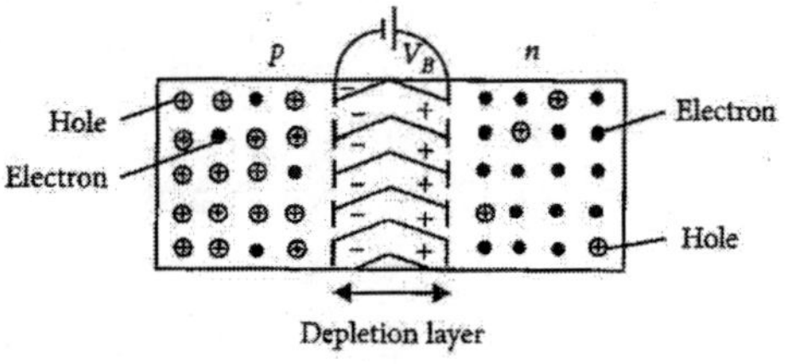

A p- n junction is shown in the figure. On account of difference in concentration of charge carriers in the two sections of $p-n$ junction, the electrons from n-region diffuse through the junction into p-region and the holes from p-region diffuse into n region.

Since the hole is a vacancy of an electron, when an electron from n region diffuses into the p-region, the electron falls into the vacancy, i.e., it completes the covalent bond. Due to migration of charge carriers across the junction, the n-region 4of the junction will have its electrons neutralized by holes from the p-region, leaving only ionised donor atoms (positive charges) which are bound and cannot move. Similarly, the p region of the junction will have ionised acceptor atoms (negative charges) which are immobile.

The accumulation of electric charges of opposite polarities in the two regions of the junction gives rise to an electric field between these regions as if a fictitious battery is connected across the junction with its positive terminal connected to n region and negative terminal connected to p region. Therefore, in a $p-n$ junction high potential is at n side and low potential is at p side.

22. **(d)**

23. **(b) :** The depletion layer in the $p-n$ junction region is caused by diffusion of charge carriers.

24. **(d) : Statement I :** Photocell/solar cell convert light energy into electric energy/current.

Statement II : We use zener diode in reverse biased condition, when reverse biased voltage more than break down voltage than it act as stablizer.

25. **(d) :** The potential drop across $p-n$ junction diode is equal when either both are in forward biased or reversed biased. so, in circuits (a) and (c) both are in forward biased.

So, correct option is (d)

26. **(d) :** Due to heating, number of electron-hole pairs will increase, so overall resistance of diode will change. Due to which forward biasing and reversed biasing both are changed.

27. **(d) :** A diode is said to be forward biased if p-side is at higher potential than n-side of $p-n$ junction.

28. **(a) :** Diode D_1 is reverse biased so, it will block the current and diode D_2 is forward biased, so it will pass the current.

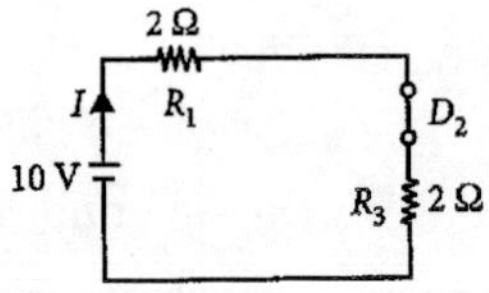

Hence, equivalent circuit becomes as shown in the figure.

Current in the circuit = Current flowing through the resistance R_1

$$= \frac{10}{2+2} = 2.5\ \text{A}$$

29. **(d) :** Here, the $p-n$ junction diode is forward biased, hence it offers zero resistance.

$$\therefore I_{AB} = \frac{V_A - V_B}{R_{AB}} = \frac{4\ \text{V} - (-6\ \text{V})}{1\text{k}\Omega}$$

$$= \frac{10}{1000}\ \text{A} = 10^{-2}\ \text{A}$$

30. **(c) :**

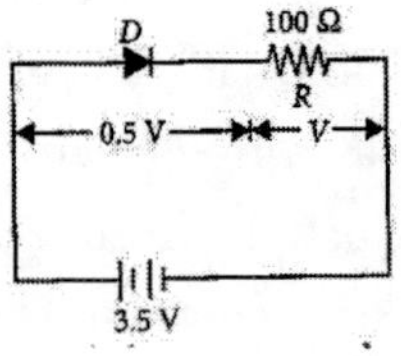

The potential difference across the resistance R is

$$V = 3.5\ \text{V} - 0.5\ \text{V} = 3\ \text{V}$$

By Ohm's law, the current in the circuit is

$$I = \frac{V}{R} = \frac{3\ \text{V}}{100\Omega} = 3 \times 10^{-2}\ \text{A}$$

$$= 30 \times 10^{-3}\ \text{A} = 30\ \text{mA}$$

31. **(b) :** Diode is forward bias for positive voltage i.e. $V > 0$, so output

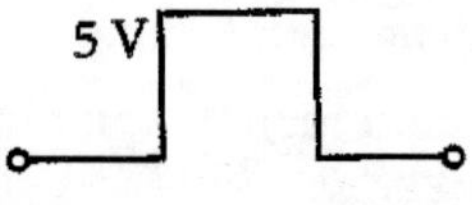

across R_L is given by as shown in figure.

32. **(d) :** In the given circuit the upper diode D_1 is forward biased and the lower diode D_2 is reverse biased. So, the current supplied by the battery is

$$I = \frac{5\ \text{V}}{10\Omega} = \frac{1}{2}\ \text{A} = 0.5\ \text{A}$$

33. **(d) :** In forward biasing, the positive terminal of the battery is connected to p-side and the negative terminal to n-

side of $p-n$ junction. The forward bias voltage opposes the potential barrier. Due to this, the depletion region becomes thin.

34. **(c) :** $p-n$ junction is said to be forward biased when p side is at high potential than n side. It is for circuit (A) and (C).

35. **(d) :**

36. **(c) :** A diode is said to be reverse biased if p-type semiconductor of $p-n$ junction is at low potential with respect to n-type semiconductor of $p-n$ junction. It is so for circuit (c).

37. **(b) :** In reverse biasing, the conduction across the $p-n$ junction takes place due to minority carriers, therefore the size of depletion region (potential barrier) rises.

38. **(a) :** Barrier potential depends upon temperature, doping density and forward biasing.

39. **(a) :** In forward biasing, the resistance of p-n junction diode is very low to the flow of current. So practically all the voltage will be dropped across the resistance R, i.e., voltage across R will be V.

In reverse biasing, the resistance of p-n junction diode is very high. So the voltage drop across R is zero.

40. **(b) :** $D_1 \rightarrow$ reverse biased

and $D_2 \rightarrow$ forward biased.

Equivalent circuit is

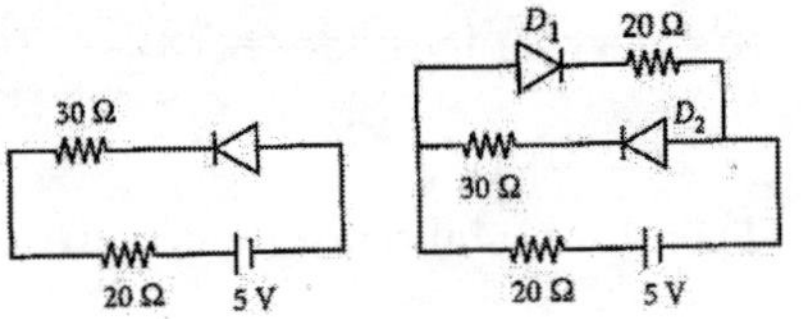

$$I = \frac{5\text{ V}}{(30+20)\Omega} = \frac{5}{50}\text{ A}$$

41. **(a) :** A diode is said to be forward biased if p-type semiconductor of $p-n$ junction is at positive potential with respect to n-type semiconductor of $p-n$ junction. It is so for circuit (a).

42. **(b) :** In forward biasing, the conduction across $p-n$ junction takes place due to migration of majority carriers (i.e., electrons from n-side to p-side and holes from p-side to n-side), hence the size of depletion region decreases.

43. **(d) :**

44. **(d) :**

45. **(c) :** On reversing the polarity of the battery, the $p-n$ junction is reverse biased. As a result of which its resistance becomes high and current through the junction drops to almost zero.

46. **(c) :** Voltage drop across diode $(V_D) =$ 0.5 V;

Maximum power rating of diode $(P) =$ $100\text{ mW} = 100 \times 10^{-3}\text{ W}$

and source voltage $(V_S) = 1.5\text{ V}$

The resistance of diode (R_D)

$$= \frac{V_D^2}{P} = \frac{(0.5)^2}{100 \times 10^{-3}} = 2.5\Omega$$

And current in diode $(I_D) = \frac{V_D}{R_D} = \frac{0.5}{2.5} =$

0.2Ω

Therefore total resistance in circuit (R)

$$= \frac{V_s}{I_D} = \frac{1.5}{0.2} = 7.5\Omega$$

And the value of the series resistor =

Total resistance of the circuit - Resistance of diode $= 7.5 - 2.5 =$ 5Ω

47. **(b) :** As soon as the $p-n$ junction is formed, there is an immediate diffusion of the charge carriers across the junction due to thermal agitation. After diffusion, these charge carriers combine with their counterparts and neutralise each other. Therefore correct direction of flow of carriers is depicted in figure (b).

48. **(b) :** Capacitor used to remove AC ripples from Rectifier output.

49. **(c) :**

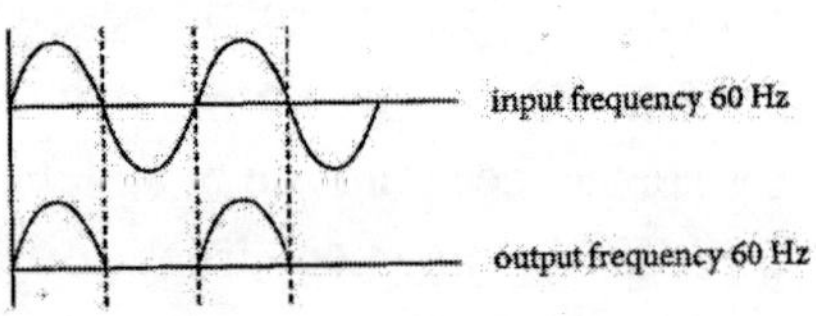

For half wave rectification, the frequency remains same as 60 Hz.

50. **(b) :** $V_{dc} = \frac{V_m}{\pi} = \frac{10}{\pi}\text{V}$

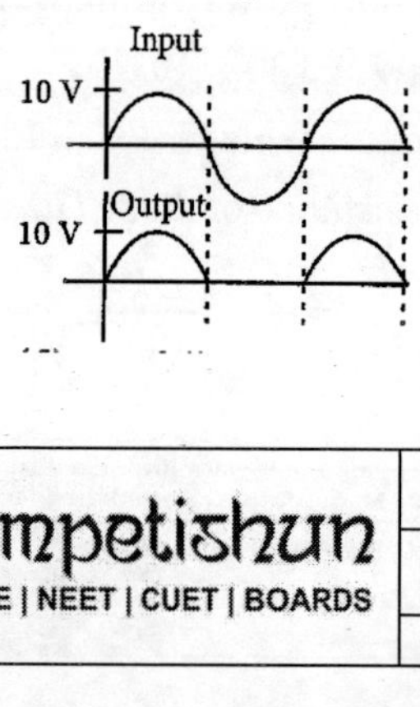

51. **(d) :** In full wave rectifier the fundamental frequency in ripple is twice of input frequency.

52. **(d) :** As a $p-n$ junction diode conducts in forward bias and does not conduct in reverse bias (current is practically zero), thus undirectional property leads to application of diode in rectifiers.

53. **(b) :** Yes, zener diode is connected in reverse bias as it is used as voltage regulator.

The potential barrier of $p-n$ junction

For Ge; $V_o = 0.3$ V; Si; $V_o = 0.7$ V

54. **(b) :** Given, energy gap = 1.9eV

Now, for the LED to operate, electrons need to cross this energy gap.

∴ Wavelength of light emitted,

$$\lambda = \frac{1242\text{eV}-\text{nm}}{1.9\text{eV}} = 654 \text{ nm}$$

55. **(a) :** The $V-I$ characteristic for a solar cell is as shown in the figure.

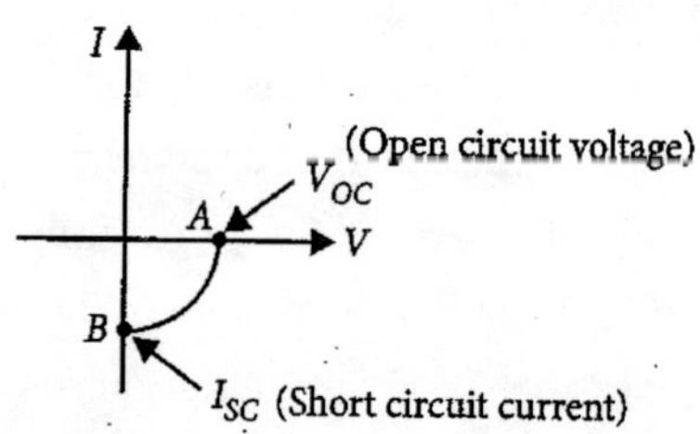

56. **(a) :**

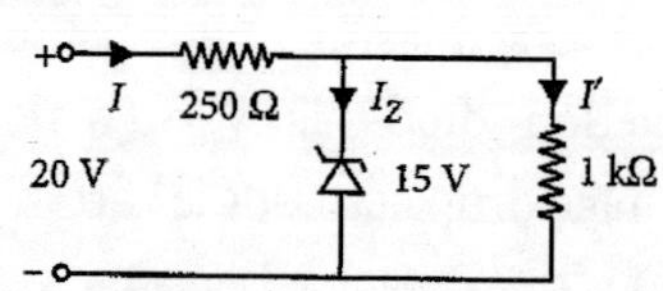

The voltage drop across $1\text{k}\Omega = V_Z =$ 15 V

The current through 1kΩ is

$$I' = \frac{15\text{ V}}{1 \times 10^{3}\Omega} = 15 \times 10^{-3}\text{ A}$$
$$= 15\text{ mA}$$

The voltage drop across 250Ω = 20 V – 15 V = 5 V

The current through 250Ω is

$$I = \frac{5\text{ V}}{250\Omega} = 0.02\text{ A} = 20\text{ mA}$$

The current through the zener diode is

$$I_Z = I - I' = (20 - 15)\text{mA}$$
$$= 5\text{ mA}$$

57. **(c) :** Band gap = 2.5eV

The wavelength corresponding to 2.5eV

$$= \frac{12400\text{eVÅ}}{2.5\text{eV}} = 4960\text{Å}.$$

4000Å can excite this.

58. **(d) :** Band gap = 2eV.

Wavelength of radiation corresponding to this energy,

$$\lambda = \frac{hc}{E} = \frac{12400\text{eVÅ}}{2\text{eV}} = 6200\text{Å}$$

The frequency of this radiation

$$= \frac{c}{\lambda} = \frac{3 \times 10^{8}\text{ m/s}}{6200 \times 10^{-10}\text{ m/s}} \Rightarrow v$$
$$= 5 \times 10^{14}\text{ Hz}$$

59. **(c) :** Zener diode is used for stabilisation while $p - n$ junction diode is used for rectification.

60. **(b) :** In photocell, photo electromotive force, is the force that stimulates the emission of an electric current when photovoltaic action creates a potential difference between two points and the electric current depends on the intensity of incident light.

61. **(a) :** $y = \overline{\bar{A} \cdot \bar{B}} = \bar{\bar{A}} + \bar{\bar{B}}$

$= (A + B)$ OR Gate

A	B	Y
0	0	0
0	1	1
1	0	1
1	1	1

62. **(c) :** Output of the given circuit is

$$C = \overline{A\bar{B}} + \overline{\bar{A}B}$$
$$= \bar{A} + \bar{\bar{B}} + \bar{\bar{A}} + \bar{B}$$
$$= \bar{A} + \bar{B} + A + \bar{B}$$
$$\Rightarrow C = \bar{B}$$

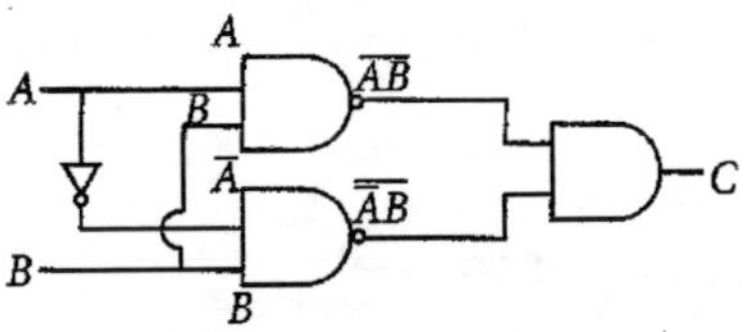

Therefore, the correct truth table corresponding to $C = \bar{B}$ is

A	B	$C=\bar{B}$
0	0	1
0	1	0
1	0	1
1	1	0

63. **(c) :**

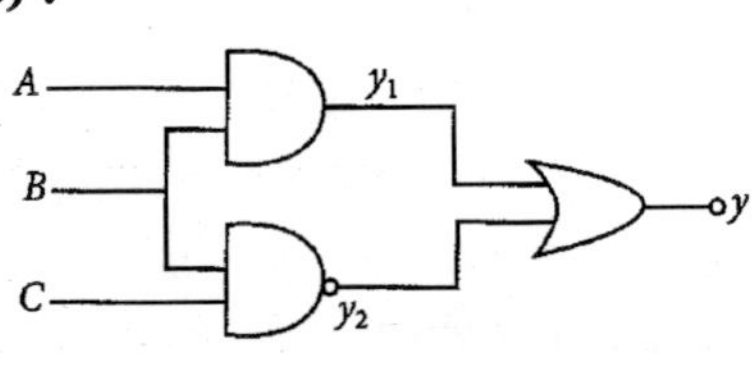

Output of combination of logic gates is given as

$$y = AB + \overline{BC}$$

A	B	C	y_1	y_2	$y = AB + \overline{BC}$
0	0	0	0	1	1
1	0	0	0	1	1
0	1	0	0	1	1
0	0	1	0	1	1
1	1	0	0	1	1
1	0	1	0	1	1
1	1	1	1	0	1

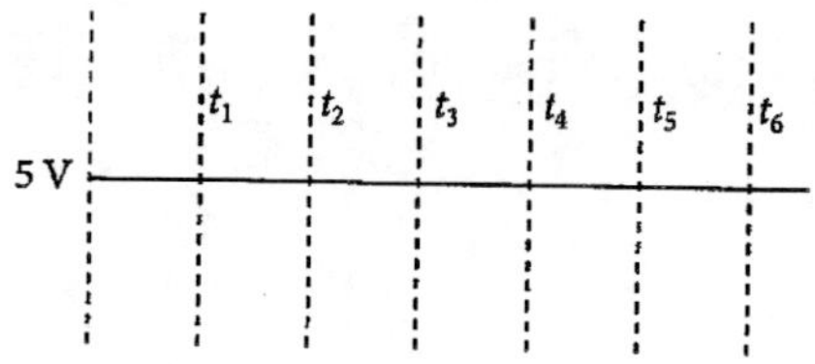

The output (y) can be represented as above.

64. **(a) :** $A \longrightarrow D^{\bar{A}}$

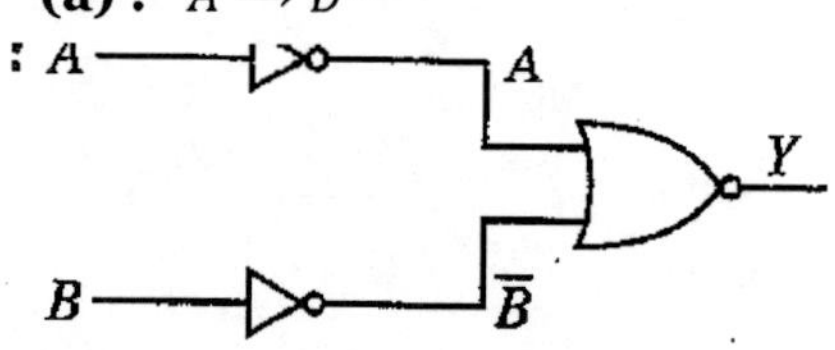

Here, $Y = \overline{\bar{A} + \bar{B}} = \overline{\overline{A \cdot B}} = A \cdot B$

This AND Gate. So, the truth table is

A	B	Y
0	0	0
0	1	0
1	0	0
1	1	1

65. **(d) :** LED bulb will light up if switch(s) A or B or both A and B is/are open. Hence it represents a NAND gate.

66. **(b) :**

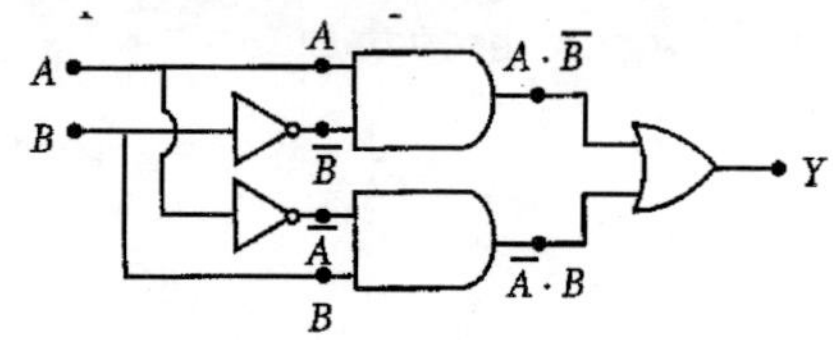

$$Y = (A \cdot \bar{B} + \bar{A} \cdot B)$$

67. **(b) :**

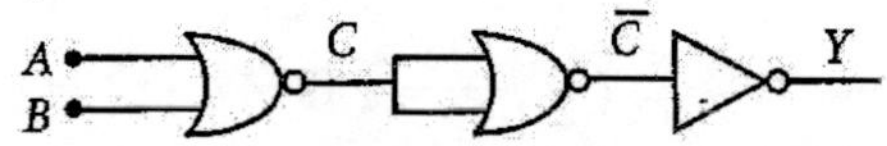

A	B	C	C^-	Output (Y)
0	0	1	0	1
0	1	0	1	0
1	0	0	1	0
1	1	0	1	0

At output, the truth table corresponds to NOR gate.

68. **(c) :**

$$Y = \overline{(AB)C} = \overline{ABC}$$

If $A = B = C = 0$ then $Y_0 = \bar{0} = 1$

If $A = B = C = 0$ then $Y_1 = \bar{1} = 0$

69. **(b) :**

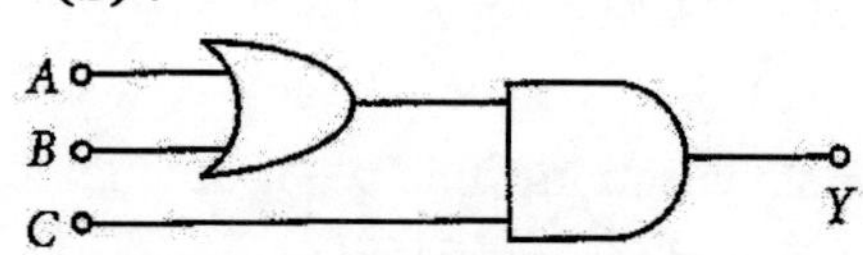

Output of the circuit, $Y = (A + B) \cdot C$

$Y = 1$ if $C = 1$ and $A = 0, B = 1$ or $A = 1, B = 0$ or $A = B = 1$.

70. **(a) :**

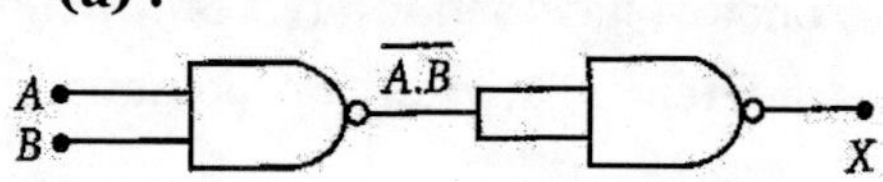

The output of the given logic circuit is

$$X = \overline{\overline{A \cdot B}} = A \cdot B$$

71. (a) :

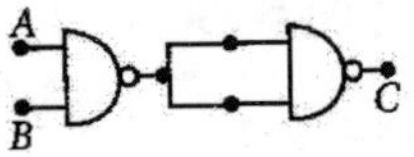

The output of the given logic gate is

$$C = \overline{\overline{A \cdot B}} = A \cdot B$$

It is the Boolean expression of AND gate.

Hence, the resulting gate is a AND gate.

72. (a) : The truth table of the given waveform is as shown in the table.

Time interval	Input A	Input B	Output C
0 to t_1	0	0	0
t_1 to t_2	1	0	1
t_2 to t_3	1	1	1
t_3 to t_4	0	1	1
t_4 to t_5	0	0	0
t_5 to t_6	1	0	1
$> t_6$	0	1	1

The logic circuit is OR gate.

73. (d) :

(i) 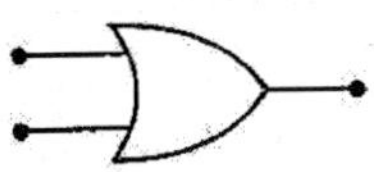

It represents logic symbol of OR gate.

(ii) 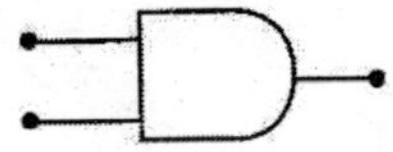

It represents logic symbol of AND gate.

(iii) 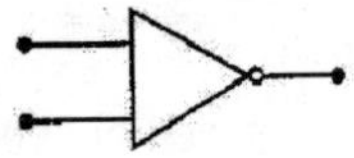

It represents the logic symbol of NOT gate.

(iv) 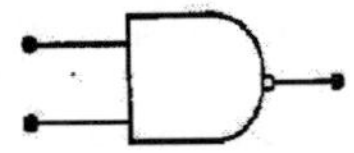

It represents the logic symbol of NAND gate.

74. (b) : The device that can act as a complete circuit is integrated circuit (IC).

75. (d) : It is clear from given logic circuit, that out put Y is low when both the inputs are high, otherwise z it is high. Thus logic circuit is NAND gate.

A	B	Y
1	1	0
0	0	1
0	1	1
1	0	1

76. (b) : (i) 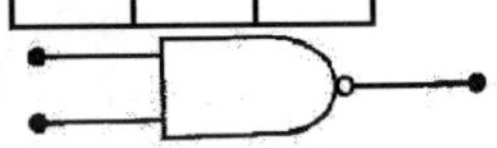

(ii) 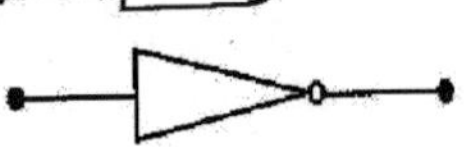

(iii) 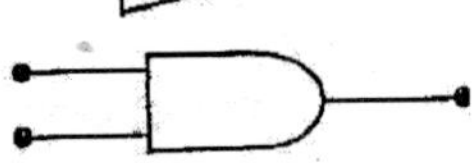

(iv) 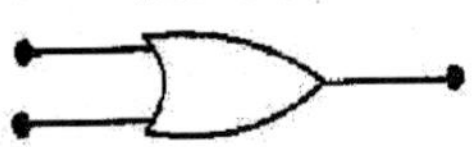

OR gate, NOT gate and NAND gates are (iv), (ii) and (i) respectively.

77. (c) :

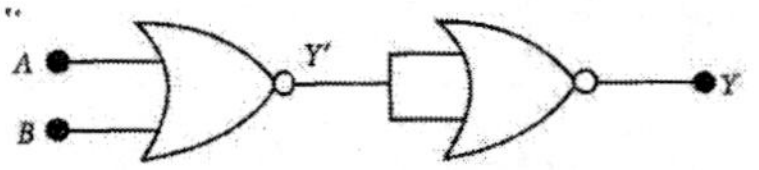

$$Y' = \overline{A+B}.\ Y = \overline{\overline{A+B}} = A+B$$

Truth table of the given circuit is given by

A	B	Y'	Y
0	0	1	0
0	1	0	1
1	0	0	1
1	1	0	1

78. (b) : The truth table corresponding to waveform is given by

A	B	C
1	1	1
0	1	0
1	0	0
0	0	0

∴ The given logic circuit gate is AND gate.

79. (b) : The truth table of OR gate is

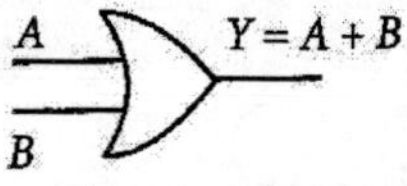

A	B	Y
0	0	0
0	1	1
1	0	1
1	1	1

From truth table we can observe that if either of input is one then output is one. Also if both the inputs are one then also output is one.

80. (a) : NAND gate is a combination of AND and NOT gate.

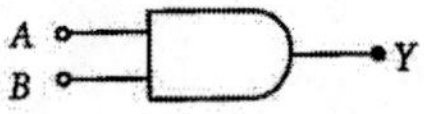

AND gate

A	B	Y
0	0	0
1	0	0
0	1	0
1	1	1

Truth table of AND gate

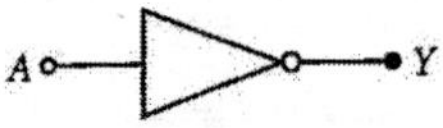

NOT gate

A	Y
0	1
1	0

Truth table of NOT gate

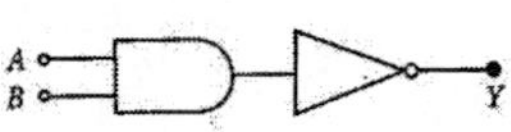

NAND gate

A	B	Y
0	0	1
1	0	1
0	1	1
1	1	0

Truth table of NAND gate

Hence the given truth table is of a NAND gate.

81. (a) :

82. (b) : For NOR gate, $Y = \overline{A+B}$.

Therefore from the given truth table

A	B	A+B	$Y = \overline{A+B}$
1	1	1	0
1	0	1	0
0	1	1	0
0	0	0	1

83. (c) : According to figure $Y = \overline{A \cdot B}$.

Therefore it is NAND gate.

84. (b) : This truth table is of identity, $Y = A + B$, hence OR gate.